Practical Homeopathy

Also by Vinton McCabe

Homeopathy, Healing, and You

Practical Homeopathy

A Comprehensive Guide
to Homeopathic Remedies
and Their Acute Uses

Vinton McCabe

St. Martin's Griffin *New York*

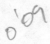

Excerpts from *The Organon of the Medical Art* by Samuel Hahnemann (Wenda Brewster O'Reilly, editor). Reprinted with permission.

Library of Congress Cataloging-in-Publication Data
McCabe, Vinton.
    Practical homeopathy / Vinton McCabe.—1st U.S. ed.
       p.   cm.
    ISBN 0-312-20669-0
    1. Homeopathy Handbooks, manuals, etc. 2. Homeopathy—Materia medica and therapeutics Handbooks, manuals, etc.   I. Title
RX73.M38 2000   99-26936
615.5'32—dc21   CIP

A Note to Readers

This book is for informational purposes only. Readers are advised to consult a trained medical professional before acting on any of the information in this book. The fact that a particular remedy, therapy, or treatment is discussed in the book does not mean that the author or publisher recommends its use.

"The physician's highest and only calling is to make the sick healthy, to cure, as it is called."

—Samuel Hahnemann,
THE ORGANON

Contents

SECTION TWO: BEING PRACTICAL

SECTION THREE: APPENDICES

Preface

Can Homeopathy
Be Practical?

Let's get this over with right up front; homeopathy is an oddball sort of medicine, one that refuses to be easily categorized or explained. In fact, the word *homeopathy* seems to be used today in so many ways that if we are to believe its common misuse in magazines and newspapers and on television, it can mean anything that is natural, from herbal medicine to witchcraft. At its best, it seems to be a form of intuitive practice that was the brainchild of a disgruntled German physician, Samuel Hahnemann, who was quite literally driven from the practice of medicine because of his beliefs. It's a form of medicine that is based not in the science of the modern technological age but in the science of two centuries ago. At its worst, homeopathy seems to be some sort of cult, one largely populated by those lacking in the finances and willingness to take advantage of the full range of modern medical discoveries from antibiotics to cloning—in other words, medical Luddites.

Homeopaths tend to be an odd breed of people as well. Often it seems that they do not play well with others. Most of those in the United States who practice homeopathy do so with medical degrees other than medical doctor. Often they are naturopaths, chiropractors, and other members of the medical fringe. The fact that in this country there is no legal or medical slot for "homeopath" may well have some bearing on this, but the complexities of medical law do not affect our understanding of homeopathy.

Given all the oddities of homeopaths and the homeopathic community—and these oddities as well as the failure of homeopaths to ever be able to gather in support of one another may well be largely responsible for the fact that homeopathy remains in most people's minds an "alternative" therapy at best—and of homeopathy as well, we have to ask the basic question "Is there any merit to homeopathy?"

I can only answer from my experience that homeopathy worked for me when nothing else had, and it appeared that nothing ever would. Like many others, I turned to homeopathy only when there was nowhere else to turn. And I was blessed by walking into the right office. There I found a practitioner who believed that the healing process is also an educational process, and who taught me homeopathy while treating me homeopathically.

While it is true that homeopathy has its roots in ancient herbal medicine and in alchemy, this is the case for all medicine, although unlike the homeopaths the practitioners of modern medicine deny this historic truth. And it is further true that homeopathy owes as much to modern chemistry and physics as it does to ancient alchemy.

For nearly two decades now I have studied homeopathy and have written about it and taught it as well. The information presented in this book is the result of those years of study and research.

But the question of whether or not homeopathy could ever be thought of as being practical or not never really occurred to me until it was thrust on me in a classroom setting. Several years ago I was teaching a course in basic homeopathic philosophy in the way that I always do. I was telling the class that homeopathy is a form of energy healing, like acupuncture, and that also like acupuncture it brings a catalyst that allows your body to heal itself. I was explaining that from a homeopathic viewpoint we have to learn to honor our disease symptoms as something native to ourselves, as an outgrowth of self, and stop just trying to stamp them out, because any symptom that is ignored, that is stamped out, will only return again, stronger than before. I explained that we have to start dealing with the root causes of our illnesses and not with the symptoms alone.

I had spent the better part of the day going over all this, teaching how the homeopath matches the symptoms to the appropriate remedy, when a hand went up. A woman asked, "Is any of this practical?"

The question rather stunned me in that the issue of practicality never really seemed important to me one way or the other. But the question had been raised and therefore needed to be dealt with.

Is homeopathy practical? And can it ever be considered practical? I guess the answer is yes—and no.

Homeopathy is based in the ancient notion of medicine—that is, medicine for the whole man. Allopathic medicine—that which would be considered Western Medicine—has taken a different evolutionary route. The allopath of ancient days saw the body, mind, and spirit as a whole unit and not as separate entities, but with the work of the Greek doctor Galen, the allopath began to see the human as a mechanism, as a form of natural construct. It was at this time, two thousand years ago, that this original notion of "wholistic" medicine—Hippocratic medicine—yielded to a form of medicine that mapped the human system differently and, increasingly, as a blend of specific chemicals and parts that together gave you a human being. What was once considered extraordinary, perhaps even miraculous, became over the centuries merely the expected outcome of gene or hormone manipulation.

Only in the latter part of this century has the allopath begun to once more accept the existence of the soul and of the miraculous as part of life. That healing may take place whether or not the genes or hormones are manipulated. And so in recent years we have seen allopath after allopath writing books on the power of prayer and the mind/body connection.

But homeopathy has developed differently. For the homeopath, today or two hundred years ago, the human being is a single unit—mind, body, and spirit—just as he was two thousand years ago for Hippocrates. There has been no search for a mind/body connection because that connection was never severed in the first place. Therefore, the practice of homeopathy today is much as it has always been, a search for the energy medicine that in its action is most similar to the disease situation at hand.

In practice, this can seem most impractical. The person who seeks help for a skin rash may well be asked what he dreams about at night or how thirsty he is. It all seems pretty roundabout and at times those learning homeopathy are made to feel that everything they have ever learned about medicine—and everything they have ever thought about healing—is wrong.

This, in fact, may well be true. If our allopathic education is not totally wrong, it is at least backward. And each of us who owns a television set or who reads a magazine or looks at the ads in a newspaper has already received a complete indoctrination, if not an education, in allopathic methodology and thought.

In fact, our allopathic education begins before birth. Perhaps no other period in life is so allopathy-intensive as the prenatal period. While still in the womb, we hear all about what is expected of us in terms of our health and health care.

Because of this I am amazed whenever any of us can be moved to consider that perhaps there is another philosophy of health and healing that can be effective and safe in the treatment of those who have disease. And given the fact that the homeopathic philosophy is in so many ways counter to the allopathic, it is even more surprising to me that anyone ever puts the time and effort into learning enough about homeopathy to actually make successful use of any of its remedies.

But something is speaking to the hundreds and thousands of us who find ourselves at this moment in time quite willing to at least explore our options. I think that it is too simple to put the blame on the allopathic medical industry or on the insurance companies and issue such a blanket statement as, "Allopathy has failed us time and again, and we are looking for a new answer in health care." And yet, if I will not make this statement, I have surely heard it made by many others.

There has been a shift in people's thinking, however, that began a few years ago, with just a disgruntled few, and now seems to be reaching the general public as well. Just as only the radical few shopped at health food stores a handful of years ago and now millions of us shop in health food supermarkets that have grown larger than the A&P, so, too, have we seen an amazing increase in the number of middle-class, middle-aged, college-educated citizens turning their attention to new ways of looking at health and disease, and new methods by which they might seek a cure.

So, back to practicality. How do we take something as philosophical as homeopathy and make it practical? How do we take what Hahnemann has written and put it into practice in our lives, on a day-to-day basis?

I think that we start with the admission that homeopathy is impractical in its nature. It demands that, like the dancer who is new at the barre, we learn to use a whole new set of muscles. The focus of homeopathy is different from the focus of allopathy. Allopathic medicine is site-specific. It demands that we zero in on the specific symptom, or group of symptoms that we term disease, and that we work on removing these symptoms. The belief is that if we can just remove these symptoms and leave everything else alone, then the patient will be well.

The homeopath is trained to look at the whole person, the person who has the symptoms, and to place those symptoms within the context of the patient's whole being. This is much more difficult to do than focusing solely on the patient's symptoms. If you believe that those painful symptoms are a part of the whole and not something foreign to it, then you can't just work against those symptoms and expect them to go away without changes—and, often, negative changes—to the whole. Instead, the homeopath works with the whole, giving a remedy based on the totality of the symptoms with the belief that given the opportunity the patient's system will heal itself.

So the homeopathic remedy is only a spark. A healing spark. A catalyst that can move the patient—and not just his symptoms—toward healing. Thus homeopathic treatment will leave the patient not just symptom-free (which it what allopathic treatment, at its most successful, has to offer), but actually stronger and healthier than before. It can do this because it works with and treats the whole person and refuses to zero in on a few choice symptoms. It does this because it recognizes first and foremost that those symptoms are there for a reason, and, secondly, that you cannot medically work on one part, or on one set of symptoms, without impacting the whole. But by working with the whole, you can radically change for the better the working set of symptoms.

It sounds odd, I know. And impractical too, at least if practical means easy. Or if practical means that a given set of symptoms always gets a given medicine. This may be a "practical" approach to medicine, always treating allergies with antihistamines, but it simply is not effective. The "impractical" approach is to acknowledge up front that each person is unique and will need whatever medicine is indicated for just that individual. It is the task of the practitioner, then, to find that medicine. While I acknowledge that it is somewhat impractical to approach medicine in this way, throwing out the map with each new case and having to find your way in the wilderness of that patient's particular system, it seems that this is the only method that gets you anywhere.

The homeopathic method forces the practitioner to pay attention to the patient, since it is believed that the patient, and not the practitioner, has the solution to the problem. The practitioner just has to help get that information from the patient, since the patient may not even be aware that he has the information, much less what to do with it. Therefore, right from the first meeting, the practitioner and patient meet as equals and teammates and not as expert and victim.

The homeopathic method demands that the practitioner know his remedies, that he know the full range of the homeopathic pharmacy, which contains thousands of remedies. In this way, allopathy is fairly simple—if you have certain symptoms, you take this medicine. And the doctor has only to stay up to date with the new medicines to keep current. In homeopathy however, since we cannot conclude even that two patients with colds need the same remedy, since there is no such thing as a "cold remedy," the task is more difficult—and, therefore, more impractical.

But, if by practical, we mean, Is homeopathy effective in the treatment of the patient? or is it cost effective? or is it a safe method of self-treatment for household emergencies? the answers are yes, yes, and yes.

Homeopathy—when properly practiced—is shown to be a safe and effective form of treatment on a daily basis in this country and around the world. Hundreds of thousands use homeopathy for the treatment of every sort of condition, from coughs and colds—for which homeopathic remedies are simply chosen and far more effective than their allopathic equivalents—to HIV disease and cancer. And homeopathy is far less costly than is allopathic medicine. The difference is largely one of technology. While allopaths are forever investing in the newest machine, homeopaths are still reaching for their books, their Materia Medica and their Repertory.

And finally, in the home, there is perhaps no safer, simpler, or more effective means of self-treatment in minor emergencies than that offered by homeopathy. The practitioner or layperson who learns the basics of homeopathic philosophy and practice can do a great deal of good for himself and his loved ones.

I believe that in the long run this was what that student was actually asking: Can any of this information ever be really useful to me? People want to know if they can ever really learn homeopathy, if they ever will be able to select the correct remedy for an emergency situation.

My answer here is, yes, absolutely. It will take a little work, and a willingness to look at that situation somewhat differently than an allopath would, but it is not only practical but feasible for an average person to learn enough homeopathy to know what to do for the little emergencies that arise in all our homes.

That's the whole purpose of this book. In it I have tried to write the book that I always hoped someone else would write—a single volume that would give an overview of homeopathic philosophy and a plan to follow for homeopathic practice; it would also give solid diagnostic tools for homeopathic practice and a key for the remedies that are most commonly used in acute practice, as well as their doses and potencies. I wrote this book to fill the need for such a reference guide for home treatment, so that the philosophy of homeopathy handed down by Samuel Hahnemann might take its place alongside a listing of the basic homeopathic remedies and their uses. That's what puts the practical in *Practical Homeopathy*.

But, most important, I have written this text because I believe in homeopathy, in both its philosophy and its practice. And because of this simple reality: When I am in pain, I do not want a practical medicine; I want a miraculous medicine. I want a form of medicine in whose core philsophy is the notion that healing is always possible and is, in fact, an innate part of my nature.

That medicine for me is homeopathy. A most practical medicine.

Author's Note

In this volume, the references to particular paragraphs from Samuel Hahnemann's work *The Organon* are taken from *The Organon of the Medical Art*, as it has been newly translated by Steven Decker and edited and annotated by Wenda Brewster O'Reilly. To my knowledge it is the finest edition of Hahnemann's writing that has ever found its way into the English language. All those who consider themselves to be serious students of homeopathy should make use of this volume as their basic educational tool.

As this new translation states, if we are to make homeopathy practical, if we are to grasp the intricacies of its philosophy and practice, we must adhere to the Latin motto *aude sapere*. We must "dare to know."

Homeopathic Remedies Commonly Used in Acute Situations (with Remedy Sources)

While the homeopathic pharmacy consists of literally thousands of medicines taken from animal, vegetable, and mineral sources, there are some remedies that are used more commonly than others. Some are more helpful in acute situations; others, in chronic conditions.

The remedies listed here are those that are used throughout this book. They form the backbone of this text in that they are the remedies which, in my opinion, are most commonly used in acute situations and are probably, again in my opinion, the most important of the remedies for home use. Among them are some of our most important homeopathic remedies.

Some remedies listed here are among those that homeopaths call *polycrest* remedies, remedies that speak to a wide range of symptoms and are of therefore many and varied uses. Others, like Spongia Tosta, are small remedies, remedies that work within a small sphere of action and speak to a short list of remedies. But all the remedies listed here are basic in their use and can be very important in times of acute illness.

Because each of us is an individual, we will each find in our own lives that some remedies work better for us than do others. It will be apparent to each reader over time which of the remedies listed here are most important in his own life and in the lives of his loved ones. Some may prove to be very important; others may not speak to any symptom you ever experience. In the same way, a remedy not listed here may be of ongoing importance in your life. But I do believe that the following list is a good and balanced gathering of the remedies that should be found in your home kit. They are also the remedies that beginning consumers of homeopathy would do well to first study and understand.

Suggested Remedies for the Home Kit

1. Aconitum Napellus (Wolfsbane)
2. Allium Cepa (Red Onion)
3. Antimonium Tartaricum (Tartar Emetic)
4. Apis Mellifica (Honey Bee)
5. Arnica Montana (Leopard's Bane)
6. Arsenicum Album (White Arsenic)
7. Belladonna (Deadly Nightshade)
8. Bellis Perennis (Daisy)
9. Bryonia Alba (White Bryony, Wild Hops)
10. Calcarea Carbonica (Calcium Carbonate)
11. Calendula Officinalis (Marigold)
12. Camphora (Camphor)
13. Carbo Vegetabilis (Vegetable Charcoal)
14. Causticum (Caustic Lime)
15. Chamomilla (Chamomile)
16. China/Cinchona (Peruvian Bark)
17. Cina (Wormseed)
18. Cocculus (Indian Cockle)
19. Coffea Cruda (Crude Coffee)
20. Colocynthis (Bitter Cucumber)
21. Drosera Rotundifolia (Sundew)
22. Dulcamara (Bittersweet)
23. Eupatorium Perfoliatum (Thoroughwort)
24. Euphrasia (Eyebright)
25. Ferrum Phosphoricum (Iron Phosphate)
26. Gelsemium (Yellow Jessamine)
27. Graphites (Graphite, "Pure Black Lead")
28. Hepar Sulphuris (Sulphuret of Lime)
29. Hypericum (Saint-John's-Wort)
30. Ignatia Amara (Saint Ignatius Bean)
31. Ipecacuanha/Ipecac (Cephaelius Ipecacuanha)
32. Kali Bichromicum (Potassium Bichromate)
33. Lachesis (Venom of the Surukuru or Bushmaster Snake)
34. Ledum Palustre (Marsh Tea)

35. Lycopodium (Club Moss)
36. Magnesia Phosphorica (Phosphate of Magnesia)
37. Mercurius (Quicksilver)
38. Natrum Muriaticum (Sodium Chloride)
39. Nux Vomica (Strychnos Nux Vomica)
40. Petroleum (Petroleum)
41. Phosphorus (Phosphorus)
42. Phytolacca (Poke Root)
43. Podophyllum (Mayapple or American Mandrake)
44. Pulsatilla (Windflower)
45. Rhus Toxicodendron (Poison Ivy)
46. Rumex Crispus (Yellowdock)
47. Ruta Graveolens (Rue)
48. Sabadilla (Cevadilla Seed)
49. Sepia (Cuttlefish Ink)
50. Silicea (Flint)
51. Spigelia (Indian Pink)
52. Spongia Tosta (Roasted Sponge)
53. Staphysagria (Stavesacre)
54. Sulphur (Sulphur)
55. Symphytum (Comfrey)
56. Thuja Occidentalis (Arbor Vitae)
57. Urtica Urens (Stinging Nettle)
58. Valeriana (Valerian)
59. Veratrum Album (White Hellebore)
60. Rescue Remedy (Bach Flower Mixture)

Hahnemann's Quantum Leap

Introduction

THE STORY OF HOMEOPATHY is largely the story of one man, Samuel Hahnemann. While he is not the "inventor" of homeopathy, or the principles of homeopathic treatment, he is the person who managed to flesh out those principles that had been in place for more than two thousand years. His function was largely that of a detective. Just as a good detective will put together numerous small clues to build a fully rounded picture of an event, Hahnemann worked for years to test the theories of the past and to blend them with cutting-edge technologies of his day. We can only imagine what he might be up to if he lived today, blending ancient philosophies of medicine with empirical experience of the methods by which the body heals itself, combined with modern physics and computer graphics. Many of us mistakenly think of Hahnemann as a man who held with the conventions of the past. But this simply is not true. In practice as well as in philosophy Hahnemann was on the cutting edge.

Christian Samuel Hahnemann was born on April 10, 1755, in Meissen, East Germany. The year of his birth was the year in which the preacher, alchemist, and great lover Casanova was imprisoned for espionage. It was also the year Benjamin Franklin published his "Observations Concerning the Increase of Mankind," which somewhat predicted Malthus' later treatise on overpopulation and its impact on the global environment. And it was the year before Frederick the Great of Prussia invaded Saxony and set off the Seven Years' War, while in the New World, the French and Indian War paralleled the European conflict.

During the eighty-odd years of Hahnemann's lifetime, innovation was in the air. In the field of medicine, the concept of inoculation was hot. In 1760, Benjamin Franklin again published, this time a work called "Some Account of the Success of Inoculation for the Smallpox in England and America," which predated both Hahnemann's and Jenner's work in the field of microdosing with toxic substances, and of using those microdoses of poisons in the treatment and prevention of disease. In medicine, European culture also saw the creation of a new discipline with the 1762 publication of *The Diseases of Children and Their Remedies*, by Swedish doctor Nils von Rosenstein, which created an entire new field of medical practice—pediatrics.

It was also the era—1780, to be exact—that saw the opening of London's Temple of Health. The Temple was the brainchild of James Graham, who was himself the son of a Scottish saddler. Graham had studied medicine but had no formal degree with which to practice. He had left his native Edinburgh to travel to the United States, where he heard about Benjamin Franklin's experiments in electricity. He took the information he obtained to London, where he opened his Temple. Within its doors, patients were assaulted with incense burners in the shape of fire-breathing dragons. They also saw the device that they had come for: the Celestial Bed, which was built to stand upon forty glass pillars and numerous electrical devices. Patients came to lie down upon the bed and be treated with gentle electrical shocks for impotence or infertility. For a while, the Temple was quite a hit, with wealthy clients coming from around the globe to lie upon the Celestial Bed. But within a few years, despite its initial chic, and the hiring of a beautiful young dancer, Emma Lyon, to dress in robes and impersonate the "goddess of health," the doors to the Temple would close. For all its splendor, the Temple's treatments simply did not work.

Inventions of the time included roller skates (1760), the steam engine (1765), the steamboat (1787), and "Bushnell's Connecticut Turtle" (1776), the first submarine designed for warfare. Another invention of the time was the hot-air balloon, which first ascended as a mode of transportation in 1782, when the Montgolfier Brothers gave a public demonstration of their invention with a ten-minute ascent. In 1785, John Jeffries did them one better by crossing the English Channel in a hot-air balloon. Discoveries included the planet Uranus in 1781, which was the first planet to have been discovered since the prehistoric times in which human culture was dominated by the nation of Babylonia.

There was a general feeling of expansion at this time. It seemed that there were infinite possibilities for scientific advancement; and for physical and geographical discovery as well, as the settlers of the New World soon found. Once they ventured beyond the area of the original colonies, they discovered that they were dealing with far more than they had imagined. And Samuel Hahnemann, very much at home in this time, also was finding a new way of working medically, one that proved to be far greater and deeper a discovery than was first imagined.

Hahnemann was born into a conservative family in a conservative culture. But he was also born into a family with some standing in the community. Because his father was an artist—a painter of fine German china— Hahnemann was given the opportunity to study, to have the education of a gentleman. While medicine was his mother's choice of a proper career for a young man of means, but not his own, he honored his parents' wishes, and with the financial support of local royals, he set off for the University of Vienna.

Here he expected to receive his education in medicine. But what he found instead horrified him. In the medical pharmacy of the day, doctors made regular use of such substances as arsenic in the treatment of disease. Further, this was the era of leeching, with millions of leeches used each year for the purposes of bleeding patients, all in the name of healing. Hahnemann concluded that all too often the treatments were more toxic than the diseases.

This belief would guide Hahnemann for the next fifty years, as he performed his own clinical experiments in search for treatments that, while not toxic, were powerful as curative tools. His search for these substances would lead him back to the dawn of medicine, and would also cause him to take a giant leap ahead of the other medical scientists of his day.

Hahnemann, in his search for a more benign medicine, began with what he knew—the herbal pharmacy of his day. This pharmacy, the use of plants and mineral substances in the creation of medicines, could largely be traced back to Dioscorides, a Greek herbalist who traveled with the Roman legions in order to learn the use of healing herbs from the witch doctors, barbers, and midwives whom he met during his long march through the known world. These he gathered into a book that he termed a "Materia Medica," a gathering together of all the knowledge he had gained of medical materials, which he left behind him as his legacy for those physicians who would follow in his path.

Hahnemann came to understand that while these medicines were able to create a tremendous change in the human system, that change was often not for the better. And in order to create a more benign drug, he began to dilute his medicines. Certainly, other practitioners had tried mixing their belladonna with a little water, but Hahnemann set up a system of dilutions that left only the slightest trace of the original substance in place in the medicine.

In using these diluted medicines, Hahnemann found something mysterious: as a medicine became more and more diluted it became less toxic and more powerful, more efficacious in the treatment of disease.

With his discoveries in medicine, Hahnemann became quite revolutionary, but I think this was certainly never his goal. He began his work as a doctor with the intent of pleasing: pleasing his parents, his family, his community. He sought originally only to practice the medicine of the day to the best of his ability. However, like the original settlers of these United States who thought that they were sitting on a landmass roughly the size of England, he was ultimately shocked by the immense implications of his medical experiments. But his evolution from conservative Lutheran youth to medical revolutionary was a task thrust upon him, one that he never sought. Take a moment and look at his life in terms of your own. He, like the rest of us, went through life with no plan, doing his best to raise a huge family—he and his wife had nine children—and please his increasingly upset and disappointed first wife, Johanna. You can't help but empathize with his trying to do his best for his family, while at the same time, feeling he had had an actual visionary experience of sorts, one to which he felt he also had to be true. So for the majority of his adult life, Hahnemann found himself in a delicate balancing act, between his responsibility to his family and his equally keen responsibility to his work.

We love to make movies about people like this—Norma Rae kind of people, who, although they themselves never early on seem like the firebrands they will prove to be, somewhere along the way receive an insight that transforms their life. In Norma Rae's case, the insight had to do with factory work conditions, and she ended up becoming a union organizer. In Hahnemann's case, he was a loving, concerned doctor who could not turn away from his patients when they reached out to him in pain and sorrow. He could not avoid the conclusion that the treatments that the doctors of his day were using were not only not ending the patients' suffering, but in many cases were actually causing it.

What is surprising is not that Hahnemann noticed the reality of the medical treatments of his day and their implications, but that no one else seemed to. Even when he pointed it out to them, they seemed angrier at him for speaking out than they were at any of the accepted medical practices.

But Hahnemann continued to speak out—and not because it would get him anywhere. In fact, it all but ended his ability to practice medicine and to support his family in the only way he knew how. No, he did it because he felt that any decent person had to speak out at the wrongs he saw around him. For instance, it was common practice at this time to prescribe arsenic as a treatment for disease.

And it is important to remember that the discoveries Hahnemann made, the insights to which he was witness, all fit within the context of the education he received at the University of Vienna, perhaps the best school of his day, and within the context of his medical viewpoint. Indeed, some of the most important insights into medical practice can and should be used equally by homeopaths and allopaths, in that they are insights into *practice* and not into the goal or method of treatment.

But let's examine Hahnemann's great shifts in the philosophy and practice of the healing arts.

For years I told my students that while he must be considered the father of the homeopathic method, Hahnemann was not really the father of homeopathy, that he was making use of information that had been collected and considered as far back as the Hippocratic School of Medicine. And this is true. But while Hahnemann's work was in the exploration and evolution of Hippocrates' philosophy, he also made some rather staggering discoveries of his own. The irony is that he often does not get any credit for these—instead, he is credited, wrongly, with the "discovery" of homeopathy.

Homeopathic philosophy began the day that Hippocrates told his students that when you were faced with a patient with symptoms, with aches and pains that he wanted to be rid of, there were only two things you could do with those symptoms. You could work against them, and, in doing so, say in essence that those symptoms came about for no reason, that they have no message for us, and that they should merely be removed from the body. Or you could work with the symptoms. In doing this, you are really saying that the symptoms are there for a reason, that they mean something. In working with the symptoms, you are trusting Nature, and believe that the symptoms bring some message.

That lecture of Hippocrates was really the "invention" of both allopathic and homeopathic medicine, although those terms were never used. Hahnemann himself coined both the word *homeopathy* and the word *allopathy*.

So, from that day forward, you are going to see those concepts come up again and again. Every healing modality, every form of medicine from every part of the world, will contain both concepts. And most will make use of both, save modern Western medicine, which, in placing all bets on the allopathic color black on the roulette wheel of life, completely forgets that very often the homeopathic color red comes out the winner.

But, back to Hahnemann. And to his genius as both a practitioner and a philosopher. And to those discoveries of his that, surprisingly, have equal impact upon both the allopathic and homeopathic traditions.

First there is the insight he had into the nature of medicine itself. Allopathic *or* homeopathic. Hahnemann refers to medicine as being an "Artificial Disease."

This is the term that Hahnemann gave to the effect that any medicine has on the human system. This concept will be dealt with more completely in the next section of this book. For now, consider Artificial Disease to describe the full impact that any medicinal substance has on the body, mind, and spirit of its user, all the many symptoms that a medicine creates. In our culture, we tend to think that medicine ends symptoms rather than creates them. But stop and think about this for a moment: think about what would happen if you, in a state of total health and wellness, took an over-the-counter medicine for a few days. Your sinuses would dry up, you would grow sleepy, very sleepy, or you would be totally unable to sleep. Your breathing and heart rate would be affected, as would your digestion, your sense of balance, even your mood. There would be some changes in your day-to-day life that if they happened totally on their own without your having taken anything to cause them, you would think of as a disease state. That's an Artificial Disease.

Notice that in this Artificial Disease state we have not just one symptom but several. Hahnemann found that medicines—and, again, this applies equally to all types of medicine—create more than one symptom. They all create many changes in the human system. In allopathic medicine, medicines are considered to have one action and many side effects. In Hahnemann's philosophy, the action of any medicine includes many different effects, all of which are taken into account in the use of that medicine.

Another of Hahnemann's insights concerned the manner in which he tested his medicines in order to see what their specific actions in the human system might be. In Hahnemann's day, most medicines were tested on the sick and dying. If a treatment worked in one crisis, then it was used in another. If over a series of treatments it was found to be more useful than harmful, then it became part of the doctor's pharmacy of medicines. But Hahnemann reasoned that if a medicine were truly to be thought of as an Artificial Disease, then it could not be tested on a human in whom a Natural Disease was already present. If it were tested in that manner, Hahnemann reasoned, you could only measure the impact that the medicine had on the disease and not on the person with the disease. And Hahnemann wanted to know—and felt the need for all doctors to know—exactly what the medicine did to the whole human system, what its total range of actions might be shown to be.

So he began working only with healthy people. Since he knew that the action of a medicine was to create an Artificial Disease, and since he knew that through the process of dilution, he had removed the toxicity from the original substances, he felt quite safe using his medicines in this manner. He began testing these medicines by having healthy people ingest them and then keeping track of exactly what happened, what changed in their bodies and in their minds, their perceptions. In giving the medicines to a number of healthy persons, all of whom kept complete diaries of their experiences, Hahnemann was able to track exactly what the Artificial Disease state created was like, what would be the likely changes caused by this medicine, and what might be termed the whole sphere of action of this particular medicine. In this way, he knew the changes in state of being that were created by the medicine, instead of just knowing the physical changes that the medicine could cause and therefore treat.

This is the only form of testing that could be appropriate to homeopathy because this is the only form of testing by which Hahnemann could assess the type of *person* that his medicines could treat, instead of the type of *disease*; because it is central to the philosophy of homeopathy that it is always the person with the disease who is to be treated, and never the disease itself.

But Hahnemann's method of testing his remedies is practical and sensible not only for the homeopath but also for the allopath. Think about it. Hahnemann came to use his medicines not just for a handful of symptoms that the patient didn't like, but for the totality of symptoms—good, bad, and benign—experienced by the patient. Instead of giving a patient one medicine for headache and another for stomachache, he matched the remedy that had both symptoms, as experienced by the patient, within its sphere of action.

This, too, could be employed by the allopaths. In their PDRs, they have a listing of every known medicine and its every action. In allopathic medicine, of course, they are listed by their principal action and their side effects. And they are given based on the principal action only. Some doctors may warn their patients about the side effects, those other, equal parts of the Artificial Disease, but some may not. But in Hahnemann's method of testing and using medicines, there were no such things as side effects of medicines, because all effects were considered equally. If allopathic medicines were considered and given in the same way, they might be far more effective, and have far less troublesome impacts upon the patient's system.

Since, unlike the other doctors of his day, Hahnemann saw a medicine as not bringing about one primary change in the human system with any number of pesky side effects, but saw a medicine instead as having a complete sphere of activity, he came to believe that no doctor should give more than one medicine at a time. He felt that *polypharmacy,* the giving of more than one medicine, would create multiple Artificial Diseases within that human system, making it quite impossible to determine which had brought about what change specifically. Further, he felt that while it was quite possible to predict what changes were likely to occur by the use of one medicine, thanks to his impeccable form of testing, it was quite impossible to predict what the combination of medicines could do within the system, or even if they might set up a new Artificial Disease by their combination that would be permanent and incurable. Where Hahnemann found that, in his healthy test subject, the symptoms of Artifical Disease would simply fade when the subject stopped taking the medicine, he was in no way sure that the symptoms would ever fade if medicines were given in combination. And certainly the experience of modern polypharmacy would seem to bear him out. Modern medicine now must include terms for those many diseases that are caused, not by nature, but by medical treatments themselves.

And so, Hahnemann's insights into the nature of medicine led to changes in how he both tested and used his medicines, but these all also led him to consider the changes that were necessary in the very nature of the medicines themselves. And here he somehow managed to leap two hundred years ahead of his time.

Hahnemann had to use the same deck of cards that everyone else had; he had only the basic pharmacy on hand that every other doctor of his day did—arsenic and the like; toxic substances.

And so, since he could not, with clear conscience, make use of medicines that he knew good and well were toxic, he sought another way of working and did the logical thing—he created a method of diluting those substances until they reached a point at which they could be used safely.

He found in his years of experiments in dilution—and Hahnemann did not dilute his medicines in just a glass or even a barrel of water, but instead with generation after generation of levels of dilution, each precisely measured out in hundreds of beakers in his laboratory—that there was a mystery to this process, that there was a level at which, if you diluted a toxic substance enough, the toxicity fell sway, but the ability to create the Artificial Disease remains intact; that this ability for a medicine to be a catalyst to change was not a function of its substance, but was instead a fundamental component of its very nature.

And Hahnemann used his dilutions for a period of some years, with great success. He acquired a reputation for practicing good medicine as he traveled every day in his wooden cart from door to door, visiting the sick in their own homes.

In what may be a homeopathic myth, it has been said that throughout these days of travel, Hahnemann noticed again and again that the person he visited at the end of the day seemed to get a greater benefit from his medicine than did the person whom he visited earlier in the day. Although this might have been chalked up to a heightened perception on his part in the afternoon hours, he instead looked at his remedies and reconsidered their nature. He traveled with his medicines in liquid diluted form, he reasoned, and therefore the shaking that the medicines received all day in his cart might have had something to do with their seemingly increased potency. And so he began to work with what he called *succussion*, the shaking of the medicines as a part of their potentizing process.

Soon Hahnemann was combining the stages of increased dilution with succussion and found that the result was a powerful medicine with no toxic impact to be found. He had created what he would in time refer to as a homeopathic remedy.

Now, it is the exact nature of this homeopathic remedy, how these two rather simplistic methods of diluting and shaking could create what today we call a *microdose*—which while retaining the impact of a catalyst no longer has the toxicity of the substance—that remains the central mystery of homeopathy.

Today, we have microscopes powerful enough to tell us that there are no molecules of the orginal substance left in a diluted homeopathic remedy. These are brought into play every time anyone sets out to debunk homeopathy. Usually the investigator will choose to test a homeopathic medicine and send it to a lab to see what's in it. It always comes back with the same result—there is nothing in the remedy. Nothing of a physical nature, at least.

In his day, Hahnemann had none of the tools at his disposal that he would have had today. He could only work with his test subjects, and later, after his remedies were correctly created and proven, with his patients, to see with his own eyes, again and again, the changes that his remedies could create.

In his day he also lacked the help that Einstein and the study of Quantum Physics could bring to homeopathy.

About ten years ago, I read an article in *The New York Times* Science Section that quite literally changed my life, and my viewpoint about life. But, like Hahnemann's life changes, mine was slow and quiet, so that I did not at the time think anything about it other than that it was an interesting article. Today I believe that if you are to accept this article, this information, as truth, then this truth changes everything.

The article said that scientists who were studying the smallest bits of matter, the smallest of the small microscopic bits, were finding that those bits changed their behavior when they knew that they were being watched. When I read it, I thought that it was typical—another proof that everyone, no matter how small, just wants to be on camera.

But over the years, it has come to mean much more to me: it means that there is a coherence—perhaps an intelligence—to every part of Creation. And that the behavior of that Creation, the rules by which it acts and interacts with all of the parts of Creation, just might be mutable in nature. That all Creation itself might be changing its structure and behavior around what the viewer perceives and what the viewer wants.

Now, I could go in a lot of directions with this thought, and it certainly has great implications for the creation of illness in our lives (for instance, if these particles were not mutable, it is highly likely to me that we would lack the ability to heal at all, but would instead, like Goldie Hawn and Meryl Streep in *Death Becomes Her,* have to glue our arms back on to our bodies if we were unlucky enough to break them), but let's look at it from the viewpoint of what it means for homeopathy.

In class I love to tell the story of Paracelsus. And I love to share his viewpoint of healing, how he said that when a cold person needs to light a fire in the fireplace, he does not stand there and think to himself, "Now, precisely, how much energy do I have to apply to these logs in order to cause them to ignite?" No, he simply strikes a spark and stands back as the fire catches.

Paraclesus tells us that healing is a spark. A Vital Spark. And that the proper use of a medicine is to ignite the natural healing mechanism within each of us. It is then, as Paracelsus tells us, the role of the physician to get out of the way and let the fire catch. Healing is a natural response; it is the realignment and reorganization of those tiny bits of matter throughout our whole body, returning it to a state of health. It is the rewriting of the rules of our personal universe.

In his book *The Organon,* Hahnemann even tells us that illness is conceptual, that it is, in its nature, nothing more than the tiny bits of our personal universe responding to some catalyst. And illness is the response. In the same way, he tells us, healing is a response. We live our lives in our own little portable universes, beset with ongoing catalysts to which we do or do not respond. Respond with healing or respond with illness.

So, in diluting his medicines, Hahnemann was in fact removing the obstacle that matter throws into the equation. He was making the catalyst action of the remedy more powerful by getting down to the Vital Spark itself. He was moving to the more fundamental level of energy. He was, without knowing it, making use of the living energy of substances in the creation of his dilutions. And all this was without Einstein to tell him that matter is energy, and that matter cannot be destroyed, only endlessly changed by meeting with catalysts of its own. So it is energy that makes up those tiny bits (particles and waves) that behave differently when you watch them, and it is energy that makes up the potency of homeopathic remedies and speaks to the energy in our own systems in creating a healing response.

Perhaps the most exciting part of homeopathy is that we even today lack the technology to truly measure its action. When our ability to see and to measure our bodies, our "selves," becomes sophisticated enough to measure those selves as energy beings, we will finally be able to see the exact action of a homeopathic remedy in a human being. Until that day, we, like Hahnemann, will have to make do by keeping careful track of the exact changes in that human—body, mind, and spirit—that we can see, that we can measure. And, in this way, we will hopefully be able to make better and better uses of these remedies as we hold tight to Hahnemann's discoveries.

Hahnemann, therefore, should be seen as the bridge between the ancient society of Hippocrates and the modern world of Einstein. He both made use of concepts that had been handed down from antiquity and presupposed the ideas of an atomic age.

So, for the moment, we are actually as bound as was Hahnemann himself. We, like him, can only be solid emipiricists and deal with our own clinical experience in determining the nature and practice of homeopathy. Not because it does not work, but because we still lack the technological tools to prove how it works.

We can only look to our clinical experience to show us the way. And so, in learning homeopathy, we must learn it as Hahnemann did, and as the great practitioners who have followed him did: with our own eyes and ears, with our own intellect and intuition.

In the pages that follow, I have attempted to create the most practical guide possible for these purposes, one that can replace the need for a bookshelf full of texts for the beginning student of homeopathy, and one that can be turned to again and again over the years as household crises arise.

The section that follows this introduction gives an outline of the philosophy of the practice of homeopathy, intertwined with a working definition of a physician's role in the community. To me, it is perhaps the most important section of this book in that it uses Hahnemann's own words, taken from his writings in *The Organon of Medicine* to give the principles behind any homeopathic treatment.

Following that, I have gathered together a large group of diagnostic symptoms that offer many clues in the selection of correct homeopathic remedies for any given situation. The idea for this came to me from Chinese medicine, a healing art that makes use of basic tools—reading the pulses and the tongue among them—that give practitioners a map to follow in selecting a course of action. I thought that what would work for acupuncture needles or Chinese herbs would also work for homeopathic remedies. And in the years since I first thought this, I have found that it is true. If you can learn the basic diagnostics in terms of homeopathic remedies, you can often move very quickly to the selection of a remedy.

What follows the diagnostics is a long section on the uses of homeopathic remedies in simple acute emergencies. Just as the average New England housewife a century ago owned and used a homeopathic kit for day-to-day ailments, so should we today. This section will give suggestions for appropriate remedies in household situations.

And then there is a materia medica of some sixty basic homeopathic remedies, those most often used in the home. Each listing gives an overview of the remedy and its actions, as well as the most commonly used dosage and potency.

It is not my intent in putting together this guide that anyone should take it upon himself to practice medicine on himself or others without the proper training and legal standing. It is instead meant as a guide for those who wish to self-treat simple acute illness in the home setting. I do believe that, at this level, it is a well-rounded guide that offers the reader primary education into homeopathy.

—*Vinton McCabe*
June 1999

The Role of
the Physician

Introduction

It all begins with Hippocrates. He was the one who created the philosophy by which illness would be considered, and the methods by which it would be treated.

In the treatment of illness, Hippocrates' method was in many ways the perfect example of what would later be known as "Eclectic Medicine" (as it would be practiced by American homeopath J. T. Kent), similar to what would today be considered naturopathy. The medicine practiced by Hippocrates on the Isle of Cos centered upon the methods that encouraged the natural healing process to take place, rather than any method by which this natural process was pushed aside or defeated. Therefore, Hippocrates was very concerned with his patient's life and lifestyle and saw diet, exercise or its lack, and emotional surroundings as key to whether or not that patient could be expected to enjoy good health. He was also greatly concerned by the environment—both physical and emotional—in which the patient lived and functioned on a day-to-day basis. So the patient was treated as a whole, with attention given equally to all parts of that whole.

Hippocrates was fond of the word *physis*. Physis was his term for the natural processes within the human system that allowed it to be self-healing and regenerative. Hippocrates believed that it was the function of the practitioner to work with the physis—again, often by rather passive means, such as developing a new diet or exercise regimen, or by listening to the patient talk about his dreams and the iconography of his personal archetypes—to bring about a healing. Hippocrates would have been horrified, therefore, to look at many modern medical techniques that involve "tricking" the physis into believing that there existed nothing that needed to be healed (techniques as complex as surgery for chronic digestive disorders, or as seemingly benign as allergy treatments), in that he would have believed that ultimately such treatments would exact a price far greater than the original illness.

This term *physis* is key to our study in that Hippocrates and those who came to follow his methods saw themselves as physis-ians. And thus the word *physician* was born.

So the word *physician* defines the role of the person to whom the word is ascribed. A physician is one who works with the being, with its natural ability to heal, and works in a manner that encourages that healing process. The word *physician* implies no particular training, no exact license or level of skill. Instead, it implies a philosophy, a manner of thinking and working that is as true today as it was when coined by Hippocrates.

Therefore, and this is important, every person who gives a homeopathic remedy, from the veteran prescriber to the newcomer who is opening a home kit for the first time and operating on a wing and a prayer, is a physician. It therefore also becomes most important that if we are going to place ourselves in the role of physician we really must understand the work we are taking on and know how healing works and why.

Samuel Hahnemann, the father of homeopathy, and a follower of Hippocrates' principles of treatment, left behind him a written record both of his philosophy and of his practice. This work, called *The Organon of Medicine,* evolved over years of writing and rewriting through six editions of publication. In it, Hanhemann explains what we are attempting to do—the work we are taking on. The need for definition of both the practice and the practitioner of medicine was so important to him that it was the topic of the very first aphorism in the *The Organon.* That first paragraph, in toto, states.

The physician's highest and *only* calling is to make the sick healthy,
to cure it is called.

It is both a simple and a powerful statement. By his choice—and I believe that it was a very conscious choice from a man who knew the meanings, both implied and given, of the words he chose—of the word *physician,* Hahnemann is telling us right up front that we must work by the natural method, by increasing the vital force or life energy within the individual, rather than by working against nature in eliminating disease. By first referring to this calling as "highest," he is reminding us that this method of treatment is just that: a calling. Hahnemann believed that the people who worked alongside others in the healing of disease, in setting themselves free of the boundaries of disease, were literally called by God into their work.

But to fully understand Hahnemann's words, we must look to the footnote that he included in his text. In it, Hahnemann tells us what the physician's calling is not: "to concoct so-called systems from empty conceits . . . and the origins of disease in the invisible interior of the organism," or "to make countless attempts at explanation regarding disease appearance and their proximate cause . . . while a sick world sighs in vain for help." He concludes, "It is high time for all those who call themselves physicians, once and for all, to stop deceiving suffering humanity with idle talk, and to *begin* now to *act,* that is to really help and to cure."

For a time I wondered about the use of that word *cure* in that highest of callings. It seemed to me that its presence hindered the meaning of the overall statement. It seemed to me that the physician should be wanting to "heal" and not to "cure." But then it occurred to me that because Hahnemann so clearly understood that the healing process was internal and could only be encouraged or hindered, but never controlled, or truly begun or stopped by any exterior catalyst, Hahnemann, in revealing the physician's role, could only speak in terms of curing disease. The physician has no power to heal; indeed, that is part of what makes his work so effective. The doctor who is not a physician as well may believe himself capable of healing a patient. The wise physician, who knows that the ultimate outcome of any treatment can only be hoped for and not guessed or controlled, knows that he is working on the somewhat more humble level of curing. He can only set the stage for an improvement of health and then hope for the best possible outcome.

In general the first through the fourth paragraphs of *The Organon* flesh out the role of the physician. The second paragraph is written as follows:

> The highest ideal of cure is the rapid, gentle and permanent restoration of health; that is, the lifting and annihilation of the disease in its entire extent in the shortest, most reliable, and least disadvantageous way, according to clearly realizable principles.

This too is a powerful if brief statement. In it, he is giving us three words that should be common to all cures: *rapid, gentle,* and *permanent.* In other words, the physician is to find a natural method by which he can spark a change, bring about a catalyst to change. And this change is to be for the betterment of the patient, for his improvement. Not just in terms of the specific ache or pain that brought him into the office seeking treatment, but in terms of his whole being. It is, therefore, not a successful treatment that allows your patient to be free of the ear infection that brought him to you, but to now be suffering from asthma because of the impact of your treatment upon his system. Nor is it good for your patient to ultimately recover from both his disease and his treatment, but with some question as to which was more challenging to his system, the disease or the cure. And, finally, it is not to be considered a successful treatment if it ends this ear infection but another one is in place in a matter of weeks.

We are supposed to, if we are to be true physicians, leave our patients better than we found them.

Hahneman makes sure that we understand this by telling us that we are in the business of "the lifting and annihilation of the disease in its entire extent." It is supposed to be gone, gone forever. And he continues that we are to undertake this total cure "in the shortest, most reliable, and least disadvantageous way." In other words, "first, do no harm."

Hahnemann was a very conservative physician, both in his philosophy and in his practice. He would not encourage the physician to what I call "entering the drama" of the illness as experienced by the patient. He would simply observe—compassionately, to be sure—but observe from an emotional distance, in order to look for the path through which this healing journey could be the shortest and easiest it could possibly be. He was forever reminding himself of the word *gentle.* Nothing in his methodology would trade this concept of gentle medicine for medicine that fulfilled the other two categories of treatment: rapid or permanent. Therefore, we must also be prepared to work more slowly, or to work day-by-day, taking what success we can achieve, in order that the journey toward total health be ultimately as brief as it can be, and as permanent as life will allow, but at every moment as gentle and loving as possible.

Hahnemann concludes his second paragraph with a short phrase. He tells us that the treatment must also be carried out "according to clearly realizable principles." In other words, we have to be able to have a philosophy to follow. We have to have a plan. And this is most important: it is clear from Hahnemann's writing that he does not insist that every physician be a homeopath, but does insist that every physician follow an organized plan of action. Hahnemann realized that there are many modalities of treatment and that there are two basic methods of treatment: the allopathic, which works against symptoms by giving a treatment that counters the natural symptoms; and the homeopathic, which works with the symptoms, believing that there is a reason for their existence, by giving a treatment that would, in a healthy person, create the symptoms that are naturally occurring in the patient's system.

What Hahnemann insists is that each physician must make a decision, a rational and well-thought-out decision as to how he is going to treat the patient and why. While Hahnemann would strongly disagree with the practice of allopathy, he would have far more respect for the rapid allopath who has thought through his philosophy and practice and then proceeded with his method of treatment. What he could not respect was the practitioner of any sort who simply treats as he has been taught to treat, without wrestling through the process of forming a personal philosophy of practice and treatment.

In this vein, Hahemann also tells us that the physician cannot allow himself to be placed in the role of "reactor," of always reacting to the drama of the illness and the pain of its sufferer. Instead, the physician must look to his position, to his knowledge and his skill, in order to keep his patient on a healing path.

Paragraph 3 of *The Organon* has more to tell us about the knowledge and skill that is required of the physician. He writes:

To be a genuine practitioner of the medical art, a physician must:
1. clearly realize what is to be cured in diseases, that is, in each single case of disease (*discernment of the disease, indicator*),
2. clearly realize what is curative in medicines, that is, in each particular medicine (*knowledge of medicinal powers*),
3. be aware of how to adapt what is curative in medicines to what he has discerned to be undoubtedly disease in the patient, according to clear principles.
   In this way, recovery must result.

So Hahnemann is telling us that the physician must have some method of looking at disease, and at medicine. There has to be a framework for his thought. And, in a sort of juggling act, he has to be able to take what the medicine has to offer in the way of cure, and match it correctly to what he understands to be the nature of the illnesses that already exist in his patient. And again, he needs some path to follow, some way of working that has been shown clinically to work. That has stood the test of time.

It is of vital importance that Hahnemann has not yet, in aphorism number 3, said in any way that the homeopathic method is better than is the allopathic. Instead, he insists that each physician must have an understanding of an underlying philosophy of treatment and must work from that philosophy in a manner that can clearly be shown to spring from the core philosophy. In this manner, Hahnemann is showing the role of the physician, and not of the homeopath (and, sadly, it is quite possible that we will have homeopaths who are not fulfilling the role of physician, just as we have physicians who know nothing of homeopathy. But give me the true physician who has no understanding of homeopathy any day over that practitioner steeped in homeopathic knowledge who is in no way a true physician. I can supply the homeopathic knowledge for the one, if need be, but can only suffer under the treatments of the other).

In aphorism number 3, Hahnemann continues:

Adapting what is curative in medicine, according to what is diseased in patients, requires that the physician be able to:
1. adapt the most appropriate medicine, according to its mode of action, to the case before him (*selection of the remedy, that which is indicated*),
2. prepare the medicine exactly as required,
3. give the medicine in the exact amount required (the right *dose*),
4. properly time the repetition of doses.

Finally, the physician must know the obstacles to recovery in each case and be aware of how to clear them away so that the restoration of health may be permanent.

If the physician has this insight, discernment, knowledge and awareness then he understands how to act expediently and thoroughly and he is a genuine practitioner of the medical art.

So, again, Hahnemann sets no easy task. He is saying that whatever the type of medicine this physician practices, he has to know about his medicines. He has to stay current; he has to be thorough in his knowledge. He is putting the knowledge of the pharmacy at hand, what the homeopath calls his Materia Medica, above and beyond the rest. If you do not have a solid knowledge of medicines available to you—the catalysts that spark the cure—you cannot be a physician. For me this means, if you don't know your Materia Medica, if you have not already grasped the philosophy of homeopathy (or any other form of medicine, for that matter), then you should not be handing out medicines. While this should be so obvious, I have, time and time again, seen people who want to rush out and buy a homeopathic kit and start using it before they bother to read a book or attend a class. They want to place themselves in the role of physician before they even understand what that role is.

So the physician must know his pharmacy. He must understand what medicines he has to work with and the uses and potential abuses of each. He must also know how these medicines are made. Now, I know that we can no longer expect a homeopath to create his or her own remedies any more than we can expect our allopath to be whipping up a batch of Prozac in his back room, but Hahnemann tells us that both the allopathic and the homeopathic physician must understand how the medicine is made, and why it is made as it is made.

Next, he tells us that the physician must know how to give his medicines in the right potency and dose. This, I know, is something of a Catch-22: You can only know what potency and dose of a remedy to use if you have used it in the past and have some basis of personal experience from which to work, but you are apparently supposed to only give the remedies if you already know how to give them. Tricky. But again we must, especially as beginners—whether laypersons or medical professionals new to homeopathy—turn again to our philosophy. Our Materia Medica study will give us guidelines as to the appropriate potency and dosage of particular remedies. And the writings of past masters of the art will also give us guidelines for usage until we can develop our own. (The best rule of thumb is to remember that Hahnemann was conservative in his use of remedies. He always started with one dose and waited to see what it would do. And he always gave that dose of medicine in the lowest possible potency that he believed could have some impact upon the case.)

Finally, Hahnemann makes a statement that gives deep insight into the role of the physician. He says that "the physician must know the obstacles to recovery in each case and be aware of how to clear them away so that the restoration of health may be permanent."

The physician's role, as identified by Hippocrates, is to work with the natural healing mechanism and to encourage healing. He is to be a catalyst, to spark some change within his patient's life that allows that patient to at least begin a true healing process. And that concept of change is paramount to understanding the healing process.

Healing is all about change. If we did not need to change, if we were not stuck in some way, at some level of being—physical, mental, or emotional—we would not need a healing. We would be in perfect health. But we are not, we are not totally free of aches and pains, and even with the best treatment, we will not stay free of our aches and pains, our limitations and doubts, unless the physician can somehow spark us to begin true change in our lives and in our very natures. Now this change may be as simple as moving out of our basement appartment to one on the second floor (see paragraph number 77 of *The Organon* for Hahnemann's insights into this sort of change), or as profound as a newfound willingness to be well. But change must happen. And, as Hahnemann tells us, it is part of the physician's role to have the discernment to help identify where this change needs to take place.

Hahnemann concludes with paragraph number 4:

> He is likewise a sustainer of health if he knows the things that disturb health, that engender and maintain disease, and is aware of how to remove them from healthy people.

So, it is not enough that the physician be able to identify and to treat disease, but, Hahnemann tells us, he must also have a methodology that allows for the sustaining of health, once health has been achieved. This certainly feeds into the notion that healing is an ongoing process, that it is a function, not of being sick, but of being alive.

The physician must have a working philosophy, a method of treatment that is at once practical and philosophically sound. He or she must know what is to be treated and how to treat it. Further, he or she must know what changes need to occur in a given life in order for the patient to both become well and stay well. Not an easy task.

In our society we have confused the terms *physician* and *doctor*. *Doctor*, as a term, relates to a level of formal education. The word itself is meant to be an honorific. It is a word by which we can set aside those who have done the work and earned the honor, but it in no way recognizes whether or not the persons who have earned the title have any true understanding of healing, or of curing. It only supposes that they have an understanding of sickness, and, perhaps, that they only understand that on the most basic physical level.

Our term *physician*, however, demands more. It demands everything that Hahnemann insists upon. But it does not demand a medical license or a particular legal standing. Instead, it demands a deeper understanding, a Road to Damascus experience almost, that gives the practitioner, layperson, or medical professional a means of working that creates an environment in which healing can take place. That is the role of the physician, whether that physician be a mother who is rocking her sick infant throughout the night or the medical practitioner with a full-service clinic and a BMW in the garage. Both have equal requirements placed upon them by Hahnemann, and by Hippocrates before him, in the role of physician and in the service of man.

Disease

Most people think that there is no need to pause even for a second to consider the nature of that which we call "disease." They are likely to tell you that they may not really know what a disease is or what causes it, but that they know when they have one, sort of like the person who says, "I may not know good art from bad art, but I know what I like."

But Hahnemann, in wrestling with the role of the physician, insists that we have to stop and consider the nature of disease, that if we cannot understand what a disease is, and where it comes from in the human system, then we can never truly find a satisfactory method of treating disease.

Aphorisms numbers 4 and 5 of *The Organon* give us Hahnemann's insights into the nature of disease. They speak particularly well of the aspects of acute disorders, which are the focus of this work.

In paragraph number 4, Hahnemann writes:

> It will help the physician to bring about a cure if he can find out the data of the most probable *occasion* of an acute disease, and the most significant factors in the entire history of a protracted wasting sickness, enabling him to find out its *fundamental cause*. . . . In these investigations, the physician should take into account the patient's
> 1. discernible body constitutions (especially in cases of protracted disease),
> 2. mental and emotional character,
> 3. occupations,
> 4. lifestyle and habits,
> 5. civic and domestic relationships,
> 6. age,
> 7. sexual function, etc.

Now, most of this will be of more importance later in his work, but it is important to note here that Hahnemann is already giving us a clue to the fact that the physician's work in multitiered. That ailments can be classified into acute, chronic (protracted), and miasmic (genetic).

But it is in paragraph number 5 that Hahnemann actually defines the term *disease*:

> The unprejudiced observer . . . perceives nothing in each single case of disease other than the alterations in the condition of the body and soul, *disease signs, beffallments, symptoms,* which are outwardly discernable through the senses. That is, the unprejudiced observer only perceives the deviations from the former healthy state of the now sick patient, which are:
> 1. felt by the patient himself,
> 2. perceived by those around him, and
> 3. observed by the physician.
>
> All these perceptible signs represent the disease in its entire extent, that is, together they form the true and only conceivable gestalt of the disease.

Ah, now here the trouble begins. Hahnemann, predicting the conclusions that would be drawn a century later, insists that we cannot even decide what a disease is without teamwork. He states, like modern linguists, that information is divided into four parts: the information I know, the information you know, the information we both know, and the information neither of us knows. And Hahnemann is saying that we need to gather what we can from all four categories to get to the bottom of whether or not a disease is present.

It seems obvious, then, that the disease state can largely be called a subjective one. That one person displaying a set of symptoms will call them "growing pains," while another will call them "flu." There is not one moment at which we will all consider ourselves to be sick. Gender, age, vital force, weight, and so many other factors come into play in this seemingly simple task of deciding whether we are to stand with the group under the "diseased" sign, or line up with the "healthy."

So, Hahnemann is saying that you are sick if you, your family, and your doctor all think you are sick. And they base this decision upon symptoms. But, in reality, we are all experiencing symptoms at all times, some good and some bad, some neither good nor bad. So the disease state could logically be concluded to be the moment at which the painful symptoms outweigh the good and neutral ones.

In *The Organon*, paragraph number 9, Hahnemann himself writes:

> In the healthy human state, the spirit-like life force (autocracy) that enlivens the material organism as dynamis, govern without restriction and keeps all parts of the organism in admirable, harmonious, vital operation, as regards both feelings and functions, so that our indwelling, rational spirit can freely avail itself of this living, healthy instrument for the higher purposes of our existence.

And, in paragraph number 11:

> When a person falls ill, it is initially only this spirit-like, autonomic life force (life principle), everywhere present in the organism, that is mistuned through the dynamic influence of a morbific agent inimical to life. Only the life principle, mistuned to such abnormality, can impart to the organism the adverse sensations and induce in the organism the irregular functions we call disease . . .

Hahnemann concludes in paragraph number 12: "It is the disease-tuned life force alone that brings forth diseases."

Thus, we are to conclude that disease is dynamic—energistic—in its nature. If the vital force bonds the soul to the body and allows all of the body's functions to take place, then disease must be considered a disruption of that energy that displays itself on the physical, rather than the dynamic, level of being.

This does not perhaps overturn the "germ theory," but states simply that something must first occur on the energistic level for the patient to be susceptible to the germ and for the immune system to be weakened to the point that the disease can take hold.

Homeopath Elizabeth Wright Hubbard took a more positive stance when it came to the subject of disease. In that the vital force was manifesting symptoms, she felt that disease was actually a positive, if painful thing. Elizabeth Wright Hubbard, in a memorable phrase, gives us homeopathy's concept that disease *is a protective explosion manifesting in an individual as a particular set of symptoms.*

In other words, the disease itself is a sign that the patient's vital force is attempting to clear itself and put all things right, that the healing process is already begun, and not that the patient's vital force is weakened, although his body may well be. Therefore, the task of the physician is to work with the vital force in the healing process by encouraging the illness to work itself through. Anything that at this point suppresses the symptoms of the illness will also suppress and weaken the vital force itself; therefore that which suppresses specific symptoms of pain also suppresses the total health of the individual.

The modern-day Greek homeopath George Vithoulkas often speaks of the three planes (mental, emotional, and physical) of being which are impacted upon by disease. In doing so, he gives us insight into this definitions of health and disease. He writes:

> Health is freedom from pain in the physical body, having attained a state of well-being; freedom from passion on the emotional level, having as result a dynamic state of serenity and calm; and freedom from selfishness in the mental sphere, having as a result total unification with Truth.

In giving us a working definition of comparative levels of sickness and health, Vithoulkas writes:

> What is the parameter that defines, for instance, whether an individual with rheumatoid arthritis is in better health than another one suffering from depression? The parameter which enables such measurement of health is creativity. By creativity, I mean all those acts and functions which promote for the individual himself and for others their main goal in life: continuous and unconditional happiness. To the extent that an individual is limited in the exercise of his creativity, to that degree he is ill. If the rheumatoid arthritis patient is crippled to the extent that his ailment prevents him from being creative more than the patient with depression, then the rheumatoid arthritis patient is more seriously ill than the depressed one . . .
>
> A healthy mind should be characterized in its functions from the following three qualities: clarity, coherence and creativity. To the extent that any or all of these qualities are reduced or missing, the person is ill . . .

This statement can be a little shocking to those who have long ago decided that any illness of the mind and spirit must be a more important illness than anything that the physical body can contain, but it seems to be, nevertheless, very true. We must consider that the patient's system will break down at its weakest point, wherever that point may be, at whatever level of being. And so, we should use the ideas of freedom and restriction in assessing the health of a patient.

I have found Vithoulkas' measuring stick of clarity, coherence, and creativity to be an excellent method of considering health and disease. The healthier the patient, the more he or she is able to live and work in a world of freedom, a world that is largely defined by one's will and imagination. To the extent the patient becomes ill, that world becomes defined by the illness, even to the point at which the illness can become the patient's career, and, even, calling in life.

Finally, there is homeopath Stuart Close's excellent consideration of the classifications of the causes of disease. Close looks at the situation from a less philosophical, and more clinical point of view, giving us a working jargon for disease classification. He writes:

(1) *Mechanical* causes of disease include injuries, foreign bodies, extraneous substances, many congenital defects, osteopathic lesions, amputations, or growths. . . . Hahnemann repeatedly instructed homeopaths first to remove the exciting cause or foreign agent that may be present in any diseased condition. For example, parasites, when their presence gives rise to disease, must be expelled, either by mechanical means or by such medicines as would be capable of weakening or destroying them, without in any way endangering or adversely affecting the patient.

(2) *Chemical* causes of disease are acids, alkalis, salts, alkaloids, a large number of poisons, and the like. . . . In such cases the use of chemical or physiological antidotes is required, combined, in some cases, with the means for the physical expulsion of the injurious substance (e.g., stomach pump). Thereafter, homeopathic treatment is necessary for the correction of the functional derangements which remain or follow.

(3) *Dynamical* causes of disease, which influence the reactive functions of the total patient, are very numerous: they may be emotional, environmental, electro-magnetic, radiation-induced, atmospheric; they may be found in diet, contagion, lack of hygiene, infection, allergic predisposition, the use and abuse of all hard drugs and medications, or result from previous constitutional resistance to the pathogenetic effects of specific toxins exuded by certain microorganisms. With regard to the last named, homeopathy is on

record as consistently being highly successful in treating "serious" disease associated with resistance to bacteria, protozoa, and viruses whenever large epidemics permitted statistically significant comparisons with comparable non-homeopathic approaches.

Note here that the term *dynamic* for Close refers to ailments closest in terms of onset and symptom picture to the usual "inflammatory disease." Hahnemann would have us believe that all illness is caused by a disruption of our vital force, and not just those diseases that usually fall into the category of infectious disease. But Close gives us some slots to consider in our study of disease, and some words for naming those slots. These slots, however, affirm Hahnemann's original findings. While it certainly is true that each of us is vulnerable to physical trauma, we may be beaten, shot, or stabbed and will have the struggle with the effects of that trauma, and each of us may be poisoned, either quickly or slowly, by substances present either in food or in our environment, it is most importantly true that all other diseases of any sort are energistic in nature and have to do with the presence of, and blocking of, our own vital force. And that the human system's reaction even to physical trauma and to poisoning of all sorts is exactly the same as is its reactions to infectious disease states. In the case of poisonings and physical trauma, the catalyst to disease is simply an act of aggression or the impact of a toxin, instead of a an internally developed block of the vital force, but the catalyst still sends the being into a state know as disease. Since that is the case, it must be remembered that for Hahnemann the treatment of the person who has been beaten or poisoned would still follow the same general pattern of homeopathic medicine: letting like cure like, and that the patient who has been beaten or poisoned would still be given the remedy that in a person who has not been beaten or poisoned would create the same symptom picture that we are already seeing in the patient.

In considering disease, therefore, we must be considering vital force, in that Hahnemann was himself a "vitalist" and believed strongly in the invisible dynamis that inhabits all living things—all things natural to our planet. Illness then must be manifested in the body only after a disruption of this vital force, but what that term *disruption* might mean, from toxic environment to negative thoughts, still remains to be seen.

Medicine and "Artificial Disease"

In seeking to understand Hahnemann, his methods and his practice, we have to remember two key facts about his philosophy. Hahnemman was a vitalist; further, he was an empiricist.

While the vitalist movement and vitalism in general have been dealt with in more detail in my previous book, it is important to note here that Hahnemann held strong for the philosophy of vitalism. He believed that each of us has a vital force inside, that this invisible, intangible energy animates our bodies and keeps our minds and bodies unified for all our days on this earth.

Further, vitalists hold with the idea that all illness must begin with a disruption on the level of vital force. And while each individual vitalist would have his own philosophical model as to just how and where this disruption takes place, all would agree that illness begins within this life force and must be healed upon this energistic level.

Finally, vitalists would hold with the notion that all things natural to this earth and to all Creation are vital; that all things, animate or seemingly inaminate, contain the same vital force; and it is the vital force of the substance—animal, vegetable, or mineral—that, in harmonizing with our own, brings about the healing on the energy level.

In homeopathy, therefore, we believe that in the process of making the remedies, of diluting toxic substances into microdoses, we are both removing the toxins and freeing the vital force, the pure energy pattern of the substance, making it more helpful in assisting our own energy healing than it ever could be in its natural form.

But Hahnemann was also an empiricist. He believed in the practice of medicine that was based in what could be experienced on the level of the human senses; therefore, when he defined disease, he did so on the level of what could be seen and recognized by the patient, the doctor, and the patient's loved ones.

So Hahnemann placed the experience of disease and the experience of the healing process in the realm of the senses. Thus, when he begins to work upon the development of homeopathy and the creation of a homeopathic pharmacy, he tests his medicines upon human subjects, upon those who may assist him actively and directly in recognizing the outcome of the medical trials.

Empirical medicine, however, is not just limited to homeopathy. It is, instead, a method of treatment that has today been somewhat supplanted by technological medicine, but nevertheless gives a solid methodology to follow.

While they had a solid philosophy and a strong viewpoint of health and disease, the empiricists lacked one thing: a statement as to the actions of medicines. In fact, the practice of any form of medicine long lacked an actual statement of exactly what medicine is and what it does.

The great and eccentric healer of the Middle Ages, Paracelsus, tells us that "all things are poison," that anything has the ability to bring about damage to the system, that it was just a matter of quantity. There is even such a thing as drinking too much water, and a point at which the presence of too great an amount of water in our system can cause harm.

Classic homeopaths have also told us that "the stronger the poison, the stronger the cure," and so complete Paracelsus' statement. Everything is poison then, and everything therefore can be a tool toward cure. It becomes a matter of what we shall use in our curative process, and how we shall use it, and how much of it is needed.

Indeed, the value of any supposed medicine comes from its ability to create any change in the human system. Thus, there is in actuality no difference between poison and medicine, or, rather, the difference has more to do with the circumstances surrounding the use of the poison or medicine and not with the substance itself; whether a substance that creates diarrhea in the human system would be a poison or a medicine, depending upon whether you yourself are suffering from constipation or diarrhea. (And, of course, whether you are involved in the practice of homeopathy or allopathy.)

All disease and all medicine are simply a process of catalyst and response. The germ, it must be remembered, is not the disease. The presence of a cold virus in your system does not cause your nose to run or your eyes to water. It is, instead, your body's own immune system, in seeking to flush out that germ, that causes the symptoms of the illness. The germ is the catalyst, the illness the response.

In the same way, the medicine is used as a catalyst as well, one that will hopefully (if used homeopathically) create a healing response in the human system. That is why anything that causes a strong response, anything that is a strong catalyst, may be considered a medicine.

Hahnemann describes this principle in aphorism number 19 of *The Organon*:

> Since diseases are nothing other than alterations of condition in healthy people which express themselves through disease signs, and

since cure is likewise only possible through an alteration of the patient's condition into the healthy state, then it is easily seen that medicines would in no way be able to cure if they did not possess the power to differently tune the human condition that resides in feelings and functions. Indeed, it is evident that the curative power of medicines must rest solely upon this, their power to alter the human condition.

Hahnemann refuses to limit the ability of a medicine to bring about a change. He will not say that this change is purely physical. He insists that it can be functional and emotional as well. The catalyst, therefore, might well be considered an insight of sorts—that the patient sees, through this catalyst, some essential truth, the understanding and recognition of which allows for a cure to take place.

He extends this notion into the realm of the spirit, and returns to his empirical roots in aphorism number 20:

This hidden spirit-like power in the inner wesen of medicines to alter the human condition and thus to cure diseases is, in itself, in no way discernible with mere intellectual exertion. It is only by experience, only through its manifestations while it is impinging on the human condition that we can distinctly perceive it.

I especially enjoy the use of the word *wesen* in aphorism number 20. The authors of the newest translation of *The Organon*, Wenda Brewster O'Reilly and Steven Decker, in retranslating Hahnemann's work from the original German to modern English, have, with their great love for words, reminded us of Hahnemann's specific intent here. In their notes, they give the following information on the word *wesen*:

"Wesen" is a multi-faceted term which can mean any of the following: essence, substance, creature, living thing, nature, or entity. There is no single English word that adequately translates Wesen. In almost every instance in *The Organon*, Hahnemann uses the term to refer to that entity which is the essential unchanging esse of something: its being, its quintessence.

Thus this vital force, this spiritlike spark of life present in everything, is also present in medicines. And it is the wesen, the core truth of that medicine, if you will, that determines the catalytic action of the medicine.

Hahnemann states that we can only identify our medicines if we can identify the impact of that medicine upon the human system, only if we can assure ourselves as to what sort of catalyst this is.

And this is true for all forms of medicine and for anything that may be considered medicinal. Virtually all of modern medicine is rooted in the ancient herbal Materca Medica. Herbalists were treating diseases with internal and external plant medicines in the period before Christ. And even today we make use of these remedies, not only in their natural herbal state, but allopathically in chemical equivalents and in a potentized state in homeopathy.

But what constitutes medicine is still tricky. Just ask the FDA or the Congress, which still, from time to time, tries to decide just what a medicine should be. Some things are fairly easy to categorize, but others . . . well, what should we do with garlic or onion, both of which are considered foods, but both of which are also decidedly medicinal in their actions? So even today we cannot decide what is medicine and what is not.

This makes all the more important Hahnemann's findings in this arena. He give us a new term to use, and this term may well be, all things considered, his greatest contribution to the science of medicine.

Hahnemann tested his medicines on healthy people because he wanted to measure the impact of the medicine on the patient as a whole being and not on the symptoms of his disease. He is the only medical pioneer to have worked in this manner. And through the findings of medical trials he coined the word *"Arneikrankheit,"* to explain the impact of his medicines.

The term itself means "drug disease," and references the fact that Hahnemann found again and again that as medicines are given they themselves created Artificial Diseases, sets of multitiered symptoms that are fully comparable to "natural" diseases, which are those that occur spontaneously in the human system. And the symptoms of the Artificial Disease, he found again and again, are totally indistinguishable from the symptoms created or brought on by a germ or infection.

This is so important, not just to homeopathy, but to all medicine, because it led Hahnemann to his next conclusion.

Again, in that Hahmenmann was an empiricist, his findings were based in observable results. And again and again, in observing his patients and the impact of medicines upon their systems, he found that *all* medicine, all things that may be said to act in a medicinal way, have not just one but two actions within the human system.

Hahnemann gives us a term for this discovery as well. He calls it *hormesis,* which relates to the biphasic action of all medicines—medicinal action that takes place in two distinct phases or steps. In an essay in 1796, he wrote: "Medicines have more than one action: the first a direct action which gradually changes into the second (which I call the indirect secondary action). The latter is generally a state exactly the opposite of the former."

In stating this, Hahnemann was putting into medical terms one of our basic laws of physics: for every action there is an equal and opposite reaction. And, in recognizing this biphasic action, he was finally once and for all giving us a reason why both homeopathy and allopathy act in the human system as they do.

Allopathy is the medicine of action. Medicines are given to the patient based upon the initial action of the substance; therefore, if you cannot sleep, you are given a sleeping pill.

Homeopathy, however, is the medicine of reaction. Your original symptoms are considered, far from being a bad thing, as a sign that your vital force is working. The physician considers that he or she must work with the symptoms and honor their existence. There is a reason for this illness, whether or not we shall ever uncover that reason. Therefore, the patient who cannot sleep is given a remedy that in a totally well person (remember, Hahnemann always tested his remedies upon healthy people) would create the symptoms of sleeplessness that the patient is already experiencing.

The immediate result, in both cases, is sleep. But, let's see what happens over time.

The patient of the allopath, as days and weeks pass, will find that he cannot sleep at all now without taking more and more of the medicine that puts him to sleep. As his body's own equal and opposite reaction is called into place, his system works against the medicine's action with its own reaction: sleeplessness. Thus the patient will in time be worse off than he was before.

The homeopathic patient was and is sleeping through the night. Why?

Hahnemann tells us that all medicine, allopathic or homeopathic, creates an action and a reaction. He tells us that we should think of this action of the medicine—again, both allopathic and homeopathic—as an "Artificial Disease." That this change in symptoms brought on by the medicine is to be considered to be a disease state that you have willfully taken into your system for hopefully curative purposes. And, as a disease state, it is to be thought of as a group of symptoms. No medicine known to man has a single action. All medicines—all catalysts to change—have a sphere of actions in which many changes take place, and on many levels of being—mental, emotional, and physical. Therefore, it is an allopathic illusion that we might take a medicine and it will have only a single action. This fact of our physical realm gives credence to the homeopathic precept that we should base our use of any medicine upon the totality of symptoms, and never upon the presence of a single symptom. Whether working allopathically or homeopathically, medicines should be given on the basis of all their actions and never on the hope that they have a single action.

Look in a *Physician's Desk Reference* and you will see under the listing of any allopathic drug a primary action for that drug and then a list of all the other actions that the drug might also create. The allopath calls these "side effects." The homeopath, however, sees them as equally valid forms of impact that the drug has on the human system. Forms of impact that must be taken into consideration in the use of the drug. The listing of primary and side effects must all be taken together into consideration as the sphere of impact of that drug and it must be matched against the totality of symptoms that the patient is experiencing. Only this can be the wise use of a medicine.

To return to the idea of medicine as "Artificial Disease," Hahnemann tells us that when you take a homeopathic remedy you are willfully placing an Artificial Disease within your system. This Artificial Disease has been selected based upon the known sphere of activity of that homeopathic remedy and its similarity to the Natural Disease state, expressed in the totality of symptoms already at hand. He says that, to work best, the Artificial should be slightly more potent than the Natural Disease state, so that when the bump of the original remedy fades, when your body rises up against it in an equal and opposite reaction, your body's response will not, as in allopathy, be to go deeper into the original disease state, but will be to make itself well. The natural symptoms and artificial symptoms (both of which are following the same symptom portrait) will together be expressed and expelled from the system when the system's own healing reaction takes place.

This is what Hahnemann has given us here in his identification of the action/reaction qualities of medicines: a plan of treatment of disease than cannot fail, if followed completely, to bring about a curative response.

Symptoms

Symptoms are good, bad, and indifferent. We have them every day. They are a sign that vital force is still present in our bodies. They are a sign of life.

Each day we come into contact with catalysts and potential catalysts. Everything that happens to us has the potential to cause a change both in our overall state of being and in the symptoms that we are, in that moment, expressing.

On a very simple level, when we are driving on the highway, and another car cuts us off, we are being offered a catalyst to change. We can choose to turn on the radio and relax, glad that we didn't have an accident. Or we can choose to chase the bastard down and run him off the road. Those are among the many choices we can make, but there are other changes that occur that we cannot so easily control. We have an increased heartbeat, or a feeling of shortness of breath that accompanies a near-miss. And we may even have to get off the road at the next exit and relax a moment before continuing.

So everything is a catalyst for change, or, at least a potential catalyst. As homeopath and Jungian analyst Edward Whitmont said, that which is absorbed on a psychological level does not lead to illness. That which cannot be absorbed on the psychological level becomes disease. In saying this, he is reminding us that, in terms of homeopathy, the germ, or the car that nearly misses us, is not the issue. What we do when faced with the germ, or the speeding car, is the issue.

So, given that we are all expressing symptoms at all times, and given that, according to Hahnemann, it is going to take a team of people—the subjective person, the patient, and the objective observers—to determine illness, how are we going to make sense of symptoms and how are they going to help us get anywhere in the treatment of the patient?

Good question. To answer that, we have to go a bit deeper into our philosophy.

In understanding symptoms, we need to take just a moment to remind ourselves from the physician's point of view that we are all, as patients, both unique beings and whole beings. This means that as individuals our symptoms mean what they mean to us. In other words, Patient A and Patient B both have a cold. When looking at the symptoms expressed by each of them, we must remember that the fact they have received the diagnosis of having a cold is nearly meaningless in terms of what remedy they might need. We do not have, in our homeopathic pharmacy, a single remedy that should be considered a cold remedy. We have, instead, remedies for patients, for patients who have colds, for patients who have sore throats, and so on and so on.

So, when we look at the patient, no matter his symptoms, we look at him as a unique individual. We can in no way make a plan for treatment until we look at his symptoms and at how he is reacting to them.

Patient A may be totally overwhelmed by his or her symptoms. Patient B may still be getting up and going to work. Yet both have colds. Both have received a disease diagnosis from our team of subjective and objective observers. The difference in the cold is the difference in the individuals who have the cold. The difference in vital force, largely. But also the difference in emotional response to the idea of being sick, the difference in how they were treated as children when they got sick, and so on.

So the symptoms, the cluster of things that put together have been given a particular name that we call disease, have to be put into the context of the individual as a whole being. The illness must be individualized. That is one method by which the homeopathic viewpoint of the patient and the disease is miles ahead of the allopathic one. The homeopath's patient always is guaranteed individualized treatment.

Now that patient, as stated above, is also whole. There are three states of being—body, mind, and spirit—and these are intertwined. The fact that a particular patient has cold feet, a hot head, and a sore throat must be interrelated. They must all be taken into account in some way or other in the treatment of that patient. All the symptoms must be placed into context. All are part of the ongoing whole.

Thorson's Encyclopedic Dictionary of Homeopathy offers the following statement concerning symptoms:

> Symptoms and signs are used by the homeopath to be guided in the choice of a truly homeopathic medicine applicable to the individual patient. That means he chooses the medicine's symptom picture that would evoke the identical symptom picture, though some (or even most) may well be subjective symptoms. In this the peculiar, unexpected, striking, or unaccountable symptoms are taken to be of pre-eminent significance.

And homeopath William Boericke gives us a term for the homeopathic method of placing the individual symptoms presently being expressed by a patient into the context of that patient's whole and unique being. He, like other classic homeopaths, calls it *"the totality of symptoms."*

Boericke writes:

> The totality of the symptoms consists in the systematic ascertaining of all the symptomatic facts necessary to determine the curative remedy. The totality of symptoms includes every change of state in body and mind that we can discover or have observed, or that has been reported to the physician; thus, every deviation from health. It includes every subjective symptom that the patient can describe correctly and every objective symptom the physician can discover with his senses, aided by all diagnostic instruments. In examining the patient, a definite, systematic plan should be followed.

So once we have twisted our way through the sheer language of the above, we find that a symptom is always a part of the greater network of being. Therefore, we should consider that there are, in reality, two kinds of symptoms: *symptoms of being* (in that we always have shifts and changes in what is normal for us, and the fact that one person is, generally speaking, thirsty and sweaty and another person is, in general, not) and *symptoms of disease*. Both have objective and subjective texts, in that we all have knowledge of ourselves that no one else has, and we all have blank spots in our self-knowledge that others can access easily. In fact, it is the shifts in our symptoms of being that represent our symptoms of disease.

The Dictionary of Homeopathic Medical Terminology has pages of information on symptoms, but the definition is short and sweet: "A symptom is basically an abnormal sensation experienced by a person as a whole or in a part of the body."

Now, these "abnormal sensations" may be painful or pleasant. An increase in energy at a given time of day or season of year is as important a symptom as is a headache or sore throat. What we are in the business of doing is learning to be in touch with ourselves and the changes in our minds, bodies, and emotions.

And by learning to work with the symptoms, whether they represent specific pain or not, we are learning to improve the general health of the patient and to prevent future illness. In other words, as the physician is, whether he wants to be or not, a great and powerful catalyst in the life of the patient, we must seek always to be a catalyst to betterment and never to bring about the overall weakening or destruction of the patient.

The Philosophies of Treatment

The only way in which a physician can *not* be a catalyst in the life of the patient is for that physician to do nothing. Sometimes even the act of listening to the patient, to taking the case without recommending a specific remedy or action, will be enough in itself to elicit a change in the life of that patient. Many patients are in need of being heard, of being paid attention to on such a fundamental level that just by letting them talk to you, you have already begun treatment. So, really, about the only thing you can do when enacting the physician's role to not have an impact on the patient is to not answer your phone when it rings.

So when we look at the patient and the whole range and context of his symptoms, the next thing we have to do is decide what we are going to do about these symptoms, and about this patient.

The null set approach to the situation is to do nothing. To leave it to God. This was largely the medical approach of ancient man, who willfully turned over the life-and-death decisions to the Creator. And offered instead prayers that, if it be the Creator's will, the patient should recover.

The moment the physician did anything, put a blanket around the patient, or covered his open wound with a leaf, treatment had begun.

And, as it was two thousand years ago, when Hippocrates first sat down to consider treatments, so it is today. There are only two things that you can really do, two pathways to take, when you enter the arena of treatment.

THE ALLOPATHIC METHOD

Allopathic medicine, first and foremost, is the medicine by which the patient's symptoms are treated by substances which, in their first action, will push the symptoms in a direction other than that in which they are presently flowing. The runny nose, therefore, will be treated by a substance that causes a healthy nose to dry up. Implicit within this philosophy is the notion that we can work in a vacuum, that we can treat one symptom or a specific set of symptoms without changing the unified system as a whole.

Allopathic medicine is the medicine of action. It works by the initial action of the medicine given, and the subsequent reaction is all but ignored. Also, rather than being given based upon the totality of the symptoms of the patient, it is given based upon one, two, or three symptoms.

When an allopathic medicine it tested, it is tested for a specific action as well. All the other changes created within the human system by the drug are considered "side effects," and not important either to the overall healing of the patient or in terms of considering the impact of the drug upon the system.

But there is more to allopathic philosophy that must be considered. First we need to understand that allopathic treatments came about by a shift in human thinking. It involves a fundamental shift in the consideration as to just what a human being is.

For Hippocrates, the human was a whole and unique being. He could not be affected upon on any level without all levels being affected.

But Hippocrates' philosophy, which more or less saw the human being as just that, a being, a solid entity created and enlivened as a whole, was supplanted by the philosophy of the Roman doctor Galen, who, through his experiments on animal corpses, came to a different and startling conclusion.

Where ancient man had seen humans as whole beings, and had created tools for those beings that fit into the hands, like simple hammers and knives, Galen saw man as a mechanism. And this concept of man as machine changed not only the practice of medicine but the concept of society as well.

Just as this notion gave rise to the idea that a patient was the sum total of his various organs and parts, it too gave rise to the idea of tools that, instead of being held and used in the hand, mimicked the human mechanism. Pulleys and weights and spinning wheels replaced the basic tools. Ultimately, the idea of man as machine was expressed in science fiction as robots, machines whose interior artificial parts mimicked our own internal organs.

It was this idea of man as machine that gave rise to the allopathic belief that we can, in medical terms, treat one organ or system of the body and not touch any other part in that treatment. It also gave rise to the notion of surgery as the ultimate expression of allopathic medicine.

So we have a system of medicine that tells us that we are not whole but are instead a machine. It also tells us that our symptoms are not messages to us but are rather a form of invasion within our bodies. The allopathic method has for centuries mimicked the military in its approach to medicine.

The allopath is in the business not of treating patients but of defeating diseases. Diseases are seen as the direct result of an attack on our system by a specific germ. Forget the fact that we have, at any given moment, hundreds of thousands of so-called germs in and on our bodies. Our illness, says the allopath, is the result of a germ invasion. We were in the wrong place at the wrong time. If we had only been able to dodge the bullet of that specific germ we would not be sick right now. (The homeopath would likely consider that if not that catalyst to illness, another would have likely done just as well.)

All of which gives rise to the notion of treatment based upon depletion. You are given a drug because you "need" that drug. Thus we have the huge industry created by allopathic treatments for depletions of all sorts, most notably hormone-replacement therapy. We treat the lack of a substance in the body by giving the body that substance artificially.

A good deal of allopathic treatment also centers on pain relief. Think of the multibillion-dollar painkiller industry. Think of a headache. If you take a painkiller for a headache, does it actually cure that headache? Of course not, it merely separates you from the sensation of your pain. In fact, that is the basis of a good many allopathic treatments. Cold medicine does the same thing for colds—it in no way ends the cold or prevents the next one; instead, it just keeps you briefly from experiencing the cold you already have.

So the irony of allopathic treatments is that in reality they actually rely upon the body's own healing mechanism to kick in and take care of the disease. Given all the technology, and all the so-called advances in medicine, we are still waiting for our own vital force to clear away the illness.

It is important to remember our homeopathic principles at this point, and be reminded that with each new television campaign promising a drug is "now stronger than ever," it means that drug is now more powerful, that there is more substance to it, or a stronger substance has replaced a weaker, so that as each "new and improved" substance is given more and more often, through the suppression of the original disease, the patient's overall vital force is weakened.

Obviously, Boericke, like Hahnemann before him, sees little value in allopathic treatments. About these, he lists the following objections:

1. It is merely symptomatic treatment attacking some prominent single condition, instead of the disease as a whole, and necessarily leads to polypharmacy in the endeavor to meet different conditions at the same time.
2. The transient amelioration is followed by an increased aggravation of the very condition to be removed, necessitating increasing dosage.
3. Drug diseases are established that complicate hopelessly the original disease of the patient; the possibility of harm by the

introduction of the necessary large dosage of drugs and foreign substances always being very evident.

None of these therapeutic methods are curative in the true sense by directly modifying the vital activities of the organism. In the cases where such treatment is ultimately successful (and certain temporary beneficial results cannot be denied), the homeopathic method is more direct, safer, more radical and with no possible harm to the patient.

Boericke says it better than I could. The reason to object to allopathic treatment is that it invariably has a boomerang effect. At first the patient will feel better as the symptom is suppressed deep into his system. Because suppression—the opposite impact of the allopathic drug on the human system already experiencing disease—is the very nature of allopathic treatment. But suppression of disease symptoms has nothing whatsoever to do with the actual treatment of disease.

But, the symptoms will return—they have, remember, not been cured, but only suppressed. And they will return worse than before their suppression and will require a stronger allopathic treatment the second time in order to suppress them once more. Or worse, the suppression of the first system will lead to a new and deeper ailment.

Think about it: since the allopathic treatment did not at any point actually deal with the cause of the disease on the energistic (or even the physical) level, that cause is still active and able to create further disease states. It will flow to the weakest part of the patient's being. If the suppression of the original ailment is deep enough, the cause of the disease will in the place of the first disease create a second disease. (Think of the infant whose diaper rash is treated with antibiotic creams, and who no longer has diaper rash but now has an ear infection.) And, unfortunately for the patient, most allopathic practitioners will not consider the second ailment an offshoot of the first, but will instead treat it as some new invader to the system that now must be attacked and defeated.

But worse still is the impact of the allopathic suppression on the patient's whole system. With each suppression, the overall vital force, the overall immune system of the patient, is weakened. And the stronger the allopathic drug, the stronger the suppression and the stronger the impact on that immune system. Thus we have a generation of patients for whom antibiotics are no longer effective, and a generation of disease for which antibiotics are now a joke. We are losing our war on disease, because the very idea of winning a war against disease is something of a joke itself. If the disease is our response to the presence of a catalyst, then, when we are making wars against diseases, we are making wars against ourselves. And the victims in this warfare are our immune systems, which have received repeated scud missile attacks in the form of antibiotics and the like.

Therefore, in concluding this brief study of allopathic philosophy and treatment, we must note that though allopathy offers a coherent and systematic approach to the treatment of disease, it offers this treatment at an overall cost to the patient as a whole. The treatment that cures the specific symptom does so by weakening the vital force as a whole.

THE HOMEOPATHIC METHOD

Here our manner of thought and mode of treatment are quite the opposite, and while homeopathic medicine may be said to be a throwback to ancient practices, it must also be considered, in the light of modern scientific discoveries, to be the most modern form of medicine.

Allopathy belongs to the body mechanism as first described by Galen, and to Newton's universe. Homeopathy belongs to the unified whole being of Hippocrates and to Einstein's universe.

In the twentieth century, mankind saw the view of self and of the surrounding universe once again shift. And again this shift was shown most clearly in the tools that mankind invented and used.

Einstein tells us that the whole of the universe and everything in it is made up of the same substance—energy—and that we are in reality simply energy beings. As such, we are truly whole beings; and, as such, we must be medically treated as whole beings.

As for our tools, we have taken the mechanical tools, the typewriter, the calculator, and such, and replaced them with computers, with machines in which the mechanism and the working parts are beside the point. They fit our imaginations more than they do our hands, and their function in no way mimics the functions of our bodies. Instead they mirror the function of our minds.

So, the rules have changed and our view of the world has changed with them. And this is the setting in which we once again look to homeopathic medicine as the philosophy and practice of medicine that actually works, that actually allows us to become well.

To do this, we must always treat the person and never treat the disease. To treat a disease is to be instantly transported back to allopathic medicine. In homeopathic medicine, we are constantly aware that anything you do to the smallest tissue in the body you do to all the tissues in the body. And anything that impacts upon the physical body must also impact upon the mind and the emotions, and upon the spirit as well.

To treat homeopathically, you must recognize what the allopaths call "the Wisdom of the Body." That means that our vital force, along with our physical body, is ever in the process of reaching for and maintaining health; that our symptoms have meaning, whether or not it is important at this moment to know exactly what that meaning is.

So we treat people, patients, as whole beings. We treat their symptoms by respecting them first, and recognizing that there is a reason that they exist in the first place. And then we work reactively—by giving the remedy that in a well person would create the totality of symptoms that the patient is already experiencing. That is the heart of the homeopathic method and practice. We call it *similarity*. It is the principle of treatment with which Hahnemann revolutionized medicine. And it is a principle of treatment that dates all the way back to Hippocrates.

He introduces us to the concept of homeopathy in aphorism number 24 of his work:

> There remains, therefore, no other manner of medicinal application promising aid against disease, except the homeopathic one. In homeopathy, a medicine is sought for the totality of symptoms of the disease case, with regard for the originating cause (when it is known) and for the accessory circumstances—a medicine is sought which (among all medicines whose condition-altering abilities are known from having been tested in healthy individuals) has the power and tendency to engender the artificial disease state most similar to that of the case of disease in question.

The homeopathic method of treatment demands of us several things. First it demands that we understand the somewhat subjective nature of disease, that we know when to treat and when not to treat; that physicians enter into a partnership with patients, in which each lends his or her own expertise to the case.

Second, it demands that we never allow ourselves to be caught up in the drama of the case, that we never allow ourselves to treat the disease and not the person with the disease. After all, since the disease state represents that patient's reaction to a catalyst that leads him or her into disease, can we ever treat any disease in any way other than by treating the person with the disease?

Next we must, if we are to be both physicians and homeopaths, learn to look for the totality of symptoms of disease. We must realize that no disease exists in a vacuum, that no single symptom of pain can exist in the human system without other symptoms existing as well. We have to learn to understand that particular patient's symptoms, their origins, their changes, their flow. We have to have an understanding of what the state of health means for that patient, and how that state may be attained. We have to learn what changes must occur in the patient's mind, body, and spirit in order for an individual to be in the state that he or she thinks of as health.

And more, we have to learn to leave patients in better shape than they were when we found them. Too often, allopaths settle for leaving their patients in a shape that is only different from the one in which they found them. In some cases, different may actually be worse overall, but the fact that they are in different shape is taken for a success.

So as physicians and homeopaths, we may actually have to help the patient to redefine what health is—to reach for a goal that is beyond the one he originally had. Many of us, when we ourselves are patients, set very shortsighted goals. Fear-oriented goals. We just want the pain to stop.

Indeed, many of us have never in our lives had a period in which we could truthfully say that we were totally healthy. There always seems to be something wrong with us. We always seem to be suffering some limitation of some sort. It may be the role of the physician in such a case to allow the patient to actually come to see that he or she might become totally well, totally free to live life. The redefinition given by the homeopath, however, must always be an enlarging of the goal and never an idea of settling for less.

And then, once the need for treatment and the goal of treatment are established, the physician and the homeopath must work with the totality of the patient's symptoms, and locate the remedy that in its total sphere of activity most nearly matches the disease state at hand. And the homeopath must be skillful in the potency of his or her remedy as well, using the remedy to establish an artificial disease state that is slightly stronger, slightly more potent than the natural disease state at hand, so that the remedy will have the power to remove the natural disease.

But remember that the homeopathic method is a reactive method. It is the job of the remedy to act as a catalyst. As the body's own immune system rises up against the remedy in equal and opposite reaction, the reactive force moves the patient from a state of disease to a state of health. This is a simplified statement of the homeopathic method.

Methods of Diagnosis

Homeopathic diagnosis, while it can certainly make use of any modern medical test or disease diagnosis that the practitioner might want to utilize, is as unique to a case as is its treatment.

When the homeopathic physician gathers all the available information from the objective and subjective team, he or she then pulls together the symptom portrait from the totality of the symptoms. This information is then, through the process of *repertorization* (see the section on acute case taking and treatment), refined and, ultimately, matched to the information that has previously been gathered—through the process known as "proving"—for each of the individual homeopathic remedies. One remedy is finally selected. And from that moment of selection onward, the case (and, usually, the patient) is described in terms of the remedy used. Thus, the physician may well say that the case is "A real Phosphorus case," or that the patient is "A real Nux type."

This is what is known as the *drug diagnosis,* and it is this method of diagnosis that separates homeopathy from other forms of medicine. The case is named by the remedy that is curative to it. And so it will be known, with the name changing as the case itself and the remedy called for changes.

The drug diagnosis is, in one specific situation, used in terms of the disease, most especially of an infectious disease that quickly multiplies to a large number of cases. That is the medical situation known as epidemic. In the case of an epidemic, you have a catalyst for change that you know works to the detriment of the persons who fall under its impact. Further, you know you have a catalyst that is going to have impact on a huge number of human systems, perhaps in the majority of systems. Therefore in this situation, you must treat the whole community as an individual. You will have large numbers of persons falling under the sway of the illness in a fairly short span of time, in a situation that may be very serious, and quite possibly deadly. You must find the range of symptoms (I hesitate to use that term *totality*) that are most common in the greatest number of cases and then treat the individuals based on the symptoms within this community pool. These symptoms are called the "general" or "absolute" symptoms, since these are the symptoms that, in any given situation, are common to all those who are a part of that group. The fact that all of us will experience less severe symptoms means that the use of general symptoms in the treatment of patients is not the strongest way to go, but in the case of an epidemic, it is the best method we have. It may not even be said to be pure homeopathy, since we are not taking the time to take the individual case or repertorize it, but clinical experience shows us that this is, at a time in which our resources are likely to be taxed to the limit, often the best we can do.

It will even be true that each fall, as the first patients begin to collapse with the season's flu, practitioners will be sharing their findings in order to be sure to have on hand, in many different potencies, the remedy or remedies that are most suggested by the situation at hand.

In the case of fast-moving epidemics, the drug diagnosis can almost be said to speak for the disease instead of the patient. But, more truthfully, it should be said that the drug diagnosis will speak to the general population and not to its individual members.

So this side trip into the realm of the consideration and treatment of epidemics aside, it may be said that the classic homeopath does not at any point diagnose a disease. The disease name, to the classic homeopath, gives us no real information. Indeed, it can lead us astray, in that once we have given the patient a disease diagnosis, we will be ever more tempted to treat the disease and not the patient.

The disease diagnosis is so important to allopathic medicine that in giving the correct disease diagnosis the practitioner is also giving an immediate plan of action. It is important that we treat any disease—cancer is a great example—by a set plan of attack, and the allopath feels that his work is half done by the successful disease diagnosis. The homeopath, however, would consider that this disease diagnosis can only tempt him to the knee-jerk response of giving "cancer remedies," if such a thing were possible, and can only create a climate of panic within the mind of the patient. (The patient is a whole being, and anything that causes a panic on the level of the mind disrupts the body as well, which is the last thing that that patient needs at that moment.)

So, just as the view of the patient and the symptoms are in opposition in allopathy and homeopathy, so, too, are the methods of diagnosis. Today, we are seeing more and more homeopaths who diagnose a case in a method that could only be described as allopathic. We are seeing many who are giving homeopathic remedies on the basis of need, of deficiency; who are testing specific tissues within the human system for specific pathology; and, finding the existence of that pathology, are giving homeopathic remedies for the specific purpose of attacking that pathology and removing it.

While these practitioners may call themselves doctors, we should not see them in the physician's role. They have abandoned the physician's task of working with the patient as a whole and encouraging the natural healing process. In so doing, they have lost the right to call themselves physicians.

The Homeopathic Pharmacy

The creation of the homeopathic pharmacy, the collection of remedies in specific and unique potencies, is perhaps Hahnemann's greatest technical achievement. Indeed, as valuable as the homeopathic philosophy is, without the remedies that add the spark of fire to the dry kindling of disease, there could be no such thing as homeopathic healing.

In making his remedies, Hahnemann was pulling together all the strings of his work in homeopathy. First, the pharmacy was based in the herbal tradition of natural medicine that could be traced all the way back to Hippocrates and could through empirical methods be shown to work clinically in hundreds of cases. The substances that we selected for the first remedies were selected because they, in their substance form, had already been shown to be medicinal.

The homeopathic pharmacy also responded to the philosophy of vitalism in that the remedies, in a dilute form, worked at all. And, as we have been taught that "the stronger the poison, the stronger the cure," it has been found that many remedies, such as Arsenicum from arsenic, have powerful curative powers because they have such toxic impact in their natural state.

What likely came as a surprise to Hahnemann and to those who followed his methods of proving new remedies was that many substances in their natural material state seem to be totally benign or inert but become so powerful in their energy state. Remedies like Natrum Mur from regular table salt and Lycopodium (from club moss, which had been ground up into a white powder that was used for years to coat pills to make them easier to swallow) prove that the vital force unleashed cannot be predicted in its potency.

But the inherent irony of the homeopathic pharmacy and one of the central mysteries of homeopathic philosophy has to do with the act of dilution itself. This irony is best expressed in the *Arndt-Schultz law,* which gives insight into the biological activity of drugs. The law states that small doses of drugs will actually encourage life activity in general. Large material doses of drugs impede life activity in general, and very large doses of drugs will actually destroy life activity.

This obviously substantiates Paracelsus' notion that "everything is poison." You can overdo any substance and, when overdone, that substance becomes toxic. Therefore, the American notion of "the more the better" is not true by natural law. And it was the observation of this natural law that led Hahnemann to the creation of the homeopathic pharmacy.

While still a student at the University of Vienna, Hahnemann noticed in his clinical studies that the patients were, in his opinion, getting sicker from their treatments than they were from their diseases. He noted that the arsenic, for instance, that was being given to patients was just too toxic in the amounts in which it was given for the patients' systems to bear.

So, when he himself became a doctor and began to give medicines, he did the only thing he could think to do: he diluted the medicine. He figured that, if one gram was too much, give half a gram, then try a tenth of a gram, and so on.

Hahnemann began to dilute his remedies in water. First in one part of the original substance with nine parts water and then one part substance to ninety-nine parts water. And what he found was entirely in keeping with the Arndt–Schultz law. Not only were the remedies as powerful in their diluted states, but they were more curative. The toxic impact of the substance had fallen away and its curative powers were enhanced. The patient, in general, was made better by the use of the minute amounts of the remedy, which we now call *microdoses*. Most mysteriously, there seemed to be an invisible barrier at which the substance seemed to fall away completely and the energy pattern that remained became totally benign and totally curative.

To this process of dilution, Hahnemann began to add a second level of preparation of the remedies, which he called *succussion*. Succussion is a process of systematically shaking the remedy while it is still in its liquid form. Hahnemann, through his empirical approach to medicine, found again and again that the remedies that had been shaken during their process of dilution were more potent than those that were not. He concluded that each remedy had to be both diluted and succussed in a set pattern of activity in order to be properly prepared as a homeopathic.

And through his clinical observations, both Hahnemann and the homeopaths who followed him noticed the actions specific to each remedy— the totality of the actions, which would be matched to the totality of the patient's symptoms—and in what potency, what level of dilution and succession, it seemed to work most effectively. All of these observations they gathered together in books called "materia medicas," which listed the total action of each individual remedy, from its major mental and emotion impact, down to its most specific physical symptom.

The term *materia medica* was borrowed from the ancient herbalists, who called their documentations of herbal impacts the same thing, which is taken from the Latin for "medical materials." While the remedies listed inside had changed in their nature from physical to energy, and from allopathic to homeopathic, the structure of the book itself largely remained the same.

Before he died, Hahnemann created dozens of remedies, some, like Camphor, taken from the standard pharmacy of his day. Others, like Sepia, were created in response to the needs of a specific patient, and were later proven as general homeopathic remedies.

In today's world, we now have thousands of homeopathic remedies available. And more are being made and proven all the time. Everything that occurs naturally in Creation can potentially become a homeopathic remedy. Even energy forms, like sunlight and X rays, have been potentized, been made into remedies. Also the north and south magnetic poles have been shaped into remedies.

Further, things that are artificial in their nature, such as chemical toxins, can be made into remedies, although these will speak only to undoing the toxins themselves in an isopathic manner and are not to generally be considered constitutional remedies.

Out of the thousands of remedies at our disposal, there are still only about four dozen that can be considered polycrests. They speak both to a wide range of ailments and to more than one miasm as the underlying cause of disease. These are still the remedies that it is most important that we understand and use correctly, as they are the foundation of the homeopathic pharmacy.

The Goals of Treatment

We all know the difference between acute and chronic illnesses. The first, the acute, tend to come on comparatively quickly and are self-limiting. The illness itself will contain its own beginning, middle, and end. While most tend to be simple ailments, like colds, that will take care of themselves in time, even without treatment, some, like the flu epidemics of the last century, can result in the death of the patient.

Chronic diseases can be more difficult to recognize. They may—most especially if they are functional in nature, rather than being pathological—

take years to develop, but once the chronic condition is in place, it is likely that there will be little that allopathic medicine can do to remove it.

In the same way, homeopaths have different levels of treatment, from the simple acute to the transformational miasmic. And the homeopath, in selecting the level of treatment that will be used in a given case, is largely determining the goal of the treatment and the possible ramifications of the remedies given.

Acute homeopathy has as its goal the restoration of status quo. It says that a week ago before the flu hit, you were a healthy person, and that, by the use of homeopathic remedy or remedies, you can be returned to the state you were in a week ago: healthy.

Therefore the acute case is fairly easy to take and to manage. You concern yourself primarily with what has changed in the patient's nature and system in a relatively brief period of time. You look at his symptom portrait of a week ago, before the flu, and compare it with the situation at the present moment, during the flu. So the whole case taking may involve only four or five symptoms that have changed with the onset of flu, and the remedy prescribed is given with the sole intent of retaining the status quo. The practitioner is looking to remove a pebble from the patient's shoe.

In *constitutional homeopathy* the practitioner is looking to fundamentally shift the patient from a position of weakness to a position of greater strength. The purpose of the remedy chosen is not just to clear up some unpleasant symptoms the patient is now experiencing that have driven him to seek treatment; no, the remedy is chosen because it speaks to the totality of the patient's symptoms—good, bad, and neutral—and not just to the symptoms of pain. Therefore, the purpose of the treatment is to strengthen the patient's vital force, and to lift him above his present illness and help to keep him from becoming ill again. Here you are trying to remove a number of rocks from the patient's path.

Finally, there is *miasmic homeopathy* in which the practitioner is working with the patient to strengthen the patient's predisposition to illness or illnesses. The work here is very deep, and the changes brought about are permanent in nature. The practitioner needs as much information as possible in order to select the remedy. You need to know not only the patient's particular symptoms, but also the symptoms that are common in the patient's family. You are working on a genetic level, really, with the goal of truly changing the patient's lifetime patterns of weakness and illness, or truly setting the patient free. Here you are trying to remove a boulder from the patient's back.

I love the fact that as you move from acute to constitutional to miasmic treatments, you are actually moving toward giving fewer and fewer different doses of remedies with each leap. You will use more different remedies in acute medicine than you ever will in constitutional or in miasmic treatment. But you will use more different potencies of a specific remedy in constitutional treatment than you will anywhere else. And, in miasmic treatment, you will often give remedies in higher potencies, sometimes in very high potencies indeed, than you will anywhere else.

So the initial determination of what kind of treatment will be undertaken will largely determine the way in which the treatment will be enacted. Other methods of determining treatment have to do with which school of homeopathic philosophy and homeopathic practice a physician belongs to.

SCHOOLS OF HOMEOPATHIC PRACTICE

Today, much of what we call homeopathy would have been considered allopathic by the homeopathic masters of the past. Certainly, those who treat with combination remedies or who prescribe remedies based on simple pathology or on deficiency would have been considered allopaths by Kent or Hahnemann.

Yet these practitioners will attest to their love of homeopathy and are likely to ask you if you think that Hahnemann knew all that there is to know about healing, or if he even managed, in one short lifetime, to master all that there was to master in the practice of homeopathy. When you are fully backed into a corner and truthfully answered that, no, while Hahnemann was a genius, he did not in fact know all there was to know about healing, and that in fact the realization that he had not been able to bring healing to all his patients haunted him to his last day, the practitioner will get an odd little smile on his face and say that he believes he is continuing Hahnemann's own work in the modern age.

Or you will be talking with a practitioner who follows each new study of homeopathic remedies and who will insist that, according to the latest French study, there are physical conditions that yield from a combination of remedies that will not yield to any single remedy. You start saying that we can never know if this is true or not, since we homeopaths consider each individual a unique being, and that after you have already given that individual a combination remedy, we will never now be able to know what the appropriate single remedy might have done. But this kind of reply only leads to loud and angry words and just isn't worth it.

In philosophy, we can be so pure. In practice, the changes begin to muddy the water and we begin to find that under the umbrella of homeopathy there are any number of people who are using the homeopathic remedies in ways that Hanhemann never considered, but who are still huddling, trying to stay out of the allopathic storm.

Therefore, we must consider the two broad definitions of homeopathic treatment: unicists and pluralists.

1. **Unicist Homeopathy**. This is the school that makes use of only one homeopathic remedy at a time, as set forth by Hahnemann in *The Organon*. And the unicist school is itself divided into two camps, the Hahnemannian and the Kentian. While both of these styles of practice may be considered to be "classical" homeopathy, it is interesting that what most Americans think of as "classical" actually owes more to American homeopath James Tyler Kent's practice of homeopathy than it does to that of Hahnemann himself.

   A. **Pure Hahnemannian School**. The pure Hahnemannian school is empirical in its approach and treats patients based upon past experience of the remedies and the presence of tangible, sensible symptoms. It holds to the full doctrine of inductive practice.

      While this school of treatment acknowledges the existence of the "germ theory," and accepts the fact that contagion does exist as a factor in medicine, it insists that there must be a weakening of the vital force and an underlying susceptibility in order for illness to take hold. In practice, this style of treatment demands the prescription of one medicine at a time, either in a single or repeated dose.

   B. **Kentian School**. The Kentian school maintains most of the beliefs of the Hahnemannian school, but adds an ingredient of mysticism, identifying matter with spirit. This takes Hahnemann's idea of wesen and extends it, maintaining that flesh is only a mirror to spirit and that all treatment must therefore take place in the realm of the spirit. Because of this, Kentians tend to not even bother to name a disease, and will often put much less emphasis on the physical symptoms, treating only the emotional and/or spiritual element of the case.

      Generally, Kentians consider the idea of contagion to be of little or no importance in the treatment of a patient. Further, as Kent is the father of the idea of constitutional treatments, his followers tend not to administer any other remedy than those found to be constitutional in illness. In practice, look for them to prescribe one high-potency dose of the suggested remedy.

2. **Pluralist Homeopathy**. Because of the belief that we are all made up of three different levels of being—the physical, the mental, and the emotional—the pluralist homeopath will tend to want to give the patient one remedy in high potency for the mental/emotional situation, while at the same time giving another in low potency for the physical symptoms.

    This approach is based on the work of the French homeopath Nebel and is followed today primarily in Europe. In practice, various medicines are administered alternatively during the day in low potency. These remedies are given with the idea that each will impact the system in a specific manner and move the individual symptoms in a specific way.

    It must be noted here that there are many who believe that so-called pluralist homeopathy is not homeopathic at all. And the reason for this is found in *The Organon* itself.

    Hahnemann stated that any medicine, whether homeopathic or allopathic, represents an artificial disease, and any medicine, therefore, creates a range of artificially induced symptoms in the human system. He stood strongly against what has been called "polypharmacy," or the use of more than one drug at a time. If we are to believe that any medicine will induce a number of symptoms, then we must also see the logic in only using one drug at a time. If we use more than one, it is impossible to know exactly what each drug is doing and what changes it is making in the patient's system. We also cannot know how the drugs themselves may combine to create a new level of illness—one caused by the drugs themselves and in no way natural to the patient. The use of polypharmacy at best will make the case more complicated. At worst, it will render the patient incurable.

SCHOOLS OF HOMEOPATHIC PHILOSOPHY

We must be also note that there are two distinct schools of homeopathic philosophy, the anthropomorphic and the biochemical, and that these schools of thought determine the method by which remedies are used.

The Anthropomorphic School considers constitutional treatments as the bedrock of homeopathic treatments. Adherents believe that the remedies, especially constitutional remedies, represent states of being that encompass personality as much as they do any other factor, including the painful symptoms that are usually categorized as disease. Therefore, the anthropomorphic school treats with a good deal of emphasis on personality and on the other "invisible" parts of the human system. It also gives a personality to the remedies it uses, stressing the emotional motivations of remedies used. Therefore the Phosphorus patient would be seen as more emotional and more sensitive to the needs of others than would the Sulphur patient.

The Biochemical School stresses the physical and visible parts of the patient. Here the disease, and the cause of the disease (whether germ, lifestyle, or genetic build), is of much more importance than in the former school of thought. Deficiency is of great importance to the biochemical practitioner. A homeopathic remedy made from healthy adrenal tissue, therefore, would likely be given to a patient with a weakened or diseased adrenal gland. The biochemical school mirrors much more the practice of the allopathic physician, relying upon the results of any number of tests to determine what to prescribe, while the anthropomorphic physician may give Phosphorus simply because the patient "is" a Phosphorus.

In looking at these divisions of homeopaths, it is important, for this course of study, to try to guess which methods Hahnemann himself would have employed. Since he was a unicist himself, I stand firm in believing that Hahnemann might well have accepted Kent's unicist practice, but would never have agreed with those following the pluralist method.

It seems to me that in accordance with what Hahnemann wrote in *The Organon,* he would have been more interested in the need for each physician to *have* a philosophical basis of treatment, rather than by controlling what that basis would be. Therefore, the important thing to remember about all these approaches to homeopathy is that they all work, one way or another, and that the practitioners of the various methods, from the pure Kentian who only works with transformational medicine to the biochemical acute prescriber, all have their share of successes to report.

The Acute Case

So, having dealt with the principles of homeopathic treatment as defined by homeopathic philosophy and the ways in which we consider disease, symptoms, medicines, and patients, we are now ready to deal with the patient himself. If a person needs some help, now is the time to take our homeopathic philosophy and put it into a clinical setting.

THE TOOLS OF THE TRADE

When we are in the process of selecting a homeopathic remedy for a particular patient in a particular situation, we must turn to two different kinds of text that will guide us along the way (of course, it goes without saying that we have already studied *The Organon* before ever making direct use of any remedy).

The first book that we need by our side is a *materia medica*. As noted before, this reference book documents the actions of specific homeopathic remedies. It will give us in toto the history and uses of the remedy, in both substance and homeopathic form, if possible. The materia medica often represents specific hands-on information on remedies as they have been used and experienced by a given practitioner. Therefore, some list more remedies than do others, and some are far more dependable than are others. So it is to be strongly advised that serious students of homeopathy make sure to buy as many different materia medicas as they can afford. Each will give a valuable viewpoint, and by studying these viewpoints together, you can best discover all the facets of a remedy's action.

Remember, too, that all homeopathic prescriptions must be made from the materia medica. Too many today are made from instinct, or from the repertorization process. But it is the materia medica that will give the total picture of a remedy, and it is from this total picture that the prescription must be made.

The other book is the *repertory*. While the materia medica is an ancient book, and certainly not unique to homeopathy, the repertory is a modern book that was created solely as a tool for the homeopathic prescriber. In the mid–1800s at more or less the same time, several homeopaths identified the need for another volume to work alongside the materia medica.

The repertory is a dictionary-style listing of the individual symptoms that the patient is experiencing. These are placed within individual listings called *rubrics* that are structured to begin with a general symptom, like headache, and then, as the listings under this category continue, to become more and more specific in the type of headache that the patient may be experiencing.

Like materia medicas, there are many different repertories on the market. The leading volume is probably still Kent's repertory, which transcended the others with its impeccable organization and 1,500 pages of information. While this is still an excellent resource in which to find the right remedy other more modern repertories in recent years have supplanted Kent's work in that they contain rubrics for modern illnesses that simply did not exist in Kent's day.

Unlike the materia medicas, I do not suggest that serious students of homeopathy rush out and buy many different repertories. In fact, I think that you are better off buying the one repertory, Kent's or otherwise, that you think will be of the most help to you. Look at all the different types and compare their structures. Find the one that you think will be easiest for you to use, one that is structured in a manner you find particularly helpful. Then do your best to become as familiar as possible with that one repertory. You will find in the long run that you are far better off by really learning how to use one repertory than by using two or three different ones and never being able to find anything easily.

Honestly, the investment in materia medicas and repertories can easily run into hundreds of dollars, since most of these books are published by micropublishers and individual books can cost a hundred dollars or more. Therefore it becomes especially important in the case of the repertories that you shop around and find what's right for you.

BEGINNING THE CASE TAKING

We are dealing here with the concept of the acute case, and are, therefore, seeking only to reestablish the status quo of the patient's health. Therefore if he, in his state of typical "good health," has low blood sugar and fits of anger, he is likely to still have these at the end of this treatment. What he will not have is that cold or flu or bump on his head for which he sought help.

Remember, in agreeing to even mention a possible homeopathic remedy to a friend, you are taking on the physician's role. You are stating that you are willing to go the whole distance with your friend or loved one, and you are pledging to do as much work as is possible in the clearing of the case.

So, how do we begin?

We must begin by defining our roles. If you are the parent or friend of the patient, then you are taking on two different roles. You are the physician and you are the objective observer. This means that things will be pretty simple, since you are already experienced with the status quo. This means that it will be fairly simple for you to examine the patient, ask a few questions, and then select the appropriate remedy. As Hahnemann puts it in aphorism #83, case taking "demands nothing of the medical-art practitioner except freedom from bias and healthy senses, attention while observing and fidelity in recording the image of the disease."

EXAMINING THE PATIENT

Certainly the physical examination here for an acute case will be far more taken into account for the selection of the remedy than it will in a constitutional or miasmic case.

Start the case taking as it is always started. Ask, "How may I help you?" or some other simple question that will allow the patient to start talking. Telling you what is wrong, as Hahnemann puts it, "The patient complains of the process of his ailments."

While the patient is talking, the job of the physician is to listen to what he is saying. Do your best not to flip through books or take too many notes. Really do your best not to ask leading questions. Just listen. And as you listen, make a few notes that outline the case. Wherever possible, take the notes in the actual words of the patient. If he says, "My throat burns like hot coals," that means something different from writing down "sore throat." So keep the notes short, but keep them specific.

Hahnemann writes about this process in aphorism #84. He writes: "The physician sees, hears and notices through the remaining senses what is altered or unusual about the patient . . . the physician keeps silent, allowing them to say all they have to say without interruption, unless they stray off to side issues. Only let the physician admonish them to speak slowly right at the outset so that, in writing down what is necessary, he can follow the speaker."

As the patient is speaking, in the acute case particularly, you might want to work the physical examination into the initial stages of case taking. You may want to note the patient's flushed cheeks or glassy eyes as he talks. You may want to look at the sore throat as he finishes describing it to you. In the case of a young child, you may want to work this into the game of case taking. Talking for a moment and then stopping while Mommy takes a look at that sore ear. In that many of the symptoms you repertorize later may not at any point be discussed by the patient, it is vital in the acute case that you learn to gather as much information as possible by looking at the patient.

Make use of those who have accompanied the patient, most especially if they are a parent or other relative. Have that person fill in any gaps of information that still exist. Ask them how they think that the patient has changed since the onset of the illness.

You will find in time that you can also gather a great deal of information from a patient's eyes or tongue and that the repertory will be of great help in leading you to the right remedy based on this knowledge, as will the materia medica, which will give many visual tips to a remedy. I have included a section of diagnostic symptoms in the section that follows, to help those learning homeopathy to deal with the specific symptoms of tongue coatings, ear color, etc.

When the patient is finished—and in the acute case, you will run into the problem of the patient finishing too soon, rather than taking too long a time in telling you his case (as can be common in constitutional prescribing)—you then will have to fill in the gaps of the information you lack.

With each individual symptom, it is important that you gather some basic information. And it is important that you get as complete a picture of each individual symptom as possible. Ask:

- The **location** of each pain. By this I mean specifically where does it hurt? It is obvious that a headache hurts in the head, but where in the head? The forehead? The occiput? Does it hurt in a broad area over the head, or does it hurt only in a very small spot? Specifically, where does it hurt?

- The **sensation** of pain. How does it hurt? Does it throb or ache or burn? Be careful not to ask the questions that I just wrote above. Instead ask, "What kind of pain is it?" and let the patient give you the information.

- The **duration** of the pain. How long have you had it? When did it begin? How did it begin? Try to find out if this pain came on in a specific order after or before another pain. Try to find out if this pain has changed in any manner since it came on. Has it moved? If so, how? Has it grown better or worse? Have you ever had this pain before?

- It is important at this point that you also find out what other **treatments** that the patient has already undergone in trying to rid himself of the illness. The patient who has already tried three or four other homeopathics, or who has already undergone deeply suppressive allopathic treatment, may just have to ride out the illness. If you are related to the patient, you again will have the advantage here, as you will already know what other treatments have been tried. If not, you must gather this information.

MODALITIES

In order to be able to find the right remedy, you will need to know what makes the symptoms feel better and what makes them feel worse. We call this the **modalities** of the case. So, start again with the first symptom given and ask the patient about the modalities for that symptom. Ask in general what makes this pain feel better or worse. If the patient is not helpful in his reply, ask:

- The time of day or night that symptoms are made better or worse.
- The environmental conditions by which symptoms are made better or worse: the temperature, weather conditions, etc.
- The body positions and how they affect the pain. Does the patient wish to lie down, or sit up, or move about?
- The specifics of his food cravings. How does drinking liquids affect the symptom? The modalities of food and drink can be very important to the case and should not be overlooked.
- The impact that sleep has on the symptom. Does the patient want to go to sleep? What side does he sleep on? Does he feel refreshed by sleep? Does he dream? If so, what are the dreams like?
- The temperature that makes him feel better or worse. Does the patient want to be heavily wrapped up or does he want to stick his feet out from under the bed covers. If you cannot tell by looking at him, ask if he feels hot or cold. Ask if he wants to be kept warm, what temperature he would like the room to be. Ask if he wants air moving, or if that would be chilly for him.
- The sort of attention he wants. Does this patient want you to stay in the room with him, or does he want to be alone? Notice the emotional modalities. Notice his mood and the manner in which he answers your questions. If a normally sweet child is curt and angry in answering your questions, you have a strong indication of a remedy.

If you do not know the normal condition of this patient, you will now have to get an indication of what has changed from the norm. The easiest way is to go back over the list of modalities, and to ask, now how do you usually feel about cold water, to the patient who is presently drinking it by the gallon.

In completing this process, you will have gathered the information central to the case and to the selection of the correct remedy. But first you must gather the information together in an organized and coherent manner.

WORKING WITH THE SYMPTOMS

Symptoms are all equally good to the homeopathically minded, in that they are all signs of a vital force that is itself attempting to rise up to defeat an illness, but not all symptoms are equally helpful in leading a practitioner toward a cure. Homeopathically, symptoms can be said to break down into several categories:

Absolute (Also Called General and Common): These symptoms live up to their names. Headache. Stomachache. Nightmares. All are symptoms that are so common to our lives that they, in and of themselves, are not helpful in leading to a curative remedy. Check out *Kent's Repertory* for headache if you don't believe me. The listing must be a page long and holds over 100 remedies listed as curative for headache. Therefore, it does us little good to fill the pages of a notebook with common or general symptoms.

Specific: These really are refinements of the common symptoms above. Usually these will not be reported directly, but will be refined through questioning. Here you have the headache in the forehead that begins on the left and moves to the right. This is much easier to repertorize than is the general "headache."

If you are planning to do a thorough repertorization, it helps to list your general complaint, headache for instance, and then follow that heading with all the refinements: better for cold, pain in the forehead, appears at 4 P.M., etc. This way, your listing of the symptoms will more or less follow the flow of the repertory.

Concomitant Symptoms: These are symptoms that appear simultaneously with other important symptoms (example: "I never get a headache without breaking out in a cold sweat up and down my spine"). Concomitants may also precede or follow another symptom regularly ("I know that I'm about to get a headache because I see gray spots in front of my eyes"). The symptoms may be of equal intensity or one may be the more troubling symptom. Either way, this is another way of refining the common symptoms to make them a bit more unique, and to find rubrics with a dozen or fewer remedies.

Alternating Symptoms: Most common may be diarrhea alternating with constipation in this day and age of irritable bowel syndrome. But here we are looking for one symptom that clears entirely and another symptom that takes its place until it itself clears, making way again for that first symptom to reappear. That is the difference between these and the concommitants. Again, by combining symptoms in this way, we are refining general symptoms into something more useful in finding the remedy.

Keynotes: As common symptoms give the general nature of the illness, keynote symptoms give specific information used in the locating of the proper curative remedy. These are the symptoms that are unique to a very few remedies and that, when discussed, seem to be most peculiar to a specific patient or illness. One example might be that one becomes nauseous when placing one's hands in warm water. This is keynote to Phosphorus. And, the symptom, when discovered, helps lead the practitioner to that correct remedy. Keynotes, while helpful, should not be relied upon too much in the selection of remedies. Remember, we are treating the person, not the disease, and the keynote represents only a small part of that being. Depending too heavily upon specific keynotes leads to allopathic treatment—treatment of the parts and not of the whole.

The tempting thing about keynotes is that these rubrics will have only two, three, or four remedies listed. Therefore, we are often tempted to make keynotes where they really do not exist. Do not ask leading questions in order to convince the patient that he really ought to have an answer in the keynote category. Instead, think of these as really beautiful seashells that you find while walking on the beach. They are treasures to be appreciated, but they can't be found where they do not exist.

The problem in doing that is, because the rubrics will have a very few remedies, you will exclude what might be the best remedy simply because it is not listed here. Remember, in selecting the right remedy, we are looking for the one that speaks to the totality of the symptoms, and not just to some weird little symptom.

SYMPTOMS AND MATERIA MEDICA

Now, have a look at your organized symptoms. Check to see, first of all, what are the general states. Say the patient has headache, sore throat, runny nose, general chills, and night sweats. We have a pretty good idea of what is going on here in terms of a disease diagnosis.

But do we have any idea what is going on in terms of a drug diagnosis?

Look through your refinement of the case. Look at the specific symptoms, look at the alternating symptoms, etc. Is there a flow of a certain remedy or remedies to the case? Does it, for instance, suggest Lycopodium or Arsenicum? Read those remedies in your materia medica and compare their actions. Consider the behavior of your patient versus the behavior pattern of the remedy portrait.

All homeopathic prescriptions are made through the materia medica. All of them. The repertory is a tool in prescribing, and a valuable one, but there is more to the decision of the prescription than the mathmatics of repertorization. As you look up the rubrics that are incorporated into the case, you are seeing the flow of the symptoms and what remedies that flow suggests. But you are not getting a final word on the case. The Materia Medica is the final word. That's why I suggested that you own as many good ones as possible; in this way, you can have the wisdom of the homeopathic masters on hand to guide you.

If, when you look at your case as you took it, you find a solid picture of a remedy, and you are convinced that this is the remedy for the case, your work is done. In many acute cases, the remedy will be obvious, and while repertorization is always required in the constitutional and the miasmic case, it is often simply not needed in the acute. You will find people with food poisoning who simply need Arsenicum. You will find people who have been stung by a bee who need Apis. Most of the work in the first acute prescription can be handled very quickly and easily by the person who knows his acute materia medica, who knows the keynotes of the remedies and can recognize them when he sees them.

That is often the fun part, when you recognize a remedy for the first time. I find that the best way to practice this is through film and fiction. Read the materia medica and then try to spot the types in popular culture. When you actually realize on a visceral level that Felix Unger is indeed an Arsenicum through and through, you will be able to celebrate the fact that homeopathy is moving from being philosophy to being a usable and practical skill in your life.

So, if you want to ultimately find that there is such a thing as "practical homeopathy," you must study the materia medica. Only by nailing that information, by knowing the basic remedies and how they are appropriately used, will you ever be able to fulfill the physician's role.

SYMPTOMS AND THE REPERTORY

Kent says, "Any man who desires to avoid this careful method should not pretend to be a homeopathic physician." Learning to use the repertory correctly is just that important. So, excepting the simple acute cases that are crying out their remedy, you are going to have to learn to repertorize. And there are no simple ways to learn it. That's why I strongly suggest that you look through several of them before you find the one that works best for you. And then I suggest that you just use it and use it and use it. You don't have to be repertorizing a case in order to use the repertory. Just look through it. See how the symptoms are listed and how the whole book is organized. See how the symptoms are refined from very general to very specific. Most beginning students make the mistake of waiting until there is some emergency before they try to use the repertory. The secret is looking through it again and again before you need it, so that, when it is needed, you will know where to look for food cravings (and the location will differ a bit from repertory to repertory—remember, these are the notes of one specific homeopathic physician who is trying to share his research with you, but you are going to have to learn to think like him; he is likely dead and can't now learn to think like you).

I think that it is important that, especially in the beginning, you write out the entire case as you look it up. Write out all the remedies, so that you get a feel for the flow of the case, and so that you are becoming familiar with the names of the remedies. This hard work early on will pay off again and again over the months and years.

Then, once you have the whole thing written out, look it over again. See what you have here. In your case taking, you likely got an idea of the disease diagnosis. Now, through your repertorization, you have been given the idea of the drug diagnosis. Look to see what remedies are running all through the case. Look to see how strongly (by the typeface, bold is the strongest, italic the second, and plain type third) the remedy is suggested in each rubric. Look to see what remedies make the most sense in the case.

Don't try to use the repertorization to make the final decision. Instead, use it to narrow down your choices from thousands to five or six. Then get out the materia medica. Look at the five or six remedies and ask yourself which seems most called for by the patient, which is most similar to the case.

Now, having done all of this, you have your remedy in mind and are ready to open your kit. I realize that it seems like a great deal of work to go through, and that the temptation exists to just run and get one of the acute guides to get you through, but this is the better way.

Certainly the acute guides, which list a few remedies for a great many emergency situations, can be of great help, especially for those who are only now learning homeopathy. We have all used them when the dog is throwing up, when a child is screaming in pain from an ear infection. And often they do work quite well. But, remember, no guide like that can list all the remedies that may be of help to you in a given situation. Out of the list of twelve remedies, you may need the thirteenth, the one that was cut out due to lack of space.

In the section that follows I have tried to gather together the best suggested remedies for all sorts of common household emergencies, always trying to include as many remedies as might be needed for a given situation. But no guide can ever really take the place of a well-used repertory.

So while I certainly advise beginners to have these guides and use them when needed, I also advise that you learn to take the case and to repertorize. And while it seems like such a lot of work, remember that in most acute situations, the case taking takes only a few seconds. There are only a handful of symptoms to consider. Sore throat, rash. Nothing too taxing.

In the same way, the repertorization takes only a few minutes, if you have to do it at all. As I said before, you will be your own best emergency guide if you have put the time in and learned the materia medica. If you can recognize the remedy needed, you are all set. If not, especially if you have put the time in with the repertory before the emergency took place, you will only have to spend a very few minutes looking things up.

Either way, by taking and considering the case, you are now ready to treat.

The Acute Treatment

Honestly, I am always a little frightened by those who approach the physician's role with a disorganized manner. Sooner or later they make a very serious mistake due to their lack of organization.

In the case taking and repertorization, you have taken the original notes of the case and rewritten them twice. First you organized the symptoms for repertorization, and then, in repertorizing them, you organized them for prescription.

Now, take those notes and put them into a folder. And in that folder also place a piece of paper. And on that paper keep track of what remedy you have given, the time, the date, the potency, etc.

Then as the case unfolds, keep notes on what takes place. Keep coherent notes as to what happens to the patient's symptoms as you give doses of the remedy.

This organized approach will not only keep you from making the most common mistake of giving the remedy too often; it will also help you learn more about the materia medica as you see how the patient responds to the remedy. It is especially helpful to the worried mother, as it shows her directly that progress is being made. If the 104-degree fever is now down by two degrees, she will be comforted by the improvement.

So if you are going to enact the physician's role, once again you will have to take the physician's responsibility and take the situation seriously.

If you originally had more than one remedy in mind, note it. Your other choices may have to be called into play if the first remedy fails, or if it needs a followup remedy.

Your organized note taking will be especially helpful in general if you need a second remedy. Because the second remedy will be selected on the basis of what has shifted from the first remedy, only if you have these notes to refer to will you be sure that you know what has shifted and how.

THE LAWS OF CURE

This seems a very good time to remind you of just how homeopathy is practiced. We have three Laws of Cure, given to us by Hahnemann, that together will shape our use of the remedies and our practice of homeopathy. They are:

The Law of Similars: Like cures like. The disease picture of a case—the totality of the symptoms—is matched against the remedy picture, or full range of symptoms that a specific remedy treats. When these two match, cure takes place. Cure, as stated above, is the total removal of symptoms, the complete and gentle and permanent restoration of health. The Law of Cure is often stated with the Latin, *Simila similibus curentur*—"Like cures like."

Now, in applying this law to the acute case, it reminds us that we are not treating a sore throat, but are instead treating the person who has the sore throat. The specific pain symptoms have to be placed in the context of the person's total being. Therefore, the patient's behavior while he has the sore throat may be more important to finding the right remedy than will the sore throat itself. Don't let yourself be tricked—by the patient's pain and by your own desire to help—into treating a disease. That is allopathy, pure and simple, and you will do little good in practicing homeopathy in an allopathic manner.

The Law of Simplex: Very simply, this law states that the wise homeopath gives one remedy at a time. Period.

This principle can be hard to stick with in an acute case, but unless you are in a true life-or-death situation, a car accident in which you may have to quickly alternate between Arnica and Aconite until the ambulance arrives, the Law of Simplex is the best way to go. Not only is it philosophically sound; it is also the most practical way to treat the patient. Imagine we are in a period of war. Think of these remedies as spies, each of which has a very important message to carry. And each of these messages has to get through to the right person, the one who knows what to do with the information in the message. So you, as the spy chief, have to get the right message to the right person. If you give the right remedy in the acute situation, you are giving the right message to the right person, but, if you panic and send all the messages to one person, he becomes overwhelmed with information, and cannot know what particular information he is to act on. Instead, he does nothing, or he does everything, and the whole cause is lost.

In the same way, even though we were raised to believe that more is better, in homeopathic practice we have to come to terms with the idea that what we want to do is create the least change in the human system that can bring about a healing response. Giving too many remedies is a sure way to confuse a case, and ultimately to ruin it. If you want your patient to stay in pain and to have to go through an illness without the help of the remedies, just give too many remedies. As each one works, you will no longer be sure of just what was the original disease, or what are the artificial diseases that you have set in place. It is not a smart thing to do.

In the acute case, choose the remedy that is best suited. Give that remedy, that one remedy. Then wait. If you have a simple acute, a cold or flu, wait overnight if possible. See how the patient is in the morning. Look for improvement and note it. If there is no improvement in a few hours, or if the situation declines, note that too and look to your other remedies. Again refer to the materia medica. And consider a second remedy.

If you are a beginner, don't give yourself more than two chances with remedy choices. If the first didn't work at all, you may, if you still feel sure in your choice, give a second dose. You may even want to slightly increase the potency. Then wait again.

If you were not sure of the remedy, or if you were torn between two remedies and the first didn't have any impact, give the other remedy after a few hours have passed. Again, wait. Look for improvement. If there is improvement, do nothing. The case is in the process of working itself out.

It is vital that you know your own limits here, your own level of expertise. Of course, you should never be treating constitutional cases at all. This includes maladies like seasonal allergies, conditions that may not seem all that complicated, but, because of the depth of the illness and its chronic nature, are really quite complicated.

In the same way, you should never keep going on a case if you know in your heart that you do not understand it. If no remedy is indicated in your understanding, give no remedy. Call a practitioner. If you have tried the remedy that made sense and it didn't work, call the practitioner. The fact that you have taken the case and that you have organized the information will be of great help to the practitioner, who will likely, based on your excellent information, be able to help you over the telephone with the choice of a remedy. You will have still done a great deal of good for your loved one by your work on the case. (And keep notes on what the practitioner told you and what happens from the remedy he suggests. Not only is this part of your learning process; it may also turn out to be information important to the case.)

The Law of Minimum: The third Law of Cure states that the properly selected remedy should be given in the lowest potency possible to effect cure, and in the least number of doses possible.

This is so important in the acute case. We have been trained in allopathic treatments and we think that we have to give more and more medicine in order for it to work. Instead, we have to learn to really watch the patient, look for change in his or her behavior, in the symptoms, and let these changes be our guide to doses.

I think that homeopathic doses are very like commas. Our grammar teachers all taught us about commas, "When in doubt, leave it out." That made our written communications cleaner and clearer.

In the same way, leave out as many doses as possible while still moving the case forward.

You have given the first dose. Say Phosphorus 30C. You have to wait and you do wait. The patient seems better. He has gotten his voice back a bit and seems to be resting peacefully. Do you give another dose? Of course not. Everything is fine.

Do you give another dose in three hours, or in four? When the hell do you give another dose?

Maybe never. As long as the general improvement continues, leave it alone. And I do mean "general" improvement. Many cases are ruined because the physician, instead of giving the remedy and letting it work as it needs to work, had a plan in mind of which symptoms should change and when, and, when the patient did not react as the physician demanded, gave the remedy again and again until no one could tell what was the natural disease and what was the artificial.

We truly give homeopathic remedies as needed. Now, does this mean that we are doing something wrong if we use the Phosphorus 30C like an allopathic and give it every four hours until improvement begins? No, it's not the worst thing you can do. In most cases, you will see the improvement set in and it will do no harm, but it is not good homeopathy either.

To properly time the doses, you have to watch your patient. You have to keep track of the improvment in the case. You have to watch for a returning of the original symptoms, in which case you will likely have to repeat the remedy (or even consider the original remedy in a higher potency to clear away the symptoms altogether), or for a change in the symptom pattern, in which case you will likely have to move on to a new remedy.

THE SECOND PRESCRIPTION

Kent tells us that while the first prescription is easy, the second prescription is hard. And while Kent was talking in terms of constitutional prescribing, there is still some truth to the statement in the acute arena.

First, let me say that if you have been organized and have been keeping good notes, the change to the second remedy is not all that difficult. If you have waited until this moment to try to remember what you have already given and why you gave it and what it did in the case, then you should probably just call a practitioner and try to give him the information to the best of your knowledge, and let it go at that.

If you have kept your notes and are aware of the ongoing changes in the patient's case, before you consider a second remedy give a thought first to trying the original remedy in a higher potency. This can be a tricky call, and largely depends upon exactly what is happening in the case at the moment.

If the patient's symptoms, the character of his sore throat, his cravings, etc., have not really changed very much in toto even though he has been helped in general by the remedy, but the remedy does not keep the improvement going for very long and the patient keeps relapsing into his symptoms ("My throat hurts again!"), you have a sign of the right remedy having been given too low a potency. You should consider staying with the remedy in a higher potency, or you should at least attempt that higher potency before changing remedies.

If, however, the patient's symptoms have changed, if he wanted cold water before and now wants hot tea and his throat no longer hurts but the pain has moved into his chest, etc., it is time to retake the case. This now is a simple process. Just ask the same questions you did at the outset and compare the patient's answers now with the answers first given. These answers are giving you the information you will need to find the next remedy.

Use the materia medica and the repertory as you did before and find the indicated remedy. Be happy in the fact that you are on the track to success. Often the newly indicated remedy will be complementary of the old one. Check the listing in your materia medica for the first remedy you gave to see what are its comparisons with other remedies. This will give you a clue as to what you may next need.

Just one note of warning. Be sure that in the changing of the symptoms, there is a solid sign of general improvement. Look at the patient's face to see if there is a sign of brightness in the eyes. Look to see whether the patient is increasing his vital force or draining it. In other words, you must know the signs of improvement.

THE SIGNS OF IMPROVEMENT

Constantine Hering, a German-born homeopath and contemporary of Hahnemann's who moved his practice to Philadelphia, has given us **Hering's Law**, which traces a general pattern for how healing takes place. While it is not a set pattern in every case, it gives us a general way of looking at the healing process so that we can tell if a patient is improving as he ought.

In general, look for healing to take place as follows:

- From the top of the head down to the bottom of the feet
- From the inside of the body to the outside (from the most important organs—heart, lungs, etc.—to the least important one—the skin)
- From the most recent symptoms to the most long-term (chronic) ones

So, if your patient had a headache and it is now gone, but he has pains in his feet, that is a good sign. If the baby's earache seems to be gone now—he is no longer screaming—but a diaper rash appears, that is a good sign. And if the sore throat that was the first symptom of illness has finally gone away, the patient is well on the road to recovery.

Hering's law is an important gift to homeopaths. It gives us insight into how healing takes place. But, remember, the very fact that you are a whole and unique being may well outweigh Constantine Hering's notion as to just how this whole thing was supposed to play out. In other words, you may or may not experience healing as Hering thought you should. As long as you are experiencing healing—increased clarity of mind, increased energy, lessened symptoms of illness—then you should be happy.

There are some other general signs of improvement to watch for. One of the best is sleep. I have found again and again that when the right remedy is given, the patient with an acute ailment will fall into a deep, restful sleep and will awaken feeling much improved. This is, to me, an infallible sign of cure.

Also look for general improvement. This can be somewhat more difficult to pin down. The patient may report that, while his throat still hurts, he can "handle it better now." In other words, the specific pains associated with the illness may not be better; in fact, they may be worse—more on that in a minute—but the patient is feeling stronger and more capable of dealing with the illness now. His vital force has been strengthened and he feels better in general. If this occurs, you need not give another dose of any remedy; look for the symptoms of pain to start to fall away.

You may not be able to trust your patient to tell you of the changes that the remedy has brought. Some remedy types, like Lycopodium, will incorporate into the picture the need to insist that the remedy is doing nothing at all. Others, like Phosphorus, will tend to want to please you and will say that they are much better, even when it is clear that they are not. In these cases, it is important that you have your notes and can review their list of symptoms with them. Both you and your patient may find yourselves amazed at how the case has been improved by the remedy when you take it one symptom at a time.

Hahnemann tells us, in aphorism #253 of *The Organon,* that the emotional state of the patient will often give us much information as to his improvement. He writes:

> In all diseases, especially the rapidly arising (acute) ones, the patient's emotional state and entire behavior are the surest and most enlightening of the signs showing a small beginning (not visible to everyone) of amelioration and aggravation. When there is an ever-so-slight beginning of improvement, the patient will demonstrate a greater degree of comfort, increasing composure, freedom of spirit, increased courage—a kind of returning naturalness. When there is an ever so slight beginning of aggravation, the patient will demonstrate the opposite of this, exhibiting a more self-conscious, more helpless state of emotional mind, or the spirit, of the whole behavior and of all attitudes, postitions and performances—a state which draws more pity to itself. This can be easily seen if one observes with exact attentiveness, but it cannot be easily described in words.

I tend to want to ask about improvement in terms of percentage. And, if I find that the patient is telling me that a simple symptom is 20 percent improved, and that a difficult symptom is even 10 percent improved upon the initial dose, I will be pleased that I am on the right track.

Sometimes you will learn about the improvement that the remedy has brought on by watching the patient and by noticing his mood. The patient who wanted quiet and rest will suddenly turn on the TV. He will suddenly tell you that he is bored (that is a wonderful sign, in my experience). He will become hungry. These are indications that you are on the right track.

I find that craving food and drink can be very important to the acute case. I do not think that the patient under acute care should be put on a specific diet, but he should, rather, be fed the things that he craves. (This is not true for the patient whose condition is chronic, as many chronic conditions are the result of bad eating and/or lifestyle habits.) These cravings should be noted and used in the selection of remedies. Therefore, the patient who craves ice cream should be given it. And the patient who feels too sick to eat should be allowed to skip a few meals (unless this fast itself becomes a problem). If you can trust the overall healing process, you will work with the body's own wisdom in illness and allow the patient the diet that he craves.

Hahnemann bears me out in this in paragraph #263 of his work. That aphorism, in part, reads as follows: "The cravings of the acutely ill patient with regard to edible delectables and drinks is, for the most part, for things that give palliative relief. These are not, however, actually of a medicinal nature and they are only appropriate for the current need." In other words, that bit of ice cream may be well and good for the child with a sore throat, but the child who eats too much ice cream too often may be opening the door to other health issues above and beyond the sore throat at hand.

AGGRAVATIONS

When you give a homeopathic remedy, the patient may at first experience a temporary worsening of symptoms. This flare-up of symptoms is called an aggravation.

In his writings, Hahnemann tells us that an aggravation is a sign of cure in acute situations. (Again, the same is not true for chronic conditions.) In acute cases, sore throats may be a bit more sore before they rapidly get better, and so on. The aggravation is, in reality, the primary action of the medicine—it shows that the medicine is working. The symptoms grow worse because the medicine that has been selected on the basis of its similarity to the symptoms occurring naturally has actually bumped the symptoms up to a worse state. Once the system reacts against the medicine, these symptoms quickly abate.

Acute aggravations, therefore, should never last more than a few hours. And they should be accompanied by a general improvement in the patient's being. So while that sore throat may be worse for the remedy, the patient's emotional state and general energy should be improved. Look for the signs of cure to inform you that what you are seeing is a simple aggravation and not a wrongly selected remedy.

And while many modern homeopaths use these aggravations as a guidepost to having selected the correct remedy, and while these aggravations are certainly not dangerous, they are almost always a sign that while the correct remedy was given, it was given in too high a potency. But after you have created an aggravation, what can you do about it? Do you give the remedy again in a lower potency? No, in most cases, you do nothing further and the symptoms will disappear in a few hours. The patient will feel much better and his vital force will be strong throughout.

You need only be concerned about aggravations if the vital force becomes weaker as the symptoms increase, if the patient seems to be growing worse. In this very rare occurence, it is a good idea to antidote the remedy. You do this by looking up the remedy in the materia medica. Under the category "antidotes" it will list them for you. Most homeopathics can be antidoted by the remedy Nux Vomica. One dose does it. And the actions of homeopathic remedies can be blunted by the substance camphor. But never hesitate to call in an experienced practitioner; don't ever risk your patient.

If you find that your homeopathic practice seems to be riddled with aggravations, perhaps you should spend more time with your materia medica. It is a sign that your practice is a bit too heavy-handed, and perhaps a lighter touch—and a lower potency—is called for. Remember, we are seeking cures that are "rapid, gentle and permanent," and while in some cases aggravations are almost inevitable, they can be most unpleasant for the patient and should be avoided if possible.

CASE FAILURES

To this point, we have rather assumed that if you have followed the plan as set forth, you will surely succeed in finding the needed remedy on the first try.

I wish this were true.

Often, especially in beginning our study and use of homeopathy, we will have far more failures than successes.

In aphorism #249, Hahnemann tells us what we should do if the remedy we have given does not work:

> Every medicine prescribed for a case of disease which, in the course of its action, brings forth new and troublesome symptoms that are not peculiar to the disease to be cured, is not capable of engendering true improvement. Such a medicine is not deemed as homeopathically selected.
>
> 1. If the aggravation is significant, it should be partly extinguished by an antidote, given as soon as possible. Then the next means should be given, which has been more precisely selected according to its similarity of action.
> 2. If the troublesome symptoms are not all-too-violently adverse, then the next means should be administered at once, to take the place of the incorrectly selected one.

So Hahnemann tells us that there is no shame in having to antidote our selected remedy. To do this, the simplest and best method is to take camphor (a skin rub like Tiger Balm works very well), and rub it on the pulse points of the patient's wrists. Have the patient breathe the camphor smell in order to antidote or blunt the action of the remedy.

Then stop and look at the case again. You have obviously missed something important. The remedy you selected was not similar enough in its action to bring about improvement. In fact, it may have aggravated the case. New symptoms may have been created by the remedy. It is best after antidoting to let the patient rest while you look the case over and let several hours pass before giving the next remedy.

But, especially in acute situations, you may not have hours to wait. As Hahnemann writes in aphorism #250, your failure to find the correct first remedy may lead to something of an emergency. He writes:

> In urgent cases, after six, eight or twelve hours, it may already be revealed to the sharp-sighted medical-art practitioner who accurately investigates according to the disease state, that he has misselected the medicine last given. The patient's state grows distinctly (even if only ever-so-slightly) worse from hour to hour, as new symptoms and ailments arise. In these cases, it is not only permitted but the physician is duty-bound to make good the mistake he has made by selecting and administering a homeopathic remedy which is not merely tolerably fitting, but which is the most appropriate possible for the present disease state (i.e., the disease state as it now appears, with the old symptoms that remain and the new symptoms).

So when we look over the case once more, we now must also take into account the changes in the case that have been caused by the incorrect remedy. We have to gather all that information together to find our most appropriate remedy choice.

This is the moment at which we must be sure of ourselves and never work beyond our skill level. Should you, after having given a remedy and finding that it does not work for the situation at hand, have a solid second remedy to turn to, then it is appropriate to do so, but should you only be making a stab in the dark, or should you have already given that second remedy, only to find that it, too, has failed to work, it is surely time now to call a professional practitioner.

Any true physician, be he professional or lay, knows when to ask for help, when to seek the wise counsel of others in the practice of medicine.

It is important to remember that Hahnemann tells us that it is quite all right to move on to the second remedy if the first has not worked, but he does not suggest a third or a fourth. Should the second remedy fail, then the case is surely beyond the skill level of the physician at hand and another voice needs to be heard. In cases of life-and-death situations, head for the emergency room and to seek allopathic help. While allopathic medicine is always to be considered suppressive, in times of true emergency even an antibiotic, wisely selected and used, is of greater value than is a poorly selected homeopathic remedy.

A final thought is this: If you are waiting for an emergency in order to open your materia medica or your repertory, or even to look at the pages of a simple home guide, then you have waited too long. Few of us are clear-sighted and clear-headed in an emergency. Open those books now. Learn homeopathic philosophy and practice now, so that when an emergency occurs, you will be in the best position to deal with it.

CONCLUDING THE ACUTE TREATMENT

Whether you have selected a correct remedy yourself, or have turned to those with greater medical skills for help, even once you have seen a solid improvement in the patient, you cannot afford to ignore your proper case management. It is important that you note the changes in the case that are brought about with each new dose of the remedy. It is vital that you note any changes in the remedy's potency, or the selection of a new remedy. You have to look at the case both subjectively and objectively. Subjectively, your heart is filled with joy that this loved one feels better and is rapidly moving toward a state of health. Objectively, you have to see this case as a learning experience, whether you solved the puzzle easily yourself or had to seek the help of others.

Since you have only been giving the patient the single remedy required and only in the required potency and doses, you should have no trouble ending the treatment. When no further doses of the remedy are called for, when the patient's vital force no longer dips and there are no more increases of symptoms, then no more remedy is needed—and none is given.

But there are few situations in which it is appropriate to give the patient "one for the road." A case in which it might be called for is a flu that in its epidemic sweep has been known to cause many relapses. In this case, you may give the patient one final dose of the called-for remedy a couple days (anywhere up to a week) after the final suggested dose, to act as a preventative to relapse. But, in most cases, when you are done, you are done.

What you have left to do is to organize your information. Complete your notes. Make sure that you have all of your experience mapped out. What you have learned this time will make you that much more effective next time. And it will make you a better physician in the long run.

Section Two

Being
Practical

~~~~~~~~~~~~~~~~

Diagnostic
Symptoms

Introduction

AS IT IS a matter of great importance to the homeopathist to be familiar with the proper method of forming a diagnosis, so as to be able to take advantage of every possible circumstance that will aid him in a knowledge of disease, we will give a few diagnostic signs by which he may be assisted in his investigation."

So wrote Dr. I. D. Johnson more than a century ago in his *Homeopathic Family Guide* as an introduction to a section on specific diagnostic symptoms. And, as arcane as his language may be, his point is sound. In the search for the remedy, the person fulfilling the role of the physician, whether he or she be a professional practitioner or a concerned parent, may all too often become dependent upon the statements of the patient concerning the patient's symptoms, to the point that he or she recognizes the symptoms that the patient's own body is providing. In this section, we will consider how a remedy may often be discovered without having to ask the patient a single question if we can learn to make use of the symptoms of visible result. The practitioner who has learned to use his or her own eyes, ears, and nose is the practitioner who will be of greatest use to the patient.

In all cases for the symptoms that follow I have listed the most important remedies first—that is, the remedy or remedies that most often speak to that specific symptom. I then follow with other remedies, from the most common to the least common, for the specific symptoms. The remedies listed here are not exhaustive (more complete lists of symptoms are to be found in the individual rubrics of the repertory) but speak to the most commonly used home remedies.

Finally, it is important to note that in making correct use of these diagnostic symptoms, we must always place them within the framework of the totality of the patient's symptoms and being in order to make the correct assessment of the case. To give a person a remedy based solely upon the fact that his skin has a bright red tone is as faulty a use of homeopathics as to give a patient the remedy Rhus Tox simply because his back hurts—without coming to understand how that back hurts and how that specific pain fits within the context of the totality of symptoms.

General Diagnostic Symptoms: States of Being

MODALITIES: INDICATORS
Environment: Air

For the patient who is made worse by being in contact with open air, consider: **Aconite, Hepar Sulph, Nux, Rumex**, and **Silicea**. Also: **Sulphur**. Also: **Kali Bi, Mercurius, Lachesis, Bryonia, Dulcamara**, and **Calcarea**.

If cold air aggravates, consider: **Aconite, Arsenicum, Hepar Sulph, Nux, Rhus Tox, Rumex, Sepia**, and **Silicea**. Also: **Calcarea, Dulcamara**, and **Hypericum**.

If the patient is averse to cold, open air, consider: **Arsenicum, Calcarea**, and **Nux**. Also: **Silicea, Hepar Sulph**, and **Belladonna**.

If the patient is aggravated by cold, open air that contains frost, consider: **Calcarea**. Also: **Sepia, Pulsatilla**, and **Mercurius**. Also: **Sulphur**.

If the patient craves cold air, consider: **Apis**. Also: **Pulsatilla** and **Carbo Veg**.

If the patient cannot bear the draft of cold air in a warm room, consider: **Nux**. Also: **Calcarea** and **Rhus Tox**. Also: **Sulphur** and **Lycopodium**.

If a patient becomes ill after being exposed to a cold draft in a warm room, consider: **Lachesis**.

If a patient becomes ill from the cold draft in the warm room because he was perspiring, consider: **Dulcamara**.

If the patient feels better because of that draft of cold air in a warm room, consider: **Arsenicum**. Also: **Carbo Veg, Rhus Tox**, and **Silicea**.

If the night air aggravates, consider: **Mercurius**. Also: **Aconite, Sulphur**, and **Carbo Veg**.

For the patient who is improved by being in warm, open air, consider: **Arsenicum, Nux**, and **Rhus Tox**. Also: **Graphites, Phosphorus, Silicea, Spongia, Arnica, Belladonna, Hepar Sulph, Ignatia**, and **Lycopodium**.

If the patient is improved by moving from a cool place into a place of warm air in general, consider: **Arsenicum, Rhus Tox**, and **Nux**. Also: **Silicea, Dulcamara, Hepar Sulph, Belladonna**, and **Ignatia**.

For the patient who is made worse by being in warm, open air, consider: **Pulsatilla, Mercurius**, and **Lachesis**. Also: **Natrum Mur, Sepia**, and **Sulphur**.

For the patient who is made better in the open air, consider: **Pulsatilla**. Also: **Arsenicum**. Also: **Rhus Tox** and **Sulphur**.

If the patient is improved by cold, open air, consider: **Drosera, Ledum, Carbo Veg**, and **Allium Cepa**.

For the patient who craves open air, consider: **Carbo Veg**. Also strongly consider: **Pulsatilla, Lycopodium, Sulphur, Lachesis, Apis**, and **Spigelia**. Also: **Graphites**.

For the patient who is averse to the open air, consider: **Nux, Rumex, Silicea**, and **Sulphur**. Also: **Mercurius, Lachesis, Natrum Mur**, and **Lycopodium**.

For the patient who is aggravated by being indoors, consider: **Pulsatilla**. Also: **Phosphorus, Natrum Mur, Spongia, Aconite, Arnica**, and **Sulphur**.

For the patient who is made better by being indoors, consider: **Nux, Silicea**, and **Calcarea**. Also: **Ruta, Rhus Tox, Spigelia, Staphysagria, Belladonna, Ignatia**, and **Ipecac**.

Environment: Temperature

COLD

For the patient who feels chilly, consider: **Arsenicum, Calcarea, Nux**, and **Silicea**, Also consider: **Dulcamara, Spigelia**, and **Ipecac**. Also: **Natrum Mur, Lycopodium**, and **Ignatia**.

For the patient who feels deeply cold, consider: **Arsenicum** and **Nux**.

If the patient has a hot head and cold feet, consider: **Arnica**. Also: **Calcarea** and **Sulphur.**

If the patient has a cold head and cold, wet feet, consider: **Calcarea.**

If the patient takes on illness from becoming cold and wet, consider: **Rhus Tox** and **Dulcamara.**

If the patient becomes ill after taking cold drink while his body is over-heated, consider: **Bryonia** and **Rhus Tox**.

If the patient becomes ill after his feet become cold, consider: **Silicea**.

If the patient becomes ill after his feet become cold and wet, consider: **Calcarea.**

If the patient becomes ill from a cold, damp spring day, consider: **Allium Cepa**.

If the patient becomes ill after exposure to dry, cold air, consider: **Aconite.**

For the patient who becomes aggravated in his symptoms when feeling cold, consider: **Nux, Rhus Tox, Hepar Sulph, Silicea, Sepia**, and **Arsenicum.** Also: **Kali Bi, Calcarea, Phosphorus**, and **Thuja.**

If the patient's symptoms are worse after the patient becomes cold, consider: **Belladonna, Calcarea, Mercurius, Nux, Phosphorus, Pulsatilla, Sepia, Silicea,** and **Spigelia**. Also: **Veratrum, Thuja, Kali Bi, Aconite**, and **Coffea.**

If a patient's symptoms are made worse from his becoming cold, specifically when he is perspiring, consider: **Aconite**. Also: **Dulcamara**.

If the patient's symptoms are improved by the patient becoming cold, consider: **Lycopodium** and **Pulsatilla**. Also: **Ledum, Chamomilla, Apis**, and **Graphites.** Also: **Natrum Mur.**

If a patient's symptoms are made worse by a single part of the body becoming cold, consider: **Hepar Sulph, Calcarea, Rhus Tox**, and **Silicea**. Also: **Phosphorus** and **Ledum.**

If by the hands becoming cold, consider: **Hepar Sulph** and **Rhus Tox**. Also: **Silicea.**

If by the feet becoming cold, consider: **Silicea**. Also: **Lachesis, Nux, Pulsatilla**, and **Calcarea.**

If by the head becoming cold, consider: **Silicea**. Also: **Hepar Sulph, Belladonna**, and **Sepia**. Also: **Nux.**

HEAT

For the patient who feels worse from becoming hot, consider: **Pulsatilla, Bryonia**, and **Silicea**. Also: **Natrum Mur, Phosphorus, Arnica**, and **Belladonna**.

For patients who cannot bear the heat of the sun, consider: **Belladonna**. Also: **Bryonia, Aconite, Gelsemium**, and **Natrum Mur**.

For patients who crave the heat of the sun, consider: **Arsenicum** and **Ignatia.**

For patients who get a headache from becoming heated, consider: **Belladonna, Lycopodium**, and **Carbo Veg**. Also: **Apis, Aconite, Ipecac, Natrum Mur, Pulsatilla**, and **Phosphorus.**

If the patient becomes weaker from becoming heated, consider: **Sulphur**. Also: **Pulsatilla, Lachesis**, and **Carbo Veg**.

For patients who become ill in hot weather, consider: **Sulphur, Pulsatilla, Apis**, and **Lachesis**. Also: **Aconite, Gelsemium, Natrum Mur**, and **Bryonia.**

For patients who feel worse in warm temperatures, consider: **Apis, Pulsatilla, Sulphur**, and **Lachesis**. Also: **Gelsemium, Natrum Mur**, and **Phosphorus**.

For patients who feel better in warm temperatures, consider: **Arsenicum, Dulcamara, Hepar Sulph, Rhus Tox, Nux**, and **Mercurius**. Also: **Silicea, Sepia**, and **Veratrum**. Also: **Spigelia, Spongia**, and **Lycopodium**. Also: **Ignatia**.

For patients who are made worse from being in a warm bed, consider: **Apis, Drosera, Ledum, Sulphur, Pulsatilla**, and **Chamomilla**. Also: **Graphites, Lycopodium, Rhus Tox**, and **Spongia**.

For patients who are made better from being in a warm bed, consider: **Nux, Arsenicum, Bryonia, Hepar Sulph, Silicea**, and **Rhus Tox**. Also: **Phosphorus, Lycopodium, Dulcamara**, and **Rumex.**

For patients who are made worse by wearing warm clothing, consider: **Apis, Belladonna, Lachesis, Lycopodium, Pulsatilla**, and **Sulphur**.

For patients who are made better by wearing warm clothing, consider: **Nux, Silicea**, and **Hepar Sulph**.

For patients who are worse in a warm, closed room, consider: **Pulsatilla**. Also: **Sulphur, Lycopodium, Carbo Veg, Graphites**, and **Thuja**.

For patients who are better in a warm, closed room, consider: **Nux, Hepar Sulph**, and **Silicea.**

WET

For the patient who, in general, feels worse from the sensation of wetness, consider: **Rhus Tox, Arsenicum, Calcarea**, and **Dulcamara**. Also: **Sulphur, Thuja, Pulsatilla**, and **Ruta**.

For the patient who feels worse from having wet applications on the body, consider: **Calcarea, Sulphur**, and **Rhus Tox**. Also: **Spigelia, Mercurius, Belladonna**, and **Lachesis**. Also: **Lycopodium**.

For the patient who feels better from having wet applications on the body, consider: **Pulsatilla**. Also: **Euphrasia, Nux, Spigelia**, and **Arsenicum**.

If cold, wet applications are a problem, consider: **Calcarea, Rhus** Tox, and **Sulphur**. Also: **Bryonia** and **Phosphorus**.

If cold, wet applications are a help, consider: **Ledum** and **Pulsatilla**. Also: **Apis**.

If warm, wet applications are a problem, consider: **Apis, Ledum**, and **Pulsatilla**.

If warm, wet applications are a help, consider: **Hepar Sulph, Lachesis, Rhus Tox**, and **Silicea**. Also: **Thuja, Kali Bi**, and **Bryonia**.

If the patient is worse in a damp room, consider: **Pulsatilla, Dulcamara**, and **Arsenicum**. Also: **Thuja, Sepia**, and **Calcarea**.

If a patient is worse at the seashore, consider: **Natrum Mur**.

If the patient is worse from perspiring, consider: **Rhus Tox**. Also: **Bryonia, Aconite**, and **Sepia**.

If the patient is worse from damp clothing or sheets, consider: **Calcarea, Arsenicum**, and **Rhus Tox**.

If the patient becomes ill from sitting on damp ground, consider: **Rhus Tox**. Also: **Arsenicum** and **Dulcamara**. Also: **Nux**.

DRY

For patients who are worse from the combination of dry and cold, consider: **Hepar Sulph, Nux, Aconite**, and **Ipecac**. Also: **Pulsatilla, Rumex, Silicea**, and **Veratrum**.

For patients who are worse from the combination of dry and warm, consider: **Carbo Veg, Kali Bi**, and **Lachesis**.

For patients who are improved by the combination of dry and warm, consider: **Sulphur** and **Rhus Tox**.

Environment: Weather

For patients who are worse from any change in weather, consider: **Dulcamara, Phosphorus, Rhus Tox, Causticum, Bryonia**, and **Silicea**. Also: **Calcarea, Ipecac, Hepar Sulph, Pulsatilla**, and **Rumex**.

For patients who become ill from changes in weather, consider: **Dulcamara**. Also: **Carbo Veg**.

For the patient who is sensitive to any change in temperature, consider: **Mercurius**. Also: **Arsenicum**. Also: **Spongia, Pulsatilla, Phosphorus, Carbo Veg**, and **Dulcamara**.

For patients who are worse for changes in weather from cold to warm, consider: **Bryonia, Sulphur**, and **Lachesis**. Also: **Lycopodium, Lachesis**, and **Natrum Mur**.

For patients who are worse for changes in weather from warm to cold, consider: **Rhus Tox**. Also: **Sepia, Pulsatilla**, and **Chamomilla**.

For patients who are worse in extreme temperatures, either hot or cold, consider: **Mercurius**. Also: **Natrum Mur, Sulphur, Silicea**, and **Graphites**.

For patients who are worse during the times of year in which the days are hot and the nights are cold, consider: **Aconite, Dulcamara**, and **Rumex**.

For the patient who is sensitive to any change in the barometric pressure, consider: **Phosphorus**. Also: **Dulcamara** and **Mercurius**.

If the patient is made worse by wet weather, consider: **Rhus Tox, Arsenicum, Calcarea**, and **Dulcamara**. Also: **Ruta, Silicea, Sepia, Mercurius**, and **Lycopodium**. Also: **Carbo Veg** and **Gelsemium**.

If the patient feels better in wet weather, consider: **Nux, Causticum, Hepar Sulph**, and **Bryonia**. Also: **Ipecac, Belladonna**, and **Spongia**.

If the patient is worse in wet, cold weather, consider: **Calcarea, Dulcamara, Rhus Tox, Silicea**, and **Arsenicum**. Also: **Spigelia, Sulphur, Thuja, Lachesis**, and **Kali Bi**. Also: **Gelsemium** and **Apis**.

If the patient feels worse in warm, wet weather, consider: **Lachesis, Sepia**, and **Carbo Veg**. Also: **Silicea, Gelsemium, Ipecac**, and **Kali Bi**.

If a patient feels worse in dry weather, consider: **Aconite** and **Nux**. Also: **Belladonna** and **Bryonia**.

If a patient feels better in dry weather, consider: **Calcarea, Dulca-**

mara, **Rhus Tox**, and **Ruta**. Also: **Carbo Veg, Pulsatilla, Spigelia, Staphysagria**, and **Sulphur**. Also: **Veratrum**.

If a patient feels better in dry, warm weather, consider: **Sulphur** and **Rhus Tox**.

If a patient feels worse in dry, warm weather, consider: **Lachesis, Kali Bi**, and **Carbo Veg**.

For the patient who is worse in windy weather, consider: **Hepar Sulph, Nux, Pulsatilla, Phosphorus**, and **Spongia**. Also: **Chamomilla, Rhus Tox**, and **Euphrasia**. Also: **Aconite** and **Silica**. Also: **Natrum Mur**.

For the patient who is made worse from a cold wind, consider: **Aconite, Belladonna, Rhus Tox, Spongia**, and **Nux**.

For the patient who feels worse in foggy weather, consider: **Hypericum** and **Rhus Tox**. Also: **Thuja, Silicea, Staphysagria**, and **Gelsemium**.

For the patient who feels worse in clear weather, consider: **Nux, Bryonia**, and **Hepar Sulph**.

For the patient who feels worse in sunny weather, consider: **Pulsatilla, Nux, Natrum Mur**, and **Veratrum**. Also: **Belladonna** and **Bryonia**.

If the patient becomes ill from exposure to the sun, consider: **Belladonna**. Also: **Pulsatilla, Lachesis**, and **Bryonia**. Also: **Natrum Mur** and **Carbo Veg**.

For the patient who feels worse in cloudy weather, consider: **Rhus Tox**. Also: **Pulsatilla** and **Sepia**.

For the patient who feels worse in snowy weather, consider: **Sepia**. Also: **Calcarea, Sulphur, Silicea, Phosphorus**, and **Lycopodium**.

For the patient who feels worse in rainy weather, consider: **Sulphur, Dulcamara**, and **Rhus Tox**. Also: **Thuja**.

For the patient who feels worse in stormy weather, consider: **Phosphorus**. Also: **Silicea, Sepia**, and **Lachesis**. Also: **Bryonia** and **Gelsemium**.

For the patient who feels worse at the approach of a storm, consider: **Phosphorus, Sepia**, and **Rhus Tox**.

For the patient who feels worse after a storm, consider: **Rhus Tox** and **Sepia**.

If the patient improves during a storm, consider: **Sepia**. Also: **Lycopodium**.

For the patient who is worse during the spring, consider: **Belladonna, Lycopodium, Lachesis, Calcarea**, and **Gelsemium**. Also: **Sulphur, Silicea, Kali Bi**, and **Natrum Mur**. Also: **Rhus Tox**.

For the patient who is worse during the summer, consider: **Bryonia** and **Sulphur**.

For the patient who is worse during the autumn, consider: **Rhus Tox, Dulcamara**, and **Kali Bi**. Also: **Mercurius, Calcarea, Graphites**, and **Lachesis**.

For the patient who is worse during the winter, consider: **Aconite, Arsenicum, Veratrum, Nux, Pulsatilla**, and **Hepar Sulph**. Also: **Dulcamara, Bryonia, Ignatia, Ipecac, Mercurius**, and **Kali Bi**.

Motion and Position

For the patient who is aggravated by motion, consider: **Nux, Ledum**, and **Bryonia**. Also: **Sulphur** and **Belladonna**. Then consider: **Spigelia** and **Natrum Mur**. Also: **Apis, Kali Bi**, and **Staphysagria**.

If the patient is aggravated after motion, consider: **Rhus Tox**. Also: **Pulsatilla** and **Ruta**. Also: **Carbo Veg, Arsenicum**, and **Spongia**.

If the patient is aggravated especially upon the first motion, or on the beginning of a motion, consider especially: **Rhus Tox**. Also: **Lycopodium** and **Pulsatilla**. Also: **Euphrasia**. Also: **Silicea** and **Phosphorus**.

If the patient is aggravated by continued or repeated motion, consider: **Euphrasia, Pulsatilla**, and **Rhus Tox**. Also: **Silicea, Sabadilla**, and **Drosera**.

For the patient who is made worse, in general, by physical exertion, consider: **Rhus Tox, Calcarea, Bryonia, Arsenicum Arnica, Gelsemium**, and **Natrum Mur**. Also: **Sepia, Spongia, Spigelia, Pulsatilla**, and **Phosphorus**. Also: **Nux, Lachesis**, and **Kali Bi**.

If the patient is made ill from physical exertion, consider: **Arnica**. Also: **Silicea**. Also consider: **Rhus Tox, Ruta, Sulphur, Calcarea**, and **Carbo Veg**.

For the patient who, in general, is made better by physical exertion, consider: **Rhus Tox, Sepia, Ignatia**, and **Hepar Sulph**. Also: **Kali Bi**.

If the patient feels better only on an emotional level from physical exertion, consider: **Rhus Tox**.

If the patient has a particular part of the body that is aggravated by motion, consider: **Ledum, Spigelia, Arnica, Bryonia**, and **Rhus Tox**. Also: **Lachesis, Mercurius, Arsenicum, Belladonna**, and **Sulphur**. Also: **Pulsatilla**.

If a particular body part is improved by motion, consider: **Rhus Tox, Sulphur, Dulcamara**, and **Sulphur**. Also: **Kali Bi** and **Sepia**.

For the patient who is, in general, improved by motion, consider: **Rhus Tox, Pulsatilla, Euphrasia, Sulphur**, and **Lycopodium**. Also: **Gelsemium**.

If the patient is improved by continued motion, consider: **Rhus Tox, Pulsatilla, Euphrasia**, and **Drosera**. Also: **Lycopodium** and **Ruta**.

If the patient is improved by slow motions, consider: **Pulsatilla**. Also: **Sulphur**.

If the patient is improved by rapid motions, consider: **Arsenicum**. Also: **Sepia** and **Bryonia**.

If the patient is improved by sudden motions, consider: **Sabadilla**.

If the patient is improved by violent motions, consider: **Arsenicum** and **Sepia**.

If the patient is improved by motions in the open air, consider: **Pulsatilla**. Also: **Rhus Tox**.

For the patient who desires motion, consider: **Chamomilla** and **Rhus Tox**. Also: **Aconite, Arnica, Coffea**, and **Arsenicum**.

For the patient who is averse to motion, consider: **Bryonia**. Also: **Ruta, Nux, Sulphur, Lachesis, Arsenicum**, and **Calcarea**. Also: **Ignatia, Carbo Veg**, and **Natrum Mur**.

If motion is, in general, difficult, consider: **Bryonia**. Also: **Sepia**. Also: **Lycopodium, Belladonna**, and **Rhus Tox**.

For the patient who, in general, is awkward in motion, consider: **Calcarea, Lachesis, Ipecac**, and **Apis**. Also: **Ignatia, Natrum Mur, Pulsatilla**, and **Nux**.

If the patient's legs are awkward, consider: **Silicea** and **Veratrum**.

If the patient knocks into things while he is in motion, consider: **Ipecac, Natrum Mur**, and **Nux**.

If the patient is awkward when walking and stumbles into things, consider: **Ipecac**. Also: **Calcarea, Lachesis, Phosphorus**, and **Ignatia**. Also: **Natrum Mur**.

If motion is awkward, consider: **Mercurius**.

If motion is exaggerated, consider: **Ignatia**.

If the patient's motions are all very slow, consider: **Pulsatilla**. Also: **Sulphur**. Also: **Calcarea**.

For the patient who, in general, is aggravated by ascending motion, consider: **Bryonia, Arsenicum, Calcarea**, and **Spongelia**. Also: **Phosphorus, Ruta, Sepia, Spigelia**, and **Sulphur**. Also: **Natrum Mur**.

If ascending to a very high place aggravates, consider: **Calcarea**. Also: **Silicea, Spigelia**, and **Sulphur**.

If ascending improves the patient's condition, consider: **Belladonna, Coffea, Lycopodium, Ruta**, and **Sulphur**.

For the patient for whom descending motions aggravate, consider: **Gelsemium**. Also: **Ruta, Veratrum, Lycopodium**, and **Sulphur**. Also: **Aconite, Rhus Tox, Sepia**, and **Bryonia**.

For the patient for whom the motion of bending aggravates, consider: **Belladonna, Bryonia, Spongia**, and **Calcarea**. Also: **Nux, Pulsatilla, Thuja**, and **Staphysagria**.

If bending backward aggravates, consider: **Rhus Tox, Staphysagria, Sepia, Pulsatilla, Chamomilla**, and **Thuja**. Also: **Sulphur, Calcarea**, and **Nux**.

If bending forward aggravates, consider: **Belladonna, Coffea**, and **Thuja**. Also: **Nux**.

If bending sideways aggravates, consider: **Belladonna, Calcarea**, and **Natrum Mur**. Also: **Lycopodium** and **Staphysagria**.

If bending the painful part of the body aggravates, consider: **Calcarea**. Also: **Arnica**. Also: **Lycopodium, Pulsatilla, Nux, Rhus Tox, Sepia, Spigelia**, and **Spongia**.

For the patient for whom the motion of bending backward is helpful, consider: **Drosera**. Also: **Lachesis, Thuja, Ignatia**, and **Belladonna**. Also: **Chamomilla**.

If bending forward is helpful, consider: **Gelsemium**.

If bending double is helpful, consider: **Sulphur, Rhus Tox, Sepia, Thuja**, and **Calcarea**.

For patients who are, in general, made worse by kneeling, consider: **Sepia**.

For patients who become ill from kneeling, consider: **Calcarea, Pulsatilla, Sepia**, and **Spigelia**.

For patients who are, in general, made better by kneeling, consider: **Euphrasia**.

For patients who, in general, are made worse by the motion of sitting, consider: **Rhus Tox, Phosphorus, Dulcamara, Euphrasia, Arsenicum, Sepia**, and **Lycopodium**. Also: **Pulsatilla, Bryonia, Ruta, Savadilla**, and **Spigelia**.

If the patient is worse on first sitting down, consider: **Spigelia**. Also: **Spongia, Coffea**, and **Bryonia**.

If the patient is worse from sitting erect, consider: **Ignatia, Lycopodium, Spigelia, Spongia, Staphysagria**, and **Mercurius**.

If the patient is made worse by sitting in a cool place, consider: **Nux**. Also: **Rhus Tox, Belladonna, Dulcamara, Sepia**, and **Silicea**.

For patients who, in general, are made better by the motion of sitting, consider: **Nux**. Also: **Graphites, Coffea, Dulcamara**, and **Mercurius**.

If the patient is improved on first sitting down, consider: **Sulphur, Rhus Tox, Sepia, Nux**, and **Euphrasia**. Also: **Belladonna** and **Carbo Veg**.

If the patient is improved by sitting erect, consider: **Dulcamara, Arsenicum, Nux, Phosphorus**, and **Pulsatilla**. Also: **Aconite**.

For the patient who desires to sit down, consider: **Phosphorus**. Also: **Nux, Graphites, Sepia**, and **Mercurius**. Also: **Natrum Mur**.

For the patient who is averse to sitting down, consider: **Arsenicum**. Also: **Lachesis**.

For the patient who, in general, is made worse by standing, consider: **Sulphur**. Also: **Pulsatilla**. Also: **Sepia, Kali Bi, Bryonia, Euphrasia**, and **Ruta**.

For the patient who, in general, is improved by standing, consider: **Belladonna**. Also: **Arsenicum**. Also: **Nux** and **Spigelia**.

For the patient who finds standing impossible, consider: **Kali Bi**. Also: **Nux, Staphysagria**, and **Aconite**. Also: **Gelsemium**.

For the patient who, in general, is made worse by the motion of lying down, consider: **Rhus Tox**. Also: **Rumex, Sulphur, Pulsatilla, Euphrasia, Chamomilla**, and **Apis**. Also: **Ruta, Phosphorus**, and **Dulcamara**.

If the patient feels worse when trying to lie down, consider: **Rhus Tox**. Also: **Dulcamara** and **Lycopodium**. Also: **Pulsatilla** and **Sepia**.

If lying down in bed makes the patient worse, consider: **Phosphorus, Lycopodium, Mercurius, Lachesis, Rumex, Silicea**, and **Sepia**. Also: **Sulphur, Spigelia, Rhus Tox**, and **Drosera**.

If lying on the back aggravates the patient, consider: **Nux** and **Phosphorus**. Also: **Arsenicum** and **Silicea**.

If lying on the side aggravates the patient, consider: **Aconite, Bryonia, Calcarea, Phosphorus**, and **Rhus Tox**. Also: **Ignatia** and **Lycopodium**.

If lying on the left side aggravates the patient, consider: **Phosphorus**. Also: **Pulsatilla**. Also: **Aconite**.

If lying on the right side aggravates the patient, consider: **Mercurius**. Also: **Nux** and **Spongia**.

If lying on the painful side aggravates the patient, consider: **Hepar Sulph, Ruta, Silicea**, and **Belladonna**. Also: **Nux** and **Aconite**.

If lying on the painless side aggravates the patient, consider: **Bryonia**. Also: **Pulsatilla** and **Chamomilla**.

For the patient who, in general, feels better from the motion of lying down, consider: **Belladonna** and **Natrum Mur**. Also: **Nux, Calcarea, Bryonia**, and **Ledum**.

If the patient feels better when lying down, consider: **Calcarea, Arsenicum, Bryonia, Nux, Natrum Mur, Pulsatilla**, and **Belladonna**.

If the patient feels better after lying down in bed, consider: **Nux, Hepar Sulph, Bryonia**, and **Natrum Mur**.

If the patient feels better lying down on his back, consider: **Pulsatilla** and **Rhus Tox**. Also: **Ignatia, Lycopodium**, and **Natrum Mur**. Also: **Thuja**.

If the patient feels better lying on his stomach, consider: **Belladonna**. Also: **Phosphorus**.

If the patient feels better lying on his side, consider: **Nux**. Also: **Phosphorus** and **Sepia**.

If lying on the painful side improves the patient, consider: **Bryonia**. Also: **Pulsatilla, Chamomilla**, and **Sepia**.

If lying on the painless side improves the patient, consider: **Belladonna, Hepar Sulph, Ruta, Silicea, Spongia**, and **Nux**.

If the pains move to the side that is laid upon, consider: **Ignatia, Bryonia**, and **Rhus Tox**.

For the patient who wants to lay down, consider: **Arsenicum, Nux, Silicea, Calcarea**, and **Sulphur**.

For the patient who does not want to lie down, consider: **Kali Bi**.

For the patient who is, in general, made worse by running, consider: **Pulsatilla, Bryonia**, and **Arsenicum**. Also: **Rhus Tox, Nux, Lycopodium**, and **Sulphur**.

For the patient who is, in general, made better by running, consider: **Sepia**. Also: **Ignatia**.

For the patient who, in general, is made worse by walking, consider: **Phosphorus, Ledum, Belladonna, Calcarea, Bryonia, Rhus Tox**, and **Sulphur**. Also: **Graphites, Natrum Mur**, and **Lachesis**.

If walking fast aggravates the patient, consider: **Belladonna, Bryonia, Sulphur, Phosphorus, Silicea**, and **Pulsatilla**.

If walking in the wind aggravates the patient, consider: **Belladonna, Nux**, and **Sepia**. Also: **Lycopodium** and **Phosphorus**.

If walking in open air aggravates the patient, consider: **Nux, Spigelia, Sulphur**, and **Hepar Sulph**. Also: **Arsenicum**.

If beginning the motion of walking aggravates the patient, consider: **Euphrasia, Lycopodium**, and **Rhus Tox**. Also: **Pulsatilla, Ruta, Silicea**, and **Thuja**. Also: **Bryonia** and **Calcarea**. Also: **Carbo Veg**.

For the patient who, in general, is improved by walking, consider: **Euphrasia** and **Dulcamara**. Also: **Rhus Tox** and **Sulphur**. Also: **Sabadilla**.

If walking slowly improves the patient, consider: **Pulsatilla**. Also: **Sepia**.

If walking fast improves the patient, consider: **Ignatia**.

If walking in open air improves the patient, consider: **Pulsatilla**. Also: **Sabadilla, Sulphur**, and **Rhus Tox**. Also: **Veratrum** and **Natrum Mur**.

Time of Day

For the patient who, in general, feels worse during the daylight hours, consider: **Sulphur** and **Sepia**. Also: **Natrum Mur, Pulsatilla, Rhus Tox**, and **Euphrasia**.

For the patient who, in general, feels better during the daylight hours, consider: **Aconite, Arnica, Bryonia, Chamomilla**, and **Mercurius**.

For the patient who is worse in the morning hours in general, consider: **Nux** and **Lachesis**. Also: **Sulphur, Natrum Mur**, and **Bryonia**. Also: **Calcarea**. Also consider: **Dulcamara, Coffea, Pulsatilla, Rumex**, and **Veratrum**.

If the patient is worse at 5 A.M., consider: **Sulphur** and **Natrum Mur**. Also: **Sepia, Silicea, Apis**, and **Rumex**.

If the patient is worse at 6 A.M., consider: **Nux, Hepar Sulph**, and **Arnica**. Also: **Lycopodium, Sepia**, and **Silicea**.

If the patient is worse at 7 A.M., consider: **Nux** and **Hepar Sulph**.

If the patient is worse at 8 A.M., consider: **Eupatorium**. Also: **Natrum Mur**. Also: **Nux**.

If the patient is worse at 9 A.M., consider: **Chamomilla, Eupatorium**, and **Natrum Mur**. Also: **Bryonia** and **Kali Bi**.

If the patient is worse from 9 A.M., until 2 P.M., consider: **Natrum Mur**.

If the period just before sunrise aggravates the patient, consider: **Lycopodium**.

If the period just after sunrise aggravates the patient, consider: **Nux**. Also: **Pulsatilla** and **Chamomilla**.

For the patient who, in general, feels better in the morning, consider: **Phosphorus** and **Mercurius**. Also: **Aconite**.

For the patient who, in general, is worse in the late morning, consider: **Natrum Mur** and **Sulphur**. Also: **Hepar Sulph, Sepia**, and **Bryonia**.

If the patient is worse at 10 A.M., consider: **Sulphur** and **Natrum Mur**. Also: **Arsenicum, Phosphorus**, and **Rhus Tox**.

If the patient is worse at 11 A.M., consider: **Sulphur** and **Natrum Mur**. Also: **Gelsemium, Rhus Tox, Nux, Sepia**, and **Phosphorus**.

For the patient who, in general, is better in the late morning, consider: **Lycopodium**.

For the patient who, in general, is worse at noon, consider: **Nux, Natrum Mur, Eupatorium**, and **Silicea**.

If the patient, in general, has symptoms that grow worse during the morning hours but begin to decrease at noon, consider: **Hepar Sulph, Natrum Mur**, and **Nux**. Also: **Aconite** and **Gelsemium**.

For the patient who, in general, is worse in the afternoon, consider: **Lycopodium**. Also: **Belladonna, Rhus Tox, Sepia, Silicea, Dulcamara**, and **Euphrasia**.

If the patient is worse at 1 P.M., consider: **Lachesis, Arsenicum**, and **Pulsatilla**. Also: **Phosphorus**.

If the patient is worse from 1 until 2 P.M., consider: **Arsenicum**.

If the patient is worse at 2 P.M., consider: **Eupatorium**. Also: **Lachesis, Arsenicum, Calcarea**, and **Pulsatilla**.

If the patient is worse at 3 P.M., consider: **Belladonna**. Also: **Apis, Thuja**, and **Sulphur**.

If the patient is worse at 4 P.M., consider: **Lycopodium**. Also: **Nux, Apis**, and **Sepia**.

If the patient is worse from 4 until 6 P.M., consider: **Sepia**.

If the patient is worse from 4 until 8 P.M., consider: **Lycopodium**.

If the patient is worse at 5 P.M., consider: **Thuja** and **Pulsatilla**. Also: **Lycopodium, Nux, Hepar Sulph**, and **Gelsemium**.

For the patient who, in general, feels better in the afternoon, consider: **Sepia** and **Rhus Tox**.

For the patient who, in general, feels worse during the evening hours, consider: **Lycopodium**. Also: **Euphrasia, Lachesis, Pulsatilla, Phosphorus**, and **Bryonia**. Also: **Carbo Veg, Chamomilla, Lachesis, Rumex, Silicea, Sulphur, Sepia, Calcarea**, and **Thuja**.

For the patient who is, in general, worse at twilight, consider: **Phosphorus** and **Pulsatilla**. Also: **Calcarea, Arsenicum**, and **Natrum Mur**.

If the patient is worse at 6 P.M., consider: **Nux**. Also: **Pulsatilla, Rhus Tox, Sepia**, and **Silicea**.

If the patient is worse from 6 to 7 P.M., consider: **Hepar Sulph**.

If the patient is worse at 7 P.M., consider: **Hepar Sulph** and **Nux**. Also: **Sepia, Lycopodium**, and **Pulsatilla**.

If the patient is worse at 8 P.M., consider: **Sulphur**. Also: **Rhus Tox**.

If the patient is worse at 9 P.M., consider: **Bryonia**. Also: **Gelsemium**. Also: **Arsenicum** and **Sulphur**.

For the patient who, in general, is better in the evening, consider: **Sepia**. Also: **Pulsatilla**.

For the patient who, in general, is better at twilight, consider: **Phosphorus** and **Bryonia**.

For the patient who, in general, is worse at night, consider: **Aconite, Arnica**, and **Arsenicum**. Also: **Mercurius, Rhus Tox, Rumex, Coffea, Calcarea, Graphites**, and **Kali Bi**.

If the patient is worse at 10 P.M., consider: **Arsenicum** and **Graphites**. Also: **Ignatia**. Also: **Pulsatilla** and **Lachesis**.

If the patient is worse at 11 P.M., consider: **Sulphur**. Also: **Arsenicum, Calcarea, Rumex**, and **Silicea**.

If a patient is worse at midnight, consider: **Aconite**. Also: **Arsenicum, Rhus Tox**, and **Drosera**.

If a patient is worse at 1 A.M., consider: **Arsenicum**. Also: **Carbo Veg**.

If a patient is worse at 2 A.M., consider: **Kali Bi** and **Hepar Sulph**. Also: **Graphites, Drosera, Pulsatilla**, and **Silicea**. Also: **Natrum Mur**.

If a patient is worse at 3 A.M., consider: **Natrum Mur, Bryonia**, and **Sulphur**. Also: **Thuja, Arsenicum**, and **Rhus Tox**.

If a patient is worse at 4 A.M., consider: **Lycopodium** and **Nux**. Also: **Arnica, Pulsatilla**, and **Apis**. Also: **Sulphur**.

For the patient who, in general, is better at night, consider: **Pulsatilla**. If the patient is better at midnight, consider: **Lycopodium**.

BASIC DRIVES: INDICATORS
Hunger

Constitutional types for which issues of hunger are most important as indicators: **Nux, Pulsatilla**, and **Sulphur**. Also: **Natrum Mur, Lycopodium**, and **Calcarea**. Also: **Silicea, Arsenicum, Graphites, Veratrum**, and **Phosphorus**.

For the patient who, in general, has a decreased appetite, consider: **Lycopodium, Lachesis**, and **Coffea**.

For the patient who, in general, has totally lost his appetite, consider: **Nux, Phosphorus, Lycopodium, Natrum Mur, Pulsatilla, Sepia, Silicea, Calcarea**, and **Arsenicum**. Also: **Spigelia, Mercurius, Kali Bi, Coffea, Cina, Bryonia, Arnica**, and **Aconite**.

If the patient loses his appetite at the sight of food, consider: **Sulphur**. Also: **Phosphorus**.

If the patient loses his appetite at the smell of food, consider: **Sepia**. Also: **Nux**.

If the patient loses his appetite in the morning, consider: **Sepia**. Also: **Ignatia, Lachesis**, and **Belladonna**. Also: **Phosphorus** and **Euphrasia**.

If the patient loses his appetite at noon, consider: **Sulphur, Phosphorus, Ruta, Rhus Tox**, and **Carbo Veg**.

If the patient loses his appetite in the evening, consider: **Hypericum, Carbo Veg, Graphites, Sulphur, Silicea**, and **Arsenicum**.

If the patient loses his appetite, but is very thirsty, consider: **Sulphur**. Also: **Spigelia, Phosphorus, Calcarea**, and **Lycopodium**.

For the patient whose appetite, in general, is increased, consider: **Calcarea, Lycopodium, Sulphur, Veratrum, Pulsatilla**, and **Phosphorus**. Also: **Natrum Mur** and **Graphites**.

If the patient has an increased appetite in the morning, consider: **Calcarea**. Also: **Silicea, Rhus Tox**, and **Hypericum**.

If a patient has an increased appetite in the late morning or just before noon, consider: **Sulphur**. Also: **Natrum Mur**.

If a patient has an increased appetite at noon, consider: **Natrum Mur**. Also: **Sulphur** and **Lycopodium**.

If a patient has an increased appetite in the afternoon, consider: **Lycopodium** and **Nux**.

If a patient has an increased appetite in the evening, consider: **Natrum Mur** and **Sepia**.

If a patient has an increased appetite during the night, consider: **Lycopodium** and **Phosphorus**. Also: **Ignatia, Pulsatilla**, and **Bryonia**.

If a patient has an increased appetite after he has already eaten, consider: **Lycopodium** and **Phosphorus.** Also: **Mercurius, Natrum Mur, Staphysagria**, and **Silicea**. Also: **Calcarea**.

If a patient has an increased appetite until he sees food, consider: **Sulphur**. Also: **Phosphorus**. If that appetite disappears upon tasting the food, consider: **Silicea.**

If a patient has an increased appetite with fever: **Phosphorus**. Also: **Eupatorium**.

If a patient has an increased appetite with a chill, consider: **Arsenicum** and **Silicea**. Also: **Eupatorium** and **Staphysagria**.

If a patient has an increased appetite with headache, consider: **Phosphorus**. Also: **Sepia**. Also: **Sulphur, Silicea, Ignatia, Nux, Bryonia, Dulcamara**, and **Lycopodium**. If a patient's appetite is increased just before a headache, consider: **Calcarea** and **Phosphorus**. Also: **Dulcamara** and **Sepia**.

If a patient has an increased appetite with a cough or a cold, consider: **Nux** and **Hepar Sulph**. Also: **Allium Cepa**.

If a patient has an incredible, insatiable appetite, consider: **Lycopodium**. Also: **Sepia** and **Spongia**. Also: **Staphysagria**.

If a patient alternates between a large appetite and no appetite at all, consider: **Calcarea**. Also: **Phosphorus** and **Thuja**. Also: **Arsenicum, Pulsatilla, Silicea, Nux**, and **Natrum Mur**. Also: **Drosera**.

For the patient who is worse while eating, consider: **Sulphur** and **Carbo Veg**, Also: **Graphites, Pulsatilla, Rumex, Hepar Sulph**, and **Sepia**. Also: **Natrum Mur** and **Phosphorus**.

If a patient is worse before eating, consider: **Phosphorus**. Also: **Sulphur, Calcarea**, and **Lycopodium**.

If a patient is worse after eating, consider: **Lycopodium**. Also: **Sulphur, Silicea, Nux, Natrum Mur, Rumex, Kali Bi, Calcarea**, and **Bryonia**. Also: **Arsenicum, Apis, Graphites**, and **Rhus Tox**.

If the patient is worse after eating only a very small amount of food, consider: **Lycopodium**. Also: **Bryonia** and **Phosphorus**. Also: **Ignatia** and **Nux.**

If the patient is worse after overeating, consider: **Pulsatilla, Nux**, and **Lycopodium**. Also: **Coffea, Ipecac**, and **Ignatia**.

For the patient who is made better, in general, by eating, consider: **Phosphorus**. Also: **Spongia, Sepia**, and **Gelsemium**. Also: **Hepar Sulph** and **Ignatia.**

For the patient who is made worse, in general, by eating cold things, consider: **Dulcamara, Lycopodium, Arsenicum, Nux, Lachesis, Rhus Tox**, and **Silicea**. Also: **Spigelia, Staphysagria**, and **Pulsatilla**.

If the patient desires cold food, consider: **Pulsatilla, Phosphorus**, and **Veratrum**. Also: **Ignatia, Bryonia**, and **Arsenicum**. Also: **Lycopodium.**

For the patient who is made better, in general, by cold food, consider: **Pulsatilla, Phosphorus**, and **Veratrum**. Also: **Bryonia, Lycopodium**, and **Ignatia**.

For the patient who is made worse, in general, by warm food, consider: **Bryonia, Phosphorus, Lachesis**, and **Pulsatilla**. Also: **Rhus Tox, Belladonna, Carbo Veg**, and **Euphrasia**.

If the patient is averse to warm food, consider: **Phosphorus, Pulsatilla**, and **Graphites**. Also: **Calcarea, Belladonna, Ignatia, Lycopodium, Silicea, Veratrum**, and **Lachesis**.

If the patient desires warm food, consider: **Arsenicum**. Also: **Bryonia, Lycopodium**, and **Silicea**.

For the patient who is made better, in general, by warm food, consider: **Lycopodium**.

For the patient who is made worse, in general, by hot foods, consider: **Lachesis, Bryonia, Pulsatilla**, and **Sepia**. Also: **Mercurius** and **Belladonna**.

If a patient is averse to hot foods, consider: **Petroleum.**

If the patient desires hot foods, consider: **Lycopodium**. Also: **Arsenicum**.

For the patient who is made better, in general, by hot foods, consider: **Lycopodium, Nux, Rhus Tox**, and **Arsenicum**. Also: **Natrum Mur, Graphites, Spigelia**, and **Silicea.**

Thirst

For the patient who, in general, is thirsty, consider: **Natrum Mur, Sulphur, Rhus Tox, Phosphorus, Mercurius**, and **Aconite**. Also: **Arsenicum, Silicea**, and **Bryonia**.

For the patient who exhibits an extreme thirst, consider: **Aconite,**

Phosphorus, Veratrum, Calcarea, Arsenicum, Sulphur, and **Natrum Mur**.

If the patient has a great thirst for small quantities of liquid, consider: **Arsenicum** and **Lycopodium**. Also: **Lachesis, Rhus Tox**, and **Sulphur**.

If the patient has a constant desire for small quantities of liquid, consider: **Arsenicum**. Also: **Belladonna** and **Sulphur**.

If the patient has a thirst for large quantities of liquid, consider: **Bryonia, Sulphur, Natrum Mur, Phosphorus**, and **Veratrum**. Also: **Aconite**.

If the patient drinks seldom, but when he does he desires large quantities, of liquid consider: **Bryonia**. Also: **Sulphur**.

If the patient desires large quantities of water very often, consider: **Phosphorus**. Also: **Natrum Mur, Belladonna**, and **Aconite**. Also: **Rhus Tox**.

If the patient is thirsty during a fever, consider: **Aconite, Belladonna, Eupatorium, Nux, Natrum Mur**, and **Thuja**. Also: **Arsenicum, Rhus Tox**, and **Hepar Sulph**.

If the patient is thirsty during a chill, consider: **Apis, Nux, Veratrum, Natrum Mur, Ignatia**, and **Eupatorium**. Also: **Aconite, Arnica, Cina, Ledum**, and **Silicea**.

If the patient is thirsty during a headache, consider: **Bryonia.** Also: **Natrum Mur** and **Veratrum**.

If the patient is thirsty during perspiration, consider: **Natrum Mur**. Also: **Arsenicum, Veratrum Bryonia, Bryonia, Coffea**, and **Rhus Tox**.

If the patient is thirsty in the morning, consider: **Nux, Graphites**, and **Veratrum**.

If the patient is thirsty in the afternoon, consider: **Calcarea**. Also: **Sulphur** and **Phosphorus**.

If the patient is thirsty in the evening, consider: **Allium Cepa, Natrum Mur**, and **Thuja**. Also: **Lycopodium, Bryonia**, and **Phosphorus**.

If the patient is thirsty during the night, consider: **Silicea**. Also: **Arsenicum**. Also: **Calcarea, Silicea, Phosphorus, Spongia, Rhus Tox, Sulphur, Coffea, Lachesis, Mercurius**, and **Hepar Sulph**.

For the patient who is thirstless, consider: **Pulsatilla**. Also: **Apis** and **Staphysagria**.

If the patient is thirstless and yet desires liquids, consider: **Arsenicum**. Also: **Camphora**.

If the patient is averse to drinking, consider: **Nux**. Also: **Pulsatilla**. Also: **Belladonna** and **Ignatia**.

For the patient who is made worse by cold drinks, consider: **Rhus Tox** and **Sepia**. Also: **Nux, Silicea, Sulphur, Arsenicum**, and **Belladonna**. Also: **Carbo Veg** and **Graphites**.

For the patient who is made better by cold drinks, consider: **Veratrum** and **Arsenicum**.

For the patient who desires cold drinks, consider: **Phosphorus**. Also: **Mercurius, Bryonia, Eupatorium, Cina**, and **Arsenicum**.

For the patient who is made worse by warm drinks, consider: **Rhus Tox, Sulphur, Phosphorus, Lachesis**, and **Pulsatilla**.

For the patient who is made better by warm drinks, consider: **Rhus Tox**. Also: **Arsenicum** and **Nux**. Also: **Lycopodium** and **Natrum Mur**.

For the patient who is averse to warm drinks, consider: **Phosphorus** and **Pulsatilla**. Also: **Veratrum**.

For the patient who desires warm drinks, consider: **Arsenicum** and **Bryonia**. Also: **Lycopodium** and **Hypericum**.

For the patient who is made worse by hot drinks, consider: **Phosphorus, Pulsatilla**, and **Bryonia**. Also: **Belladonna** and **Chamomilla**.

For the patient who is made better by hot drinks, consider: **Arsenicum, Nux**, and **Lycopodium**.

Sleep: Insomnia

For the patient who, in general, has insomnia, consider: **Belladonna, Arsenicum, Lachesis, Nux, Hepar Sulph, Mercurius, Rhus Tox, Staphysagria**, and **Thuja**. Also: **Kali Bi, Bryonia, Calcarea, Pulsatilla**, and **Sepia**.

For the patient who has insomnia from anxiety, consider: **Arsenicum**. Also: **Bryonia, Kali Bi, Silicea, Lachesis**, and **Sepia**.

For the patient who has insomnia from daily cares and worries, consider: **Calcarea**.

For the patient who has insomnia from excitement, consider: **Coffea, Nux**, and **Pulsatilla**. Also: **Calcarea, Lachesis**, and **Lycopodium**.

For the patient who has insomnia from news, consider: **Coffea**.

For the patient who has insomnia from humiliation, consider: **Staphysagria**. Also: **Calcarea** and **Ignatia**.

For the patient who has insomnia from anger, consider: **Natrum Mur, Coffea, Aconite**, and **Lachesis**. Also: **Gelsemium**.

For the patient who has insomnia from grief, consider: **Natrum Mur**. Also: **Ignatia** and **Sulphur**. Also: **Gelsemium**.

For the patient who has insomnia because of fear, consider: **Aconite**. Also: **Phosphorus**. Also: **Arsenicum, Pulsatilla, Ignatia, Bryonia**, and **Rhus Tox**.

For the patient who has insomnia from nervousness, consider: **Arsenicum**. Also: **Gelsemium, Nux**, and **Aconite**.

For the patient who has insomnia from mental exhaustion and over-work, consider: **Arsenicum**.

Also: **Calcarea, Coffea, Lycopodium**, and **Nux**. Also: **Lachesis**.

For the patient who has insomnia from great fatigue, consider: **Gelsemium**.

For the patient who has insomnia from hunger, consider: **Ignatia** and **Phosphorus**. Also: **Sulphur** and **Lycopodium**.

For the patient for whom the bed feels too hard to sleep, consider: **Arnica**.

For the patient who has insomnia from too much coffee, consider: **Coffea**. Also: **Nux** and **Mercurius**.

For the patient who has insomnia from too much alcohol, consider: **Nux**. Also: **Gelsemium** and **Arsenicum**.

If insomnia occurs for no apparent reason, consider: **Sulphur**. Also: **Spigelia**.

If fever accompanies insomnia, consider: **Sulphur, Apis**, and **Rhus Tox**. Also: **Phosphorus, Bryonia, Calcarea, Cina**, and **Petroleum**.

If chills accompany insomnia, consider: **Hepar Sulph, Lachesis**, and **Pulsatilla**.

If insomnia is accompanied by difficult breathing, consider: **Chamomilla**. Also: **Arsenicum**.

If insomnia is caused by coughing, consider: **Apis, Phosphorus, Rhus Tox**, and **Sulphur**. Also: **Eupatorium** and **Pulsatilla**.

If insomnia is caused by cramps, consider: **Calcarea**.

If insomnia is caused by headache, consider: **Sulphur**. Also: **Pulsatilla, Lachesis, Coffea**, and **Mercurius**.

If insomnia is caused by hiccups, consider: **Nux** and **Ignatia**.

If insomnia is caused by itching, consider: **Sulphur, Pulsatilla, Apis, Arnica**, and **Gelsemium**.

If insomnia is caused by digestive distress, consider: **Nux**. Also: **Pulsatilla** and **Lycopodium**. Also: **Lachesis**.

For the patient who cannot sleep due to pain, consider: **Chamomilla**. Also: **Lachesis, Mercurius, Aconite**, and **Sulphur**.

For the patient who cannot sleep due to pain in the head, consider: **Sulphur**. Also: **Spigelia, Lachesis**, and **Silicea**.

For the patient who cannot sleep due to pain in the limbs, consider: **Pulsatilla**. Also: **Belladonna** and **Hepar Sulph**.

For the patient who cannot sleep due to pain in teeth, consider: **Sepia**. Also: **Silicea, Staphysagria,** and **Mercurius**.

For the patient who cannot sleep due to pain in back, consider: **Dulcamara**.

For the patient who is too restless to sleep, consider: **Arsenicum** and **Aconite**. Also: **Apis, Pulsatilla**, and **Coffea**. Also: **Ignatia**.

For the patient who is sleepy but who cannot sleep, consider: **Gelsemium**. Also: **Pulsatilla, Sepia, Chamomilla, Belladonna**, and **Phosphorus**.

Sleep: Position

For the patient who sleeps on his back, consider: **Rhus Tox, Bryonia,** and **Pulsatilla**. Also: **Ignatia** and **Lycopodium**.

For the patient who sleeps with hand over the head consider: **Pulsatilla**.

For the patient who sleep with the hand tucked under the back of the head, consider: **Nux**.

For the patient who sleeps on his abdomen, consider: **Pulsatilla**. Also: **Belladonna, Natrum Mur, Sulphur,** and **Phosphorus**.

For the patient who sleeps on his left side, consider: **Sulphur**. Also: **Aconite, Bryonia**, and **Calcarea**.

For the patient who sleeps on his right side, consider: **Phosphorus**. Also: **Lachesis**. Also: **Arsenicum, Lycopodium**, and **Ignatia**.

For the patient who sleeps in a sitting position, consider: **Arsenicum**. Also: **Rhus Tox, Lycopodium**, and **Sulphur**.

PHYSICAL MECHANISMS: INDICATORS
Breathing

For the patient who, in general, has difficulty breathing, consider: **Mercurius, Apis, Arsenicum, Carbo Veg, Phosphorus, Pulsatilla, Sulphur**, and **Veratrum**.

If the patient has trouble breathing in open air, consider: **Rhus Tox** and **Sulphur**.

If the patient breathes more easily in open air, consider: **Carbo Veg, Pulsatilla**, and **Bryonia**.

If the patient has trouble breathing in, consider: **Aconite, Phosphorus, Calcarea**, and **Arsenicum**. Also: **Ignatia**.

If the patient has trouble breathing out, consider: **Ipecac**. Also: **Gelsemium, Sepia**, and **Drosera**.

If the patient feels that he cannot get enough air and wants to be fanned, consider: **Carbo Veg**. Also: **Pulsatilla**. Also: **Apis, Arsenicum, Sulphur**, and **Antimonium Tartaricum**.

If the patient has trouble breathing while sleeping, consider: **Lachesis**. Also: **Kali Bi, Carbo Veg**, and **Sulphur**.

If the patient has trouble breathing after sleeping, consider: **Lachesis** and **Spongia**. Also: **Phosphorus** and **Sepia**. Also: **Apis** and **Belladonna**.

If a patient must be awakened in order not to suffocate, consider: **Sulphur**.

If the patient has trouble breathing when chilled, consider: **Apis**. Also: **Natrum Mur**.

If the patient has trouble breathing while perspiring, consider: **Sepia** and **Sulphur**.

If the patient has trouble breathing while having a nosebleed, consider: **Aconite**. Also: **Belladonna, Carbo Veg**, and **Phosphorus**.

If the patient has trouble breathing after physical exertion, consider: **Calcarea** and **Arsenicum**. Also: **Ipecac, Natrum Mur, Silicea**, and **Lycopodium**.

If the patient has trouble breathing while lying down, consider: **Apis, Graphites**, and **Arsenicum**. Also: **Carbo Veg**.

If lying down ameliorates the symptom, consider: **Nux**. Also: **Euphrasia** and **Lachesis**.

If lying on the back ameliorates the symptom, consider: **Lycopodium**. Also: **Hypericum, Phosphorus, Pulsatilla, Silicea, Sulphur, Arsenicum**, and **Spigelia**.

If the patient has trouble breathing while sitting, consider: **Lachesis, Lycopodium**, and **Phosphorus**. Also: **Rhus Tox**.

If sitting ameliorates the symptom, consider: **Apis, Arsenicum**, and **Pulsatilla**. Also: **Nux**.

If the patient has trouble breathing while walking, consider: **Arsenicum, Calcarea**, and **Sulphur**. Also: **Carbo Veg, Ignatia, Phosphorus**, and **Sepia**.

If the patient is worse from walking in the open air, consider: **Carbo Veg** and **Lycopodium**. Also: **Graphites**.

If the patient is better from walking in the open air, consider: **Drosera** and **Bryonia**.

If the patient is worse after running, consider: **Silicea**.

If running does not aggravate the patient but slow movement does, consider: **Sepia**.

If the patient has trouble breathing in the morning, consider: **Nux, Phosphorus, Sepia, Lachesis**, and **Silicea**.

If the patient has trouble breathing in the afternoon, consider: **Sulphur** and **Lachesis**. Also: **Lycopodium**.

If the patient has trouble breathing in the evening, consider: **Rhus Tox** and **Sulphur** Also: **Arsenicum, Nux, Lachesis, Pulsatilla**, and **Carbo Veg**.

If the patient has trouble breathing during the night, consider: **Arsenicum, Lachesis, Phosphorus**, and **Sulphur**. Also: **Antimonium Tartaricum, Spongia, Rhus Tox**, and **Thuja**.

If the patient has trouble breathing at 10 P.M. consider: **Phosphorus**.

If the patient has trouble breathing from 10 P.M. until 10 P.M., consider: **Ipecac**.

If the patient has trouble breathing at 11 P.M., consider: **Natrum Mur** and **Sulphur**.

If the patient has trouble breathing at midnight, consider: **Arsenicum**. Also: **Aconite** and **Rhus Tox**. Also: **Calcarea** and **Pulsatilla**.

If the patient has trouble breathing just after midnight, consider: **Drosera, Graphites**, and **Spongia**. Also: **Arsenicum**.

If the patient has trouble breathing from 1 to 2 A.M., consider: **Spongia**.

If the patient has trouble breathing at 2 A.M. and after, consider: **Kali Bi**. Also: **Rumex**.

If the patient has trouble breathing at 3 A.M., consider: **Antimonium Tartaricum**. Also: **Natrum Mur**.

If the patient has trouble breathing at 4 A.M., consider: **Kali Bi**.

For the patient whose breathing has a gasping sound, consider: **Carbo Veg, Apis**, and **Lycopodium**. Also: **Spongia, Phosphorus, Drosera**, and **Antimonium Tartaricum**.

For the patient whose breathing has a rattling sound, consider: **Antimonium Tartaricum, Hepar Sulph, Dulcamara, Pulsatilla**, and **Lycopodium**. Also: **Ipecac, Arsenicum**, and **Kali Bi**.

For the patient whose breathing has a sighing sound, consider: **Bryonia, Carbo Veg, Ignatia**, and **Ipecac**.

For the patient whose breathing has a wheezing sound, consider: **Ipecac, Carbo Veg**, and **Arsenicum**. Also: **Cina, Lachesis**, and **Natrum Mur**.

For the patient whose breathing had a whistling sound, consider: **Arsenicum, Sulphur, Antimonium Tartaricum, Silicea**, and **Spongia**.

For the patient whose breathing is troubled and loud, consider: **Calcarea, Kali Bi, Lachesis, Sulphur**, and **Veratrum**. Also: **Carbo Veg, Rhus Tox**, and **Spongia**. Also: **Phosphorus**.

For the patient who is panting, consider: **Aconite**. Also: **Phosphorus**. Also: **Antimonium Tartaricum, Cina, Silicea**, and **Spongia**.

If the patient stops breathing while coughing, consider: **Arsenicum, Drosera, Ipecac**, and **Nux**. Also: **Lycopodium** and **Aconite**.

Pulse

For a patient with a rapid pulse, consider: **Aconite**. Also: **Apis, Belladonna, Veratrum, Mercurius, Ignatia**, and **Rhus Tox**. Also: **Spigelia, Nux**, and **Gelsemium**. Also consider: **Arnica**.

Consider the following remedies for specific beats per minute:

  80 beats: **Phosphorus**.
  85 beats: **Lachesis**.
  90 beats: **Antimonium Tartaricum** and **Mercurius**.
  100 beats: **Ignatia**.
  120 beats: **Ignatia, Lachesis**, and **Lycopodium**. Also: **Rumex** and **Sulphur**.
  125 beats: **Sulphur**.
  130 beats: **Silicea** and **Mercurius**.
  140 beats: **Cina**. Also: **Sulphur**.
  150 beats: **Veratrum** and **Mercurius**.
  160 beats: **Veratrum**.

If the pulse seems to be more rapid than the heartbeat, consider: **Rhus Tox** and **Spigelia**. Also: **Aconite** and **Arnica**.

If the pulse is rapid and indistinct, so that it cannot be counted, consider: **Antimonium Tartaricum, Lachesis, Lycopodium**, and **Mercurius**.

If the pulse is rapid during fever, consider: **Ruta**.

If the pulse is rapid during croup, consider: **Aconite**. Also: **Antimonium Tartaricum, Belladonna**, and **Hepar Sulph**.

If the pulse is rapid in a patient with diarrhea, consider: **Sulphur**.

If the pulse is rapid in a patient with pneumonia, consider: **Antimonium Tartaricum**. Also: **Mercurius, Sulphur**, and **Nux**.

For the patient who has a slow pulse, consider: **Gelsemium** and **Veratrum**. Also: **Sepia, Natrum Mur, Antimonium Tartaricum**, and **Camphora**.

If the pulse is slow but jumps to high with slight exertion, consider: **Arnica**.

For the patient who has an irregular pulse, consider: **Veratrum, Lachesis, Natrum Mur**, and **Kali Bi**. Also: **Rhus Tox, Sulphur, Spigelia, Mercurius, Gelsemium, Hepar Sulph**, and **Phosphorus**.

If the pulse is irregular in a patient with heart disease, consider: **Arsenicum**.

For the patient whose pulse is hard and pounding, consider: **Aconite, Belladonna, Bryonia**, and **Graphites**. Also: **Allium Cepa, Lachesis, Ledum, Phosphorus, Mercurius, Dulcamara**, and **Hepar Sulph**.

For the patient whose pulse is hard and fast, consider: **Dulcamara**.

For the patient whose pulse is accompanied by pneumonia, consider: **Antimonium Tartaricum**. Also: **Veratrum**.

For the patient whose pulse is faint and almost imperceptible, consider: **Carbo Veg**. Also: **Aconite, Camphora**, and **Gelsemium**. Also: **Spongia, Pulsatilla, Rhus Tox, Apis, Arsenicum**, and **Ipecac**. Also: **Ledum** and **Lachesis**.

For the patient whose symptoms are accompanied by pneumonia, consider: **Phosphorus**.

For the patient with an irregular pulse, consider: **Arsenicum, Lachesis**, and **Natrum Mur**. Also: **Spigelia, Silicea, Phosphorus, Kali Bi, Hepar Sulph**, and **Gelsemium**.

If the pulse is irregular in a patient with heart disease, consider: **Arsenicum** and **Lachesis**.

If the pulse is irregular in a patient with a fever, consider: **Lachesis** and **Mercurius**.

PHYSICAL SENSATIONS: INDICATORS
Physical Symptoms and Sides of the Body

For the patient who, in general, has symptoms that either originate or are dominant on only one side of the body, consider: **Bryonia, Lycopodium, Arsenicum**, and **Sulphur**. Also: **Calcarea, Spigelia, Staphysagria**, and **Pulsatilla**.

For the patient whose symptoms either originate or are dominant on the left side, consider especially: **Sulphur** and **Lachesis**. Also: **Cina, Euphrasia, Sepia**, and **Phosphorus**. Also, to a lesser extent, consider: **Mercurius, Dulcamara, Bryonia**, and **Calcarea**. Also: **Spigelia, Graphites**, and **Silicea**.

For the patient whose symptoms either originate or are dominant on the right side, consider especially: **Lycopodium** and **Arsenicum**. Also: **Apis, Pulsatilla**, and **Nux**. Also, to a lesser extent, consider: **Drosera, Staphysagria, Belladonna**, and **Arnica**.

If the symptoms alternate sides, consider: **Lachesis** and **Lycopodium**. Also: **Pulsatilla, Phosphorus, Cina**, and **Sepia**.

If the symptoms are located crosswise, upper right to lower left, consider: **Phosphorus**. Also: **Calcarea, Euphrasia**, and **Silicea**.

If the symptoms are located crosswise, upper left to lower right, consider: **Ledum** and **Rhus Tox**. Also: **Arnica, Thuja**, and **Veratrum**.

Sensations (in General)

For the patient who has a general physical sensation of uneasiness, consider: **Chamomilla**. Also: **Calcarea, Bryonia, Dulcamara, Sepia, Apis,** and **Spigelia**. Also: **Hepar Sulph** and **Camphora**.

For the patient with a general sensation of sickness, consider: **Aconite, Gelsemium**, and **Nux**. Also: **Arsenicum, Bryonia, Sulphur**, and **Spongia**.

For the patient who has an internal sensation of heaviness, consider: **Aconite, Gelsemium, Calcarea, Natrum Mur**, and **Pulsatilla**. Also: **Sepia**. Also: **Nux** and **Petroleum**.

For the patient with has the external sensation of heaviness, consider: **Belladonna, Gelsemium, Sulphur**, and **Rhus Tox**. Also: **Bryonia**. Also: **Sepia, Thuja**, and **Staphysagria**.

For the patient who has a general feeling of lightness, consider: **Arsenicum** and **Coffea**.

For the patient with an internal sensation of constriction, tightness, or of a band tightening internally, consider: **Pulsatilla, Silicea**, and **Sulphur**. Also: **Natrum Mur, Spigelia, Mercurius**, and **Graphites**.

For the patient with an external sensation of constriction or tightness, consider: **Rhus Tox**. Also: **Nux, Graphites**, and **Mercurius**. Also: **Aconite, Lycopodium, Phosphorus, Spongia, Veratrum, Sulphur**, and **Pulsatilla**.

For the patient who has a sensation of looseness or that a part of the body is flabby, consider: **Calcarea, Lycopodium**, and **Ignatia**. Also: **Arsenicum, Phosphorus**, and **Sulphur**.

For the patient who has a sensation of fullness internally, consider: **Rhus Tox, Sulphur**, and **Aconite**. Also: **Phosphorus, Pulsatilla**, and **Lycopodium**.

For the patient who has a sensation of fullness externally, consider: **Arsenicum, Phosphorus**, and **Veratrum**.

For the patient who has the sensation of emptiness, consider: **Ignatia**. Also: **Lycopodium, Pulsatilla**, and **Sepia**. Also: **Phosphorus** and **Sulphur**.

For the patient with the sensation that a part of his body is swollen, consider: **Rhus Tox**. Also: **Mercurius, Spigelia, Lachesis**, and **Pulsatilla**. Also: **Aconite, Euphrasia**, and **Sulphur**.

For the patient who has the sensation that a part of his body, or his whole body, is enlarged, consider: **Belladonna**.

For the patient who has the sensation that a part of his body, or his whole body, is shrunken, consider: **Calcarea**. Also: **Nux, Sulphur**, and **Aconite**.

For the patient with a tingling sensation, consider: **Phosphorus** and **Aconite**.

For the patient with a throbbing sensation, consider: **Belladonna**. Also: **Ledum, Hepar Sulph, Sulphur, Phosphorus, Calcarea**, and **Antimonium Tartaricum**.

For the patient with a crawling sensation, consider: **Arsenicum, Calcarea, Sulphur**, and **Belladonna**. Also: **Sepia**.

For the patient with a general sensation of heat, consider: **Arsenicum, Rhus Tox, Veratrum**, and **Carbo Veg**. Also: **Calcarea** and **Sulphur**.

For the patient with the general sensation of internally being tied in a knot, consider: **Sulphur** and **Lachesis**. Also: **Spigelia**. Also: **Arsenicum** and **Rhus Tox**.

For the patient with a strangling sensation, consider: **Sulphur**.

For the patient with a prickling sensation, consider: **Drosera**. Also: **Phosphorus, Belladonna**, and **Calcarea**. Also: **Hepar Sulph**.

For the patient with a sinking sensation, consider: **Dulcamara** and **Phosphorus**.

For the patient with a sensation of electricity or electrical shock, consider: **Aconite, Arsenicum**, and **Veratrum**. Also: **Phosphorus, Nux, Ruta**, and **Lycopodium**.

For the patient with a stinging sensation, consider: **Apis**. Also: **Gelsemium** and **Ledum**.

For the patient who has the sensation that everything, particularly his bed, is too hard, consider: **Arnica**. Also: **Silicea, Rhus Tox**, and **Arsenicum**.

For the patient with an internal sensation of a ball, consider: **Ignatia, Sepia**, and **Lachesis**. Also: **Bryonia, Arnica, Belladonna, Pulsatilla**, and **Nux**.

For the patient with an internal sensation of a plug, consider: **Kali Bi** and **Thuja**. Also: **Ignatia, Hepar Sulph, Ruta, Nux, Sulphur**, and **Spigelia**.

For the patient with an internal sensation of a stick or splinter, consider: **Hepar Sulph**. Also: **Carbo Veg** and **Silicea**.

For the patient who gets specific sensations only in small spots on or in the body, consider: **Kali Bi**. Also: **Sulphur, Sepia, Phosphorus**, and **Natrum Mur**.

Sensations of Pain

For the patient whose pains appear suddenly, consider: **Aconite, Belladonna, Pulsatilla**, and **Arsenicum**.

If the pains appear suddenly but leave gradually, consider: **Hypericum**. Also: **Calcarea**, and **Ignatia**.

If the pains appear suddenly and leave suddenly, consider: **Belladonna**. Also: **Lachesis** and **Pulsatilla**.

For the patient whose pains appear gradually, consider: **Gelsemium, Nux**, and **Bryonia**.

If the pains appear gradually and leave gradually, consider: **Calcarea, Nux, Sepia, Spigelia, Gelsemium**, and **Natrum Mur**.

If the pains appear gradually and leave suddenly, consider: **Pulsatilla**. Also: **Rhus Tox**.

For the patient whose pains occur in a downward direction, consider: **Sepia, Coffea, Lycopodium**, and **Rhus Tox**. Also: **Silicea**.

For the patient whose pains occur in an upward direction, consider: **Belladonna, Ignatia, Phosphorus, Silicea**, and **Sepia**.

For the patient whose pains occur in an inward direction, consider: **Arnica**. Also: **Calcarea**.

For the patient whose pains occur in an outward direction, consider: **Sulphur**. Also: **Sepia**.

For the patient whose pains occur in a backward direction, consider: **Sulphur**. Also: **Sepia, Kali Bi**, and **Bryonia**.

For the patient whose pains occur in a forward direction, consider: **Spigelia**. Also: **Gelsemium**.

For the patient whose pains occur crosswise in his body, consider: **Sulphur, Veratrum, Silicea**, and **Belladonna**.

For the patient whose pains radiate about the body, consider: **Mercurius**. Also: **Apis** and **Chamomilla**.

For the patient who has the general sensation of internal soreness, consider: **Pulsatilla**. Also: **Apis, Sulphur, Nux**, and **Veratrum**.

For the patient who has a general sensation of external soreness, consider: **Rhus Tox, Ruta, Natrum Mur, Eupatorium, Bryonia, Arnica**, and **Nux**. Also: **Ignatia, Belladonna**, and **Hepar Sulph**.

For the patient who has an internally cutting pain, consider: **Belladonna, Calcarea, Veratrum, Sulphur, Mercurius, Natrum Mur**, and **Nux**.

For the patient who has an externally cutting pain, consider: **Drosera, Belladonna**, and **Calcarea**.

For the patient who has an internally sharp pain, consider: **Ignatia**. Also: **Ledum, Lachesis, Phosphorus, Arsenicum**, and **Mercurius**.

For the patient who has an externally sharp pain, consider: **Staphysagria**. Also: **Sulphur, Pulsatilla, Ledum, Rhus Tox**, and **Thuja**.

For the patient who has an internally pinching pain, consider: **Lycopodium, Ignatia, Graphites**, and **Calcarea**.

For the patient who has an externally pinching pain, consider: **Arnica, Spongia**, and **Sulphur**. Also: **Rhus Tox**.

For the patient who has an internally gnawing pain, consider: **Pulsatilla, Sepia**, and **Ruta**. Also: **Arsenicum, Calcarea**, and **Carbo Veg**.

For the patient who has an externally gnawing pain, consider: **Spongia** and **Staphysagria**. Also: **Phosphorus** and **Pulsatilla**.

For the patient who has an internally burning pain, consider: **Sulphur, Arsenicum**, and **Phosphorus**. Also: **Rhus Tox, Mercurius, Apis**, and **Belladonna**. Also: **Spigelia** and **Spongia**.

For the patient who has an externally burning pain, consider: **Apis, Arsenicum, Phosphorus**, and **Sulphur**. Also: **Carbo Veg, Natrum Mur, Mercurius**, and **Euphrasia**.

For the patient who has an internally pressing pain, consider: **Rhus Tox, Ruta, Lycopodium, Belladonna, Arnica**, and **Natrum Mur**. Also: **Spongia, Sepia, Nux,** and **Calcarea**.

For the patient who has an externally pressing pain, consider: **Rhus Tox, Ruta, Eupatorium, Drosera, Kali Bi**, and **Pulsatilla**. Also: **Sepia** and **Sulphur**.

For the patient who has a digging pain, consider: **Dulcamara** and **Spigelia**. Also: **Belladonna, Arnica**, and **Rhus Tox**. Also: **Ruta**.

For the patient who has a twisting pain, consider: **Silicea** and **Veratrum**. Also: **Rhus Tox, Bryonia**, and **Belladonna**.

For the patient who has wandering pains, consider: **Pulsatilla** Also: **Ledum** and **Kali Bi**. Also: **Arnica, Rumex, Spigelia, Lachesis**, and **Rhus Tox**.

For the patient who is very sensitive to pain, consider: **Pulsatilla, Chamomilla, Hepar Sulph**, and **Nux**. Also: **Staphysagria, Ignatia**, and **Aconite**.

Sensations of Weakness

For the patient with the general sensation of weakness, consider: **Gelsemium, Calcarea, Natrum Mur, Mercurius, Hepar Sulph**, and **Sulphur**. Also: **Arsenicum, Apis, Graphites, Silicea**, and **Carbo Veg**.

If the weakness is sudden, consider: **Graphites** and **Arsenicum**. Also: **Carbo Veg, Apis, Aconite**, and **Veratrum**. Also: **Sepia**.

If the weakness is gradual, consider: **Calcarea**. Also: **Nux** and **Lycopodium**.

For the patient with sensation of weakness in the morning, consider: **Arsenicum, Lycopodium**, and **Lachesis**. Also: **Sulphur, Nux**, and **Bryonia**. Also: **Gelsemium** and **Natrum Mur**.

If the sensation of weakness is upon waking, consider: **Lycopodium, Lachesis, Staphysagria, Dulcamara, Bryonia, Calcarea, Phosphorus**, and **Nux**.

If the sensation of weakness is while still in bed, consider: **Pulsatilla**.

If the sensation of weakness is upon rising from bed, consider: **Bryonia** and **Lachesis** Also: **Dulcamara, Sepia**, and **Lycopodium**.

If the sensation of weakness is after rising from bed, consider: **Nux** and **Lycopodium**.

For the patient with a sensation of weakness in the late morning, consider: **Bryonia**. Also: **Lycopodium** and **Sulphur**.

For the patient with a sensation of weakness at noon, consider: **Carbo Veg, Natrum Mur**, and **Thuja**.

For the patient with a sensation of weakness in the afternoon, consider: **Sulphur**. Also: **Gelsemium, Bryonia**, and **Silicea**.

For the patient with a sensation of weakness in the evening, consider: **Natrum Mur**. Also: **Sulphur, Lachesis, Graphites, Ignatia**, and **Kali Bi**.

For the patient with a sensation of weakness during the night, consider: **Silicea**. Also: **Carbo Veg, Calcarea, Nux, Rhus Tox**, and **Sulphur**.

For the patient with a sensation of weakness from heat, consider: **Pulsatilla, Lachesis**, and **Sulphur**.

If the sensation is from a warm room, consider: **Pulsatilla**.

If the sensation is from warm weather, consider: **Sulphur**. Also: **Lachesis** and **Natrum Mur**.

For the patient with a sensation of weakness from cold, consider: **Veratrum, Arsenicum**, and **Carbo Veg**.

If the sensation is from cold weather, consider: **Apis, Lachesis**, and **Arsenicum**.

If the sensation comes during a chill, consider: **Natrum Mur** and **Phosphorus**.

If the sensation comes from cold and damp, consider: **Arsenicum**.

For the patient with a sensation of weakness in the open air, consider: **Spigelia**. Also: **Calcarea** and **Veratrum**.

For the patient with a sensation of weakness from physical exertion, consider: **Arnica**, Also: **Arsenicum**.

If the weakness comes from a very slight exertion, consider: **Calcarea, Arsenicum, Spongia, Rhus Tox**, and **Bryonia**. Also: **Lachesis** and **Phosphorus**.

For the patient with a sensation of weakness following physical injury, consider: **Camphora**. Also **Arnica, Calendula**, and **Carbo Veg**.

For the patient with a sensation of weakness following the loss of bodily fluids, consider: **Natrum Mur** and **Calcarea**. Also: **Phosphorus** and **Sepia**.

For the patient with a sensation of weakness from bleeding, consider: **Hypericum, Phosphorus**, and **Carbo Veg**.

For the patient with a sensation of weakness from perspiration, consider: **Calcarea** and **Lycopodium**.

For the patient with a sensation of weakness after sex, consider: **Calcarea**. Also: **Silicea, Phosphorus, Graphites**, and **Natrum Mur**.

For the patient with a sensation of weakness from hunger, consider: **Phosphorus**. Also: **Sulphur** and **Lycopodium**. Also: **Spigelia**.

For the patient with a sensation of weakness from grief, consider: **Ignatia** and **Natrum Mur**.

For the patient with a sensation of weakness from fear, consider: **Gelsemium**. Also: **Coffea** and **Mercurius**.

For the patient with a sensation of weakness from sorrow, consider: **Ignatia** and **Natrum Mur**.

For the patient with a sensation of weakness from anger, consider: **Staphysagria**.

For the patient with a sensation of weakness from humiliation, consider: **Staphysagria**. Also: **Ignatia**.

For the patient with a sensation of weakness from talking, consider: **Silicea** and **Gelsemium**.

For the patient with a sensation of weakness from overwork, consider: **Calcarea** and **Nux**. Also: **Lycopodium** and **Silicea**.

For the patient with a sensation of weakness after recovering from illness, consider: **Gelsemium**.

Sensitivities (in General)

For the patient who is, in general, very sensitive to allopathic drugs, consider: **Sulphur** and **Pulsatilla**. Also: **Aconite, Arnica, Arsenicum, Nux**, and **Lycopodium**.

For the patient who is, in general, very sensitive to homeopathic remedies, consider: **Phosphorus**. Also: **Thuja** and **Arsenicum**. Also: **Aconite, Chamomilla**, and **Coffea**.

For the patient who, in general, would be considered to be very sensitive, or rather nervous, consider: **Coffea, Belladonna, Lachesis, Ignatia, Staphysagria, Phosphorus, Silicea**, and **Nux**. Also: **Veratrum, Arsenicum, Pulsatilla, Sulphur**, and **Aconite**.

For the patient who, in general, would be considered to be very sensitive to pain, consider: **Aconite, Arsenicum, Chamomilla, Hepar Sulph**, and **Coffea**. Also: **Nux**.

For the patient who is sensitive to noise, consider: **Phosphorus, Aconite, Nux, Ignatia**, and **Belladonna**.

For the patient who is sensitive to music, consider: **Nux, Natrum**

Mur, Sepia, and **Graphites**. Also: **Ignatia**. If the patient is made better by hearing music, consider: **Natrum Mur** and **Thuja**.

For the patient who is sensitive to the sound of the human voice, consider: **Arsenicum, Nux**, and **Silicea**.

If noise is painful to the patient's ears, consider: **Nux, Silicea, Spigelia**, and **Coffea**.

If the least noise irritates or aggravates the patient, consider: **Nux, Coffea**, and **Silicea**. Also: **Lycopodium, Phosphorus**, and **Belladonna**.

For the patient who is very sensitive to smells, consider: **Sepia, Nux**, and **Phosphorus**. Also: **Lachesis, Ignatia, Staphysagria**, and **Sulphur**.

For the patient who is very sensitive to the smell of flowers and perfumes, consider: **Nux**. Also: **Phosphorus** and **Graphites**.

For the patient who is very sensitive to foul smells, consider: **Sulphur**.

For the patient who is very sensitive to the smell of food, consider: **Eupatorium** and **Sepia**. If the sensitivity during eating, consider: **Nux**.

For the patient who is very sensitive to touch, consider: **Aconite** and **Lachesis**. Also: **Coffea** and **Cina**. Also: **Phosphorus** and **Staphysagria**.

For the patient who is very sensitive to light, consider: **Phosphorus, Nux**, and **Belladonna**. Also: **Aconite, Natrum Mur**, and **Arnica**.

For the patient in whom all senses are heightened, consider: **Phosphorus**. Also: **Lycopodium, Graphites, Sepia**, and **Arsenicum**.

For the patient who is very sensitive, in general, to all external impressions, consider: **Phosphorus**. Also: **Nux** and **Staphysagria**. Also: **Hepar Sulph** and **Lachesis**.

If sensitivity is heightened with headache, consider: **Ignatia, Nux, Belladonna, Chamomilla**, and **Silicea**.

If sensitivity is heightened during perspiration, consider: **Belladonna**.

If sensitivity is heightened during fever, consider: **Pulsatilla**. Also: **Belladonna, Natrum Mur**, and **Calcarea**.

For the patient who is very sensitive emotionally to what others think about him, consider: **Lycopodium, Natrum Mur**, and **Ignatia**. Also: **Staphysagria**.

For the patient who seems to be less sensitive in general than the average person to the situation at hand, consider: **Lycopodium**. Also: **Staphysagria** and **Euphrasia**.

General Diagnostic Symptoms: States of Mind

EMOTIONAL MOTIVATIONS: INDICATORS
Anger

For the patient who is, in general, angry, consider: **Nux, Bryonia**, and **Lycopodium**. Also: **Staphysagria, Sulphur, Natrum Mur, Ignatia**, and **Hepar Sulph**. Also: **Aconite** and **Belladonna**.

If the patient is angry when asked questions about his condition, consider: **Nux**. Also: **Arnica** and **Bryonia**.

If the patient is angry when contradicted, consider: **Sepia, Lycopodium**, and **Ignatia**. Also: **Thuja, Silica, Nux, Bryonia**, and **Veratrum**.

If the patient becomes angry when comforted, consider: **Natrum Mur** and **Ignatia**.

If illness comes on after anger, consider: **Ipecac, Ignatia, Nux**, and **Staphysagria**. Also: **Aconite, Apis, Bryonia**, and **Lycopodium**. Also: **Natrum Mur**.

If anger is due to the pain of illness, consider: **Aconite**. Also: **Chamomilla** and **Hepar Sulph**.

If anger accompanies screaming, consider: **Belladonna** and **Veratrum**. Also: **Lachesis**.

If biting accompanies anger, consider: **Veratrum** and **Camphora**.

If the patient is very strong physically when angry, consider: **Belladonna**.

If anger accompanies a cough, consider: **Staphysagria**. Also: **Antimonium Tartaricum, Chamomilla, Belladonna**, and **Arnica**.

If anger accompanies a headache, consider: **Staphysagria** and **Bryonia**.

If anger accompanies trembling, consider: **Staphysagria**. Also: **Gelsemium** and **Lycopodium**.

If the patient is violent when angry, consider: **Staphysagria, Nux, Chamomilla, Hepar Sulph, Aconite**, and **Lachesis**. Also: **Bryonia, Graphites, Lycopodium, Sepia, Arsenicum**, and **Apis**.

If the patient is verbally abusive, consider: **Chamomilla, Lycopodium, Hepar Sulph, Lachesis, Nux**, and **Ignatia**. Also: **Natrum Mur, Belladonna, Aconite, Arnica, Sepia**, and **Veratrum**.

(Note: For the victim of abuse, consider: **Staphysagria, Natrum Mur, Ignatia**, and **Sulphur**. Also: **Nux, Pulsatilla, Bryonia, Chamomilla, Lachesis**, and **Aconite**.)

If the patient is in a rage, consider: **Lycopodium** and **Nux**. Also: **Belladonna, Veratrum**, and **Lachesis**.

If the patient alternates between anger and cheerfulness, consider: **Lycopodium, Mercurius**, and **Antimonium Tartaricum**. Also: **Spigelia** and **Spongia**.

If the patient has anger which cannot be quieted, consider: **Chamomilla** and **Cina.** If the patient can only be comforted by being carried or rocked, consider: **Chamomilla**. Also: **Pulsatilla**. Also: **Arsenicum**.

Fear

For the patient who, in general, is fearful, consider: **Aconite, Arsenicum, Lycopodium**, and **Phosphorus**. Also: **Graphites, Belladonna**, and **Pulsatilla**.

If the patient's illness comes on from fear, consider: **Aconite**. Also: **Gelsemium, Ignatia, Belladonna**, and **Phosphorus**.

If the patient is afraid of illness, consider: **Phosphorus, Arsenicum**, and **Calcarea**.

If the patient is afraid of germs, consider: **Arsenicum** and **Sulphur**. Also: **Lachesis** and **Thuja**. Also: **Silicea**.

If the patient is afraid that his disease cannot be cured, consider: **Arsenicum**. Also: **Lachesis, Aconite**, and **Arnica.**

If the patient is afraid of having a stroke, consider: **Coffea.** Also: **Sepia** and **Pulsatilla**.

If the patient is afraid of doctors, consider: **Gelsemium, Aconite**, and **Arnica**. Also: **Ignatia, Sepia, Calcarea**, and **Phosphorus**.

If the patient is afraid of death, consider: **Aconite, Arsenicum, Calcarea, Nux, Phosphorus**, and **Gelsemium**. Also: **Veratrum, Rhus Tox, Spongia, Lachesis, Mercurius**, and **Apis**. Also: **Arnica**.

If the patient is afraid at night, consider: **Aconite, Arsenicum, Rhus Tox**, and **Phosphorus**. Also: **Calcarea** and **Natrum Mur**. Also: **Pulsatilla**.

If the patient is afraid of the dark, consider: **Phosphorus**. Also: **Camphora, Arsenicum, Aconite, Carbo Veg**, and **Natrum Mur**. Also: **Lycopodium**.

If the patient is afraid of going to sleep, consider: **Rhus Tox, Lachesis**, and **Ledum**.

If the patient is afraid at the moment of falling asleep, consider: **Rhus Tox**.

If the patient is afraid that he will never again be able to sleep, consider: **Ignatia**.

If the patient is afraid upon awakening, consider: **Bryonia, Natrum Mur**, and **Pulsatilla**. Also: **Nux, Spongia, Sulphur, Belladonna, Calcarea**, and **Silicea**.

If the patient is afraid upon awakening from a dream, consider: **Nux** and **Arnica**. Also: **Aconite** and **Lycopodium**.

If the patient is afraid of noises, consider: **Phosphorus**. Also: **Natrum Mur** and **Lycopodium**.

If the patient is afraid of being touched, consider: **Arnica, Chamomilla, Aconite**, and **Hepar Sulph**. Also: **Nux** and **Spigelia**.

If the patient is afraid of being alone, consider: **Arsenicum** and **Lycopodium**. Also: **Phosphorus, Camphora, Apis, Gelsemium**, and **Pulsatilla**.

If the patient is afraid of people in general, consider: **Rhus Tox**. Also: **Lycopodium**. Also: **Natrum Mur, Ledum, Aconite**, and **Carbo Veg**.

If the patient is afraid of men, consider: **Lycopodium, Pulsatilla**, and **Natrum Mur**.

If the patient is afraid of strangers in general, consider: **Thuja, Lycopodium**, and **Carbo Veg**.

If the patient is afraid of being spoken to, consider: **Coffea, Pulsatilla**, and **Sepia**.

If the patient is afraid during perspiration, consider: **Spongia**.

If the patient is afraid during pregnancy, consider: **Aconite** or **Arsenicum**.

If the fear is accompanied by palpitations, consider: **Aconite, Mercurius, Phosphorus**, and **Pulsatilla**. Also: **Natrum Mur** and **Spongia**.

If the fear is accompanied by fever, consider: **Arsenicum**. Also: **Aconite, Belladonna, Phosphorus, Calcarea**, and **Spongia**. Also: **Sulphur**.

If the patient is afraid of everything, has constant fear, consider: **Lycopodium**. Also: **Calcarea** and **Pulsatilla**. Also: **Phosphorus, Arsenicum**, and **Belladonna**.

If the patient has the vague fear that something bad is about to happen, consider: **Phosphorus**. Also: **Nux**. Also: **Sulphur, Calcarea, Arsenicum, Carbo Veg, Natrum Mur**, and **Calendula**.

Worry

For the patient who, in general, is worried, consider: **Arsenicum, Calcarea, Ignatia**, and **Staphysagria**. Also: **Sulphur, Natrum Mur, Spigelia**, and **Kali Bi**.

For the patient who is worried about illness, consider: **Arsenicum, Calcarea, Phosphorus**, and **Nux**.

For the patient who is worried when alone, consider: **Hepar Sulph**.

For the patient who is worried that he will not be left alone, consider: **Natrum Mur**.

If the patient feels better when worrying, consider: **Mercurius**.

If the patient is worried about other people, consider: **Calcarea** and **Pulsatilla**. Also: **Phosphorus, Sulphur, Arsenicum**, and **Lachesis**.

If the patient is worried about loved ones, consider: **Spigelia**. Also: **Arsenicum, Hepar Sulph, Lachesis**, and **Rhus Tox**.

If the patient is worried about work, consider: **Calcarea** and **Nux**. Also: **Bryonia, Pulsatilla**, and **Lycopodium**.

If the patient is worried about house and home, consider: **Calcarea** and **Pulsatilla**. Also: **Arsenicum**.

If the patient is always worried, whether there is anything to worry about or not, consider: **Arsenicum**.

Depression

For the patient who, in general, is depressed, consider: **Gelsemium, Natrum Mur, Arsenicum, Calcarea, Chamomilla, Aconite, Mercurius, Lycopodium, Ignatia, Phosphorus, Rhus Tox, Sepia, Sulphur, Veratrum**, and **Thuja**.

If depression alternates with anger, consider: **Staphysagria**.

If depression alternates with indifference, consider: **Sepia**.

If depression alternates with fear, consider: **Arsenicum**.

For the patient who is depressed when alone, consider: **Arsenicum, Natrum Mur**, and **Pulsatilla**. Also: **Drosera** and **Calcarea**.

For the patient who is depressed when he has company, consider: **Natrum Mur** and **Lycopodium**.

If the depression accompanies headache, consider: **Pulsatilla** and **Dulcamara**. Also: **Ignatia**.

If the depression accompanies fever, consider: **Aconite, Arsenicum**, and **Natrum Mur**. Also: **Spongia, Silicea, Gelsemium, Belladonna, Calcarea**, and **Eupatorium**. Also: **Rhus Tox**.

If depression accompanies chill, consider: **Aconite, Arsenicum, Natrum Mur**, and **Ignatia**. Also: **Pulsatilla, Lycopodium, Graphites**, and **Apis**.

If depression accompanies flashes of heat, consider: **Natrum Mur**.

If depression accompanies perspiration, consider: **Aconite, Apis, Rhus Tox, Sepia, Natrum Mur, Sulphur**, and **Ignatia**.

If depression accompanies menopause, consider: **Sepia** and **Sulphur**. Also: **Lachesis** and **Veratrum**.

If depression occurs after injury, consider: **Hypericum**. Also: **Arnica**. If the injury is to the head, consider: **Natrum Sulph, Arnica, Hypericum, Rhus Tox**, and **Pulsatilla**. Also: **Sulphur**.

For the patient who is depressed from hearing music, consider: **Aconite, Natrum Mur, Graphites**, and **Thuja**. Also: **Sepia** and **Lycopodium**.

For the patient who is depressed and sighing, consider: **Ignatia, Pulsatilla**, and **Natrum Mur**. Also: **Sepia**.

For the patient who is depressed, apparently without reason or cause, consider: **Sepia**. Also: **Natrum Mur, Phosphorus**, and **Rhus Tox**.

Grief

For patients who become ill from grief, consider: **Ignatia, Natrum Mur, Phosphorus**, and **Staphysagria**. Also: **Nux** and **Lachesis**. Also: **Pulsatilla, Bryonia, Arnica, Arsenicum, Calcarea, Gelsemium, Graphites**, and **Apis**.

If a recent grief or loss leads to illness, consider: **Ignatia**. Also: **Natrum Mur**.

If the loss of a loved one leads to illness, consider: **Ignatia** and **Natrum Mur**. Also: **Staphysagria**, **Nux**, and **Lachesis**. Also: **Sulphur**.

Indifference

For the patient who, in general, is indifferent to circumstances, consider: **Staphysagria, Sepia, Pulsatilla, Calcarea**, and **Natrum Mur**. Also: **Graphites, Thuja, Sulphur**, and **Nux**. Also: **Gelsemium**.

For the patient who seems indifferent to illness, consider: **Arnica**. Also: **Apis** and **Veratrum**.

If the patient seems sleepy as well as indifferent, consider: **Antimonium Tartaricum**. Also: **Arsenicum** and **Aconite**. Also: **Lycopodium** and **Ipecac**.

If the patient seems bored as well as indifferent, consider: **Nux**. Also: **Lachesis, Sulphur**, and **Lycopodium**.

If indifference alternates with anxiety, consider: **Natrum Mur** and **Antimonium Tartaricum**.

If indifference alternates with anger or irritability, consider: **Chamomilla**.

If indifference alternates with weeping, consider: **Phosphorus**.

For the patient who seems indifferent to his loved ones, consider: **Sepia**. Also: **Phosphorus**. Also: **Aconite, Mercurius, Arsenicum**, and **Belladonna**.

For the patient who seems indifferent to work, consider: **Ignatia, Silicea, Lachesis**, and **Staphysagria**.

For the patient who seems indifferent to pleasure, consider: **Natrum Mur** and **Sulphur**. Also: **Chamomilla, Pulsatilla, Sepia**, and **Arsenicum**.

For the patient who seems indifferent to everything, consider: **Staphysagria, Carbo Veg**, and **Natrum Mur**. Also: **Sepia, Pulsatilla, Nux, Gelsemium**, and **Ignatia**. Also: **Mercurius** and **Lycopodium**.

EMOTIONAL REACTIONS AND RESPONSES: INDICATORS
How the Patient Answers Questions About His Case

When you are taking a homeopathic case, often you can get more of an indication of what remedy might be helpful by the manner in which the patient is speaking, rather than by the meaning of the words that are actually spoken. It is important that we use these indicators as the very helpful tools they are.

For the patient who speaks loudly, consider: **Lachesis**. Also: **Belladonna**. Also: **Arnica** and **Arsenicum.**

For the patient who speaks rapidly, consider: **Hepar Sulph, Lachesis**, and **Sulphur**. Also: **Mercurius, Sepia, Thuja, Ignatia**, and **Belladonna**. Also: **Camphora** and **Lycopodium**.

For the patient who is abrupt in speech, consider: **Arsenicum, Chamomilla**, and **Sulphur**.

For the patient who is confused in speech, consider: **Lachesis, Nux, Gelsemium, Natrum Mur**, and **Lycopodium**.

For the patient who speaks hesitatingly, consider: **Pulsatilla**. Also: **Mercurius, Lycopodium, Staphysagria**, and **Thuja**.

For the patient who is forgetful while speaking, consider: **Arnica**. Also: **Thuja, Lachesis, Nux, Lycopodium**, and **Sulphur**.

For the patient who speaks incoherently, consider: **Lachesis, Phosphorus, Rhus Tox, Bryonia, Camphora**, and **Sulphur**. Also: **Apis, Belladonna**, and **Gelsemium**.

For the patient who speaks as if drunk, consider: **Nux** and **Gelsemium**. Also: **Lycopodium** and **Natrum Mur**.

For the patient who is delirious, consider: **Belladonna**. Also: **Sulphur** and **Bryonia.** Also: **Coffea**.

For the patient who cannot finish a sentence, consider: **Arsenicum, Lachesis**, and **Thuja**.

For the patient who cries when speaking, especially when describing his symptoms, consider: **Sepia** and **Pulsatilla**.

For the patient who laughs when speaking, consider: **Phosphorus, Ignatia, Belladonna, Coffea**, and **Calcarea**. Also: **Natrum Mur** and **Sepia**.

If the patient both jokes and cries at the same time, consider: **Ignatia**.

For the patient who jokes when speaking consider: **Rhus Tox** and **Ignatia**. Also: **Lachesis**.

If the patient is averse to jokes, consider: **Aconite, Mercurius**, and **Cina**.

If the patient simply can't take a joke, consider: **Aconite**. Also: **Lycopodium, Mercurius**, and **Nux**. Also: **Natrum Mur** and **Pulsatilla**.

If the patient both laughs and cries at the same time, consider: **Pulsatilla**. Also: **Staphysagria**.

If the patient jokes only at the expense of others, consider: **Lachesis**.

For the patient whose speech is very serious, consider: **Arsenicum**. Also: **Staphysagria, Euphrasia, Ledum**, and **Mercurius**. Also: **Cina**.

For the patient whose speech is inappropriate or lewd, consider: **Lachesis, Belladonna**, and **Nux**. Also: **Camphora, Phosphorus, Veratrum**, and **Calcarea**.

For the patient who screams when speaking, consider: **Camphora** and **Veratrum**. Also: **Lycopodium, Gelsemium, Ignatia, Apis**, and **Antimonium Tartaricum**.

For the patient who sighs when speaking, consider: **Ignatia** and **Bryonia**. Also: **Nux, Pulsatilla, Rhus Tox, Sepia, Graphites, Ipecac**, and **Eupatorium**.

If the patient sighs in his sleep, consider: **Sulphur**. Also: **Belladonna, Camphora, Arsenicum**, and **Pulsatilla**.

Talking (in General)

For the patient who talks too much, consider: **Lachesis**. Also: **Camphora, Belladonna, Phosphorus, Nux**, and **Veratrum**.

For the patient who tends to make speeches, consider: **Lachesis**. Also: **Arnica, Ignatia**, and **Chamomilla**.

For the patient who tends to speak little but once he gets started talks on and on, consider: **Natrum Mur**.

For the patient who takes great pleasure in his own talking, consider: **Sulphur, Lachesis**, and **Natrum Mur**.

For the patient who talks to himself, consider: **Staphysagria, Lachesis**, and **Nux**. Also: **Antimonium Tartaricum** and **Kali Bi**.

For the patient who speaks only when alone, consider: **Nux** and **Lachesis**.

For the patient who talks about nothing but his aches and pains, consider: **Nux**.

For the patient who talks only about unimportant things, consider: **Lachesis**.

If the patient alternates between talking and laughing, consider: **Belladonna**.

If the patient alternates between talking and silence, consider: **Ignatia** and **Belladonna**.

For the patient who talks incoherently, consider: **Lachesis**. Also: **Phosphorus, Bryonia**, and **Ignatia**.

For the patient who raves, consider: **Veratrum**. Also: **Apis, Lachesis**, and **Staphysagira**. Also: **Belladonna**.

For the patient who is eager to speak about others, to gossip, consider: **Bryonia, Arsenicum**, and **Nux**. Also: **Sepia**.

For the patient who speaks too little, or who seems disinterested in communicating, consider: **Pulsatilla, Phosphorus**, and **Sulphur**. Also: **Veratrum, Natrum Mur, Arnica**, and **Aconite**.

If the patient seems too sad to speak, consider: **Arsenicum** and **Pulsatilla**. Also: **Ignatia** and **Veratrum**.

If the patient seems silent over his sufferings, consider: **Ignatia**.

For the patient who talks in his sleep, consider: **Lachesis, Belladonna**, and **Sulphur**. Also: **Gelsemium, Natrum Mur, Rhus Tox**, and **Pulsatilla**. Also: **Nux, Ledum, Calcarea, Arnica**, and **Cina**.

If the patient speaks loudly during sleep, consider: **Arnica, Belladonna, Sulphur, Sepia, Silicea**, and **Spongia**.

If the patient speaks quietly all night long, consider: **Camphora**.

If the patient speaks excitedly, consider: **Nux** and **Sulphur**.

If the patient reveals secrets during sleep, consider: **Arsenicum**.

If the patient talks about work during sleep, consider: **Rhus Tox** and **Sulphur**.

If the patient confesses crimes during sleep, consider: **Belladonna**.

Specific Diagnostic Symptoms: The Face

THE FACE: INDICATORS
Indications of the Face (in General)

DISCOLORATIONS

A face that has taken on an ashy or pale color during illness should lead you to consider: **Arsenicum** or **Phosphorus**. Also: **Sulphur**. Also: **Kali Bi** and **Veratrum**.

A face that is spotted black and blue should lead you to consider: **Lachesis**. Also: **Arnica, Phosphorus**, and **Rhus Tox**.

A face that is bluish should lead you to consider especially: **Arsenicum, Belladonna, Carbo Veg, Lachesis**, and **Veratrum**. Also: **Apis** or **Nux**.

If the skin is discolored a bluish/red, consider: **Belladonna** or **Bryonia**. Also: **Aconite, Apis**, and **Hepar Sulph**.

If the face is discolored brownish, consider: **Sepia** or **Sulphur**.

A face that has taken on a clay-colored or earthtone suggests: **Mercurius** or **Sepia**. Also consider: **Arnica, Natrum Mur, Pulsatilla**, and **Bryonia**. Also: **Phosphorus**.

A face that looks greenish should lead you to consider: **Carbo Veg**. Also: **Pulsatilla** or **Arsenicum**.

A face that looks grayish in color should lead you to consider especially: **Lycopodium**. Also: **Arsenicum** or **Carbo Veg**.

For a patient whose face is grayish yellow, consider especially: **Lycopodium**. Also: **Carbo Veg**.

A red face suggests especially: **Aconite, Apis, Belladonna, Bryonia, Nux, Phosphorus, Rhus Tox**, or **Sulphur**.

A face that alternates red and pale should lead you to consider: **Aconite**. Also: **Belladonna, Ignatia, Nux,** and **Rhus Tox**.

A face that has one cheek red and the other pale suggests: **Chamomilla**.

A face that has two bright red cheeks suggests: **Belladonna**, especially if the face feels hot and dry to the touch.

A face that is red across both cheeks and the bridge of the nose suggests: **Sulphur**.

A face that is yellow suggests especially: **Lycopodium, Nux, Sepia,** and **Sulphur**. Also: **Arsenicum, Carbo Veg, Calcarea, Natrum Mur**, and **Phosphorus**.

A face that seems to continually change color suggests: **Ignatia** or **Phosphorus**. Also: **Aconite, Pulsatilla**, and **Nux**.

DISTORTIONS

For a swollen face, consider especially: **Aconite, Belladonna, Rhus Tox**, and **Hepar Sulph**. Also consider: **Bryonia, Lycopodium, Natrum Mur, Sepia, Veratrum, Calcarea**, and **Lachesis**.

If the swelling is one-sided, consider: **Arsenicum**. Also: **Mercurius, Phosphorus, Bryonia**, and **Belladonna**. Also: **Pulsatilla, Sepia**, and **Spigelia**.

If the left side of the face is swollen, consider: **Lachesis**. Also: **Natrum Mur**.

If the right side of the face is swollen, consider: **Arsenicum** and **Calcarea**. Also: **Mercurius**.

For swelling in the area of the forehead, consider: **Rhus Tox, Ruta, Sepia, Nux**, and **Phosphorus**.

For swelling around the eyes, consider: **Apis** and **Rhus Tox**. Also: **Phosphorus, Arsenicum**, and **Ferrum Phos**. Also: **Urtica Urens** and **Spigelia**.

For swelling above the eyes, consider: **Lycopodium**. Also: **Ruta, Pulsatilla**, and **Sepia**.

For swelling below the eyes, consider: **Apis, Arsenicum**, and **Sulphur**. Also: **Nux** and **Phosphorus**.

If the cheeks are swollen, consider: **Mercurius**. Also: **Arnica, Calcarea, Silicea**, and **Spongia**. Also: **Sepia, Nux, Pulsatilla**, and **Belladonna**.

If the area around the mouth is swollen, consider: **Nux**.

If the chin is swollen, consider: **Carbo Veg**.

If the glands under the chin are swollen, consider: **Belladonna, Calcarea, Hepar Sulph, Mercurius, Rhus Tox**, and **Sulphur**. Also: **Natrum Mur, Lycopodium**, and **Silicea**. Also: **Lachesis**.

If the swollen face is pale, consider: **Apis, Arsenicum**, and **Calcarea**. Also: **Graphites** and **Lycopodium**.

If the swollen face is red, consider: **Aconite** and **Arnica**. Also: **Belladonna, Nux, Rhus Tox**, and **Sulphur**.

If the swollen face is shiny, consider: **Apis** and **Arnica**.

If the swollen face feels stiff, consider: **Rhus Tox**.

If a swollen face also itches, consider: **Rhus Tox**.

If the face has a sensation of being swollen, consider: **Belladonna** and **Natrum Mur**. Also: **Phosphorus** and **Pulsatilla**.

If the swelling is accompanied by toothache, consider: **Mercurius, Lachesis, Sepia**, and **Silicea**. Also: **Calcarea, Hepar Sulph, Spigelia**, and **Allium Cepa**.

If the swelling occurs in the morning, consider: **Arsenicum**. Also: **Hepar Sulph, Sepia, Spigelia**, and **Lycopodium**. Also: **Phosphorus**.

If the swelling occurs in the afternoon, consider: **Arsenicum**. Also: **Belladonna** and **Phosphorus**.

If the swelling occurs in the evening, consider: **Arsenicum, Rhus Tox, Sulphur**, and **Lycopodium**.

If the swelling occurs at night, consider: **Lachesis**.

Indications of the Eyes

DISCOLORATIONS

Bluish circles around or under the eyes especially suggest: **Arsenicum, Lycopodium, Nux, Phosphorus**, or **Rhus Tox**. Also: **Belladonna, Pulsatilla**, and **Veratrum**.

An earthtone discoloration around the eyes suggests: **Pulsatilla**. Also: **Silicea**.

A greenish discoloration around or under the eyes suggests: **Carbo Veg**. Also: **Arsenicum** and **Veratrum**.

DISTORTIONS

For swelling in the region of the eyes, consider especially: **Rhus Tox, Apis**, and **Sepia**. Consider also: **Hepar Sulph, Aconite, Ignatia, Ipecac**, and **Nux**. Also consider: **Mercurius, Lachesis, Dulcamara**, and **Lycopodium**.

For swelling of the upper lids, consider: **Apis**. Also: **Ignatia, Sulphur**, and **Bryonia**. Also: **Thuja**.

For swelling of the lower lids, consider: **Phosphorus**. Also: **Rhus Tox** and **Sepia**.

For swelling under the lids of the eyes, consider: **Apis, Phosphorus**, and **Arsenicum**. Also: **Hepar Sulph**.

For swelling around the margins of the eyelids, consider: **Euphrasia**. Also: **Phosphorus** and **Mercurius**.

For swelling in the area of the tear duct, consider: **Silicea**. Also: **Calcarea, Natrum Mur**, and **Pulsatilla**.

If the eye itself is swollen, consider: **Calcarea**. Also: **Belladonna, Bryonia**, and **Mercurius**. Also: **Silicea.**

If the retina is swollen, consider: **Apis.**

If the swelling takes place in the morning, consider: **Sulphur**. Also **Sepia** and **Bryonia**. Also: **Silicea.**

If the swelling takes place in the afternoon, consider: **Bryonia**, and, especially, **Euphrasia**.

If the swelling takes place in the evening, consider: **Hepar Sulph** and **Sepia**.

If the swelling takes place at night, consider, **Hepar Sulph**.

If the left eye is swollen, consider: **Carbo Veg**.

If the right eye is swollen, consider: **Lycopodium**.

DISTORTIONS OF VISION

If vision is blurred, consider especially: **Natrum Mur**. Also strongly consider: **Gelsemium**. Also: **Aconite, Phosphorus, Ruta**, and **Nux**. Also: **Rhus Tox**.

If vision blurs after close work, consider: **Ruta**.

If vision blurs with the onset of a headache, consider: **Kali Bi, Sepia**, and **Sulphur**.

If vision blurs when the patient tries to read, consider: **Natrum Mur, Ruta**, and **Silicea**. Also: **Aconite** and **Belladonna**.

If vision blurs so that the letters in a word seem to run together, consider: **Ruta**.

If vision blurs so that objects seem to run together, consider: **Calcarea**.

If vision is dimmed, consider especially: **Ruta, Lachesis, Euphrasia, Calcarea**, and **Gelsemium**. Also consider strongly: **Hepar Sulph** and **Mercurius**. Also: **Pulsatilla, Sepia, Silicea**, and **Sulphur**.

If vision of distant objects dimmed, consider: **Sulphur** and **Gelsemium**.

If vision dims with headache, consider: **Iris, Sulphur**, and **Belladonna**. Also: **Natrum Mur, Phosphorus, Gelsemium**, and **Arsenicum**.

If vision dims when reading, consider: **Sulphur, Ruta**, and **Natrum Mur**. Also: **Phosphorus** and **Silicea**. Also: **Hepar Sulph** and **Apis**.

If dimmed vision is accompanied by vertigo, consider: **Gelsemium**,

Nux, and **Sulphur**. Also: **Aconite, Belladonna, Apis, Kali Bi, Phosphorus**, and **Sabadilla**.

For double vision, consider: **Natrum Mur** and **Gelsemium**. Also: **Belladonna, Pulsatilla**, and **Sulphur**. Also: **Veratrum** and **Thuja**.

If double vision occurs when reading, consider: **Graphites**. Also: **Thuja**.

If double vision occurs when writing, consider: **Graphites**.

If double vision occurs during headache, consider: **Gelsemium**.

If double vision is accompanied by vertigo, consider: **Belladonna**.

If double vision occurs after injury to the eye, consider: **Arnica**.

For farsighted vision, consider: **Calcarea, Silicea**, and **Sepia**. Also: **Lycopodium, Nux, Drosera**, and **Belladonna**.

For nearsighted vision, consider: **Phosphorus** and **Pulsatilla**. Also: **Natrum Mur, Ruta, Sulphur, Carbo Veg**, and **Thuja**.

For weak vision, and for the physical weakness of the eyes, consider: **Phosphorus**. Also: **Gelsemium** and **Ruta**. Also: **Sulphur, Nux, Mercurius, Lachesis, Arsenicum**, and **Spigelia**.

If the patient sees bright colors before his eyes, consider: **Nux**. Also: **Graphites, Kali Bi, Ipecac, Pulsatilla**, and **Belladonna**.

If the patient sees darkness before his eyes, consider: **Pulsatilla**.

If this is accompanied by vertigo, consider: **Dulcamara**.

If the patient sees shades of blue before his eyes, consider: **Belladonna, Bryonia**, and **Lachesis**. Also: **Lycopodium**.

If the patient sees blue spots before his eyes, consider: **Aconite**.

If the patient sees shades of gold before his eyes, consider: **Belladonna**.

If the patient sees shades of green before his eyes, consider: **Phosphorus** and **Arsenicum**. Also: **Ruta**.

If the patient sees shades of gray before his eyes, consider: **Silicea** and **Phosphorus**. Also: **Lachesis** and **Lycopodium**.

If the patient sees shades of red before his eyes, consider: **Belladonna** and **Phosphorus**. Also strongly consider: **Sulphur**. Also: **Hepar Sulph**.

If the patient sees red spots before his eyes, consider: **Lycopodium**.

If the patient sees shades of white before his eyes, consider: **Arsenicum** and **Sulphur**. Also: **Thuja** and **Belladonna**.

If the patient sees white spots before his eyes, consider: **Sulphur**. Also: **Arsenicum**.

If the patient sees shades of yellow before his eyes, consider: **Kali Bi** and **Sepia**. Also: **Belladonna**.

If the patient sees yellow spots before his eyes, consider: **Phosphorus**.

Indications of the Nose

DISCOLORATIONS

A blackish discoloration suggests **Mercurius**.

A blue or purple nose suggests the remedy **Lachesis**.

A nose that turns purple only when the patient is out in the cold air suggests the remedy **Phosphorus**.

A nose that is brown suggests the remedy **Sepia**. Also: **Lycopodium**.

A nose that is copper-colored suggests **Arsenicum**.

A red nose suggests **Sulphur**. If only the tip of the nose is red, **Sulphur** still remains the leading remedy, but also consider: **Calcarea, Belladonna, Lachesis**, and **Rhus Tox**. Also: **Carbo Veg, Natrum Mur**, and **Phosphorus**. Also: **Sepia** and **Silicea**.

A yellow nose suggests **Sepia**.

DISTORTIONS

For a swollen nose, consider: **Apis, Arnica**, and **Sulphur**. Also: **Arsenicum, Mercurius, Sepia, Hepar Sulph**, and **Calcarea**.

If the inside of the nose is swollen, consider: **Calcarea, Lachesis, Mercurius**, and **Sepia**. Also: **Kali Bi, Ignatia**, and **Silicea**. Also: **Belladonna** and **Rhus Tox**.

If the tip of the nose is swollen, consider: **Sulphur, Bryonia, Belladonna**, and **Sepia**. Also **Lycopodium** and **Mercurius**.

If the wings of the nose are swollen, consider: **Sulphur**. Also: **Lachesis, Phosphorus**, and **Natrum Mur**.

If the left side of the nose is swollen, consider: **Calcarea** and **Natrum Mur**. Also: **Mercurius** and **Lachesis**.

If the right side of the nose is swollen, consider: **Kali Bi** and **Mercurius**.

If the nose is both swollen and shiny, consider: **Sulphur**. Also: **Phosphorus**.

If the nose is both swollen and painful to the touch, consider: **Phosphorus**. Also: **Natrum Mur** and **Calcarea**.

DISTORTIONS OF SMELL

For an increased sense of smell, consider: **Aconite, Belladonna, Coffea, Phosphorus**, and **Nux**. Also consider strongly: **Ignatia, Lycopodium**, and **Sepia**. Also: **Sulphur, Hepar Sulph**, and **Arsenicum**.

A decreased sense of smell indicates: **Calcarea, Pulsatilla**, and **Silicea**. Also: **Sepia, Natrum Mur**, and **Lycopodium**. Also: **Rhus Tox, Mercurius**, and **Nux**.

The loss of the sense of smell indicates: **Hepar Sulph, Mercurius, Natrum Mur**, and **Pulsatilla**. Also strongly indicates: **Phosphorus, Silicea**, and **Calcarea**. Also: **Sulphur, Arsenicum, Bryonia, Ipecac, Kali Bi**, and **Chamomilla**.

If the sense of smell is distorted, so that one smell seems like another, consider: **Sepia**.

If a patient is very sensitive to odors, consider: **Nux, Sulphur**, and **Phosphorus**. Also **Belladonna, Coffea, Lycopodium**, and **Graphites**. Also consider strongly: **Ignatia**. Also: **Sepia, Aconite**, and **Bryonia**.

If a patient is sensitive to the smell of coffee, consider: **Lachesis**.

If a patient is sensitive to the smell of food cooking, consider: **Sepia**.

If a patient is sensitive to the smell of flowers and perfumes, consider: **Nux** and **Phosphorus**. Also: **Graphites**. Also: **Lycopodium**.

If a patient is sensitive to the smell of gasoline and petroleum products, consider: **Nux** and **Phosphorus**.

If a patient is sensitive to the smell of peaches, consider: **Allium Cepa**.

If a patient is sensitive to the smell of tobacco, consider: **Ignatia**. Also: **Nux, Pulsatilla, Sepia**, and **Belladonna**.

If a patient is beset with imaginary odors, consider: **Nux, Phosphorus**, and **Sulphur**. Also: **Belladonna, Sepia, Kali Bi**, and **Pulsatilla**.

For imagined offensive odors, consider: **Calcarea, Sulphur**, and **Phosphorus**. Also: **Arsenicum**.

For the imagined smell of something burning, consider: **Sulphur, Nux**, and **Graphites**.

For the imagined smell of sour things, especially sour beer, consider: **Thuja** and **Belladonna**.

For the imagined smell of sulphur or rotten eggs, consider: **Sulphur, Nux**, and **Arsenicum**. Also **Calcarea**.

For imagined sweet odors, consider: **Nux**.

For the imagined smell of tobacco, consider: **Pulsatilla**.

For the imagined smell of fish, consider: **Belladonna** and **Thuja**.

For the imagined smell of coffee, consider: **Pulsatilla**.

For the imagined smell of cheese, consider: **Nux**.

Indications of the Ears (External)

DISCOLORATIONS

Red ears especially indicate: **Apis** and **Pulsatilla**. Also: **Belladonna, Carbo Veg, Kali Bi, Lycopodium, Natrum Mur, Phos, Rhus Tox**, and **Sulphur**.

One-sided redness suggests: **Ignatia**. Also consider: **Natrum Mur, Carbo Veg, Calcarea**, and **Sepia**.

A red right ear suggests: **Calcarea**.

A red left ear suggests: **Sepia**.

A reddish discoloration all around the area of the ear suggests: **Arnica**.

An ear that is red only in the afternoon suggests: **Natrum Mur**.

An ear that is red in the evening especially suggests: **Carbo Veg**. Also consider: **Rhus Tox**.

DISTORTIONS

For a swollen ear, consider: **Calcarea, Graphites**, and **Pulsatilla**. Also: **Aconite, Belladonna, Kali Bi, Rhus Tox, Sepia, Silicea**, and **Natrum Mur**. Also: **Spongia, Arnica, Lycopodium, Urtica Urens**, and **Arsenicum**.

For swelling of the glands around the ear, consider: **Calcarea** and **Mercurius**. Also: **Belladonna**.

For swelling in front of the ear, consider: **Calcarea** and **Mercurius**. Also: **Bryonia.**

For swelling behind the ear, consider: **Hepar Sulph, Graphites, Silicea**, and **Lachesis**. Also: **Rhus Tox, Calcarea, Bryonia**, and **Lycopodium**.

For swelling below the ear, consider: **Allium Cepa**.

For swelling inside the ear, consider: **Calcarea** and **Pulsatilla**. Also: **Silicea, Sepia**, and **Lachesis**. Also: **Thuja** and **Bryonia**. Also: **Aconite**.

For swelling of the ear lobes, consider: **Rhus Tox**.

For swelling of the left ear, consider: **Graphites** and **Rhus Tox**.

For swelling of the right ear, consider: **Belladonna** and **Calcarea**.

DISTORTIONS OF HEARING

For very sensitive or acute hearing, consider: **Belladonna, Nux**, and **Lachesis**. Also: **Silicea**. Consider also: **Coffea, Hepar Sulph**, and **Spigelia**. Also: **Sulphur**.

If hearing alternates between very acute and very dull, consider: **Sulphur**.

If hearing is very sensitive during headache, consider: **Aconite, Bryonia**, and **Coffea**.

If hearing is very sensitive to music, consider: **Aconite** and **Nux**. Also: **Coffea, Lycopodium**, and **Sepia**.

If the patient cannot bear to hear music, consider: **Aconite** and **Nux**. Also: **Sepia, Chamomilla, Lycopodium**, and **Sepia**.

If hearing is very sensitive during fever, consider: **Nux, Belladonna, Ipecac**, and **Lycopodium**.

If sensitive hearing alternates with cracking in the ears, consider: **Graphites.**

If the patient seems very, very sensitive to noise and overreacts, to it, consider: **Nux**. Also: **Aconite, Belladonna, Lycopodium**, and **Lachesis**. Also: **Ignatia, Coffea, Calcarea**, and **Phosphorus**.

If the patient reacts to noise with fear, consider: **Phosphorus, Aconite**, and **Belladonna.**

If the patient reacts to noise with anger, consider: **Nux**. Also: **Lycopodium**.

If the patient reacts to noise with anxiety, consider: **Silicea**.

If the patient actually reports physical pain from hearing noises that are not loud enough to cause pain, consider: **Coffea, Silicea**, and **Spigelia**. Also: **Arnica.**

For deafness or dulled hearing in general, consider especially: **Sulphur**. Also: **Lycopodium** and **Graphites**. Also: **Hepar Sulph**. Then consider: **Pulsatilla, Spigelia**, and **Natrum Mur**.

If hearing is dulled during fever, consider: **Euphrasia, Calcarea, Apis, Arsenicum**, and, especially, **Belladonna**.

If hearing is dulled after fever, consider: **Arnica**.

If hearing is dulled during a cold or flu, consider: **Sulphur** and **Pulsatilla**. Also: **Gelsemium, Natrum Mur**, and **Mercurius**. Also: **Belladonna**.

If hearing is dulled when there is a discharge from the ear, consider: **Pulsatilla** and **Hepar Sulph**. Also: **Lycopodium** and **Mercurius**.

If hearing is dulled in left ear, consider: **Sulphur**. Also: **Pulsatilla**.

If hearing is dulled in right ear, consider: **Calcarea** and **Arnica**.

If the patient hears noises in the ear (tinnitus), consider: **Pulsatilla, Sulphur**, and **Calcarea**. Also: **Graphites** and **Lycopodium**. Also strongly consider: **Belladonna**. Also consider: **Lachesis, Mercurius, Ignatia, Arsenicum, Arnica**, and **Natrum Mur.**

If the patient hears buzzing, consider: **Nux, Lycopodium**, and **Sulphur**. Also: **Phosphorus.**

Buzzing in the left ear: **Coffea**.

Buzzing in the right ear: **Sulphur**.

If the patient hears cracking sounds, consider: **Rhus Tox, Graphites, Calcarea**, and **Lachesis**. Also: **Pulsatilla** and **Natrum Mur**.

Cracking sounds in the right ear: **Hepar Sulph**.

If the patient hears fluttering sounds, consider: **Spigelia**. Also: **Sulphur** and **Mercurius**.

If the patient hears hissing sounds, consider: **Nux, Graphites**, and **Lachesis**.

If the patient hears humming, consider: **Lycopodium, Sepia**, and **Phosphorus**. Also: **Aconite, Belladonna**, and **Drosera.** Also: **Graphites, Spigelia**, and **Sulphur**.

If the patient hears a ringing in the ears, consider: **Calcarea, Sulphur**, and **Pulsatilla**. Also strongly consider: **Belladonna, Carbo Veg, Lycopodium, Sepia**, and **Spigelia**. Also: **Silicea** and **Nux**.

A ringing in the left ear, consider: **Nux**. Also: **Staphysagria** and **Arnica.**

A ringing in the right ear, consider: **Lycopodium**. Also: **Thuja** and **Spongia**.

If the patient hears a roaring in the ears, consider: **Carbo Veg, Pulsatilla, Sulphur**, and **Spigelia**. Also strongly consider: **Silicea, Graphites, Belladonna**, and **Nux**. Also: **Calcarea, Bryonia, Arsenicum, Drosera, Hepar Sulph**, and **Natrum Mur**. Also: **Phosphorus** and **Sepia**.

A roaring in the left ear, consider: **Bryonia, Graphites, Thuja**, and **Natrum Mur**.

A roaring in the right ear, consider: **Silicea**. Also: **Phosphorus** and **Mercurius**.

If the patient hears voices, consider: **Phosphorus**.

If the patient hears a whispering in the ears, consider: **Dulcamara.**

If the patient hears a whistling in the ears, consider: **Nux**. Also: **Veratrum, Belladonna**, and **Lycopodium**.

If the patient hears a whizzing sound in the ears, consider: **Lycopodium**. Also: **Sulphur, Hepar Sulph, Lachesis**, and **Rhus Tox**.

If every noise seems to echo in the patient's ears, consider: **Lycopodium** and **Phosphorus**. Also strongly consider: **Sepia**. Also: **Graphites, Pulsatilla, Nux**, and **Lachesis**.

If the patient experiences vertigo accompanied by a distortion in hearing, consider: **Phosphorus**. Also: **Silicea.**

Indications of the Mouth

DISCOLORATIONS

If the mouth is purple, consider: **Mercurius**.

If the mouth is bluish, consider: **Mercurius**.

If the mouth is reddish/blue, consider: **Arsenicum**.

If the mouth is red, consider: **Apis, Kali Bi**, and **Mercurius**.

DISTORTIONS

For swelling in the region of the mouth in general, consider: **Mercurius**. Also: **Belladonna** and **Aconite**. Also: **Nux, Silicea, Sepia, Lycopodium, Carbo Veg**, and **Dulcamara**.

If the skin around the corners of the mouth is cracked, consider: **Phosphorus**. Also: **Silicea, Sepia, Mercurius**, and **Natrum Mur**.

Indications of the Gums

DISCOLORATIONS

Black gums suggest: **Mercurius**.

Bluish gums suggest: **Lachesis**. Also: **Lycopodium**. And also consider: **Mercurius**.

Brownish gums suggest: **Phosphorus**.

Purple gums suggest: **Mercurius**.

Red gums suggest: **Apis, Belladonna, Calcarea, Lachesis, Nux**, and, especially, **Mercurius**.

If the gums are dark red, it suggests especially: **Sepia.**

If the margins of the gums are bright red, it suggests especially: **Mercurius**.

Pale gums suggest, especially: **Mercurius**. Also: **Nux** and **Phosphorus**.

DISTORTIONS

For swelling of the gums, consider: **Arsenicum, Sulphur, Mercurius, Lachesis**, and **Calcarea**. Also: **Lycopodium, Apis, Hepar Sulph, Sepia, Silicea**, and **Natrum Mur**. Also: **Phosphorus, Kali Bi**, and **Staphysagria**.

For swelling of gums on the right side of the mouth, consider: **Mercurius**.

For swelling of the gums around decayed teeth, consider: **Calcarea, Carbo Veg, Phosphorus**, and **Natrum Mur**.

For swelling that is accompanied by pain, consider: **Bryonia** and **Sulphur**. Also: **Belladonna, Calcarea, Silicea**, and **Staphysagria**.

For swelling and pain after dental surgery, consider: **Arnica**. Also: **Silicea**.

For a sensation of swelling in the gums, consider: **Chamomilla**. Also: **Pulsatilla** and **Spongia**.

Indications of the Lips

DISCOLORATIONS

For bluish lips in general, consider: **Arsenicum, Apis, Lachesis, Lycopodium**, and **Nux**. Also think of **Calcarea**.

If there are bluish lips in a very cold patient, think especially of **Arsenicum** and **Nux**. Also consider: **Natrum Mur**.

If the lips have a blackish discoloration, especially consider: **Phosphorus, Arsenicum**, and **Carbo Veg**. Also consider: **Mercurius**.

Brown discoloration of the lips suggests: **Arsenicum, Carbo Veg, Phosphorus**, and **Veratrum**. Also consider **Bryonia** and **Rhus Tox**.

If the lips are very red, consider: **Apis, Belladonna**, and, especially, **Sulphur**. Also consider: **Bryonia** and **Carbo Veg**. Also: **Mercurius**.

If the lips are very pale in color, consider: **Arsenicum** and the **Kalis**. Also consider: **Calcarea, Apis, Ferrum Phos**, and **Pulsatilla**.

DISTORTIONS

For swelling of the lips, consider: **Apis** and **Belladonna**. Also: **Bryonia** and **Sepia**. Then consider: **Calcarea, Natrum Mur, Sulphur, Silicea, Carbo Veg, Arsenicum**, and **Lachesis**. Also: **Mercurius**.

If the lower lip is swollen, consider: **Natrum Mur**. Also: **Sepia, Mercurius, Lycopodium**, and **Sulphur**.

If the upper lip is swollen, consider: **Apis, Belladonna, Hepar Sulph, Natrum Mur, Staphysagria**, and **Sulphur**. Also: **Phosphorus, Bryonia**, and **Mercurius**.

If the lips are cracked, consider: **Calcarea, Natrum Mur, Lachesis, Sulphur**, and **Bryonia**. Also: **Arsenicum**. Then consider: **Arnica, Chamomilla, Mercurius, Rhus Tox**, and **Phosphorus**. Also: **Silicea** and **Veratrum**.

If the lower lip is cracked, consider: **Natrum Mur**. Also: **Sepia**. Then consider: **Phosphorus, Sulphur**, and **Bryonia**.

If the lower lip is cracked in the middle, consider: **Natrum Mur**. Also: **Nux** and **Hepar Sulph**. Then consider: **Pulsatilla, Phosphorus**, and **Drosera**.

If the upper lip is cracked, consider: **Natrum Mur**. Also: **Calcarea.**

If the upper lip is cracked in the middle, consider: **Natrum Mur** and **Hepar Sulph.**

If the lips are chapped, consider: **Calcarea, Carbo Veg, Sulphur**, and **Natrum Mur**. Also: **Kali Bi, Phosphorus**, and **Graphites**. Also: **Arsenicum** and **Hepar Sulph**.

Indications of the Tongue

DISCOLORATIONS

A pale tongue suggests especially: **Mercurius**. Also: **Arsenicum, Natrum Mur, Sepia**, and **Veratrum**. Also consider: **Phosphorus**.

A black tongue suggests especially: **Carbo Veg, Mercurius**, and **Phosphorus**. Also: **Arsenicum, Lachesis, Lycopodium**, and **Nux**.

A blue tongue suggests especially: **Arsenicum**. Also: **Antimonium Tartaricum, Iris**, and **Thuja**.

A brown tongue suggests especially: **Bryonia, Lachesis, Phosphorus**, and **Rhus Tox**. Also: **Belladonna, Carbo Veg, Nux, Sulphur**.

A gray tongue suggests especially: **Phosphorus**. Also: **Pulsatilla**.

A red tongue suggests especially: **Apis, Arsenicum, Belladonna, Mercurius, Phosphorus**, and **Rhus Tox**. Also: **Sulphur, Carbo Veg, Calcarea, Lachesis, Lycopodium**, and **Veratrum**.

If the tongue is red in the center, consider: **Phosphorus** and **Rhus Tox**.

If the tongue is red at the base only, consider: **Bryonia**.

If the tongue is red on the edges, consider especially: **Arsenicum, Mercurius**, or **Sulphur**. Also: **Aconite, Gelsemium, Kali Bi, Phosphorus**, or **Rhus Tox**.

If the tongue is bright, fiery red, consider: **Apis** or **Belladonna**.

If only the tip of the tongue is red, consider: **Rhus Tox**. Also: **Arsenicum** and **Sulphur**.

If the tongue is red and shiny, consider: **Apis, Phosphorus, Rhus Tox**, and especially **Kali Bi**.

A white tongue suggests especially: **Belladonna, Bryonia, Calcarea, Kali Bi, Mercurius, Pulsatilla**, and **Sulphur**. Also: **Arnica, Carbo Veg, Lycopodium, Natrum Mur**, and **Rhus Tox**.

A tongue with a white center suggests: **Bryonia**. Also: **Gelsemium, Phosphorus**, and **Sulphur**.

A milky white tongue suggests: **Belladonna**.

A tongue that is white only in the morning suggests: **Pulsatilla**.

A tongue that is so white that it seems to have been painted suggests: **Arsenicum**.

A pale white tongue suggests: **Phosphorus**.

A tongue that is white only on one side suggests: **Rhus Tox**.

A tongue that is silvery white suggests: **Arsenicum**.

A yellow tongue especially suggests: **Mercurius** and **Rhus Tox**. Also: **Bryonia, Gelsemium, Hepar Sulph, Ipecac, Lachesis, Lycopodium, Pulsatilla, Sepia**, and **Sulphur**.

A tongue that is yellow at the base suggests: **Mercurius** and **Nux**.

A tongue that is bright yellow suggests: **Apis**.

A tongue that is dirty yellow suggests: **Mercurius**.

A tongue with a thick yellow coating suggests: **Mercurius, Pulsatilla**, or **Sulphur**. Also: **Bryonia** and **Carbo Veg**. Also: **Nux**.

If the tongue is very pale, consider: **Arsenicum, Ipecac, Natrum Mur, Sepia**, and **Veratrum**. Especially: **Mercurius**.

If the tongue is very clean, consider: **Ipecac** and **Rhus Tox**.

For a coated tongue, consider: **Bryonia** and **Nux**. Also: **Mercurius, Phosphorus, Pulsatilla**, and **Sulphur**.

If the tongue is coated diagonally, consider: **Rhus Tox**.

If the coating is one-sided, consider: **Rhus Tox**.

If the tongue is coated white, consider: **Arsenicum, Belladonna**, and **Pulsatilla**. Also consider: **Sulphur**. Also: **Phosphorus, Mercurius, Calcarea**, and **Kali Bi**.

If the tongue is coated yellow, consider: **Bryonia**. Also: **Mercurius, Rhus Tox**, and **Spigelia**.

DISTORTIONS

If the tongue is very dry, consider especially: **Aconite, Apis, Arsenicum, Belladonna, Bryonia, Calcarea, Lachesis, Mercurius, Pulsatilla, Rhus Tox**, and **Sulphur**. Also: **Ipecac, Phosphorus**, and **Natrum Mur**.

If the tongue is dry in the center only, consider especially: **Phosphorus**. Consider also: **Lachesis, Veratrum**, and **Aconite**.

If the tongue is dry at the tip, consider: **Carbo Veg, Nux**, and **Rhus Tox**. Also: **Belladonna, Pulsatilla**, and **Phosphorus**.

If the tongue is dry at the root, consider: **Allium Cepa**.

If the tongue is cracked, consider especially: **Arsenicum, Phosphorus**, and **Rhus Tox**. Also consider: **Belladonna, Bryonia, Calcarea, Lachesis**, and **Lycopodium**. Also: **Mercurius, Sulphur**, and **Veratrum**.

If the tongue is cracked down the middle, consider: **Bryonia** and **Rhus Tox**.

If the tongue is cracked across the middle, consider: **Lachesis** and **Mercurius**.

If the tongue is cracked down the edges, consider: **Nux** and **Lachesis**.

If the tongue is cracked on the tip, consider: **Lachesis**.

If a tongue is swollen, consider especially: **Apis, Aconite**, and **Mercurius**. Consider also: **Arsenicum, Belladonna**, and **Lachesis**. Also: **Phosphorus, Dulcamara**, and **Natrum Mur**.

If the base of the tongue is swollen, consider: **Arsenicum**.

If the center of the tongue is swollen, consider: **Phosphorus**.

If the tip of the tongue is swollen, consider: **Natrum Mur**.

If only one side of the tongue is swollen, consider: **Silicea**. Also: **Apis** and **Mercurius**.

If the left side is swollen, consider: **Lachesis**.

If the right side is swollen, consider: **Apis**. Also: **Thuja**.

If the tongue has the sensation of being swollen, consider: **Nux**. Also: **Pulsatilla** and **Gelsemium**.

If the tongue is swollen and feels as if it has been stung by an insect, consider: **Apis**. Also: **Aconite, Belladonna, Natrum Mur**, and **Mercurius**.

A very moist mouth with increased saliva suggests: **Mercurius**.

Bleeding from the tongue suggests: **Lachesis** and **Mercurius**. Also consider: **Calcarea, Arsenicum, Kali Bi, Lycopodium, Nux,** and **Phosphorus**. Also: **Sepia** and **Natrum Mur**.

If the bleeding comes from the tip of the tongue, consider: **Lachesis** and **Phosphorus**.

DISTORTIONS OF TASTE

For a general loss of taste, consider: **Belladonna, Natrum Mur, Pulsatilla**, and **Silicea**. Also: **Sulphur, Sepia, Veratrum, Bryonia, Calcarea**, and **Nux**. Also: **Hepar Sulph** and **Mercurius**. Especially consider: **Phosphorus**.

If the sense of taste is increased, consider: **Belladonna, Coffea**, and **Lycopodium**.

A bad taste on the tongue suggests especially: **Calcarea, Mercurius, Nux V, Pulsatilla**, and **Sulphur**. Also: **Gelsemium** and **Kali Bi**.

For a bad taste in the mouth after eating, consider: **Lycopodium**.

For a bad taste in the mouth every morning, consider: **Nux V** and **Pulsatilla**. Also: **Calcarea** and **Natrum Mur**.

If the tongue tastes of flour in the morning, consider: **Lachesis**.

If the tongue tastes of rotten eggs, consider: **Mercurius, Arnica**, and **Silicea**. Also: **Thuja, Hepar Sulph**, and **Kali Bi**.

A bitter taste in the mouth especially suggests: **Aconite, Arsenicum, Bryonia, Carbo V, Mercurius, Natrum Mur, Nux V, Pulsatilla**, and **Sulphur**. Also: **Apis, Calcarea, Chamomilla, Hepar Sulph, Ignatia**, and **Rhus Tox**.

If the tongue tastes bitter during eating, especially consider: **Pulsatilla**. Also: **Ignatia, Bryonia**, and **Rhus Tox**.

If the tongue tastes bitter after eating, consider: **Arsenicum** and **Pulsatilla**. Also: **Phosphorus, Natrum Mur, Bryonia**, and **Carbo Veg**.

If the tongue tastes bitter every morning, consider especially: **Nux V** and **Pulsatilla**. Also: **Bryonia, Lycopodium, Phosphorus**, and **Sulphur**.

If the tongue tastes bitter and sour together, consider: **Lycopodium, Sulphur, Rhus Tox**, and **Sepia**.

If the tongue tastes bitter and putrid, consider: **Euphrasia**.

If the tongue tastes of bitter milk, consider: **Belladonna**.

If all food tastes bitter on the tongue, consider: **Aconite**.

If food tastes bitter, consider: **Natrum Mur** and **Silicea**. Also: **Lycopodium** and **Hepar Sulph**. Also: **Sulphur**.

If the tongue tastes bloody, consider: **Belladonna, Arsenicum, Ipecac**, and **Sulphur**. Also: **Thuja** and **Aconite.**

If the tongue tastes burnt, consider: **Pulsatilla, Nux V**, and **Sulphur**. Also: **Bryonia**.

If there is a metallic taste on the tongue, consider: **Mercurius** or **Rhus Tox**. Also: **Arsenicum, Lachesis, Lycopodium, Nux**, and **Sulphur**. Also: **Arsenicum**.

If the tongue tastes salty, consider: **Mercurius** or **Natrum Mur**. Also: **Pulsatilla, Carbo Veg, Calcarea, Phosphorus, Sepia**, and **Sulphur**.

If the tongue tastes sour, consider especially: **Ignatia, Calcarea, Nux**, and **Phosphorus**. Also: **Hepar Sulph, Mercurius**, and **Sulphur**.

Indications of the Throat (Internal)

DISCOLORATIONS

A copper-colored throat suggests: **Mercurius**.

A purple throat suggests: **Mercurius, Pulsatilla**, and **Nux**. Also: **Kali Bi** and **Sulphur**.

A yellow throat, or a throat with yellow spots, suggests: **Lycopodium**.

A red throat especially suggests: **Aconite, Belladonna,** and **Lycopodium**. Also: **Apis, Arsenicum, Calcarea, Gelsemium, Ignatia, Lachesis, Mercurius,** and **Phosphorus**.

If the throat is very dark red, it suggests: **Apis, Lachesis, Rhus Tox**, and **Pulsatilla**.

If the throat is a bright, shiny red, it suggests: **Apis**. Also: **Belladonna** and **Phosphorus**.

DISTORTIONS

For swelling of the throat, consider: **Apis, Belladonna**, and **Lachesis**. Also: **Hepar Sulph, Mercurius**, and **Lycopodium**. Also: **Sulphur** and **Spongia**.

Indications of the Tonsils

DISCOLORATIONS

If these glands seem infected, or a general infection is present with the swelling, consider: **Mercurius, Calcarea**, and **Silicea**. Also: **Hepar Sulph** and **Sulphur**.

If the tonsils are gray, think of: the **Kalis**, especially of **Kali Mur**.

Also: **Mercurius** and related remedies.

If the tonsils look purple, think especially of: **Lachesis**.

DISTORTIONS

For swelling of the tonsils, consider: **Calcarea, Belladonna, Sulphur, Phosphorus, Silicea**, and **Lachesis**. Also: **Lycopodium, Hepar Sulph, Mercurius, Apis**, and **Graphites**. Also: **Gelsemium, Dulcamara**, and **Staphysagria**.

For swelling of the left side, consider: **Lachesis**. Also: **Apis, Sepia**, and **Sulphur**.

For swelling of the right side, consider: **Lycopodium**. Also: **Belladonna, Mercurius, Hepar Sulph**, and **Apis**.

Indications of the Throat (External)

DISCOLORATIONS

For a general discoloration of the external throat (neck), consider: **Kali Bi** and **Rhus Tox**.

If the throat looks blue/purple, consider **Lachesis** as a remedy.

If the throat is brown, think of the **Kalis** as remedies, and, if it is brown only in specific spots or areas, think of **Sepia**.

If the throat looks white in spots, think of the **Natrums**, especially **Natrum Carbonicum**.

If the throat is red, think of **Apis** and **Rhus Tox**. If it is red only in spots, think of **Belladonna**. If the external throat is mottled with red spots, consider: **Lachesis**.

If the throat is yellow, think of **Arsenicum**. If the neck is yellow only in spots, consider: **Lycopodium**.

DISTORTIONS

For the general swelling of the external throat, consider: **Rhus Tox** and **Lycopodium**. Also: **Mercurius, Belladonna**, and **Spongia**. Also: **Sulphur** and **Phosphorus**.

For the general swelling of the whole neck, consider: **Phosphorus**. Also: **Nux**.

For the general swelling of the sides of the neck, consider: **Belladonna** and **Rhus Tox**. Also: **Apis**. Also consider: **Lycopodium** and **Lachesis**.

For the swelling of the veins in the neck, consider: **Silicea** and **Thuja**.

For the swelling of the glands in the throat, consider: **Mercurius, Calcarea**, and **Lycopodium**. Also strongly consider: **Rhus Tox, Staphysagria, Sulphur, Graphites**, and **Belladonna**. Also: **Lachesis, Natrum Mur, Pulsatilla**, and **Phosphorus**. Also: **Carbo Veg** and **Dulcamara**.

If the swollen glands are hard to the touch, consider: **Silicea**. Also: **Calcarea** and **Lycopodium**. Also: **Mercurius**.

THE FACE: DISCHARGES
Discharges from the Eye

FOR A DISCHARGE OF MUCUS (PUS)

For a general discharge of pus from the eye, consider: **Calcarea, Euphrasia, Mercurius**, and **Pulsatilla**. Also consider: **Hepar Sulph, Sulphur, Nux, Natrum Mur, Apis, Ferrum Phos, Ipecac, Graphites,** and **Lycopodium**. Also: **Arsenicum, Carbo Veg, Dulcamara, Phosphorus, Rhus Tox**, and **Sepia**. Also consider: **Thuja**.

If the discharge is bloody, consider: **Hepar Sulph, Mercurius, Pulsatilla** and **Silicea**. Also: **Lachesis, Lycopodium, Arsenicum, Carbo Veg, Rhus Tox, Sepia, Thuja**, and **Sulphur**.

If the pus is clear, consider: **Ipecac**.

If the pus is green, consider: **Mercurius**.

If the pus is yellow, consider: **Pulsatilla, Silicea**, and **Kali Bi**. Also consider: **Calcarea, Euphrasia, Mercurius, Sepia, Sulphur**, and **Thuja**. Also: **Arsenicum, Carbo Veg**, and **Lycopodium**.

If the discharge is thick, consider: **Natrum Mur**. Also: **Silicea, Lycopodium, Pulsatilla, Euphrasia**, and **Kali Bi**. Also think of: **Sulphur** and **Sepia** and **Thuja**.

If the discharge is thin, consider: **Graphites**.

If the discharge appears only in the morning, consider: **Sulphur**. Also consider: **Arsenicum, Sepia, Kali Bi**, and **Sepia**.

If the discharge appears only in the evening, consider: **Phosphorus**.

FOR DISCHARGE OF TEARS

For tearing of the eyes, consider: **Natrum Mur, Euphrasia, Mercurius, Phosphorus, Rhus Tox, Pulsatilla, Belladonna, Lycopodium, Calcarea**, and **Sulphur**. Also consider: **Aconite, Apis, Arsenicum, Carbo Veg, Ferrum Phos, Graphites, Hepar Sulph, Nux, Ruta, Sepia, Silicea, Thuja,** and **Veratrum**.

For tearing in the open air, consider: **Calcarea, Phosphorus, Sulphur**, and **Silicea**. Also consider: **Pulsatilla, Ruta, Rhus Tox, Graphites**, and **Thuja**. Also: **Natrum Mur, Dulcamara, Belladonna, Bryonia, Euphrasia**, and **Veratrum**.

For tearing when the patient is in cold air, consider: **Pulsatilla**. Also: **Sepia**, and **Silicea**. Also consider: **Sulphur, Thuja, Lycopodium**, and **Phosphorus**.

For tearing from light, consider: **Pulsatilla**.

For tearing in the morning, consider: **Pulsatilla, Sulphur**, and **Calcarea**. Also consider: **Sepia**. Also: **Rhus Tox, Phosphorus, Belladonna**, and **Mercurius**.

For tearing at night, consider: **Apis**. Also: **Arnica, Arsenicum, Gelsemium, Hepar Sulph**, and **Phosphorus**.

Discharges from the Nose

FOR A DISCHARGE OF MUCUS

If the discharge is blood-streaked, consider: **Phosphorus**.

If the discharge is bloody, consider especially: **Allium Cepa, Arsenicum, Belladonna, Hepar Sulph, Mercurius**, and **Phosphorus**. Also: **Calcarea, Carbo Veg, Kali Bi, Nux V**, and **Sulphur**.

If the discharge is bloody only in the morning, consider: **Lachesis**. Also: **Calcarea**.

If the discharge is bluish, consider: **Kali Bi**.

If the discharge is totally clear, consider: **Aconite** and **Natrum Mur**. Also: **Phosphorus** and **Sulphur**. Also: **Arsenicum**.

If the discharge is gray, consider: **Lycopodium**.

If the discharge is greenish, consider especially: **Kali Bi, Mercurius, Pulsatilla**, and **Thuja**. Also: **Phosphorus, Sepia, Rhus Tox, Bryonia**, and **Carbo Veg**.

If the discharge is greenish and bloody, consider: **Phosphorus**.

If the discharge is greenish/yellow, consider especially: **Kali Bi, Mercurius, Pulsatilla**, and **Thuja**. Also: **Hepar Sulph, Phosphorus**, and **Silicea**.

If the discharge is orange, consider: **Pulsatilla**.

If the discharge is white, consider especially: **Natrum Mur**. Also: **Nux V** and **Lycopodium**.

If the discharge is yellow, consider especially: **Calcarea, Hepar Sulph, Kali Bi, Lycopodium, Pulsatilla, Sepia**, and **Sulphur**. Also: **Natrum Mur, Phosphorus**, and **Thuja**.

If the discharge is copious, consider especially: **Allium Cepa, Arsenicum, Natrum Mur**, and **Phosphorus**. Also: **Kali Bi, Pulsatilla**, and **Sulphur**.

If the discharge is watery, consider especially: **Allium Cepa, Arsenicum, Euphrasia, Mercurius, Natrum Mur**, and **Nux V**. Also: **Aconite, Carbo Veg, Bryonia, Kali Bi**, and **Sulphur**.

If the discharge is thick, consider: **Arsenicum, Kali Bi, Pulsatilla**, and **Thuja**. Also: **Calcarea, Natrum Mur, Phosphorus, Rhus Tox**, and **Sulphur**.

FOR A DISCHARGE OF BLOOD

For a nosebleed in general, consider: **Aconite, Belladonna, Phosphorus**, and **Sulphur**. Also: **Mercurius, Calcarea, Ipecac, Lachesis, Ar-**

nica, and **Pulsatilla**. Also think of: **Apis, Arsenicum, Carbo Veg, Ignatia, Lycopodium, Natrum Mur, Silicea, Sepia, Veratrum, Thuja, Ruta**, and **Kali Bi**.

If the blood is bright red, consider: **Phosphorus** and **Belladonna**. Also: **Ipecac**. Then consider: **Aconite, Calcarea, Bryonia, Lachesis, Sulphur, Sepia, Silicea, Dulcamara**, and **Mercurius**.

If the blood is dark red, consider: **Nux, Lachesis**, and **Carbo Veg**. Then consider: **Pulsatilla, Belladonna, Arnica, Kali Bi, Sepia**, and **Phosphorus**.

If the blood is a pale red, consider: **Carbo Veg, Sulphur, Graphites**, and **Arnica**. Also: **Belladonna, Lachesis, Phosphorus, Pulsatilla**, and **Rhus Tox**. Also: **Ledum** and **Dulcamara**.

For a blood flow in the morning, consider: **Sulphur**. Also consider: **Phosphorus, Nux, Rhus Tox, Sepia, Natrum Mur, Lachesis, Bryonia**, and **Calcarea**. Also: **Aconite, Kali Bi, Apis**, and **Arnica**.

For a blood flow in the evening, consider: **Phosphorus, Pulsatilla, Sepia, Sulphur, Lachesis**, and **Graphites**. Also: **Thuja** and **Coffea**.

For a blood flow at night, consider: **Carbo Veg**. Also: **Rhus Tox, Pulsatilla, Belladonna**, and **Mercurius**. Also think about: **Veratrum, Calcarea, Arnica**, and **Bryonia**.

For a blood flow during sleep, consider: **Mercurius**. Also: **Bryonia, Nux**, and **Veratrum**. Also: **Belladonna** and **Graphites**.

Discharges from the Ear

FOR A DISCHARGE OF MUCUS (PUS)

For a discharge of pus in general, consider: **Mercurius** and **Pulsatilla**. Also consider: **Lycopodium, Calcarea, Carbo Veg, China, Allium Cepa, Natrum Mur, Petroleum**, and **Silicea**.

For a discharge containing earwax, consider: **Thuja**. Also consider: **Lycopodium, Mercurius, Pulsatilla**, and **Natrum Mur**.

If the discharge is brownish, consider: **Carbo Veg**.

If the discharge is clear, consider: **Bryonia**.

If the discharge is flesh-colored, consider: **Carbo Veg**.

If the discharge is green, consider: **Mercurius, Hepar Sulph**, and **Lycopodium**.

If the discharge is white, consider especially: **Natrum Mur**. Also: **Hepar Sulph**.

If the discharge is yellow, consider: **Pulsatilla** and **Kali Bi**. Also: **Arsenicum**. Also: **Lycopodium, Mercurius,** and **Phosphorus**.

If the discharge is yellow/green, consider: **Pulsatilla**.

If the discharge is chronic in nature, consider: **Silicea**.

If the discharge is periodic in nature, reoccurring at regular intervals, consider: **Sulphur**.

If the discharge comes only at night, consider: **Sepia**.

If the discharge comes on only when the patient is in bed, consider: **Mercurius**.

If the discharge is from the left ear only, consider: **Graphites**.

If the discharge is from the right ear only, consider: **Lycopodium**. Also: **Silicea** and **Thuja**.

If the discharge is thick, consider: **Pulsatilla** and **Kali Bi**. Also: **Calcarea** and **Silicea**. Also: **Lycopodium** and **Carbo Veg**. Then think of **Natrum Mur** or **Sepia**.

If the discharge is sticky like glue, consider: **Natrum Mur** and **Kali Bi**.

If the discharge is thin, consider: **Sulphur**. Also: **Silicea**. Also consider: **Sepia** and **Arsenicum**.

If the discharge is watery, consider: **Silicea**. Also: **Sulphur, Carbo Veg**, and **Mercurius**.

If the discharge is bloody, the first remedies to consider are **Calcarea, Lachesis, Mercurius**, and **Silicea**. Others to consider are **Hepar Sulph, Carbo Veg, Sulphur, Pulsatilla, Causticum**, and **Belladonna**. Also: **Arsenicum, Lycopodium, Petroleum, Phosphorus, Rhus Tox, Sepia**, and **Bryonia**.

If the discharge is painful to the ear, consider: **Sulphur**. Also consider: **Mercurius, Hepar Sulph, Lycopodium, Natrum Mur, Phosphorus**, and **Pulsatilla**.

Discharges from the Mouth

FOR A DISCHARGE OF MUCUS

For mucus from the mouth, consider: **Natrum Mur**. Also: **Calcarea, Ignatia, Mercurius, Nux, Pulsatilla, Rhus Tox, Silicea**, and **Sulphur**. Also think about: **Arnica, Lycopodium**, and **Veratrum**.

If the mucus is present only in the morning, consider: **Belladonna** and

Pulsatilla. Also consider: **Sulphur** and **Sepia**. Think also of: **Ignatia, Lycopodium, Mercurius, Silicea**, and **Thuja**.

If the mucus is present only at night, consider: **Sulphur**.

FOR A DISCHARGE OF BLOOD

If there is a discharge of blood, consider: **Phosphorus** and **Hepar Sulph**. Also: **Arsenicum, Lachesis, Mercurius, Nux,** and **Rhus Tox**. Also consider: **Belladonna, Ipecac, Ferrum Phos**, and **Carbo Veg**.

If the blood is black, consider: **Carbo Veg** and **Lachesis**.

For discharge of blood after dental surgery, consider: **Phosphorus**.

If there is a great deal of blood being discharged, consider: **Phosphorus**. Also: **Lachesis** and **Mercurius**. Also consider: **Rhus Tox**.

For a discharge of blood that accompanies fits of coughing, consider: **Nux** and **Ipecac**.

For bleeding gums, consider: **Carbo Veg, Calcarea, Lachesis, Mercurius, Natrum Mur, Sepia**, and, especially, **Phosphorus**. Also consider: **Apis, Belladonna, Hepar Sulph, Nux, Silicea**, and **Sulphur**. Finally think of: **Ferrum Phos, Lycopodium, Ruta**, and **Spigelia**.

For bleeding from the lips, consider: **Arsenicum, Bryonia, Ignatia**, and **Lachesis**.

For bleeding from the palate, consider: **Phosphorus** and **Lachesis**.

FOR A DISCHARGE OF SALIVA

For frothy saliva, consider: **Apis, Bryonia, Ignatia**, and **Pulsatilla**. Consider also: **Aconite, Dulcamara, Kali Bi, Lachesis, Lycopodium, Phosphorus**, and **Spigelia**. Also: **Sulphur**.

If saliva is brown, consider: **Belladonna**.

If saliva is coppery colored, consider: **Mercurius**.

If saliva is white, consider: **Arsenicum** and **Ipecac**.

If saliva is yellow, consider: **Gelsemium** and **Spigelia**. Also consider: **Lycopodium** and **Mercurius**. Also: **Rhus Tox**.

If saliva is thick, consider: **Arsenicum**. Also: **Belladonna** and **Rhus Tox**.

If saliva flows concomitant to or in combination with other symptoms, consider: **Mercurius**.

If saliva flows in the afternoon, consider: **Phosphorus**.

If saliva flows in the forenoon, consider: **Calcarea**.

If saliva flows at night, consider: **Mercurius**. Also consider: **Ignatia, Natrum Mur**, and **Rhus Tox**. Also: **Nux** and **Phosphorus**. Also: **Sulphur, Pulsatilla**, and **Veratrum**.

If saliva flows while the patient is lying down in bed at night, consider: **Mercurius** and **Belladonna**.

If the saliva flows while the patient is asleep, consider: **Mercurius**. Also consider: **Arnica, Lycopodium, Sulphur, Phosphorus, Pulsatilla**, and **Rhus Tox**. Also: **Ipecac** and **Lachesis**.

If saliva flows in the morning, consider: **Graphites**. Also: **Lycopodium** and **Sulphur**. Also consider: **Rhus Tox** and **Veratrum**.

If saliva flows during a headache, consider: **Mercurius**. Also: **Ignatia**. Also consider: **Phosphorus, Sepia**, and **Veratrum**.

If saliva flows during nausea, consider: **Sulphur, Lachesis**, and **Ipecac**. Also: **Veratrum**.

If saliva flows during toothache, consider: **Mercurius**. Also: **Dulcamara**. Also consider: **Belladonna, Calcarea, Graphites, Natrum Mur**, and **Sepia**.

If saliva flows during menses, consider: **Mercurius** and **Pulsatilla**.

If saliva flows during pregnancy, consider: **Natrum Mur**. Also: **Arsenicum, Coffea, Mercurius, Sepia**, and **Sulphur**.

Specific Diagnostic Symptoms:
The Body

THE BODY: INDICATORS
Indications of the Skin (in General)

DISCOLORATIONS

If the skin has a black or blackish tone, consider especially: **Arsenicum**. Also: **Apis, Carbo Veg**, and **Lachesis**. Also: **Spigelia**.

If the black skin appears only in spots, consider: **Arsenicum** and **Lachesis**. Also: **Rhus Tox**.

If the skin has a bluish tone, consider especially: **Carbo Veg** and **Veratrum**. Also: **Nux** and **Lachesis**. Then consider: **Arsenicum**. Also: **Thuja, Ipecac, Apis, Mercurius, Rhus Tox, Silicea**, and **Sulphur**.

If the bluish area also has a burning sensation, consider: **Arsenicum** and **Lachesis**.

If the bluish area is from a physical trauma, consider first: **Arnica**. Also consider: **Belladonna, Ledum, Lachesis, Calcarea**, and **Pulsatilla**.

If the bluish area of the skin appears only in spots, consider: **Arnica, Lachesis, Phosphorus**, and **Arsenicum**. Also consider: **Bryonia, Carbo Veg, Hepar Sulph, Ledum, Lycopodium, Nux**, and **Pulsatilla**. Also: **Rhus Tox** and **Ruta**.

If the skin has brown spots (often called liver spots), consider: **Lachesis, Lycopodium, Sepia, Mercurius**, and **Sulphur**. Also consider: **Thuja, Arsenicum, Carbo Veg, Dulcamara, Nux**, and **Phosphorus**. Also: **Rhus Tox, Ruta, Silicea, Arnica**, and **Veratrum**.

If these brown spots itch, consider: **Sulphur**. Also: **Lycopodium**.

If the skin has a copper-colored tone, consider: **Carbo Veg**.

If the skin has a gray tone, consider: **Lycopodium**.

If the skin has a green discoloration, consider: **Arnica, Lachesis**, and **Carbo Veg**. Also: **Sepia** and **Veratrum**.

If the skin has a purple discoloration, consider: **Lachesis**.

If the skin has a red discoloration, consider: **Belladonna, Apis**, and **Rhus Tox**. Also consider: **Mercurius, Graphites**, and **Sulphur**. Also: **Arnica, Aconite, Bryonia, Pulsatilla, Nux, Phosphorus**, and **Lycopodium**. Also: **Ruta, Ledum**, and **Carbo Veg**.

If the skin becomes red after scratching, consider: **Rhus Tox**. Also:

Belladonna, Natrum Mur, Graphites, and **Mercurius**. Also: **Pulsatilla, Lycopodium**, and **Nux**.

If the skin is discolored red only in spots, consider: **Calcarea, Phosphorus, Sulphur, Arsenicum**, and **Belladonna**. Also consider: **Apis, Arnica, Bryonia, Silicea, Rhus Tox, Graphites, Carbo Veg, Dulcamara**, and **Ipecac**. Also: **Veratrum, Nux, Hepar Sulph**, and **Chamomilla**.

If these red spots appear after the patient bathes, consider: **Phosphorus**.

If these spots are bluish-red in color, consider: **Belladonna** and **Phosphorus**. Also: **Arsenicum, Lachesis**, and **Apis**.

If these spots are brownish-red in color, consider: **Sepia**. Also: **Phosphorus, Carbo Veg**, and **Thuja**.

If the red spots have a coppery tone to them, consider: **Lachesis**. Also: **Arsenicum, Rhus Tox**, and **Veratrum**. Also: **Ruta, Phosphorus, Calcarea**, and **Carbo Veg**.

If the red spots are bright scarlet, consider: **Belladonna** and **Mercurius**. Also: **Arsenicum, Bryonia, Sulphur**, and **Arnica**. Also: **Aconite, Lachesis, Dulcamara, Euphrasia, Phosphorus**, and **Hepar Sulph**.

If the red spots are pale, consider: **Silicea** and **Phosphorus**.

If the red spots are rose-colored, consider: **Carbo Veg** and **Sepia**.

If the red spots have a violet tone, consider: **Phosphorus** and **Veratrum**.

For skin that is streaked red, consider: **Phosphorus**. Also: **Apis, Rhus Tox, Euphrasia, Lachesis, Calcarea, Carbo Veg**, and **Mercurius**.

For skin that is discolored with a violet tone, consider: **Belladonna**.

For skin that is discolored with a white tone, consider: **Apis** and **Arsenicum**. Also: **Calcarea** and **Carbo Veg**.

For white discoloration that appears only in spots, consider: **Silicea** and **Arsenicum**. Also: **Calcarea, Mercurius, Phosphorus**, and **Sulphur**. Also: **Sepia** and **Graphites**.

For skin that is very darkly colored, consider: **Lycopodium, Lachesis**, and **Arsenicum**.

For skin that is very pale, consider: **Calcarea, Lycopodium, Pulsatilla, Sulphur, Veratrum**, and **Belladonna**. Also: **Apis, Arsenicum, Carbo Veg, Mercurius, Natrum Mur**, and **Phosphorus**.

For skin that looks dirty, consider: **Sulphur**. Also: **Thuja, Natrum Mur**, and **Arsenicum**. Also: **Mercurius** and **Bryonia**.

For skin that looks dirty and itches, consider: **Sulphur** and **Lycopodium**.

DISTORTIONS

For skin that feels cold, consider: **Arsenicum, Rhus Tox, Sulphur, Veratrum**, and **Sepia**. Also: **Belladonna, Calcarea, Graphites, Lachesis, Nux**, and **Silicea**. Also: **Ruta, Ignatia, Ledum**, and **Lycopodium**.

If the skin is icy cold, consider: **Carbo Veg**. Also: **Calcarea, Arsenicum, Natrum Mur**, and **Veratrum**.

If the skin is icy cold only in spots, consider: **Veratrum**.

If the skin is cold, but the patient feels internally hot, consider: **Ignatia** and **Veratrum**. Also: **Ferrum Phos** and **Euphrasia**.

If the skin feels cold and clammy, consider: **Calcarea** and **Carbo Veg**.

For skin that feels hot, without fever, consider: **Lachesis** and **Graphites**. Also: **Bryonia, Belladonna, Lycopodium, Kali Bi, Rhus Tox, Sulphur, Sepia**, and **Silicea**.

For skin that is dry, consider: **Belladonna, Bryonia, Phosphorus, Sulphur, Lycopodium, Ledum, Graphites, Dulcamara, Arsenicum**, and **Silicea**. Also: **Sepia, Aconite, Arnica, Coffea, Nux, Rhus Tox, Ruta**, and **Veratrum**.

For skin that is both dry and burning, consider: **Aconite, Belladonna, Bryonia, Arsenicum, Lachesis, Lycopodium, Sulphur, Phosphorus**, and **Pulsatilla**. Also: **Mercurius, Silicea, Sepia, Coffea, Dulcamara**, and **Ledum**.

For skin that is moist or damp, consider: **Carbo Veg, Graphites, Lycopodium**, and **Rhus Tox**. Also: **Lachesis, Phosphorus**, and **Ledum**. Also: **Thuja** and **Ruta**.

For skin that is moist in specific spots, consider: **Silicea**. Also: **Sulphur**. Also consider: **Carbo Veg, Lachesis**, and **Ledum**.

For skin that becomes moist after scratching, consider: **Lycopodium**. Also: **Rhus Tox, Graphites**, and **Lachesis**. Also: **Carbo Veg, Bryonia, Calcarea, Ledum, Sepia, Silicea**, and **Natrum Mur**. Also: **Ruta** and **Mercurius**.

For rashes of the skin in general, consider: **Sulphur, Rhus Tox, Mercurius, Aconite, Belladonna, Bryonia**, and **Arsenicum**. Also: **Apis, Arnica, Calcarea, Dulcamara, Silicea, Sepia, Natrum Mur, Ipecac, Kali Bi**, and **Coffea**. Also: **Veratrum, Nux, Spongia, Euphrasia**, and **Carbo Veg**.

For a rash after a bee sting, consider: **Apis**. Also: **Sepia**.

For a rash with a blackish hue, consider: **Lachesis**.

For a rash that has a bluish coloration, consider: **Aconite** and **Lachesis**. Also: **Coffea, Ledum**, and **Phosphorus**. Also: **Sulphur, Belladonna**, and **Sepia**.

For a rash that is bright red, consider: **Aconite** and **Belladonna**. Also: **Sulphur**.

For a rash that is scarlet, consider: **Aconite, Belladonna, Bryonia**, and **Ipecac**. Also: **Coffea, Kali Bi**, and **Mercurius**. Also: **Dulcamara, Carbo Veg, Phosphorus, Rhus Tox, Sulphur**, and **Lachesis**.

For a rash that is white, consider: **Arsenicum**. Also: **Sulphur, Bryonia, Apis**, and **Phosphorus**. Also: **Nux** and **Ipecac**.

Indications of the Skin (in Wounds)

DISCOLORATIONS

If the skin around a wound has a black tinge, consider: **Lachesis**. Also: **Ledum**.

If the skin around a wound has a bluish tinge, consider: **Apis, Lachesis**, or **Ledum**.

If the skin around a wound is greenish, consider: **Lachesis**.

If the skin looks reddish, consider: **Lachesis**.

If the skin looks red and raw, like uncooked meat, consider: **Calcarea**.

If the skin around a wound looks yellow, consider: **Lachesis**.

DISTORTIONS

If the skin around a wound feels cold, consider: **Ledum**.

If the skin around a wound feels hot, consider: **Apis**.

For wounds in general, consider: **Apis, Arnica, Ledum, Lachesis, Phosphorus**, and **Arsenicum**. Also: **Natrum Mur, Pulsatilla, Bryonia, Rhus Tox**, and **Ruta**.

For wounds that bleed a good deal, consider: **Lachesis,** and **Phosphorus**. Also: **Arnica, Aconite, Euphrasia, Nux, Sulphur**, and **Silicea**.

For small wounds that bleed a great amount, consider: **Phosphorus**. Also: **Lachesis**.

For wounds that are slow to heal, consider: **Silicea**.

For the chronic effects of a wound, consider: **Ledum**. Also: **Staphysagria, Lachesis, Phosphorus**, and **Arnica**. Also: **Rhus Tox** and **Ruta**.

THE BODY: DISCHARGES
Perspiration

For hot sweat, consider: **Aconite, Ignatia, Nux, Sulphur**, and **Ipecac**. Also: **Belladonna, Rhus Tox, Phosphorus, Thuja**, and **Veratrum**.

For a cold sweat, consider: **Carbo Veg, Calcarea, Arsenicum, Lycopodium, Veratrum, Hepar Sulph**, and **Mercurius**. Also: **Arnica, Antimonium Tartaricum, Lachesis, Spigelia, Sulphur, Thuja, Graphites, Ignatia, Staphysagria, Phosphorus, Ruta**, and **Nux**.

If the skin is clammy and chilled, consider: **Veratrum**.

If the patient feels worse, in general, from sweating, consider: **Mercurius** and **Sepia**. Also: **Calcarea, Ignatia, Staphysagria, Natrum Mur**, and **Nux**. Also: **Belladonna** and **Bryonia**. Also: **Arsenicum**.

If the patient feels better, in general, from sweating, consider: **Rhus Tox, Bryonia**, and **Calcarea**. Also: **Sulphur, Thuja, Natrum Mur, Gelsemium, Arsenicum**, and **Veratrum**.

If the sweat stains the bed linen, consider: **Belladonna, Lachesis**, and **Mercurius**. Also: **Arsenicum, Calcarea, Graphites, Nux**, and **Lycopodium**.

If the stains are bloody, consider: **Lachesis**. Also: **Lycopodium, Arnica, Chamomilla, Nux**, and **Phosphorus**. Also: **Dulcamara**.

If the stains are brown, consider: **Sepia**.

If the stains are yellow-brown, consider: **Lachesis** or **Belladonna**. Also: **Thuja** or **Arsenicum**.

If the stains are yellow, consider: **Graphites, Mercurius**, or **Lachesis**. Also: **Belladonna, Ipecac, Thuja, Lycopodium**, or **Veratrum**.

If the stains are red, consider: **Arnica, Calcarea, Nux, Dulcamara, Lycopodium**, or, especially, **Lachesis**.

If the stains do not wash out, consider: **Mercurius**.

If the patient sweats in the daytime, in general, consider: **Sulphur, Lycopodium, Calcarea, Sepia**, and **Ferrum Phos**. Also: **Staphysagria, Mercurius, Bryonia, Dulcamara, Graphites**, and **Ledum**.

If the patient sweats in the night, in general, consider: **Mercurius, Lachesis, Hepar Sulph, Sulphur, Thuja, Sepia, Arsenicum**, and **Natrum Mur**. Also: **Dulcamara**. Also: **Arnica, Bryonia, Calcarea, Rhus Tox, Veratrum**, and **Silicea**.

If the patient sweats day and night without letup, consider: **Hepar Sulph**.

For morning sweats, consider: **Calcarea, Hepar Sulph, Mercurius, Veratrum, Phosphorus**, and **Silicea**. Also: **Bryonia, Carbo Veg, Lycopodium, Sepia**, and **Sulphur**.

For afternoon sweats, consider: **Natrum Mur** and **Nux**. Also: **Hepar Sulph**.

For evening sweats, consider: **Phosphorus** and **Sulphur**. Also: **Natrum Mur, Hepar Sulph, Mercurius, Rhus Tox**, and **Spigelia**. Also: **Thuja** and **Veratrum**.

For sweats after midnight, consider: **Ferrum Phos, Drosera**, and **Phosphorus**. Also: **Hepar Sulph, Mercurius, Pulsatilla, Belladonna, Aconite**, and **Arsenicum**.

For sweats of strong odor, consider: **Sulphur, Mercurius**, and **Hepar Sulph**. Also: **Sepia, Lycopodium, Nux, Pulsatilla**, and **Silicea**. Also: **Rhus Tox, Graphites, Arnica, Arsenicum, Carbo Veg, Dulcamara**, and **Lachesis**. Also, especially: **Thuja**.

For sweats with a sour odor, consider: **Sulphur, Calcarea, Arsenicum, Bryonia, Lycopodium, Sepia**, and **Silica**.

For sweat that smells like urine, consider: **Graphites, Rhus Tox, Lycopodium**, and **Natrum Mur**.

For sweat that smells sickly sweet, consider: **Thuja**.

For sweat that smells sweet and sour, consider: **Pulsatilla**. Also: **Bryonia**.

For sweat that smells like onions, consider: **Lycopodium**. Also: **Thuja, Calcarea, Lachesis**, and **Phosphorus**.

For sweat that smells like smoke, consider: **Belladonna**.

For sweat that smells like Sulphur or rotten eggs, consider: **Sulphur** or **Phosphorus**.

For sweat that smells like rotted meat, consider: **Staphysagria**.

For sweat that is pungent, consider: **Ipecac, Sepia**, and **Rhus Tox**. Also: **Thuja**.

For sweat that has a horrible, putrid smell, consider: **Carbo Veg** or **Staphysagria**. Also: **Nux, Rhus Tox, Spigelia**, or **Silicea**.

For sweat that smells sickly, consider: **Thuja**.

For sweat that smells and feels oily, consider: **Thuja** and **Mercurius**. Also: **Bryonia, Arsenicum**, and **Natrum Mur**. Also: **Nux** and **Rhus Tox**.

For sweat that attracts flies, consider: **Thuja, Bryonia**, or **Pulsatilla**.

Urine

For black urine, consider: **Lachesis**. Also: **Arsenicum, Apis, Natrum Mur**, and **Phosphorus**.

For brown urine, consider: **Arnica, Arsenicum**, or **Bryonia**. Also: **Phosphorus, Rhus Tox**, and **Pulsatilla**. Also: **Sepia** and **Lycopodium**.

For greenish urine, consider: **Ruta, Veratrum, Arsenicum**, and **Calcarea**.

For earth-colored or clay-colored urine, consider: **Sepia**. Also: **Sulphur**. Also: **Phosphorus** and **Thuja**.

For red urine, consider: **Bryonia, Sepia**, and **Mercurius**. Also: **Rhus Tox, Lycopodium, Nux, Dulcamara, Silicea, Sulphur**, and **Arnica**.

If the urine is blood red, consider: **Calcarea, Hepar Sulph,** and **Sepia**. Also: **Mercurius** and **Rhus Tox**.

If the urine is brownish red, consider: **Hepar Sulph**. Also: **Apis** and **Lycopodium**.

If the urine is dark red, consider: **Sepia**. Also: **Lycopodium, Bryonia, Apis, Belladonna, Mercurius**, and **Hepar Sulph**.

For urine that is pale in color, consider: **Ledum, Natrum Mur**, and **Mercurius**. Also: **Rhus Tox, Phosphorus, Nux, Arsenicum, Arnica, Belladonna, Bryonia**, and **Carbo Veg**.

If the urine is totally colorless, consider: **Gelsemium, Natrum Mur, Sepia**, and **Sulphur**. Also: **Phosphorus** and **Pulsatilla**.

For urine that is dark in color, consider: **Aconite, Belladonna, Mercurius, Lachesis, Veratrum, Bryonia**, and **Calcarea**.

For urine with a strong odor, consider: **Sulphur, Sepia, Arnica, Apis, Calcarea, Dulcamara, Carbo Veg,** and **Phosphorus**. Also: **Rhus Tox, Mercurius**, and **Arsenicum**.

If the urine smells acidic, consider: **Lycopodium** and **Rhus Tox**.

If the urine smells like sweaty feet, consider: **Sulphur**.

If the urine smells sweetish, consider: **Phosphorus**.

If the urine smells sour, consider: **Sepia**. Also: **Mercurius** and **Calcarea**. Also: **Hepar Sulph**.

If the urine has no smell, consider: **Belladonna** and **Spongia**.

Stool

For a black stool, consider: **Arsenicum, Mercurius**, and **Veratrum**. Also: **Calcarea, Thuja, Phosphorus**, and **Natrum Mur**. Also: **Nux, Hepar Sulph**, and **Lachesis**.

For a brown stool, consider: **Mercurius, Lycopodium, Veratrum**, and **Apis**. Also: **Arnica, Arsenicum, Lachesis, Phosphorus**, and **Bryonia**.

For a stool that is clay-colored or earth-colored, consider: **Mercurius**. Also: **Lachesis** and **Phosphorus**.

If the stool actually seems to be made from clay, consider: **Calcarea**.

For a stool that is gray-colored, consider: **Arsenicum, Phosphorus**, and **Mercurius**. Also: **Lachesis**.

For a stool that is green-colored, consider: **Mercurius, Pulsatilla, Sulphur, Phosphorus, Veratrum**, and **Ipecac**. Also: **Arsenicum, Dulcamara, Rhus Tox** and **Natrum Mur**.

If the stool is blackish green, consider: **Arsenicum, Phosphorus, Mercurius**, and **Veratrum**.

If the stool is bluish green, consider: **Phosphorus**.

If the stool is brownish green, consider: **Arsenicum, Calcarea, Sulphur, Dulcamara**, or **Veratrum**.

If the stool is green as grass, consider: **Ipecac**. Also: **Thuja** and **Aconite**.

If the stool is olive green, consider: **Apis**. Also: **Arsenicum**.

If the stool is yellow-green, consider: **Ipecac**.

For a stool that is orange, consider: **Apis**.

For a stool that is reddish-colored, consider: **Rhus Tox** and **Mercurius**. Also: **Lycopodium, Silicea, Phosphorus**, and **Sulphur**.

For a stool that is white-colored, consider: **Pulsatilla**. Also: **Belladonna, Rhus Tox, Apis, Calcarea, Dulcamara, Nux**, and **Spongia**. Also: **Phosphorus, Chamomilla**, and **Sepia**.

If the stool is white like chalk, consider: **Calcarea**. Also: **Silicea**. Also: **Belladonna, Hepar Sulph**, and **Mercurius**.

If the stool is like cooked egg white, consider: **Urtica Urens**.

If the stool is gray-white, consider: **Phosphorus**. Also: **Dulcamara**.

If the stool is gray-white and streaked with blood, consider: **Calcarea**.

If the stool is milk white, consider: **Calcarea** and **Mercurius**. Also: **Belladonna, Arnica, Sulphur, Dulcamara, Gelsemium**, and **Nux**.

For a stool that is yellow-colored, consider: **Dulcamara, Rhus Tox, Lycopodium**, and **Thuja**. Also: **Mercurius**. Then consider: **Apis, Bryonia, Hepar Sulph, Kali Bi**, and **Lachesis**.

If the stool is bright yellow, consider: **Phosphorus**. Also: **Gelsemium**.

If the stool is brownish yellow, consider: **Apis**.

If the stool is greenish yellow, consider: **Sulphur**. Also: **Pulsatilla, Apis, Mercurius, Veratrum**, and **Dulcamara**.

If the stool is saffron-colored, consider: **Mercurius**.

If the stool is whitish yellow, consider: **Sulphur**. Also: **Ignatia, Pulsatilla, Phosphorus, Aconite**, and **Lycopodium**.

For a stool that is light-colored or pale-colored, consider: **Mercurius**. Also strongly consider: **Calcarea, Arsenicum, Silicea**, and **Lycopodium**. Also: **Phosphorus, Gelsemium, Hepar Sulph**, and **Kali Bi**.

For a stool that is dark-colored, consider: **Graphites**. Also: **Rhus Tox, Nux, Bryonia, Arnica, Lachesis**, and **Arsenicum**. Also: **Veratrum** and **Carbo Veg**.

For a bloody stool, consider: **Nux, Phosphorus**, and **Arsenicum**. Also consider: **Aconite, Belladonna**, and **Rhus Tox**.

If the stool has bloody streaks, consider: **Nux** mand **Mercurius**. Also: **Rhus Tox**.

For a stool that contains what appears to be chopped foods, consider: **Aconite**. Also: **Chamomilla** and **Rhus Tox**.

If the stool looks like chopped beets, consider: **Apis**.

If the stool looks like chopped eggs, consider: **Mercurius** or **Pulsatilla**. Also: **Chamomilla** and **Sulphur**.

If a stool looks like chopped spinach, consider: **Aconite**. Also: **Chamomilla** and **Mercurius**.

For a stool that actually contains undigested foods, consider: **Bryonia, Calcarea, Phosphorus**, and **Graphites**. Also: **Lycopodium, Mercurius, Pulsatilla**, and **Sulphur**. Also: **Rhus Tox**.

For a stool that is long and thin like a dog's, consider: **Phosphorus**. Also: **Staphysagria**.

For a stool with an offensive smell, consider: **Carbo Veg, Graphites**, and **Sulphur**. Also: **Arsenicum** and **Lachesis**. Also consider: **Silicea, Phosphorus, Apis**, and **Nux**.

If the patient takes on this same offensive smell, consider: **Sulphur**.

For a stool that smells like a cadaver, consider: **Carbo Veg** and **Lachesis**. Also consider: **Arsenicum**. Also: **Bryonia, Chamomilla, Sulphur, Silicea, Phosphorus**, and **Rhus Tox**.

If the stool smells like rotting cheese, consider: **Bryonia** and **Hepar Sulph**.

If a stool smells like rotten eggs, consider: **Calcarea**. Also: **Arsenicum** and **Staphysagria**. Also: **Sulphur** and **Phosphorus**.

If the stool smells sour, consider: **Calcarea, Mercurius, Hepar Sulph**, and **Sulphur**. Also: **Arnica, Dulcamara**, and **Graphites**. Also: **Phosphorus**.

For an odorless stool, consider: **Veratrum**. Also: **Kali Bi**. Also: **Apis** and **Phosphorus**.

Acute Remedies
and Their Uses

Introduction

WHILE IT IS MOST IMPORTANT that when we study homeopathy we study materia medica, it is also true that sometimes there is a situation at hand in which there is no time to study materia medica. We just need help in finding a remedy that will be curative in that given situation.

Therefore, I have gathered together information on some of the most basic uses of the common acute remedies. And I have gathered them into some basic categories.

The first category is WOUNDS. In this section, we deal with those ailments that are classified as either mechanical illness or physical trauma, all those circumstances that come upon us from blows and bruises, and from cuts, with the site of the injury being the soft tissue of the body—most commonly, the skin.

While these symptoms of pain are forced upon us by circumstance, it is important that we interpret them and work with them as we would any other symptom of the human system. We must remember that the bruising that appears after a blow to the body is not caused by the blow itself, but by the body's response to the blow. We must continue to treat the symptoms with the Law of Similarity as always. Therefore, while the case taken for a physical trauma may be much simpler and shorter than the case taken for a flu, it must still be well taken and interpreted.

The second section of this guide deals with INJURIES TO MUSCLE, JOINTS, AND BONES. Here we continue in the realm of mechanical illness, again caused by any number of accidents. However in this case, the part of the body affected by the accident is a joint or the soft tissue that connects joints or bones. Therefore, this section will cover strains, sprains, dislocations, and fractures.

The final section for mechanical injuries is called EMERGENCIES. This is sort of a cluster category for the crises, like nosebleeds, that can come from many causes but tend to happen suddenly and take us by surprise. In this category, I have also listed both emotional emergencies and a problem that has troubled me in the past—vertigo.

When an emergency occurs—from an accident to a gash or blow—we often must look at the needs of the moment, rather than any long-term health goals, in order to save a life. In other words, it is in the domain of emergency medicine that we may have to set aside the Three Laws of Cure (specifically, the Law of Simplex) and appropriately seek to preserve life, to control the impact of injury, and to relieve pain. Whatever measures we must take to save lives—both homeopathic and allopathic—are healing gifts in that moment. Because it is in first aid and emergency medicine that homeopathy and allopathy most easily join together with the common goal of the preservation of life above all else.

In general, when we deal with a crisis situation, it is important that we keep as clear a head as possible. It also helps to remember that it is most important to know that the symptoms that the person in crisis is experiencing are signs that his vital force is still working. Also remember that it is far less important to know exactly how the symptoms were brought about—instead it is only necessary that you know what the symptoms are and what remedy speaks to those symptoms. Remember that in treating first-aid injuries. The cause is secondary; the way the body reacts to whatever has caused injury or illness is of primary importance.

Note that this is a guide to the use of homeopathic remedies and not a book of medical first aid. My goal is to assist in the correct selection and use of homeopathic remedies in acute situations. But, in some cases, I include basic information in first aid.

The next category is GENERAL ACHES AND PAINS. Here I have gathered together information on common noninfectious ailments, such as toothaches and indigestion, and supplemented them with as complete a listing of acute remedies as possible. It is important to know your limits in using any form of medicine and important to know when to call for help.

Next is the category COMMON AILMENTS. These conditions are, for the most part, contagious. Listings here are for the most common ailments and remedies for home use: colds, flus, sore throats, and the like. Also included are many illnesses that would be considered "children's" illnesses: chicken pox, measles, and related ailments.

It is important that we know what we are treating when we treat any of these common ailments, as any of these may or may not be considered acute. The child who has a cold every winter may be considered to be in an acute illness, but the child who gets three or four colds every winter needs to be considered chronically ill from a homeopathic point of view, and as such in need of constitutional treatment from a professional practitioner.

In our desire to have everything as straightforward and simple as possible, we may try to treat a constitutional situation as if it were simply acute. If we do this one of two things will happen—either the remedy selected will work less effectively with each use (in that we have selected a boy's remedy to do a man's job), or the remedy will have a much greater impact upon the person than we ever suspected it would (you have touched the constitutional situation with its constitutional remedy, which you thought to be only an acute remedy). In either of those two cases, having the telephone number of a good professional is very important.

So, to be sure that you are treating acutely, treat the acutes—bumps on the head, food poisoning, etc. If you are not sure it is an acute situation, please consider professional constitutional care.

The final section of this acute guide is called ACUTE ASPECTS OF CHRONIC COMPLAINTS. Here I list the homeopathic treatments most common for conditions such as allergies and asthma, as well as headaches and fever.

In most cases, even if they seem acute, these ailments tend to be the tips of icebergs. They are signs that all is not well with the immune system. Therefore, they are listed here as stopgap treatments, as remedies that may be considered while waiting for your appointment with your practitioner. They are the remedies to use in the dead of the night to get you through those hours until dawn. I have gathered these together for you because they tend to be among the hardest sets of symptoms to treat effectively.

In each section of this guide, I have listed first the topical remedies, if any. Then I list those remedies that are the most common in usage and are also listed in the brief acute materia medica at the back of this volume. And finally, I list any other remedies I think are important for that specific topic.

From time to time, the word *aqua* may appear in front of the name of a remedy listed for topical use. This simply refers to making a topical rub of a remedy by dissolving it in water and placing the liquid remedy at the site of the wound. This is a term that has been popularized in recent years by a homeopathic practitioner named Robin Murphy. It should be remembered that any remedy may be dissolved in water and used both topically and internally. If you are creating an aquafied version of a remedy, be sure to use a few pellets and dissolve them in pure water and store in a clean glass container. Keep that covered container in your refrigerator and the remedy will remain potent in this state for a couple of days.

Finally, I have, where possible, also listed a **REMEDY CHECKLIST**, which will, in very general terms, speak to the causation of the problem at hand and will make a suggestion of remedies to consider. I hope it will be of help.

WOUNDS
In General

Wounds are defined as any break in the overall wholeness of the soft tissues of the body. Most often, they therefore involve the skin as the principal site of the wound. They are usually produced by some mechanical agent— that is, some third party, whether it is a knife, a hard surface like pavement, or an insect's stinger. They may be classified as *incised, contused, lacerated*, and *puncture wounds.*

An *incised* wound is one made by a clean, sharp object such as a knife. It is generally the most easily treated. Stopping the bleeding is often the hardest part of dealing with such a wound. The incisions made during any form of surgery are, of course, to be considered wounds of this type and recovery from surgery might be enhanced with the use of remedies listed here.

A *contused* wound is inflicted by some blunt instrument that injures the parts underneath the skin without breaking the skin itself (see entry on bruises).

A *lacerated* wound is where the soft parts are torn asunder by violence, leaving a ragged edge. This sort of wound bleeds less than an incised wound, but may prove slow and difficult to heal.

A *puncture* wound is one made by a sharp, narrow instrument, such as a needle, thorn, or nail. In homeopathic terms, insect bites will be treated as puncture wounds as well. Puncture wounds may be slow to heal, and offer the danger of infection (see entry on puncture wounds).

While these categories of wounds may be helpful in understanding the challenges at hand presented by a specific wound, remember that in the practice of acute homeopathy we will always work in the same way: by finding the remedy that is most similar in action to the situation at hand.

In dealing with a wound, the first thing that needs to be done is to stop the bleeding. This is usually accomplished by pressure on the wound, and/ or by the raising of the limb and the application of cold water or ice. The next step is the removal of all dirt, gravel, and other matter from the wound. This is best done with running water and a clean, soft cloth. Finally, the wound should be bandaged to protect it from reinjury. In cases of extensive wounds, and those of the eyebrows, eyelids, ears, and some other parts of the body, it may be necessary to use stitches to keep the edges of the wound together and bring about a neat healing of the wound.

EXTERNAL REMEDIES

ARNICA—This remedy is to be used only in contused wounds, and in sprains and dislocations. Should Arnica be placed on open skin, the patient will experience severe pain. This is a mistake that most of us make once and only once.

CALENDULA—This used for all incised, punctured, and lacerated wounds—whenever the skin has been broken. As a natural antibiotic, Calendula helps to guard against infection, while promoting healing of the wound.

HYPERICUM—An excellent topical treatment. Use a Hypericum rub, or create Aqua Hypericum by dissolving the remedy in water and then applying the remedy to the wound. For patients who are experiencing nerve pain from their wound and who seem foggy in their response.

REMEDIES

ACONITE—For wounds that are accompanied by great fear and anxiety. When the patient is greatly debilitated by the injury. And yet, the patient will be restless. He will rave about the future and may predict the time of his own death. The patient will be greatly fearful of death. Consider this remedy when shock accompanies the wound.

ARNICA—The first remedy to be thought of in helping to heal any injury. It should be given as soon as possible after the accident. There are sore, aching pains. The injury feels bruised. The whole patient feels injured—everything on which he lies feels too hard. The patient will not want to be touched. Often, such patients will insist that they are all right, that nothing is wrong with them, and will refuse any treatment. Also an excellent shock remedy.

CHAMOMILLA—Copious infection, with severe pains; the wound is very slow to heal. Patient is very impatient, furious at his injury. The emotional actions of the patient are the best indicator here. Expect the patient to rush about. Expect him to be demanding and to throw things.

CHINA—For the case in which the patient experiences great exhaustion from loss of blood. The patient also experiences vertigo and fainting spells. The patient's face will be dreadfully pale. Look for the patient to complain of a throbbing headache from loss of blood. Consider this remedy in all cases of wounds that are difficult to stop bleeding, when the patient is rapidly losing strength from bleeding.

HEPAR SULPH—Every little cut and/or injury seems to become infected. Especially useful in patients with a tendency to injure themselves time and again. Also think of this remedy in cases in which an infected wound is slow to heal or continues to become reinfected. Think of this remedy first for any wound of any sort that has become infected.

HYPERICUM—An extraordinary remedy for lacerations of all sorts. Historically, this remedy has been used to save limbs that have been all but separated from the body, and this has been a great first choice in cases of animal bites, especially for wounds caused by the bites of rodents. Look for the patient to seem foggy. This is also a remedy for shock and for patients who are emotionally disconnected from their situation. The pain that the patient experiences will run along the nerves and radiate throughout the body.

PHOSPHORUS—The blood flowing from the wound is bright red. Every wound, no matter how small, bleeds a great deal. Given in homeopathic hospitals to stop bleeding after surgery. This is an excellent remedy to consider for any wound that bleeds a great deal. For wounds in which the bleeding is hard to stop. The patient will usually want company and will feel much better for feeling cared for.

SILICEA—Think of this remedy first for the patient who seems chronically slow to heal. Think of this remedy also for the patient in whom past wounds have developed into unhealthy scar tissue and keloids. The Silicea patient will be timid and fearful. He will have unhealthy-looking skin. He will be chilly.

STAPHASAGRIA—The first remedy to think of in cases of knife blows and wounds. In any case that involves a clean cut. The patient will be overwhelmed with pain. Will not be able to think of anything but the pain. This, along with Phosphorus, is used to speed postsurgical recovery.

WOUNDS
Scrapes and Scratches

We are here considering any break to the skin that allows blood to escape, and which may allow infection to enter. The first step is to stop the bleeding and prevent infection. Try not to touch the wound. Clean it with a sterile pad that has been soaked in a solution of Calendula. You may give Hypericum internally if there is nerve pain, or you may mix the two as a liquid tincture (not the best homeopathic method, but in an emergency it may be required to speed recovery).

From here, it is a matter of severity. Dress the wound and leave it to heal if it is not a serious condition. Proceed to the emergency room for stitches if the wound is deep.

REMEDIES

ARNICA—Useful especially for wounds that need stitches; aids healing. Be careful to only use Arnica internally in cases that involve broken skin. Applying the remedy topically to broken or cut skin will cause the patient a great deal of pain. Use Calendula topically for this sort of wound, and Arnica may be used concurrently as an internal remedy.

HYPERICUM—For scratches and scrapes that are causing the patient to experience internal nerve pain. The patient will have his senses dulled by the pain. He will seem to be in a fog. His pains will feel electrical and numb.

STAPHYSAGRIA—For wounds that are very painful. The patient will seem to be in more pain than could be possible from the injury. The patient may be very angry in his pain.

Note: Continue to soothe the wound with Calendula with each change of bandage.

WOUNDS
Puncture Wounds

In homeopathic terms, whether you have stepped on a nail or been stung by a bee, you are dealing with a puncture wound. While I will not deal with the situations surrounding the event (for instance, you should seek medical attention if you step on a rusty nail), it goes without saying that for puncture wounds, just as for any other event that breaks the skin, cleanliness is next to godliness, so clean the wound before you treat it.

Just as with any other type of wound, consider externally using Calendula or Hypericum, or a combination of both, in the form of a tincture for wounds that involve both nerve pain and broken skin.

REMEDIES

APIS—This is the usual first remedy to be considered when a puncture wound has occurred. Apis wounds are red and swollen. They feel hot to the touch, and the wound feels better for cold applications. Apis is made from the honeybee, and the feel of this wound is the feel of having been stung by a bee.

ARNICA—This remedy should never be overlooked as a solid remedy for puncture wounds. They are, after all, wounds, and will heal faster with the use of Arnica. The remedy should especially be considered for hornet stings, and for puncture wounds of all sorts that seem overwhelming, shocking to the overall system. Wounds with a degree of shock or collapse, or when the area feels bruised and sore. The area will swell but will not change color.

HYPERICUM—May be used internally for a puncture wound. Here the wound carries nerve pain with it. The pain will shoot up the arm, down the leg, etc.

LACHESIS—Used for puncture wounds (snake bites are also puncture wounds, after all, so what better remedy than snake venom?) in which the wound itches initially and only swells after it has been scratched. After scratching, the wound begins to hurt with a burning sensation. The swelling will usually be red–purple in color. Patient will feel worse for sleeping. If there is bleeding from the wound, look for the blood to be dark.

LEDUM—Here the wound is cold to the touch. Internally it also feels cold, and "squishy." And yet, the wound still is better with use of cold applications. The wound itself may be red or purple in color.

RHUS TOX—Highly useful in spider bites, when the reaction is bright red in color. The area may swell and itch (similar to poison ivy in both itch and color). Alternative remedy here is Ledum, to be considered when the spider bite feels cold. In the Rhus wound, the patient feels wound up, restless, very concerned about the wound.

STAPHYSAGRIA—Said to be a potent weapon against the mosquito. Classic homeopathic literature claims that mosquitoes will stay away if Staphysagria 12C is taken before you travel outdoors.

ALSO CONSIDER

CANTHARIS—Very helpful for punctures in which the major sensation is hard, hard burning. Look for the patient to say that it feels more like he burned his skin on a hot stove, rather than having been stung or punctured.

CROTALUS—An alternative to Lachesis, here look for rapid swelling of the skin; the skin will be discolored from blood under the skin. The patient will be very sensitive to movement and much worse for being shaken, for any jarring motion.

TARENTULA—Used in puncture wounds that may look at first like Apis. But look for the wound to have a blue color. The pain will have a burning sensation and the patient will be angry and difficult to deal with.

WOUNDS
Splinters

Another variation on the puncture wound, the splinter is a foreign object trapped in or below the skin.

Externally, the best bets are Hypericum, again for nerve pain radiating from the area of the splinter, and Calendula, to soothe the area and help keep it from becoming infected.

REMEDIES

ARNICA—May be used either internally or externally in helping the body heal. A general remedy for splinters and other punctures. But don't be too quick to use Arnica if one of the following remedies is better suited to the case.

HEPAR SULPH—Think of this remedy in the case in which the pain from the puncture is so intense that the patient cannot bear to have it touched. Think of this remedy especially in instances in which the foreign object seems to be becoming infected.

LEDUM—The most useful remedy for any deep splinters, most especially when the area has become infected. Look for swollen redness of the area and the local formation of pus. As is usual with Ledum, look for a sensation of cold in the area, and, often, a general chill to the patient. The patient will most often crave warmth for the body, but cold applications on the wound. Ledum is often alternated with Hypericum in cases in which the splinter has entered during an injury that has left part of the body crushed. Hypericum is also given as a preventative to tetanus.

SILICEA—Classical homeopathic literature is filled with stories of veterans of the world wars whose bodies shot out shrapnel with just one dose of Silicea. While your experience of the remedy may not be so extreme, be aware that it is very useful in helping to loosen any foreign object from the skin if no infection is present. Silicea may be used either externally or internally—or both. It may also be used along with Arnica to remove the splinter and promote healing. One would be used internally, one externally.

WOUNDS
Bruises

In the case of any injury in which the body has received a blow and blood flows under the skin, the discolored area is called a bruise. Most people, even those who are almost entirely unaware of the full range of possibilities that homeopathy offers, know that Arnica is the homeopathic bruise remedy. And in most cases Arnica will do the job very well—it will reduce swelling, relieve pain, and allow the body to reabsorb the bruise. And yet, in homeopathy we never have just one remedy available to us for any situation, because we must seek to personalize the situation—always treating a person in a given situation, never treating the situation (or the disease) itself.

And so we cannot take the allopathic route. We must seek to use Arnica when Arnica is called for, and other remedies for bruises when they seem appropriate.

REMEDIES

ARNICA—The usual remedy for a bruise. Bruising from bumps and blows to any part of the body. Blows to soft tissue, to skin. Bruising of any sort, with or without swelling. Look for the characteristic shock in the person who has been bruised. As if they were on "seven-second delay." They seem slow, a little frozen. For fresh bruises.
Note: Classical homeopaths considered that Arnica was of much greater use than many do today. Arnica has been used successfully to treat headaches in which the head feels bruised. Also, it has been used in the treatment of emotional "bruising" from receiving bad news and from nightmares. Constitutionally, the Arnica type has been a "Princess and the Pea" sort of person, for whom everything seems too hard—the mattress, clothing, and, even, life in general.

BELLIS PERENNIS—A remedy made from the daisy, Bellis is the correct remedy for deep bruises and bruises that Arnica fails to heal. Use Bellis for deep muscle pain and for bruises that do not improve in 24 hours with the use of Arnica.

CALCAREA—A little-known bruise remedy. Just as Calcarea is a remedy that improves digestion in general and is required by those with chronic faulty digestion, it is also a wonderful remedy for long-term bruises that have never been fully reabsorbed into the body. Arnica is a wonderful bruise remedy while the bruise still has red in it. When the bruise has moved on to the stage in which it is blue or even brownish, Calcarea will greatly speed healing.

HEPAR SULPH—For bruises that fail to heal. When the bruise becomes filled with pus. The patient will be exhausted; will feel toxic or infected. The patient will talk of the pain as the sensation of a splinter or something else caught in the skin.

LEDUM—Used for black eyes and may be considered for any other bruise (most usually to the ankle or wrist) that follows the typical Ledum formula: the bruised area is cold to the touch and the patient is chilly in general. Most often the patient wants to keep the body warm, but the injury feels better for cold applications (think of black eyes again and the cold steaks that are traditionally pressed against them). The area feels squishy both to the touch and to the person who has been injured. Often the bruised area will be numb.

RUTA—Used when the bone itself is bruised, or when the bruise is to the muscle ligaments that connect muscle to bone. Motion will be very difficult. The patient will usually also be very thirsty. This is an excellent remedy to consider for shin splints that develop after exercising on too hard a floor surface. Also for situations in which the action of rising up from a sitting position is especially difficult.

ALSO CONSIDER

CONIUM—A sort of backup remedy to be thought of when Arnica or Ruta has failed to work. For bruising that is associated with a general sensation of muscle weakness. This is a remedy for the patient with a weak body and a weak mind; whose body trembles. Especially consider this remedy for any case that involves a bruising in the area of the spine.

WOUNDS
Injuries to the Eye

While black eyes were covered in the previous section on bruising, eyes can be injured in a number of ways, and few things can be as painful as a scratch on the cornea.

It is important to note that the eye is perhaps the fastest organ in the body to heal and that most injuries to the eye will heal within 48 hours. Extreme sensitivity to light is a common symptom in eye injuries, as is ongoing tearing of the eye.

As vision is our most important sense, it is vital that we promptly turn to professionals to help us with injuries to our eyes, using the remedies listed here as an emergency treatment until help can be obtained.

EXTERNAL REMEDIES

CALENDULA—Can be used as an eyewash (10 drops of the mother tincture mixed with a pint of warm water) for foreign objects in the eye or a blow to the eye. Also excellent for cuts around the eye. Apply as needed to prevent infection and to assist healing process. Best if mixed with Hypericum in one solution.

EUPHRASIA—Mother tincture of Euphrasia can be mixed with warm water (10 drops tincture to a pint of water) to create Aqua Euphrasia to bathe an eye that has a foreign object in it. Use the eye wash every 3 or 4 hours while also giving Euphrasia, or another of the remedies listed below. This eye wash is generally soothing to the eye and can also be used for blows to the eye and for snow blindness.

HYPERICUM—Can be used in an eye wash (mix 10 drops of mother tincture with a pint of water) alone or in combination with Calendula. Excellent for nerve pain in association with a blow to the eye or foreign objects in the eye.

REMEDIES

ACONITE—For any chemical injury to the eye. Or for accidents that occur very quickly. The patient will be anxious and very frightened. The patient will be very restless, will refuse to sit down, and will pace around the room in great pain. Fever may accompany the pain, as will great thirst. It is also an excellent remedy for deep cuts around the eye. Symptoms will remain the same, with fear a major feature.

APIS—Here the major symptom is a feeling of heat in the eye and the aggravation that the eye gets from any application of heat. There will be a great deal of swelling of the eyelids. The eyeball itself may swell so that the iris of the eye can look as if it were sitting in a shallow depression. The eye will be red. Tears, like the eye itself, feel hot. Only cold brings relief.

ARNICA—For blows from blunt objects. While the remedy is not specific for the eye, it will speed the healing from any sort of blow or bruise. The remedy will work best if given immediately after the accident has taken place. Will assist in healing process. If pain persists after Arnica has been given, follow with Ledum to complete cure.

BELLADONNA—Useful for any blow to the eye, or for a scratch on the cornea. The eye will be bright red, bloodshot, and will feel hot. The pain will be throbbing in nature. Tears will flow. Major symptom will be intense sensitivity to light. The patient will likely be in such great pain that he will pace the room; he will be unable to rest, to sleep. Think of Belladonna and Apis in cases involving scratched cornea. Also a great remedy for snow blindness.

EUPHRASIA—A general remedy for the eye. Look for a great flow of tears, but the tears are acrid and will burn the face. Eye will feel as if there were dust or sand in it. Tears begin as clear, but may change to yellow, opaque material. Also a great remedy for snow blindness.

LEDUM—An excellent remedy for black eyes. The eye has been injured by a blunt object. The area of the bruise is blue in color. Keynote symptom is that the bruise feels cold and squishy to the touch, and yet the patient wants cold applications on the injury. Because of these keynotes, think of this for black eyes. They respond especially well to a dose of Arnica given right after the injury, and then Ledum given afterward to complete the cure.

MERCURIUS—Here the discharge from the eye is yellow/green. Mercurius is often used as a second remedy in the recovery from an injury to an eye. The first stage of clear tears has passed and the eye now secretes a yellow thick liquid. Light will bother the eye, which will also be worse at night in bed. Any sort of glare will cause intense pain.

PULSATILLA—A remedy for the second stage of eye injury. The tears are yellow to green in color and they are thick, although the tears do not in any way irritate the skin. A warm room makes all symptoms worse; the eye feels better when the patient goes out of doors into open air. Cold applications also make the eye feel better.

STAPHYSAGRIA—For black eyes that come on in anger during a physical fight. The patient will be very sensitive to their pain; will complain of cutting pains, pains that seem worse than the situation usually calls for. The patient will complain of bursting pains; will complain of a sensation of heat in the eyes.

SYMPHYTUM—This is the best first remedy to think of when an eye is injured by a blunt object such as a football or a fist. Look for the area around the eye to take on the traditional purplish blue color. This is, perhaps, the general "black eye" remedy. Consider this remedy for any eye pain after a mechanical injury from a blunt object.

INJURIES TO MUSCLES, JOINTS, AND BONE
Strains and Sprains (Subluxation) in General

Strains and sprains may involve muscles, tendons, or ligaments. A sprain is a violent stretching or twisting of the soft parts surrounding the joints. Here the body has attempted to do more than it safely could handle, leaving the back, the hips, or any other specific area of the body open to injury. The degree of the stretch or twist will determine whether the fibrous parts of the joint have been simply stretched or completely ruptured.

Externally, an Arnica rub should always be used, as long as the skin has not been broken in the injury. No matter what remedy or remedies may be used internally to handle the specific case, an Arnica rub will assist in removing the pain of the injury and will promote healing. After the rub has been applied, the limb should be placed in an elevated position and held perfectly still.

REMEDIES

APIS—For strains and sprains that involve redness, swelling, and stinging pains. Apis has a particular affinity for the knee and knee pain, but may also be very helpful for a sprained ankle. For general sprains and strains, Apis and Rhus Tox have a special affinity for each other and often complete each other's action.

ARNICA—This is the closest thing to allopathy that homeopathy has. Whenever there is a strain or sprain, in virtually every part of the body for every individual person, the very best first remedy is Arnica. Often the remedy will not complete the entire case and will need to be followed by a more individualized remedy, but whenever there is a strain or sprain, reach for the Arnica first, at least one dose, to begin the healing process before moving on to the next remedy.

BRYONIA—The remedy when the strain or sprain is painful with any movement. Bryonia is the major remedy for cracked ribs, and if you have ever cracked a rib, you know how painful it is to move at all—even to breathe. This is the Bryonia sensation. The patient must stay very still; even moving his eyes may be painful. And he will want to be left alone; he will not want to be helped. He may get angry if you bother him, or especially if you suggest that he try to move. Look for the patient to have great stiffness in the joints.

RHUS TOX—The most commonly used remedy for any sort of strain or sprain, particularly when someone is said to have "thrown their back out." The injury has to do with overdoing it—too much exercise, lifting too heavy a box, etc. Rhus Tox is called the "rusty hinge" remedy— the person feels that the injured part is like a rusted gate hinge. Look for the greatest pain to be on first motion, upon first getting out of a chair or out of bed in the morning, for instance. As the patient moves gently, however, the injured part feels warmed, looser, and less painful. There is a limit to this improvement, however, and as the patient continues to move, look for the injury to become more painful again. The Rhus patient is restless. He will not sit still, cannot get comfortable. Look for him to continue to shift and move in trying to get comfortable. Consider also for sprained wrists and ankles. Can also be very effective for a wounded Achilles' tendon.

RUTA—The remedy for injury to ligaments or tendons. It is wonderful for shin splints that can come on after too vigorous a workout. It is helpful for runner's knee (you may have to alternate Apis and Ruta to completely clear runner's knee) and for any knee situation in which the knee is pained when the patient tries to walk up stairs. Ruta is also a great remedy for lower back pain—pain that makes rising from a chair and getting out of a car the most difficult motions.

ALSO CONSIDER

ANACARDIUM—To be considered for a hurt Achilles' tendon when Rhus fails to work. For strained hamstrings, which hurt like hell, try Ammonium Muriaticum. And for any sprain that stubbornly refuses to heal, even though you've tried every possible homeopathic remedy, use Zinc.

INJURIES TO MUSCLE, JOINTS, AND BONES
Backache: Lumbago

Lumbago is a pain in the small of the back, usually associated with lifting too much weight or somehow straining the back. In its chronic state, lumbago is usually worse in cold or damp weather (see Rheumatic remedies). The attack may come on very suddenly; the individual may be moving about freely without any pain, and, the next moment, when in the act of stooping or rising from a sitting position, be in terrible pain. Pain may last from seven days to several weeks if left untreated.

REMEDIES

ACONITE—Sudden sharp pain, worse for exposure to cold air. The patient will be restless. Even if he is bed bound, he will toss and turn in his restlessness.

ANTIMONIUM TARTARICUM—Pain without relief or ceasing. Pain with nausea and vomiting. Worse for cold in general. Patient covered in cold sweat, very tired. Worse for eating. The patient is better for standing, which is, in general, the most comfortable position. He will tend to feel nauseous if he attempts to move while in pain.

ARNICA—The first remedy to try for severe lower back pain that comes on after an injury. This is especially called for in cases of aches and pains that have been brought on from an injury or accident. But think of this remedy when the patient describes the pain as "bruised." The patient will not be able to find a comfortable postition. He feels that every surface is too hard. Even the bed will feel too hard. He will not want to be touched and may become angry if you try to touch him.

BELLADONNA—Intense cramplike pain in the small of the back. A feeling as if the back would break, hindering any motion. Look for a red face and a hot head to accompany back pain. Look for the patient to be angry, difficult, and demanding. Pains will occur and leave very quickly and without warning.

BRYONIA—Deep pain in back, worse for any motion. Patient must lie very still, usually angry and difficult to deal with. Back feels sensitive and worse for touch, better for lying against hard object (like the floor). Constipation may accompany back pain. The patient will drink seldom, but when he does he will drink huge amounts of water. He will want to be left alone and will get angry if you don't just leave.

CALCAREA—This remedy is only to be considered in cases of chronic low back pain. Here, the patient will tell you that he has a weak back. This is especially true of the constitutional Calcarea, who tends to be heavyset and who tends to have underdeveloped abdominal muscles. Think of this remedy for lower back pain in persons of this type. Pain comes on if the feet get cold and wet.

CAUSTICUM—The patient will feel that the back is totally paralyzed. The pain will be worse in the left side of the back. The patient will not be able to walk without great pain. He will feel very heavy. The back will also feel numb and internally cold. The patient is better with warmth, especially the warmth of bed. It will usually feel as if the muscles in the back have shrunk and tightened into steel bands. The patient will feel better in rainy weather.

COLOCYNTHIS—All the muscles in the lower back and lower limbs feel constricted and shortened. It is as if all the limbs have been drawn together. The patient will feel a cramplike pain in the lower back that extends into the hip. The patient will want to lie down on the painful side of the body. The pain will run down the right thigh. Pain in the left knee.

DULCAMARA—As with Sulphur, pain is worse while stooping. Worse for exertion. Very much worse in cold, damp weather, which will bring on chronic pain. The pains will be worst during times of year in which the days are sunny and hot and the evenings cool. Worse in autumn and spring.

MERCURIUS—Symptoms worse at night and from any change in the weather. Worse from damp, cold weather. Patient sweats freely, but it does not relieve him. The patient will also be very sensitive to temperature changes, and will always be either hot or cold.

NATRUM MUR—This is a great general backache remedy if the patient wants firm support for the back. The patient will just want to go lie down (also consider Rhus Tox, Sepia). The patient's arms will feel weak during the back pain. The legs will feel cold, while the head and chest feel congested and hot. The patient will be very thirsty.

NUX—The patient is very angry, and the pain in the back is worse from any cold. Especially if the patient is in a cold draft. Pain from any movement of air. Pain in the small of the back as if bruised, worse from turning in bed. Back pain accompanied by hemorrhoids and constipation. The patient will demand alcohol or drugs to stifle the pain.

RHUS TOX—The pain comes on from overlifting or overstretching. Lower back feels stiff and bruised. Worse on first motion after rest. Worse in damp weather. Slow, steady motion improves the pain. Pain also relieved by lying on something hard. The patient may also want to take a hot shower to ease the pain. He will stay in the shower a long time, with the water beating down hot and hard on the painful part. Worse at night, particularly after midnight, worse before a storm and in damp weather.

RUTA—An excellent remedy for lumbago. Backache will be better from pressure and from lying down on the back. And yet look for the patient to complain that the pain is worse in the morning just before rising. The pain will extend down the back and into the hips and legs. The legs will give out under the patient as he tries to rise up out of a chair. The hamstrings in the legs feel shortened. Lumbago from overwork.

SEPIA—A good general remedy for lower back pain that is associated with a desire to have support on the back. The patient will feel heavy. The back will feel shortened and tightened in pain. The lower back will feel stiff and heavy. A sense of heaviness is a general quality of the remedy type. Look for a sensation of weakness in the small of the back, with pains extending through the back. A sensation of coldness between the shoulder blades.

SULPHUR—Pain is stitching in character. Worse for stooping, worse for any movement. Sensation of heat throughout the body accompanies pain. Patient is also sweaty. Worse for heat of bed. The patient will want company. He will be very hungry. He will seem so well that you may suspect that he is not in as much pain as he says he is.

ALSO CONSIDER

AMMONIUM MUR—Think of this remedy for lower backache that is worse when the patient is in a sitting postion. Patients will say that they feel like their back is being tightened in a vise when they are in a sitting postion. Pain extends to the coccyx when the patient is sitting. Look for the patient to experience coldness between the shoulder blades.

BERBERIS—A general remedy for lower back pain that radiates out to the entire body. Remedy for long-term rheumatic ailments. Aching in the small of the back that extends to the extremities. Pain in the back associated with rheumatoid arthritis. Pain will be greatest in the region of the kidneys. Wandering and radiating pains. Pain is worse from standing, from any exercise.

CALCAREA PHOS—Take a look at the listing for Calcarea under this heading. This remedy is the alternative to Calcarea Carbonica for patients who have weak abdominal muscles and chronic lower back pain, but who are slender in body type. The back pain will have a cold and numb feeling associated with it. Patients are worse in any change of weather. Pain is worse from walking, especially from walking up stairs.

KALI CARB—Especially good for pain in the lower back that occurs just before a woman's menstrual cycle. The back will suddenly feel weak. The back and legs will feel like they are going to give out. Look for a sensation of burning to accompany the pain. Also excellent for severe backache that accompanies pregnancy.

RHODODENDRON—Can look just like Rhus Tox, but patient is much worse before thunderstorm or in dry, cold weather. Pain will be especially bad on the right side of the body. Pain will disappear and reappear with changes in the weather. Pain in the bone as well as the muscle. Consider this an excellent backup remedy for Rhus Tox.

INJURIES TO MUSCLE, JOINTS, AND BONES
Backache: Sciatica

This is pressure on the sciatic nerve, which supplies the leg. Pain shoots into buttock and leg, and sometimes down all the way to the foot (following the sciatic nerve from near the hip joint down the back part of the thigh to the knee). It is usually made worse for jerking movement, like coughing or sneezing. Usually better for sitting still. Sciatica is often accompanied by digestive upset.

REMEDIES

ACONITE—Pain is so severe that patient is desperate. Great fear and anxiety accompanies pain. Vertigo when rising from a seat. Worse at night. Great restlessness accompanies pain. Worse for cold.

ARSENICUM—For chronic rheumatic states. Typical in the elderly or in invalids. Worse at night, worse for becoming cold. Improved by heat and gentle exercise. For periodic attacks of sciatica. Pain is stinging, as if skin were pierced with hot needles. Terrible pain, especially at night.

BELLADONNA—Darting or tearing pains, which come quickly and end just as quickly. Dread of noise and of light. The patient will be better if he is left in a cool, dark place in a semi-erect position. Aggravations in the afternoon. Look for the characteristic red and hot face and head.

CAUSTICUM—Think of this remedy for left-sided sciatica. The keynote for the remedy is that the sciatic pain is accompanied by numbness. The patient will feel unsteady when he tries to walk. Will feel as if he is going to fall. The ankles will feel weak. The patient will be improved by heat, especially the heat of the bed.

CHAMOMILLA—Pain causes hot perspiration about the head. Patient cries out in pain. Is furious in pain. Very impatient, can hardly speak politely when spoken to. Great sensitiveness to pain.

COLOCYNTHIS—Pain shoots down the leg all the way to the foot, feelings of numbness and weakness in leg. Pain is worse for cold, damp weather. Pain chiefly on the left side. Aggravations from motion and from touch. Great restlessness and anxiety.

GELSEMIUM—As with Rhus Tox, worse on first motion. Patient weary, confused. Pains are burning in nature and worse at night. The patient emotionally and physically very slow. Exhaustion pronounced.

KALI BI—An excellent remedy to consider in left-sided sciatica. The pain will occur in one specific spot at a time. The pain will suddenly shift from place to place. The bones will feel sore and bruised. Look for the patient to feel very weak in times of pain.

LYCOPODIUM—Pain in right leg. Pain is worse for pressure or from lying on right side. Worse at 4 P.M. Pains will have a sensation of numbness and heaviness. The leg will feel very heavy. Look for the patient to have a hot right foot and a cold left foot.

MAGNESIA PHOS—Pain in right leg. Lightninglike in character. Better for heat. The pain will have an electric quality to it. Worse for any jerking motion, like coughing. Twitching will accompany pain. Parts feel stiff and numb.

NUX—Tearing pain, with numbness of the affected parts. Patient is very angry and wants to be left alone. Especially suited to those who eat highly seasoned foods, in which stomach upset accompanies sciatic pain.

RHUS TOX—Pain relieved for movement, for heat. Worse in cold, damp weather. Worse for sitting, lying, or sleeping too long. Worse at night, particularly after midnight. The patient will feel better for a hot shower.

SEPIA—The lower limbs will feel lame and stiff. There is a sense of gravity to the body; it is hard to move the lower limbs. And yet the patient is restless, and will likely want to exercise or move to ease the pain. Better from strong motion. Pain in the heels. The legs and feet will feel cold.

ALSO CONSIDER

AMMONIUM MUR—Pain worse for sitting still, better for walking, lying down, or sleeping. The patient will be worse when sitting. Patient has difficulty straightening the knee of the painful leg because hamstring has shortened. The patient will also have a pain in the heel. Will also tend to have sweaty feet.

KALI CARB—Burning pains, shooting into the knee and foot especially. Worse from coughing, legs feels itchy. Pain worse at 3 A.M. The legs will just give out from pain. Sudden pains up and down the back. An excellent remedy for sciatica during pregnancy.

NATRUM SULPH—As there perhaps is no greater rheumatic remedy, we must consider Natrum Sulph carefully in all cases of sciatic pain. No other remedy is as sensitive to damp, and to having to live and work in damp environments, like basements. Few other remedies are as sensitive to changes in weather and are as aggravated by damp weather. The patient will have pain in the left hip joint that will travel down to the knee. Stiff knees. General sciatica that is worse on the left.

INJURIES TO MUSCLES, JOINTS, AND BONES
Neck Pain

Neck pain can be caused by anything from sleeping on a bad pillow to stress and strain to weather conditions. While we are tempted to simply treat such a condition in and of itself, it is best still to place the specifics of the neck pain within the overall context of the whole being. You most often will find relief for this condition in the rheumatic and sciatic remedies.

Neck pain, may also, of course, be the result of a physical injury. In these cases, consider our usual array of remedies for those with physical trauma: Arnica, Rhus Tox, Hypericum, and Bryonia.

REMEDIES

ACONITE—For neck pain caused by exposure to cold, dry wind, or from suppressed sweat. Sudden pain of great intensity. The patient will panic in their pain. He will be very restless and will walk the floor in pain. (*Note:* Rhus will often be required as a follow-up remedy to finish cases of neck pain that are first treated with Aconite.)

BELLADONNA—When the neck is very stiff and painful to touch. Neck pain accompanied by a sore throat, with swollen glands in the neck. Look for redness and heat to accompany the pain. The patient is very demanding.

BRYONIA—This is perhaps our most important remedy in cases of neck pain caused by whiplash. As always, the pain is worse from any movement, and worse from touch. Better from pressure. Soreness extends to the internal throat and larynx. Neck pain may come on from cough. Patient is angry. Wants to be alone.

CAUSTICUM—The neck pain typical in this remedy includes a dull pain in the nape of the neck, as well as stiffness between the shoulder blades. The neck pain is more common on the left side. The neck has a dull, achy sensation. Numbness accompanies pain. Pain may travel down the arm to the hand. Hand is numb and totally lacking in sensation. Better with wet weather. This is an excellent remedy for the condition known as torticollis.

DULCAMARA—Pain at the top of the nape. Pain that seems to come from "sleeping funny." Better for heat. Worse from cold, or becoming chilled.

These pains tend to appear during the seasons in which the weather is hot and sunny during the day, but cool at night.

HYPERICUM—This is an excellent remedy for cases of neck pain that involve a sensation of tingling. Consider this for cases of whiplash. The pain will travel along the nerves into the shoulder and back. The patient will feel numbness as well as tingling in the pain state. The patient himself will seem a little numb, a little foggy.

RHUS TOX—If neck pain is caused by becoming drenched in the rain. The pain and soreness are relieved by continually moving the neck. The pain will be improved by gentle pressure. The patient will want to rub his neck. He will also want to take a hot shower and allow the hot water to beat on his neck.

SPIGELIA—This is an excellent remedy for those with pain that is located on the left side of their neck. The neck pain will be burning in nature, as if the patient had hot needles in his skin. Often the pain will radiate out to the left shoulder and into the left arm. The left arm and hand will be numb. The limb feels tired and weak. The patient is fatigued. Look for the patient's pain to be worse during the day and to begin to improve as the sun lowers on the horizon.

ALSO CONSIDER

BERBERIS—Rheumatic pains in the shoulders, arms, hands, and fingers. Pains will extend into the fingers, with pain under the fingernails. The patient will be worse from standing.

CHELIDONIUM—The patient's neck will feel stiff. It is frozen in postion to the left. The patient will also have a pain traveling under the right scapula. The patient's head will feel cold and heavy. He will crave heat.

CIMICIFUGA—Stiff neck. Chin is fixed in a raised position. Whole of the upper spine is tender and painful. Neck feels achy, muscles sore. The head feels heavy. This general sensation of heaviness will move down the spine and into the lower limbs.

NATRUM SULPH—Another excellent remedy for cases involving neck pain as a result of physical trauma. Especially from a blow to the head. Violent pain at the base of the brain, at the back of the neck.

RHODODENDRON—An excellent remedy for stiff necks. The pain will appear in a specific spot on the neck. Worse on the right side. Worse in damp and rainy weather, especially just before a thunderstorm. The pain may move into the shoulder, the arm, even the wrist.

INJURIES TO MUSCLES, JOINTS, AND BONES
Shoulder Pain

This type of pain is usually considered as a part of the rheumatism rubric. Those are the remedies of first choice. And, in general, this is the category of remedies that speak to pain in the upper half of the body. However, pain may be caused by injury or stress as well, and some specific shoulder remedies are as follows.

REMEDIES

BRYONIA—Following its general pattern, the pain in the area of the shoulder will be worse from any motion. Further, the area of the shoulder joint will feel very dry internally, as if the internal parts of the joint were grinding together whenever motion occured.

CAMPHORA—Rheumatic pains between the shoulders. The patient will have difficulty in making any motion. There will be a sensation of numbness associated with the pain. It is keynote of the remedy that the patient will feel a sensation of coldness in the painful area, as if it were covered in ice or snow. Also, icy cold feet accompany the pain.

RHUS TOX—The pain in shoulder is burning in sensation. Worse in cold, damp weather. Worse from rest, better from gentle motion. The patient will be worse upon first motion, but will feel better and better if he moves around a bit. This is bad in that the Rhus patient will tend to overdo the motion and keep going until the pain returns, worse than ever. In general, in cases of pain in the shoulder and related areas of the body, think first of Rhus if the case involves overwork or strained muscles. In general, the pain will be relieved by gentle motion and by warm applications.

SULPHUR—Rheumatic pain in left shoulder. Shoulder feels dead, heavy. Patient brings shoulder forward to feel relief. Look for the patient to walk stoop-shouldered. The pain will tend to come on slowly and build in intensity. Pain will be accompanied by itching. Look for the patient's hands to be hot and sweaty.

ALSO CONSIDER

CHELIDONIUM—Pain in the right shoulder with headache. Pain is located in the lower part of the shoulder blade. Pain will move into arms and down to the hands. Look for the patient to have icy cold fingertips. Look for the back of the patient's head to feel cold. The head is also heavy. The neck will feel stiff and drawn to the left. The patient will have a pain that travels from the neck to under the right scapula.

FERRUM—A remedy for those rheumatic pains in the region of the shoulders. Pain may travel downward to the hips. The patient is better from slow walking. He also feels better while rising (opposite of Ruta). The patient is worse from cold, from sitting, from getting overheated. Pain is the worst at midnight.

SANGUINARIA—For cases involving a rheumatic pain in the right shoulder. The patient may also have pain in the left hip. The area of the shoulder will be frozen in place. Stiffnessness in the neck. Better for sleep, worse for any motion or pressure. The patient will want to touch the painful part and will feel better from touching it himself. He will not want you to touch it. Sensation of burning in the feet will accompany the pain.

INJURIES TO MUSCLES, JOINTS, AND BONES
Hip Pain

Again, pains located in the hips are commonly the result of a chronic rheumatic condition. However, it is also quite common that they are the result of overwork and overexercise.

As pains in this area are apt to overlap with those in the knees and lower back, it is important that you check those sections out as well before selecting a remedy.

And look to the general injury remedies for hip pains associated with physical trauma.

REMEDIES

ARNICA—Any case of hip pain from fall or injury. Alternate with Hypericum in cases of injury from a fall, which has left the area painful, but with a tingling sensation that travels along the nerves. For cases of hip pain from childbirth, start the case with Arnica, then follow up with Ruta, which will complete the cure. For cases in which Arnica fails to cure, consider Bellis.

KALI BI—As is keynote for the remedy, the pain will occur in specific spots in the area of the hips. Look for pain, swelling, and stiffness in the joint. The hip joint will crack when the patient moves. Pains will be worse on the left side. Pains will have the tendency to move about from one place to another.

RUTA—The top remedy for hip pain. Think of the motion associated with rising up out of a chair and you have a portrait of the sort of motion that Ruta finds most painful. The hip will feel weak. The legs will give out when the patient tries to rise out of a chair. The whole spine and lower limbs will feel bruised.

ALSO CONSIDER

CARBO ANIMALIS—Hip pain that is worse at night. Pain from straining and from overlifting. Pain in the whole area of the hip and the coccyx. Hip pains that are accompanied by night sweats. The patient will be worse for sweating. Weakness in the area of the hips and the wrists.

CHELIDONIUM—Rheumatic pains in the hips and thighs. The muscles surrounding the joint will feel rigid. Pain is worse on the right side. Patient will want hot things on the painful area, will also want hot food and drink.

CIMICIFUGA—Consider this remedy for hip pain that comes on during the hormonal changes associated with menopause. Look for a sensation of jerking in the hip joint and the lower limbs. The pain will be worse in the morning and worse from cold. The patient will feel uneasy and in discomfort rather than overcome by pain.

KALI CARB—Pains that centralize in the hip joint and thigh. Sharp pains that extend from the lower back, into the hips, and down into the thighs. Hip pains associated with pregnancy. Look for the patient to complain of a sensation of burning in the spine. Hip joint feels very weak, but improves with motion.

SANGUINARIA—An odd little remedy that combines a right shoulder pain with a left hip pain. The patient will want to touch or press on the pain, but will not want anyone else to touch it. The patient will have burning pains in the soles of the feet. He will feel better at rest in the dark.

Injuries to Muscles, Joints, and Bones
Coccyx Pain (Coccydynia)

Usually caused by a fall, this is an injury to the end of the spine.

As always, in cases caused by physical trauma, we will consider Arnica, Rhus Tox, Bryonia, and Bellis. The following are to be considered in addition to these.

REMEDIES

ANTIMONIUM TARTARICUM—Coccyx has heavy, dragging weight attached to it. The patient's lower limbs will tremble and twitch when the patient attempts to walk. There is also a twisting sensation in the muscles. Look for the slightest motion to bring on sensation of nausea, accompanied by a cold sweat.

CAUSTICUM—Pain has bruised feeling. The patient feels achy in general. The patient will be better in damp, cold weather. The patient will feel unsteady when he tries to walk. Look for numbness and coldness in the lower limbs to accompany the injury and pain. This is the most common remedy for the condition.

HYPERICUM—A good remedy for any pain caused by a fall. A good general remedy. The pain will radiate along the nerves. The patient will be in a foggy state and will be worse in any damp weather, especially in the fog.

KALI BI—Pain is worse for sitting or for walking. A sensation of jerking and twitching will accompany the pain. The bone will feel sore and bruised. The pain will usually occur in one small, specific spot.

SILICEA—Worse for pressure, worse for drafts. The area of the coccyx will feel heavy and distended. The patient will be afraid and lacking in vital heat. He will want to be taken care of. This remedy is especially suited to elderly patients in pain. Constipation may accompany the pain.

Injuries to Muscles, Joints, and Bones
Knee Pain

Again, the remedies for rheumatic pain listed in the end of this section should be the first considered. In addition to these, however, are the following.

REMEDIES

APIS—Used when the knee is red and swollen. The swollen area will have a shiny look to it as well. The knee feels as if stung by a bee, often with burning sensation as well. The knee will feel better for ice and any other cold application. The patient will be angry while in pain.

CAUSTICUM—For knees that crack when the patient is walking. The patient will be unsteady when he walks. He will feel as if he cannot trust the knee to hold his weight. Pain will decrease in rainy weather.

RHUS TOX—Used most often for chronic knee pain, when knee follows the traditional "rusty hinge" Rhus formula: worse on first motion, better for continued gentle motion. Look for the patient to want to take a hot shower or to soak the knee in hot water.

RUTA—Usually considered the general knee pain remedy, particularly if the pain extends from the hips to the knees. The patient will have great difficulty in rising out of a chair or in getting out of a car. The knee pains associated with Ruta are usually those of gardeners or other laborers who overwork their body.

ALSO CONSIDER

BERBERIS—Knees feel as if they have been beaten. Feel stiff and sore. The entire leg feels weary and lame. There is a sensation of external cold to the area of the knee. The patient will have a difficult time rising due to the stiffness of the joint. Look for the pain to travel up to the hip.

INJURIES TO MUSCLES, JOINTS, AND BONES
Ankle Pain

The basic remedy here, as in all first aid, is going to be Arnica—to be given when there is injury to the ankle. But the ankle is a sensitive part of the body, and many different remedies may be used for pain in the region.

REMEDIES

APIS—Look for the ankle to have the sensation of burning or stinging. Look for it to have a swollen appearance and to improve with ice and other cold applications. The affected area will be red and swollen. Apis is often used in conjunction with Rhus Tox for clearing chronic or acute knee and ankle pain.

BELLIS PERENNIS—This is to be used when Arnica fails. When the bruising of the ankle is too deep for Arnica to cure. Look for the ankle to be blue or purple in color, and for that bruised coloring to be deep and long-lasting.

CAUSTICUM—For tearing pain in the ankle, worse for cold, dry weather. The patient will not trust the ankle, and, although he will be able to walk on it, he will be afraid that it will give out under him. The ankle will crack and pop when moved.

LEDUM—The general remedy of choice for a twisted ankle. The ankle feels cold and mushy. And yet, the patient will not be able to bear putting heat on the ankle. Patient cannot put weight on ankle. The ankle will be swollen and purple/red in color.

NATRUM MUR—For the chronic weakness of the ankles. They turn easily, in a person prone to constipation and headache. This is an excellent remedy for those who have injured their ankle in the past and now find that it is vulnerable to injuries.

RHUS TOX—For cases in which the pain has gone on for a while and is in danger of becoming chronic. The condition may even seem to be arthritic in nature. The ankle hurts most on first motion, feels better for continued, gentle motion. The patient will want to apply support or pressure to the ankle. He will want to bathe it in hot water.

INJURIES TO MUSCLES, JOINTS, AND BONES
Deep Muscle Pain

What do you do when injuries that should have responded to Arnica fail too respond to Arnica alone? Consider the following remedies to complete the healing action begun by Arnica.

REMEDIES

BELLIS PERENNIS—Always consider this remedy as a completion of Arnica in any injury situation, whatever its cause. Bellis will bring the pain to an end, will cause the clearing of bruises that Arnica alone cannot cure.

COLOCYNTHIS—Removes deep pain in a specific part of the body that Arnica alone cannot cure. Look for the patient to want to put hard pressure on the injured part. Especially look for patient to ball the fist into the injury and hold with strong pressure to comfort the pain.

RHUS TOX—Often can be used to complete the work of Arnica. Most useful when the injury is nearly healed and the pain is mostly gone, but the injury never quite finishes the healing process. Look for the patient to feel restless. Look for much tossing and turning and trying to get comfortable. Much moving about. The pain, as is usual for Rhus, is most potent on first motion, better for prolonged gentle motion.

INJURIES TO MUSCLE, JOINTS, AND BONE
Cramps

Cramps are, simply put, the sudden, involuntary, and highly painful contraction of the muscles. Cramps most commonly occur in the calves of the legs and the soles of the feet. They can be caused by the sudden overuse of a muscle, by sitting or lying in an unaccustomed position, or during pregnancy.

REMEDIES

ARNICA—Consider this remedy for cramps in muscles that have been overused. Cramps associated with a state of fatigue. The patient will say that his body feels bruised.

CALCAREA—For violent cramps of the calves at night, especially when extending the legs. Feet feel damp and cold during cramps, as if one were wearing wet socks. Chronic cramping in overweight people.

CAMPHORA—Cramps in calves. Feet are icy cold. Associated with this will be icy cold feet that ache as if they were sprained. Cramps with numbness and tingling.

CARBO VEG—Cramps in the soles of the feet in the evening when lying down. Profuse sweating of the feet. Also an excellent remedy for cramps in the front of the leg that occur while walking. Patient will have to rest and rub the affected part.

CHAMOMILLA—Cramps in legs and thighs. Cramps will be worse when the patient is asleep in bed at night. Cramps will awaken the patient and drive him out of bed. The patient must move about to soothe the pain.

Will be anxious and irritable. Also foot cramp and paralysis. The patient will be unable to step on his foot.

COLOCYNTHIS—For general cramps in any part of the body that are made better by hard pressure on specific parts. If patient presses on the sore spot with a balled fist, consider Colocynthis.

MAGNESIA PHOSPHORICA—Cramps that are alleviated by heat and by warm applications (consider as a great PMS remedy). Cramps will be radiating in nature. Pain will travel to the whole of the body from the specific site of the pain. This is perhaps the best general remedy for cramping pains in muscles that are improved by heat. Cramps are often associated with trembling, especially trembling of the hands. Think of this remedy in cases of writer's cramp.

NUX—Cramps with headache. Nausea, loss of appetite. Worse at night. Cramp in the calves. Painful cramps in the soles when bending the legs. Patient is angry and wants to be alone. The remedy is well known for its cramps and twitches. Look for a spasm of a single muscle or group of muscles anywhere in the body. Chronic cramping.

SEPIA—Consider for cases of violent cramps in the calves at night when in bed, especially during pregnancy. The patient's legs will feel heavy and too short. They will twitch and jerk at night when the patient is in bed. Also consider this remedy for all cases of cramp that are attended by a downward motion of pain and a sensation of heavy gravity. The patient will be chilly when in pain.

VERATRUM—Cramps in the calves, better from massage, worse for walking. May be accompanied by diarrhea and/or vomiting; by cold sweat on the patient's face. As a general cramp remedy, Veratrum, taken at night for a few days, will usually remove the predisposition to cramp.

ALSO CONSIDER

CUPRUM—This remedy, taken from the metal copper, is perhaps our best general cramp remedy. Mostly for foot and leg cramps. Cramps that begin as twitching muscles. Also look for the cramps to begin in the toes or in the fingers and then to travel throughout the body. Cramps may be associated with convulsions. Cramps in the palms of the hands, hands will be icy cold. Cramps in the calves and soles of the feet. Cramps accompanied with jerking and twitching of muscles.

ZINC—This is a little remedy—taken from the metal zinc—that comes in handy for cases involving foot cramps occurring at night, when the patient is in bed. In this case, the patient will have to keep his feet moving to soothe the pain. The patient will cry out in his sleep from the pain. Patient may be awakened by the pain. This is also a general remedy for the cramps associated with PMS. Cramps accompanied by night sweats, shivers down the spine.

INJURIES TO MUSCLES, JOINTS, AND BONES
Restless Legs

Restless legs that jump and twitch at almost all times may be more an irritation to the person watching than the person twitching. Most of the time, restless legs do not represent a deep problem, only boredom or nervousness. However, the following remedies may help overcome the situation.

Check the previous sections on cramps for listings of other remedies associated with the situation.

REMEDIES

ARSENICUM—Consider this remedy for the patient who does not have twitching legs, but moves them in more of a restless motion. This is a remedy for the patient with a condition of general restlessness, even when he is exhausted. Anxiety accompanies the motion. There is a general sensation of coldness. An excellent remedy to consider for restlessness in general, especially in older patients.

BELLADONNA—In this remedy picture, the patient's legs are in spasm, and the patient is, in general, hot. He feels a sensation of congestion and heat in his head. But the patient's legs and feet feel very cold. The restlessness becomes worse when the patient is going to sleep.

IGNATIA—Consider for twitching of leg (or any other part of the body) that comes on after grief or romantic disappointment. Sleeplessness due to twitching. The Ignatia person feels that he will never sleep again. He feels that some part of the body is in spasm. His legs twitch and jerk.

PHOSPHORUS—A remedy to consider when the case involves twitching on the right leg. This is also a leading remedy for the restless legs of young adults, for the student who constantly and heedlessly bounces his right leg up and down. The patient is always worse for lying on the right side. Better for sleep. For similar symptoms, also consider Sulphur.

SEPIA—The patient's legs are twitching and jerking, and the symptoms are worse during the day. Better for exercise. Patients will feel that their legs cannot be trusted for support, that they will give out under them. Also consider this remedy for cases in which a pregnant woman's legs twitch and jerk when she goes to bed at night.

Injuries to Muscles, Joints, and Bones
Fractures

Fractures to bones can be either simple or compound. Basically, if the bone is broken, but the skin is left intact, the injury is considered to be a simple fracture. If the skin is broken as well, it is to be considered a compound fracture. (Compound fractures are those where, in addition to the injury done to the bone, there is a rupture of tendons, ligaments, and skin.) The break itself can be considered either a "greenstick" fracture—also called an incomplete fracture, in which the bone is not completely broken—or a complete fracture, in which case the bone has been completely snapped.

The danger of fractures is not just within the bones themselves. Splinters of bone can cut into either nerves or blood vessels. Fractures can also lead to infection of the bone, also to internal bleeding or, in the case of a compound fracture, heavy blood loss.

It goes without saying that fractures of any sort are very painful. Although some fractures—particularly of the small bones in the feet and hands—are not completely apparent and must be confirmed by X rays, most fractures are obvious. Usually, the area of the fracture is swollen and bruised, even if it is not bleeding.

Do not move the patient. Apply gentle pressure to the sides of the wound and cover the wound, if the skin has been broken, with sterile cloth. Call 911 for assistance or proceed to the hospital.

Perhaps more than any other acute situation, bone fractures require a blending of allopathic and homeopathic procedures. The bone must be X-rayed and it must be set. However, homeopathic remedies will play a large part in the gentle, rapid, and permanent healing of the injury.

Note: While homeopaths are forever trying to individualize their cases, specifically seeking the remedy that best matches the patient's own response to his ailment, the case of fractures is one in which most of us respond in the same way. Therefore, this is one of the few situations in which we can almost set down a standard method of treatment. Most often, in the case of fractures, Arnica will be given first to start the healing process and to deal with the bruises and blows associated with the fracture. Then Ledum will be given briefly to complete the work with bruising that was begun by Arnica. Then, after the bone has been set, the patient will be given Symphytum to speed the healing of the bone itself. These and other remedies associated with fractures are listed below.

REMEDIES

ACONITE—Should be thought of for any kind of trauma, both emotional and physical. Aconite will help with the shock of the situation. Aconite and Arnica can be alternated in the hours following injury to help balance the patient's energy and to begin healing.

ARNICA—As usual, Arnica is the remedy of first choice and should be begun as soon as the injury takes place. Arnica will begin the healing process, take care of the bruising and swelling. Arnica can be taken as needed until the injury is totally healed.

BRYONIA—A remedy specific to broken and cracked ribs. Remember that Bryonia is a remedy whose picture includes pain so intense that the patient cannot move because of it, and may even become angry if you suggest that he try to move. Consider Bryonia in fractures that involve intense pain that keeps the patient totally immobilized.

CALENDULA—Should be considered in cases involving compound fractures. While we usually consider this to be only a topical remedy, it is an excellent choice in potentized form, usually in a 200C or above, to be given to the patient after surgery. It not only will speed the healing of the wound but it will safeguard against infection.

HYPERICUM—May be either given internally or used externally for the nerve pain that accompanies a broken bone. Hypericum is most often called for in the case of a compound fracture. For injuries to nerves associated with compound fractures.

LEDUM—A remedy that is said to complete the work of Arnica in an injury like a fracture. Arnica should be given in the first days following the injury. After swelling and bruising have lessened and the patient is on the mend, Ledum is given to complete the healing.

SILICEA—The remedy for fractures of bones that involve splinters breaking off the bone. Silicea will help the body to reabsorb the splintered bone harmlessly. Consider this remedy especially in weakened patients who are, in general, of low vital force and slow to heal.

STAPHYSAGRIA—Must be considered in cases of abuse that have resulted in broken bones. While Arnica will assist the healing process and, in general, will soothe the patient, Staphysagria, given after the bone has healed, will assist the patient in healing emotionally, in dealing with his own anger.

SYMPHITUM—After the initial shock phase has passed, Symphytum should be alternated with Arnica. Symphytum will promote the healing of the bone itself and can be used until the injury is totally healed. *Note*: Symphytum should only be given after the bone has been set.

RESCUE REMEDY—Should be employed at the time of the fracture before other remedies are given. (Since Rescue is a Bach Flower Remedy mixture, it works in a manner that is different from the traditional Hahnemannian remedies and should not be used in conjunction with the other remedies listed here.) Rescue would be given to the patient who has been overwhelmed by the event that has taken place. For the emotional, but not the physical, trauma.

ALSO CONSIDER

CALCEREA PHOS—Consider this remedy especially in the case of an elderly patient who is having problems healing a broken bone. This remedy will complete the healing begun by Symphytum. It will also follow Bryonia quite well in the healing of cracked ribs. A sense of weariness will accompany the pain of the fracture.

INJURIES TO MUSCLES, JOINTS, AND BONES
Head Trauma (Concussion)

A concussion signifies a sudden interruption of the functions of the brain, caused by a blow, fall, or other mechanical injury to the head. Any blow to the head can lead to serious complications. Disorientation, even of only a few minutes' duration, is a sign of brain damage—although in most cases not permanent brain damage. Should the patient lose consciousness, he should be taken for immediate medical treatment.

General symptoms of concussion include dimness of vision, headache, trembling of limbs, rapid pulse, clammy skin, and chills and nausea. Look for the patient to want to go to sleep.

In more serious cases, the patient is unconscious or incoherent, the surface of the patient's skin is pale and cold, his pulse is slowed and faint, his breathing is slow and shallow. Look for deep sighing.

REMEDIES

ACONITE—Will assist the patient in dealing with shock associated with the trauma. Aconite should be given as soon as possible after the injury and will no longer be useful after the shock stage has passed.

ARNICA—As with any other blow, a blow to the head can cause bruising and internal bleeding. Arnica, taken from the moment of injury, will help to alleviate the bruising and promote the healing process. The more overwhelmed the patient seems from the blow, the higher the potency that will be required to restore balance.

BELLADONNA—The patient sees sparks in front of his eyes after trauma. Face has a furious look. Face red and bloated. Throbbing headache, patient cannot bear noise or light. Patient is sleepy but cannot sleep.

HYPERICUM—For nerve pain that may radiate throughout the skull, often as an aftermath to head trauma.

ALSO CONSIDER

NATRUM SULPHURICUM—For blows to the head that lead to a personality change. The Arnica patient may lose consciousness, may even have some memory loss. The Natrum Sulph patient, however, seems greatly changed by the accident, as if he will never return to being the person he was before the accident.

OPIUM—The patient is snoring, breathing with eyes half closed. Delirious, talking a great deal, with eyes opened wide. Face is purple and swollen. After trauma, the patient's hearing becomes very acute.

EMERGENCIES
Emotional Crisis

From time to time, we all feel overwhelmed, pushed beyond our limits. We feel as if we can no longer be held responsible for anything that we might say or do. In these times, homeopathic remedies, used acutely, can do a great deal of good. Naturally, if the crisis is long-lasting, or the emotional pain is deeply felt, the patient should consult with a professional practitioner for constitutional care.

REMEDY CHECKLIST

For a crisis of fear or fright, consider: **Aconite, Belladonna, Gelsemium, Ignatia, Mercurius, Opium, Valeriana**, and **Pulsatilla**.

For grief, consider: **Cocculus, Colocynthis, Ignatia, Lachesis, Natrum Mur, Phosphoric Acid, Pulsatilla**, and **Staphysagria**.

For a broken heart, consider: **Hyoscyamus, Ignatia, Natrum Mur**, and **Phosphoric Acid**.

For feelings of homesickness, consider: **Capsicum, Mercurius, Phosphoric Acid**, and **Staphysagria**.

For excessive joy that leads to manic behavior, consider: **Aconite, Coffea, Opium, Valeriana**, and **Pulsatilla**.

For jealousy, consider: **Hyoscyamus, Lachesis**, and **Nux**.

For feelings of having been insulted or damaged or betrayed, consider: **Belladonna, Colocynthis, Ignatia, Platina, Pulsatilla**, and **Staphysagria**.

For feelings of having be made to look foolish, consider: **Aconite, Bryonia, Chamomilla, Colocynthis, Nux, Platina**, and **Staphysagria**.

For feelings of anger and indignation, of having been wronged, consider: **Colocynthis** and **Staphysagria**.

For violent anger, consider: **Aconite, Bryonia, Chamomilla, Nux**, and **Phosphorus**.

For deep depression, consider: **Arsenicum, Aurum, Calcarea Carbonica, Lachesis, Natrum Mur, Nux**, and **Sulphur**.

For those who are depressed and withdrawn, consider: **Cocculus, Ignatia, Phosphoric Acid**, and **Pulsatilla**.

For those who are manic, consider: **Belladonna, Hyoscamus**, and **Pulsatilla** or **Valeriana**.

REMEDIES

ACONITE—The patient will be very "wound up." He will not be able to sit still or calm down. Look for him to pace the floor in fear and/or pain. Expect palpitations of the heart. The skin will be hot and dry; the pulse is rapid and full, pounding. The patient fears death, will predict the time of his death. The patient is very excited, very frightened, and easily angered. A manic patient.

ARNICA—For the angry patient. The patient who refuses to answer questions. Who insists that he is fine and that you should leave him alone. The patient is excited, cries easily. Look for the patient to have coughing fits that accompany anger. This is also an excellent remedy for shock following the receipt of bad news. For the patient who has just learned that a loved one has died. Also for those with nightmares, who awaken suddenly from sleep with fear.

BELLADONNA—One of our most excited patients. The patient is afraid, angry, or both. He screams in anger or in pain. The patient may go into convulsions, especially if the patient is a child. Look for twitching of the arms and legs. Look for the patient to have a red face, and to complain of a sensation of blood rushing to the face and head. This is an excellent remedy for those with anxiety attacks, who also experience palpitations, and a rush of heat to the head and face.

BRYONIA—A very irritable person. Everything, even your interest in his well-being, seems to make him angry. The Bryonia patient wants to be left alone, wants to stay very still. Every motion causes physical pain. Headache often accompanies emotional upset. The patient will say that his head hurts as if it were about to split open. The patient will shudder. He will have a total loss of appetite, although he may have a great thirst. Constipation may also accompany emotional upset.

CALCAREA CARBONICA—An excellent remedy for midlife crisis, and for those who, due to early retirement or divorce, find themselves starting over late in life. These patients will be very depressed, will be inclined to weep. They will have a good deal of anxiety about the future, will feel that they have nowhere to turn. They are worried about their health and will often feel palpitations or congestion around the heart. They are worried about misfortunes of all sorts, about catching diseases and about going insane. They will be very afraid that they might die. They will feel that they cannot think, that they are losing their mind. Because of the similarities between the actions of this remedy and Natrum Mur, the two work well together. Most often, Calcarea Carbonica will be used first, with Natrum Mur as the follow-up.

COFFEA—This patient is more nervous than angry, but very manic. The patient cannot stay still, cannot sleep. Excitement may come from any cause, and is as likely from excessive joy as it is from excessive grief or anger. This is a remedy for children who cannot sleep from excitement on Christmas Eve. The patient may weep and may call out his complaints. He often feels that things are not fair. Look for fainting and trembling to accompany emotional upset.

CHAMOMILLA—A remedy for those in a violent rage. The patient may become so angry that he cannot breathe. This is the leading remedy for those who have breathing problems after anger. Look for the patient to complain of a bitter taste in his mouth. He may also smash things or lash out verbally and physically. Look for indigestion to accompany emotional upset. This is an especially good remedy to know for children who throw tantrums.

COLOCYNTHIS—A remedy for those who tend to have diarrhea every time they become angry. The same holds for diarrhea with grief. The patient will experience colic from anger or grief. He will have terrible abdominal cramps. Bitter vomiting is common. Sleeplessness accompanies emotional complaints. The patient is easy to anger, wishes to withdraw. He will not want to speak, or, especially, to answer any questions.

GELSEMIUM—The patient is afraid. Look for diarrhea to accompany the fear. Look for the patient to seem too weak to cope with fear. This remedy is especially good for future-based fears, for those who feel that "something bad is about to happen." This is a great remedy for those who fear public speaking, and who are about to have to give a speech. Also for those who must take a test and who feel anxious about that.

IGNATIA—This is perhaps our best-known remedy for those who are in a state of grief. But it is important to understand that the purpose of this remedy is not to suppress or avoid grief. Grief, at the time of loss, is a natural and healthy reaction. Ignatia is helpful for either those who have suppressed their grief and refuse to experience it or those who are trapped in grief and cannot let go of it or their loss and get on with their lives. The Ignatia patient seems indifferent to everything, but anger lurks just beneath the surface. This patient sighs often, cries and laughs at odd times, and keeps everyone else off-balance with sudden emotional swings. Look for physical tics and spasms to accompany the grief. Vertigo is very common to this remedy type.

LACHESIS—A remedy for those who are deeply unhappy. Look for the patient to feel worse just after sleeping. Look for every emotional and physical symptom to be worse from sleep. This is a very talkative patient. He talks a lot but says little. He changes the subject often and avoids speaking about what troubles him. Physically, the patient will feel constricted, will not be able to bear anything tight around the throat.

MERCURIUS—A remedy for those with fear or homesickness. The patient will seem anguished and restless. Trembling is common. The patient will wake suddenly from sleep and will be very upset, will not be able to return to sleep. He will not be able to stand the warmth of the bed, will need to get up out of bed. Will thrash about. The patient will seem nervous and quarrelsome, as opposed to angry. He will have many complaints about other people, especially members of his own family. After leaving his bed, he will shiver with cold, tremble with upset. The patient will have to get back in bed to calm down. Look for night sweats to accompany emotional upset.

NATRUM MUR—This is an excellent remedy for those suffering from depression, especially after the loss of a loved one or the breakup of a love relationship. The patient will want to be alone, will refuse to be consoled, and will become angry from consolation. Deep depression. The patient will weep often, and will look to the future with total negativity. The patient will become angry very easily, especially if she perceives that someone is intruding in her privacy. Look for a loss of appetite to accompany emotional upset. The patient is worse from eating, has indigestion after eating. Natrum Mur is considered the chronic remedy for Ignatia and follows that remedy well.

NUX—The ultimate angry person. The patient may be violent and is always quick to temper. The Nux may be unpredictable in his anger, and will keep others off-balance by never letting them know what will anger him next. This is the remedy for the person who says, "See what you made me do!" The patient will be very irritable, will want to be left alone. He will feel cold, and will not be able to stand any movement of air. Noise and light are also intolerable to him. The Nux patient may be inclined to violence. He may also be suicidal. Look for tics to accompany anger. Look for constipation to accompany anger.

PHOSPHORUS—An excellent remedy for the sudden breakdown. For those who have reached the point at which they feel that they can take no more. The patient almost literally explodes with anger. Especially for anger from a person who is seldom angry. The Phosphorus will feel as if all his defenses have collapsed, as if all the walls that separate him from others are gone. The patient has reached the point of the straw that broke the camel's back and can take no more. He feels thin-skinned and wants to be cheered up and taken care of. Failing that, he wants to be left alone. Look for the depression and anger to be worse at twilight.

PULSATILLA—A remedy for those with fear. The Pulsatilla will first feel a great heat in the abdomen. Often, this will even come before he is aware of his fear. Diarrhea will often accompany this sense of heat. The patient will seem melancholy, sad. Disposed to weep for the slightest reason. He may also laugh suddenly, and for no known reason. The patient will be very concerned about his health. And will also feel the emotional upset in the region of his heart. The patient will feel disgusted by everything. The patient will feel as if he is suffocating, especially if he is in a warm room. He will want to open windows or to go outdoors. When upset, he either will go outdoors for a walk or will sit rocking, as if in a rocking chair.

STAPHYSAGRIA—A remedy that is often needed for those who have been a victim of crime, especially violent crime. For those who have been raped. Also for victims of sexual or physical abuse in childhood. These patients know that they have been wronged, even if they have suppressed the memory of that wrong. They feel a deep and even a righteous anger, and yet they do not know what to do with the anger. These patients are fearful, mistrustful, and restless. They will have trouble forming trusting relationships. Physically, they will push violently away whatever is near them. Emotionally as well. These patients will be sleepless at night, will sleep only in the daylight. They dread the future. They speak with their voice in one or two volumes: either in a feeble whisper or in a shout.

SULPHUR—These patients have a lowness of spirit. They feel impatient and anxious. They often feel that the world does not appreciate or understand them. They feel that they cannot think, that they are losing their mind. Exhaustion after mental labors. Exhaustion after perceived failure in career and achievements. This is a good remedy for those who are functionally depressed. Often this is a long-term condition. Look for digestive disorders, especially a sensation of pressure in the abdomen, to accompany the emotional distress. Constipation is also common.

VALERIANA—An excellent little remedy for emotional upset. The remedy is taken from the same source as the allopathic drug Valium and is used much in the same way. The patient is upset and given to wide swings of emotion, laughing one moment and crying the next. The patient is easily and mysteriously angered. Look for flatulence to accompany anger. Look for the patient to experience weightlessness, to feel as if he might float away during times of emotional distress.

RESCUE REMEDY—The perfect basic remedy for emotional upset. This remedy blend of five of Bach's Flower Remedies should not be combined with any of the above, but can be used in place of virtually any of them. The remedy will act in a calming and balancing manner for patients with virtually any emotional upset. It may be taken internally, applied topically, or used in a calming hot bath.

ALSO CONSIDER

CAPSICUM—An excellent remedy for those with acute feelings of homesickness. The patient will yearn for the place in which he feels most safe and at ease. Look for the patient to be unable to sleep from homesickness. Look for a feeling of external heat and for redness of the cheeks to accompany emotional upset.

COCCULUS—For the patient who is sad and who has a tendency to become suddenly startled, especially at night. The patient is exhausted, but very nervous, cannot calm down and relax, even though he longs to. There is nervous grief with worry about the future. This remedy is very helpful to those who are exhausted from attending to a sick friend or from helping others in a time of loss. Look for headache to accompany grief.

HYOSCYAMUS—For the patient who has fits of mania, and who may actually have seizures during these manic times. The patient flails his limbs wildly, makes meaningless gestures. He may also speak in meaningless syllables. The patient will be very fearful. The patient will try to remove all his clothing, wants to be uncovered, wants to be naked. The Hyoscyamus is highly suspicious of others, will suspect others of being jealous, of betraying him. The patient will especially fear being poisoned. An inability to swallow will accompany emotional upset.

OPIUM—These patients are cut off from almost all sensations. They are not sure what they are angry about, but they are angry. They rage on and on about the same thing, over and over again. They are tired, but cannot sleep. If they do sleep, look for them to snore. Loss of consciousness with delerium. The patients talk in their sleep. Will be very fearful, and will tend to startle suddenly with no apparent cause. Look for spasms in the limbs, trembling in the limbs. These spasms come on after fear. Look for a full and slow pulse. Constipation will accompany emotional distress.

PHOSPHORIC ACID—A remedy for those who are deep in grief. Also for long-lasting homesickness and for those who have, for a long time, been unhappy in love. The patient is dull, listless, depressed. He seems to take little or no interest in any aspect of his life. The patient will have trouble falling asleep in the evening, but will be very sleepy in the morning. He will want to sleep in, want to stay in bed. Look for the patient to begin to lose his hair, or for the hair to begin turning gray. Look for sweat to accompany emotional upset. The patient will complain little and will seem to have no energy or interest at all. This remedy is often used as a follow-up to Ignatia in cases of grief.

PLATINA—The patient is angry. This anger most commonly comes on after the patient has been made to feel embarrassed in public. The patient feels contempt for those who have angered him, feels emotionally withdrawn from them, superior to them. Feels misunderstood and unappreciated. Deep inside, the Platina is very sad, but does not show it. The patient displays a deep fear and dread of death.

EMERGENCIES
Shock

In dealing with an emergency situation, it is important to consider the need to treat the patient for shock. Shock occurs when the blood flow through the vital organs of the body becomes inadequate due to a loss of blood, or due to a sudden drop in blood pressure (as in the allergic reaction anaphylactic shock). The symptoms of shock are a clammy sweat on the skin, nausea, vertigo, thirst, and anxiety. As the patient feels faint, he will also grow pale. Breathing will become shallow and rapid, the pulse is fast and weak.

If possible, the patient should be on his back with the legs slightly raised. A patient with a bodily injury, however, should never be moved. Loosen clothing and cover the patient.

Shock can be very serious. If a person is lapsing into shock, call 911 right away.

Note: Emergencies that combine physical trauma with shock may require us to break the law of Simplex. In these cases, it is often best to alternate between Aconite and Arnica, given as close together as every five minutes. Any philosophical issues that the use of multiple remedies might bring up can be discussed later when the patient is safe and sound.

REMEDIES

ACONITE—The patient will be restless and very anxious. The patient is very fearful. He will predict the moment of his own death. He will be very fearful of dying. His body may feel very hot to the touch. Sometimes the patient will want to get up and move about, and will have to be convinced to stay very still. This remedy is especially useful for cases in which the trauma occurred very quickly and without warning.

ARNICA—Consider this remedy in cases in which the shock has been caused by direct injury to the body. A blow or bruise to the body. Also, as above, in cases of car accidents and other sudden physical traumas. Also think of this remedy in cases of physical abuse and of muggings and such. Often the patient will insist that he is fine and that nothing is wrong with him. He will tend to be a bit glassy-eyed and a bit slow to respond. He will not want to be touched. This is keynote—the patient may become angry or even violent if you try to touch his injury. Arnica and Aconite are often used in alternation to speed healing and calm the patient who is in shock.

CARBO VEG—Look for the patient's face to take on a bluish color, instead of pale white. That color is keynote of the remedy type. The patient is gasping for air, may want to have air fanned onto the face. Patient is yawning. In a state of total collapse. Nosebleed may accompany shock.

VERATRUM—The keynote here is that the forehead will be covered in cold sweat. Skin will feel very cold. Nausea accompanies shock. Patient may vomit. The patient will also tend to be very anxious, very wound up. He will talk. He may rave on and on incoherently.

RESCUE REMEDY—The Bach Flower Remedy, a mixture of five of Dr. Bach's floral essences, can be of great help in overcoming shock. If the patient is conscious, put the drops (4 or 5 at a time) under the tongue. If the patient is unconscious, put the drops on the pulse points of the wrist and gently rub into the skin. May be used as often as needed.

EMERGENCIES
Fainting

Fainting may come about from hunger, from emotional duress or pain. Some people faint easily and often, and, in such cases, the problems should be addressed constitutionally. For acute fainting spells, the situation is approached in a manner similar to treatments for shock.

REMEDIES

ACONITE—From fright, from hearing bad news. Also, fainting caused by violent pain.

ARNICA—For fainting after a fall or a blow.

CHAMOMILLA—When fainting comes from intense physical pain. Or from sudden overwhelming emotions.

CHINA—For fainting from loss of blood. Also, fainting during a long-term or serious disease.

COCCULUS—fainting from violent pain, pain that makes patient double up, or place hard pressure on area of pain.

COFFEA—Fainting comes on from overexcitement, from too much of any stimulant.

HEPAR SULPH—For fainting from pain in situations in which the pain is not intense, but the person faints anyway.

IGNATIA—When fainting comes on from intense emotion, from grief.

NUX—For those who faint at the sight of blood. Also for those who faint due to strong odors or perfumes.

PULSATILLA—Fainting due to lack of air, or from being in an overheated, stuffy room.

SILICEA—For those who faint at the sight of needles.

VERATRUM—Fainting in patients who have been nearly driven out of their mind with pains. Also, fainting after severe diarrhea. Fainting with a cold sweat.

ALSO CONSIDER

NUX MOSCHATA—For fainting that comes on from physical over-exertion.

EMERGENCIES
Vertigo

This sensation of dizziness and spinning may come on from many different causes, from travel sickness to anxiety to inner ear troubles. Whatever the cause, the following remedies may offer relief.

REMEDIES

ACONITE—For sudden dizziness. For vertigo that comes on when rising up from a chair, from stooping, or from looking up. The patient will feel his vision cloud over. He may faint from dizziness.

ANTIMONIUM TARTARTICUM—For vertigo that comes on after eating too much, or from eating too rich foods. Look for a white coating on the patient's tongue to accompany his dizziness. Look for the patient to alternate between vertigo and drowsiness.

ARNICA—For vertigo that is caused by a blow or any other mechanical injury. The vertigo will be accompanied by nausea. The patient will be better from lying down. The patient's head will feel hot and the rest of the body cold.

BELLADONNA—These patients will complain of a loss of sight during the bout of vertigo. They will see sparks of color in their eyes and may feel as if they will faint. Sudden vertigo that is made worse by stooping or bending. Vertigo that comes on from too much sun. Patients are very sensitive to light and will want to lie down in a cool, dark place. Vertigo accompanied by throbbing in the head, a rush of blood to the head and face. Accompanied by a sensation of heat in the face.

CALCAREA—For vertigo that is accompanied by a congestion of the head. The head also feels chilly. It may be covered with a sour, cold sweat, especially the occiputal area. Vertigo with trembling that begins before breakfast.

COCCULUS—Consider for fainting from violent pain, pain that makes patient double up, or place hard pressure on area of pain. For cases of vertigo, especially when the patient rides in a vehicle, or just sits up. The patient will say that his head feels empty. Nausea accompanies vertigo.

MERCURIUS—Vertigo in which the vision seems to be fading to black. Vertigo that comes on only in the evening. Vertigo that comes on when the patient is lying on his back in bed. The dizziness may come on any time the patient tries to raise his head from a pillow, and will be better from lying back down.

NUX—Vertigo that comes on from overwork and from mental exertion. The patient will experience a blurring of vision and a whizzing sound in the ears. Vertigo from drinking alcohol. Vertigo from eating too rich foods. Patient will feel cold, irritable. Vertigo that accompanies chronic constipation.

PULSATILLA—Dizziness after eating greasy food, or from being in a warm, enclosed place. The patient experiences vertigo when rising from a chair. Vertigo from looking upward. Vertigo accompanied by chills. Accompanied by nausea and vomiting. Vertigo worse in the evening.

RHUS TOX—For the patient who experiences vertigo when lying down on his bed in the evening. Vertigo accompanied by a fear of falling or a fear of dying.

SILICEA—Vertigo that comes on in the morning, or after strong emotion.

The vertigo will seem to begin in the back and rise up into the neck and then into the head. Vertigo accompanied by weakness and chills.

SULPHUR—For vertigo that comes on when the patient is ascending. He may be climbing stairs or taking off in an airplane. This is the classic Hitchcock vertigo, in which the staircase behind or the sky below seems to elongate and distort in the patient's senses. The patient tends to panic during bouts of vertigo. Vertigo that comes on after eating.

ALSO CONSIDER

OPIUM—Vertigo that is accompanied by a rush of blood to the head. The face will be very dark red and will be bloated. The patient will have to go and lie down. He will sleep with his eyes half closed. He will seem to be in a stupor. He will snore in his sleep. Look for a slow but full pulse. This is the best remedy for elderly patients with vertigo.

EMERGENCIES
Palpitations of the Heart

Palpitations are typified by a heaviness in the left chest that is sometimes accompanied by stinging pains. Usually, the patient is unable to lie on the left side and experiences difficulty in breathing. There is often profuse sweating as well. Palpitations may be caused by stress, by strong emotions, or by overindulgence in food and drink. Palpitations may also be common in women during pregnancy. Do not confuse palpitations with cardiac events; or if there is any question, or if palpitations persist, or if there is accompanying severe pain, seek immediate help.

REMEDY CHECKLIST

If palpitations come on from fright, consider: **Coffea** or **Opium**.

If from sudden joy, consider: **Coffea**.

If from fear, consider: **Veratrum**.

If from disappointment, consider: **Aconite, Chamomilla, Ignatia**, and **Nux**.

If accompanied by congestion of the head, consider: **Aconite, Belladonna, Coffea, Lachesis, Phosphorus, Opium**, and **Sulphur**.

If from loss of blood, consider: **Phosphoric Acid, Nux**, and **Veratrum**.

For palpitations in nervous people, consider: **Coffea, Chamomilla, Cocculus, Ignatia, Lachesis, Nux**, and **Pulsatilla**.

In young people, consider: **Aconite** and **Pulsatilla**.

In elderly people, consider: **Arsenicum** and **Lachesis**.

For those who are chronically given to palpitations, consider: **Aconite, Arsenicum, Lachesis, Phosphorus, Pulsatilla**, and **Sulphur**.

REMEDIES

ACONITE—For the patient with sudden, wild palpitations accompanied by fever. The skin is hot and dry, especially on the face. The heart beats rapidly, but the pulse is slow. There is a stitching pain in the area of the heart. The patient complains of aching and will feel as if a heavy load has been placed on his chest. The patient sweats from agony, also from pain in the region of the kidneys that is also stitching in character. The patient will be very restless, very fearful. Will be certain that he is going to die.

ARNICA—Expect the patient here to experience pains in the chest that move from left to right. The pain is accompanied by fainting. The heart feels squeezed in the chest. The patient will say that it feels as if it is quivering.

ARSENICUM—The patient will experience terrible palpitations, as if the heart were going to burst out of the chest. The palpitations are worse at night, especially around midnight. They are worse when the patient lies on his back. The patient is exhausted, drained of all strength, but very restless, very fearful. The patient may struggle to get out of bed, or might lie, utterly exhausted, without moving. The patient will be very thirsty, but will only take small sips of liquid at a time.

BELLADONNA—Palpitations that are accompanied by a rush of blood to the face and head. The patient's head and face will feel hot internally and externally. The patient will have a red face. There is a sensation of pressure in the area of the heart that will make breathing difficult. The palpitations and pains will come and go very suddenly. The patient is in great anguish, and is most often very manic. Look for vomiting, fainting, and a cold sweat to accompany the palpitations.

BRYONIA—The patient has great difficulty breathing in that the motion of breathing causes great pain. Breathing is very shallow. Stitching pains run all throughout the chest. This pain may spread down the left arm. Pain is of a cutting nature. The patient is angry, manic. Wants to lie perfectly still. Feels that it is too painful to move, talk, or breathe.

LACHESIS—The irregularity of the palpitations is key here. Both the heartbeat and the pain are spasmodic in nature. There is a constrictive nature to all pain. The patient will experience a shortness of breath from any motion, especially from any motion of the hands. The patient is very weak and feels a great heaviness in the area of the heart. The patient will be unable to lie down, in that he will feel that he cannot breathe, that he is suffocating. The patient will be worse from resting, and, especially, worse from sleep. The patient will feel that he must sit up and bend forward. The patient will want to keep on talking, even if what he is saying makes little sense. He will not allow anything to touch his throat and feels that he will suffocate and die if anything touches his throat.

MERCURIUS—The key here is that the patient keeps trying to take a deep breath, but cannot. His greatest desire is to breathe; he struggles to do so. Palpitations are accompanied by coughing. Patient may even cough blood during palpitations. There is a sensation of heat and burning in the chest. The patient sweats during palpitations.

NUX—The palpitations here are usually worse at night. They usually begin after anger, or after too much to eat or drink. The patient will feel that his clothing is too tight in the region of the chest. There is heat and burning in the chest, with a throbbing sensation. The patient will be restless, irritable, and much worse from becoming cold or being in open air.

PHOSPHORUS—The patient here experiences a sensation of tightness across the chest that makes for very difficult breathing. He may say that he feels as if a steel band were being tightened across his chest. The patient will be extremely weak. The key to this remedy is that this sensation of pain and tightness will move up into the region of the throat. The palpitations may be brought on from any strong emotion. They are worse after eating. The patient may pant in trying to breathe. He will be unable to lie on his left side.

PULSATILLA—The patient will experience a clouding of vision during the palpitation. There is a burning sensation in the region of the heart. The patient will feel that he cannot breathe, will want open, cool, and moving air to be able to breathe. The patient is unable to lie on his left side. This will be a highly anxious patient, one who will want to cling, and to be taken care of.

RHUS TOX—Palpitations that are worse from sitting still. The patient will have to move frequently and keep moving about in order to stop the palpitations. There will be a stitching pain in the region of the heart. The left arm will be numb. The patient may complain of a sensation of trembling in the heart.

SPIGELIA—The patient feels as if he is suffocating during bouts of wild palpitations. The pain in the chest is spasmodic in nature. The pain grows worse if the patient moves up to a sitting position or in any way bends his chest forward.

VERATRUM—A crampy pain in the left side of the chest is the most common symptom of the Veratrum patient. The palpitations are quite violent in nature; the patient is very anxious and fearful. The pain moves into the left shoulder and is cutting in nature. The patient is in agony.

ALSO CONSIDER

CIMICFUGA—Intense palpitations that are accompanied by a pain that moves into the left shoulder and may extend down the left arm. The left arm feels as if it were attached to the left side of the chest. The patient cannot move the left arm.

DIGITALIS—The patient will feel that the heart will stop beating altogether if he moves in the slightest. The palpitations are also made worse if the patient talks or attempts to lie down. The patient feels as if the heart were contracting in his chest. Sharp pain in the chest that comes on suddenly. Palpitations that are so violent as to be visible. The patient is in unbearable pain. Look for a cold sweat to appear on the patient's forehead.

EMERGENCIES
Nosebleeds (Epistaxis)

This is another of life's household emergencies. Nosebleeds come from many different causes, from mechanical injuries to overblowing the nose during a cold. But nosebleeds are often not simply acute situations, but a sign of deeper constitutional problems. This is true especially when a patient is faced with frequent nosebleeds or finds it difficult to stop the bleeding. Nosebleeds are most common in the Phosphorus and Rhus Tox constitutional types, although the Sulphur is known to have chronic nosebleeds as well.

Acute nosebleeds may be grouped into two categories. Those that involve bright red blood are called "active" nosebleeds. They may be caused by mechanical injury or by emotional excitement. Nosebleeds in which the blood is dark are called "passive" nosebleeds. These usually come on at the end of a cold, fever, or other acute ailment.

But in general, when dealing with a nosebleed, pinch the lower part of the nose for a few minutes. If the bleeding does not stop, pinch again for five additional minutes. If by then the nose is still bleeding, this is the time to start out for the emergency room.

REMEDY CHECKLIST

For nosebleeds that come on from a cut to the nose or from mechanical injury, consider: **Arnica**.

For nosebleeds that come on after a drinking binge, consider: **Nux.**

For nosebleeds that come on after the patient has become overheated, consider: **Aconite** or **Bryonia.**

For nosebleeds that come on after the patient overexerts himself, consider: **Carbo Veg** or **Rhus Tox.**

For nosebleeds that come on during the night, consider: **Belladona, Bryonia**, and **Rhus Tox**.

For nosebleeds that come on during the day, consider: **Carbo Veg** or **Nux**.

REMEDIES

ACONITE—For nosebleeds that come on very suddenly. The blood will be bright red. The patient will have a flushed face and will complain of a strong sensation of pulsing in the arteries. The patient will be restless and fearful.

ARNICA—This is the first remedy to think of when you walk into a door or get punched in the nose. It's for when the nosebleed comes on from an injury of any sort. Also for when the bleeding is preceded by itching of the nose and forehead.

BELLADONNA—For the nosebleed accompanied by congestion in the head. Nosebleeds that come on after the patient becomes overheated. During the nosebleed, the patient will see sparks in front of his eyes. The patient will be worse from motion, noise, and bright light. The patient is better for lying down in a cool, dark place.

BRYONIA—Nosebleed in the morning after rising. This is the first remedy to think of when the patient's nose bleeds in hot weather or from getting overheated. Summer nosebleeds in children who have been running and playing. Think of this remedy especially when a woman gets a nosebleed instead of her scheduled period. The patient will want to lie down and be very still. She will feel sure that the nose will bleed some more if she moves.

CHINA—Considered an excellent remedy for those who have frequent nosebleeds or those for whom a simple nosebleed is very long-lasting. The bleeding never seems to want to end, no matter what you do. The patient's face will be very pale. He will complain of a ringing in his ears during the nosebleed. Itching in their nose. The patient may experience vertigo during nosebleed. The patient will be weakened by the loss of blood.

IPECAC—This is a remedy for nosebleeds with bright red blood that may be accompanied by severe nausea. It is the nausea, and perhaps vomiting, that will be the guiding symptom in the selection of this particular remedy.

FERRUM PHOS—Here, too, the blood is bright red. But the patient will also feel dizzy and faint (like all those commercials on television for "iron-poor blood"). The patient's skin is pale. A throbbing sensation in the head, and especially in the nose, will accompany the bleeding.

LACHESIS—The snake-venom remedies are all to be considered in the treatment of those with nosebleeds (see Vipera below). Lachesis is a good general remedy for nosebleeds, and a common remedy as well. The nostrils will be very sensitive. The blood will be very dark red or purple. The face will also take on a dark red or purple tinge. The face will look bloated or swollen. The patient will complain of pains at the root of the nose.

NUX—This is a remedy to think of especially for nosebleeds in alcoholics and drug addicts. For nosebleeds that are accompanied by a pressing pain in the forehead. The patient will complain of the sensation of a nail being driven into his forehead. Nosebleeds will commonly occur in the morning, accompanying a hangover. The patient will feel toxic and sick. Nosebleed with headache. Also, nosebleeds from suppressed hemorrhoids. A sensation of coldness throughout the entire body will accompany the nosebleed. The patient will be irritable.

PHOSPHORUS—Also for nosebleeds with bright red blood, but there is more bleeding here, and the nosebleed often comes on from violent blowing of the nose. (Those who need Phosphorus constitutionally often have crusted blood in the nose on a daily basis, and nose-blowing always yields a little blood.) General remedy for those who get frequent nose-bleeds. Profuse bleeding that seems never to stop. A remedy specific to nosebleeds that come on when the patient is passing a stool.

RHUS TOX—Think of this remedy for the patient who is, in general, given to nosebleeds, but the nosebleeds happen only at night. This is also a remedy specific to nosebleeds from general overexertion and overlifting. From straining the body. Also for nosebleeds that come on from stooping. Look for the patient's nose to seem swollen from bleeding. Look for a red tip of the nose, red tip of the tongue.

ALSO CONSIDER

VIPERA—This is a minor and not very well-known remedy, but you should think of it as a general nosebleed remedy (with Phosphorus). For nosebleeds without specific cause or symptom picture. As Ferrum Phos is to fevers, Vipera (which is taken from the venom of the German Viper) is to nosebleeds. The patient's head will have to be elevated for the bleeding to stop.

EMERGENCIES
Burns and Scalds

Remember that burns can be caused by more than just fire: burns can be caused by heat, by friction, or by chemicals. Scalds, for our purposes, will also be considered as burns. In the treatment of burns, as in our other homeopathic treatments, we must watch how this patient's body reacts to the burn and the specific symptoms that are created in response to it. Obviously, with severe burns, get the patient to the emergency room.

The first step to treatment is to remove the cause of the burn. Take the patient's hand out of the fire, for example. Once the danger of continued burn has passed, if the skin is not broken, immerse the burn in cold water for at least 10 minutes. Add Hypericum and/or Calendula to the water to help ease the pain. If you can remove the patient's jewelry, go ahead and remove it. If clothing sticks to the wound, however, leave it alone. You will cause more pain and do more damage to the wounded area by removing the clothing than it is worth. Cover the burn to prevent infection. If blisters or boils appear, do not open them. Again, leave them alone. Give the patient plenty of water to drink.

Obviously, a condition like a burn or a scald is a natural match for topical applications of remedies. But not all topical applications will do the job well. If all you have on hand is Calendula in a petroleum-based jelly, do not use it on a burn or scald. Petroleum jelly will seal the heat into the wound and not let it escape. Aqua Calendula or Aqua Hypericum will do a much better job.

A wonderful alternative is Rescue Remedy Cream, which will soothe the burn and help it to heal. For me, I find that it works better in the long run than Hypericum and Calendula.

REMEDIES

ACONITE—For burns that are accompanied by chills, fever, dry, hot skin, and great thirst. Look for the patient to have great fear and anxiety, with much nervous excitement. Often, Aconite will alternate with Arnica in burn situations, as in other mechanical injuries.

ARNICA—Should be given immediately for the shock that accompanies the burn and to promote healing in general. Then follow up the Arnica with specifically called-for remedies that may either be used as follow-ups to Arnica, or used in alteration.

ARSENICUM—As a remedy for burns in which most of the symptoms involve a burning sensation, it makes sense that Arsenicum be considered. Look for dark, watery diarrhea to accompany burn. Look for a rapid sinking of vital force. Look for extreme thirst, although the patient drinks little. Look for great fear and anguish, with great restlessness.

CAUSTICUM—Another general burn remedy, Causticum is very helpful in clearing up the final stages of a burn, or in the case where the scar left by the healing wound is still painful.

CHAMOMILLA—Used when convulsions arise from severe burns. Patient will be furious in his pain. He will be very impatient and will hardly be able to answer your questions politely. Look for the patient to have warm sweat on his face and head.

HEPAR SULPH—If the burn becomes infected, give Hepar Sulph internally; externally, use either a Hypericum or Calendula tincture—the two may be combined to promote healing and soothe pain.

KALI BI—For second-degree, deeper, more damaging burns. The pain will occur in specific spots on the body.

SILICEA—Think of this remedy when the burn heals too slowly, or when the skin does not completely heal from the burn. When the skin looks unhealthy. When the patient is chronically weak and, in general, slow to heal from any condition.

URTICA URENS—This is perhaps our most used remedy for those with burns. Think of Uritca for burns with a strong stinging sensation to the wound (the remedy is taken from stinging nettle and a stinging sensation follows all of its pain patterns). Urtica Urens is a remedy for all burns, not just for superficial cases. It will bring about a quick healing, as long as the burns follows the stinging pattern of the remedy portrait. Urtica Urens may also be dissolved in water and applied topically. It may be used topically and internally at the same time.

ALSO CONSIDER

CANTHARIS—For general burns, with or without shock, with deep overwhelming burning sensation. For both burns and scalds. The patient will feel better from cold applications. The patient will be restless, will not be able to think of anything but the pain of the burn. Cantharis is perhaps the first remedy to think of in cases of superficial burns or scalds.
Note: Cantharis is also to be considered as an external remedy for burns. Create Aqua Cantharis by dissolving five or six pellets of the remedy in a half glass of water and apply often to the injured area of the patient's body. Make sure to keep the injured part constantly wet with the mixture, either by immersion or by covering with a cloth that is soaked with the mixture.

EMERGENCIES
Sunburn

While usually not a life-threatening emergency, sunburn is treated homeopathically very like a burn of any other kind. Remember Rescue Remedy Cream for use as a topical remedy.

REMEDIES

ACONITE—A specific remedy for those times in which the patient's head and face receive a full dose of the sun's rays. The patient will be restless and excitable. He will have a throbbing headache accompanying the sunburn. In addition, look for the patient to be very thirsty. Distortion of vision is also common: objects will seem to swim by the patient's field of vision.

BELLADONNA—For serious sunburn. The skin is red, hot, and dry. Look for the patient to have a blinding headache from the sunburn. The patient will have to lie down in a cool, dark place in order to feel better. The patient will also be greatly aggravated by noise and, especially, by light. Look for the patient to experience a sense of congestion or a rush of blood to the head. Look also for the patient to have a sense of vertigo that is made worse by stooping.

CALENDULA—Applied externally, Calendula offers a soothing balm to sunburned skin.

Note: Aqua Calendula, the potentized remedy dissolved in cool, fresh water, will be much more soothing to the sunburn than the Calendula rub. The remedy may also be taken internally, either in pellet or in liquid form for the treatment of the sunburn.

ALSO CONSIDER

GLONOINUM—The general basic sunburn remedy. Especially called for if the patient feels cold internally, even though his skin is burning hot. A congestive headache typically will accompany the sunburn. The patient will be confused. He will feel that his head is very heavy, and yet he cannot put it down on a pillow. The patient cannot bear for his head to touch anything. In general, the patient will complain of a sensation of pulsation in his body. The patient will experience vertigo with the sunburn.

EMERGENCIES
Heat Exhaustion

Heat exhaustion is a well-named ailment. It occurs when the patient's body has been exposed to too much hot weather. The body loses water and salt from sweating, becoming dehydrated, and the result is a mild form of shock in which the patient finds himself overcome with exhaustion. Expect the patient to have clammy skin and a pallid complexion. Headaches and nausea and vomiting are common. Also look for dizziness and muscle cramps. The patient's body temperature, however, will stay normal or slightly above normal. Look for a rapid pulse and rapid, shallow breathing. The entire condition will be made worse if the patient has been drinking alcohol, which further dehydrates the body, making the patient feel even worse.

As heat exhaustion is very like a mild form of shock, we will treat it as a mild form of shock.

Before selecting a remedy, make sure that the patient lies down in a cool, dark place. Apply cool, wet cloths. Add a bit of salt to a glass of water and make him sip it.

Note: Unlike heat exhaustion, heatstroke is a life-threatening emergency. It occurs most often to older persons and to people who overdo exercise on a hot summer day. The middle-aged man of sedentary habit who decides to mow his lawn on a hot August day, therefore, is a prime candidate for heatstroke.

In heatstroke, the heat-regulating mechanisms in the body have been overwhelmed and have failed. Fever results. The presence of fever is the quickest way to tell the difference between heat exhaustion and heatstroke. Often the fever can be as high as 104 degrees. And often, despite the high fever, the patient will not sweat. It is as if the heatstroke has burnt out the patient's ability to sweat. If the patient does sweat, however, look for him to be drenched in sweat. One extreme or the other is possible. The skin will be both red and hot. The pulse will be fast and pounding. The patient typically will seem confused, and may be in something of a stupor. Unconsciousness is common. The patient may complain of headache or nausea, and may also experience abrupt changes in vision.

REMEDIES

BRYONIA—A remedy for many ailments due to the heat of the summer. The typical patient will have overdone it in the heat, and will have drunk a good bit of alcohol, especially beer. The patient then feels "done in." He is irritable. He has a terrible headache, one that makes him feel as if his head would split open. The patient wants to lie down and to be left alone. He feels worse for any kind of motion. Even the motion of his eyes will make the headache worse. The Bryonia patient will not be able to sit up without feeling nauseous. He will also feel faint. The patient may, however, be very thirsty and have to sit up from time to time to drink great quantities of water.

CAMPHORA—Suggested for cases of heatstroke in which the patient responds to the heat by feeling intense chilliness. The patient will shiver.

He will feel faint. He will be very dizzy. Look for muscle cramps in the legs, arms, or abdomen to accompany the heat exhaustion.

CARBO VEG—Shows the perfect picture of heat exhaustion. Look for the patient to have clammy skin, with sweat covering his whole body. The patient will also have a sense of heaviness in the head, with a throbbing congestion being common. A headache centered in the forehead will accompany the heat exhaustion. The patient will complain of pain in his eyes. This pain is aggravated by the patient staring fixedly at any object. And, as the patient seems in a bit of a stupor, he tends to stare fixedly at many objects, thus increasing his own discomfort. The patient will have trouble breathing and will want moving air on his face. He will want to be fanned.

GELSEMIUM—The patient here is exhausted and a bit overwhelmed. He seems a little puzzled by what has happened, and a little disconnected from it. The patient may experience changes in vision. It may go a little cloudy or, more commonly, images may double. The patient's head will feel heavy. The patient will fell dizzy. He may also experience muscle pain, as if he had overexerted his body.

VERATRUM—For profuse and clammy sweat, great weakness, fainting, extreme coldness of body, especially the feet, hands, and face. The patient will have terrible nausea. Look for a rapid pulse and stiffness of the body. The patient will be anxious and afraid. He may call out as well or rant and rave wildly. In this remedy portrait, the patient is much more exhausted and depleted than above. Incredible nausea and the possibility of either vomiting or diarrhea is a keynote of this remedy.

ALSO CONSIDER

CUPRUM METALLICUM—Look for the basic symptoms of heat exhaustion as listed above, but with cramping as the dominant symptom. Patient will have jerking motions of the muscles. This is a keynote of this particular remedy's portrait for nearly all ailments. In severe cases, convulsions may accompany the sensation of cramping.

EMERGENCIES
Hypothermia (Chilblains)

Hypothermia, or, as I prefer to call it, chilblains, occurs when the core body temperature falls below 95 degrees. When the patient has for too long a time been exposed to cold temperatures, or subjected to too sudden a change in temperature.

At the point in which chilblains set in, the patient becomes somewhat foggy in his behavior, somewhat unresponsive. Like a character in a Jack London story, he no longer wishes to move. He just wants to lie down and sleep in the snow. The patient may also have cramps or numbness throughout his body.

Chilblains may occur either when the patient is out in the cold, or when he moves from being in a very cold place to a very warm one. Chilblains, as such, generally occur in the feet, hands, nose, and ears. Affected parts may take on a purple-red color and may be swollen.

In treating the situation, first bring the patient into a warm place. Give sips of hot, sweet liquids. It is not, however, a good idea to give the patient alcohol. Wrap the patient up well. Do not massage the body, not even gently. Do not put the patient in a hot bath. The most effective thing you can often do is hold the victim close and let your own body heat help warm him, just as in an old Hollywood movie.

The remedies listed here all will be equally helpful for cases in which part of the body has simply been chapped, which consists of a slight inflammation of the skin, especially on the back of the hands.

REMEDIES

ARNICA—Consider this remedy for cases in which the affected area of the skin is hard and shining red. The patient wil complain of both pain and itching of the affected parts. In this case, Aqua Arnica should be created and used topically, as well as internally, as long as the skin has not been broken or scraped.

ARSENICUM—In this remedy portrait, look for hot, shining red spots on the skin, spots that will have burning pains. Ulcerated, spreading blisters, especially on toes. Expect the patient to be restless and anxious. He will tend to be very afraid. The patient will feel chilly and will want to be wrapped up warm and tight. He will usually, however, prefer his head to be uncovered. The patient will be very thirsty for warm liquids, especially for tea with lemon; however, he will drink only small sips of liquid at any given time.

BELLADONNA—For patients in whose case the affected part of the skin is fiery red. Look for swelling of affected parts. The patient will complain of feeling of inflammation. He will complain of pulsing and throbbing pains that come and go very quickly and without warning.

PHOSPHORUS—Consider this a good general remedy for chilblains, especially in the fingers and toes. The parts have a blue-red appearance and burn and itch violently. These patients will want to be taken care of. They may be very emotional in their pain. They will want company. Also, they will tend to be thirsty for cold things.

PULSATILLA—Look at the skin as an indicator. In this remedy portrait, the affected parts are deep red or red-brown in color, and the color is particularly vivid. The effected parts of the body will burn and itch violently. The patient may cry when he tells you his symptoms. The patient will want to be comforted and paid attention to. He will be worse if you do not pay enough attention to him.

SULPHUR—This remedy is specific to chilblains of the toes, with ulcerated blisters. A wild heat or itching sensation may accompany chilblains. The patient will be greatly aggravated in general by heat. Heat and warm applications will also aggravate affected areas, increasing the itch. The patient will seem strong in his illness and able to cope with it.

EMERGENCIES
Frostbite

While frostbite is certainly similar in both impact and treatment to chilblains, frostbite is a more serious condition. Emergency medical care may be indicated. If frostbite has set in, then circulation has been cut off to a part of the body, most often to the hands, feet, nose, and ears. The affected areas of the body will have a cold and pale look.

In treating frostbite, first move the patient into a warm—but not too hot—place. Do not, for instance, put him in front of a hot fire. Instead bring the patient inside to a nice cool room and let him slowly return to his natural temperature. Give warm drinks and cover the patient up, nice and tight. Make sure to warm frostbitten parts with body heat only. It is of great importance that you do not heat the body too quickly. It is also important that you do not rub the affected areas, but just let the person slowly warm.

REMEDIES

APIS—The patient will be very cold in this remedy portrait and will want, more than anything else, to get warm. He will want a warm room and will want to sip warm liquids. But look out for severe burning pains in all affected parts of the body as those parts get warm. The patient will be irritable. The pains associated with the warming of the body will be stinging and burning in nature, like the stinging pains of the bee sting from which this remedy is taken.

ARSENICUM—As with the Apis patient, the Arsenicum patient is very cold and very much wants to be warmed. These patients will be very thirsty for warm drinks, especially for hot tea with lemon. They will only sip small amounts of the warm liquid, however. They are fussy patients, and fearful. They will not want to be left alone, as they will actually feel worse physically when left alone. These patients will want to be totally wrapped up in blankets, with the possible exception of their head. The Arsenicum, no matter how cold, tends to want to have the head unwrapped and may even want it exposed to cool air.

CARBO VEG—Think of Carbo Veg as being, in some ways, very similar to Apis. The Carbo Veg patient is also very cold and wants to get warm. He also has a good deal of pain as the body warms. But look for the severe pain to occur in the whole body, and not in specific parts, as it becomes warm. The patient may be unaware of what has happened to him; he may simply feel disconnected to the event until the pain sets in. Also look for the patient to have trouble breathing, will want air fanned on him. This symptom will guide you to the remedy.

LACHESIS—Think of this remedy in cases involving frostbite with purple discoloration of the skin. As is typical of this remedy, the affected part of the body will also be swollen. The area may itch, and will greatly swell up if scratched. This patient is very verbal and will talk a great deal. He will want to keep on talking and complaining through the entire event.

ALSO CONSIDER

AGARICUS—This is to be considered a general frostbite remedy and may be your best first choice remedy. Any situation that calls for Agaricus will be rather serious in nature. The patient will seem overcome by his exposure to cold. The patient will seem almost drunk in his stupor. He may hallucinate. Look for the patient to be of little help in answering questions. These patients tend to be rather incoherent. The patient may sing to himself, or may grow angry at being asked questions. He will be much worse from anything cold, especially cold air.

GENERAL ACHES AND PAINS
Sleep Disorders—Insomnia

Although all of us experience insomnia from time to time, from overeating or from daily stresses, sleeplessness is sometimes a symptom of some constitutional disorder. If it continues for an extended period of time it should be treated constitutionally, as it will sooner or later cause a disruption to the entire system. The appetite becomes impaired, the stomach disordered, and depression is common. Insomnia is often accompanied by headache, nervousness, and nightmares.

REMEDY CHECKLIST

For sleeplessness after being emotionally upset, or from becoming agitated, consider: **Aconite** and **Arnica**.

For sleeplessness after too much excitement or fun, consider: **Coffea**.

For sleeplessness from overwork, from mental strain, consider: **Lycopodium** or **Nux**.

For sleeplessness after overeating or drinking, consider: **Nux** or **Pulsatilla**.

For sleeplessness after a severe illness, consider: **Hyoscyamus.**

For sleeplessness caused by grief, consider: **Ignatia**.

For sleeplessness caused by fear, consider: **Aconite, Arsenicum,** or **Opium**.

For sleeplessness in children, consider: **Belladonna, Chamomilla,** or **Coffea**.

For sleeplessness in the elderly, consider: **Arsenicum** or **Opium**.

REMEDIES

ACONITE—Sleep is blocked by agitation and upsetting events. Sleeplessness accompanied by fever and anxiety. Sudden waking from nightmares. The patient thinks that he is about to die, clutches his throat, calls out in fear. This is also a remedy for restlessness at night, for tossing and turning in bed.

ARSENICUM—Sleeplessness from anxiety. The patient fears the vulnerability that sleep represents. He fears being attacked in the sleep state. The patient is restless, and yet exhausted. Walks the floor from midnight to 2 A.M. The patient will be chilly in sleeplessness. He will check corners and closets for intruders. He will hear noises in the night.

BELLADONNA—The patient is very sleepy but cannot sleep. Starts—often in a fright—on falling asleep. Sleeplessness from nightmares. These patients are startled, angry. They are worked up and they cannot calm down. The sleeplessness is worse toward morning.

CHAMOMILLA—Sleeplessness caused by drinking coffee. Patient is excited and irritable. Very impatient. The patient will want to move about, to walk the floor. He will also want to be carried. This is an excellent remedy for the sleepless child who demands total attention from the parent.

COCCULUS—Consider when the patient is used to staying up at night and now no longer feels sleepy at an appropriate time. Most often used for patients who have stayed by the side of the sick to see them through their illness. And now they cannot sleep. Individuals feel "too tired to sleep." Giddy with lack of sleep. They will be very irritable.

COFFEA—Extreme wakefulness and general state of excitability. Especially indicated in situations in which insomnia is caused by excessive joy. Sleeplessness from drinking tea. From any stimulant. Think of this as the remedy for Christmas Eve.

LYCOPODIUM—The mind is too active for sleep to come. The patient relives the day over and over. "What I should have said was . . ." Individual talks and laughs in sleep. Often the patient will fall asleep, but will awaken again at 4 A.M. and will not be able to go back to sleep. Also for chronic insomnia, for the patient who always awakens in the middle of the night.

NUX—Insomnia caused by intense mental exertion, from overwork. Insomnia from gastric distress, from drinking coffee, from eating highly seasoned food, from drinking alcohol. The first choice remedy for those with chronic insomnia that lasts until 3 A.M. Some Nux patients cannot fall asleep until the sun begins to rise. This is an excellent remedy for those who, night after night, fall asleep in a chair while watching television, only to find that they cannot sleep at all when they get into bed.

PULSATILLA—Insomnia worse in warm room, from eating rich foods. Individual falls into a light sleep, becomes too hot and kicks off covers, then becomes too cold and wakes looking for covers. Sleeps with arms overhead.

RHUS TOX—The patient's body feels too overworked to sleep. "Too tired to sleep." Sleeplessness caused by overexertion, which is accompanied by restlessness. The patient tosses and turns in attempt to find a comfortable position and to fall asleep. Especially for insomnia that involves physical pain or discomfort.

ALSO CONSIDER

OPIUM—Insomnia from fear, fright, and depression. When various figures and visions appear before the eyes of the patient and prevent him from sleeping. Suitable after severe mental exertion or long, continued night watching. In chronic Opium insomnia, senses are too elevated to allow patient to sleep. Noises too loud, bed too hot, for sleep to come.

GENERAL ACHES AND PAINS
Sleep Disorders—Nightmares

These are the moments during sleep in which the individual experiences a distressing sensation while in the dream state. The individual cannot move or speak and seems threatened with suffocation. Frequent efforts are made to cry out, but often without effect. The person wakes in terror, feeling very anxious. Nightmares are often caused by problems with digestion, and, in addition to the remedies listed below, readers should look at the remedies listed under "Digestion Upsets: Indigestion."

REMEDIES

ACONITE—The patient will awaken in shock and panic. Dr̶e̶a̶̶ ̶̶ ̶̶ ̶g̶. The patient will feel that he can predict the moment of his death. The patient clutches his throat. He is restless. He is very fearful. Look for a physical feeling of oppression in the chest to accompany fear. This is perhaps the first remedy to consider for nightmares in childhood.

ARNICA—This is the classic remedy for nightmares. For bad news of any sort. Just as Arnica soothes the body after a blow or fall, so, too, it soothes the mind after a nightmare. The remedy works best if given in a high potency. The patient will feel that he cannot get comfortable, that his body and soul are sore. The bed feels too hard. Nightmares of being chased by animals.

ARSENICUM—Here the nightmares come between midnight and 2 A.M. Sleeper dreams of robbers breaking into the house, awakens full of fear. Does not want to be left alone. The Arsenicum is always hearing noises downstairs and needs them investigated in order to feel safe. The patient may walk the floor for hours, keeping watch over the house, keeping everyone safe.

NUX—For the patient who wakens from a nightmare after overeating, and especially after drinking alcohol. Especially if he ate and drank just before going to bed. The patient will be upset and very irritable. He will not want to be comforted and may strike out at anyone who tries to awaken or comfort him.

PULSATILLA—For nightmares that come on after eating rich food. Especially after eating greasy food. The patient awakens feeling that he cannot breathe. He wants to be held and comforted. Does not want to be left alone. The patient may be clingy and weepy.

ALSO CONSIDER

AURUM—For the chronic nightmares of depressed patients. Dreams of hunger, of dying, of problems at work. Will often dream of money, of gold. The dreams are often so chronic that the patient will not want to sleep. The patient, over time, will develop a fear of sleeping.

OPIUM—The patient has a terrible nightmare, but seems unable to awaken from it. He will call out in his sleep, wave his arms and legs, but seem to still be asleep. The patient will call out in his sleep, mutter, sigh, snore. He may seem to have trouble breathing. But still he doesn't wake. The patient's body will be covered in cold sweat; his eyes will be half open. The dream will be very real to him.

GENERAL ACHES AND PAINS
Teeth: Acute Situations—Toothache

Usually, toothache is caused when tooth decay is advanced enough to cause pain. It may also be caused by sinus problems, by mechanical problems with the tooth, and by sensitivity to specific conditions. Whatever the cause, treatment is needed, and you need to get into a dentist's office. But there are acute remedies to use for the pain. In other words, the following suggestions are to help you until you get to the dentist's office, but are not offered for use instead of going to that office.

A toothache often takes more than one remedy. I have included a list of follow-up remedies where possible.

REMEDY CHECKLIST

For a toothache that comes on after the patient becomes chilled, consider: **Aconite, Belladonna, Chamomilla, Coffea, Dulcamara, Ignatia, Mercurius, Nux**, or **Pulsatilla**.

For a toothache that comes on after exposure to damp, cold air, consider: **Belladonna, Bryonia, Chamomilla, Dulcamara, Mercurius, Nux, Pulsatilla, Rhus Tox**, or **Sulphur**.

For a toothache that comes on after drinking coffee, consider: **Chamomilla, Ignatia**, or **Nux**.

For a toothache that is caused by tooth decay, consider: **Bryonia, Chamomilla, China, Mercurius, Pulsatilla, Silicea**, or **Sulphur**.

For a toothache that hurts into the bones of the face, consider: **Mercurius** or **Sulphur**.

For a toothache that hurts into the ears, consider: **Arsenicum, Chamomilla, Mercurius, Pulsatilla**, or **Sulphur**.

For a toothache that hurts into the eyes, consider: **Pulsatilla**.

For a toothache that hurts the whole head, consider: **Chamomilla, Mercurius, Nux, Pulsatilla**, or **Sulphur**.

For a toothache accompanied by a swollen face, consider: **Bryonia, Chamomilla, Mercurius, Nux, Pulsatilla**, or **Sepia**.

For a toothache accompanied by swollen gums, consider: **Aconite, Belladonna, Hepar Sulph, Mercurius, Nux**, or **Sulphur**.

For a toothache accompanied by swollen glands, consider: **Carbo Veg, Mercurius, Nux**, or **Staphysagria**.

If the toothache feels better from pressure, consider: **Belladonna, Pulsatilla**, or **Rhus Tox**.

If the toothache feels better from warmth, consider: **Arsenicum, Mercurius, Nux, Rhus Tox**, or **Sulphur**.

If the toothache feels better from cold, consider: **Bryonia** or **Pulsatilla**.

If the toothache feels worse from warmth, consider: **Bryonia, Coffea, Chamomilla, Pulsatilla**, or **Sulphur**.

If the toothache feels worse from cold, consider: **Belladonna, Nux, Rhus Tox, Staphysagria**, or **Sulphur**.

For toothache in children, consider: **Aconite, Belladonna, Chamomilla, Coffea**, and **Ignatia**.

REMEDIES

ACONITE—For toothache that comes suddenly. The patient is frantic with the pain, which is intense. Pain is throbbing or stitching. Patient is very restless, in a constant state of fear and anxiety. Look for the patient to be feverish with toothache. (Belladonna, Bryonia, Chamomilla, and Coffea all follow Aconite well in toothache.)

ARNICA—For toothache that comes on after an operation. Or from a blow to the jaw. Teeth feel bruised, sprained. Cheeks will be red and swollen. The patient will not want the jaw or mouth touched.

ARSENICUM—The patient's teeth feel elongated and may also feel loose. The patient complains of jerking pains in the teeth and the gums. Pain extends from the teeth into the ears, cheeks, and temples. Pain overwhelms the patient. Patient is restless and can only tolerate small sips of warm drinks.

BELLADONNA—Look for the face to be swollen and red. The throat will be very dry, as will the mouth. The patient is very thirsty. Toothache comes on very suddenly and can leave just as quickly. Pain worse in cold air, worse at night. Especially after the patient has gone to bed. The patient will also have red eyes. (Hepar Sulph or Mercurius most often act as a follow-up remedy, as will Chamomilla or Pulsatilla.)

BRYONIA—For pain in decayed teeth. The teeth will feel loose in the patient's mouth. They will also typically feel too long. The pain in a Bryonia toothache is worse for warm air, drink, or food. Worse at night. The patient's mouth feels very dry. The patient thirsty for great amounts of liquid. He will want to stay very still. He may experience constipation with the toothache. (Bryonia follows well after Rhus Tox, Mercurius, or Chamomilla with toothache.)

CALCAREA—The patient's tooth—and it will likely seem like all his teeth—is sore. The patient's pain is boring in nature. The pain is worse from any intake of air, warm or cold. Worse for anything warm or cold. Worse for any change in temperature at all. The patient's gums are swollen and sore, bleed easily. The face may be swollen as well, and red, especially at night. This is often the best remedy for pregnant women who have toothache.

CARBO VEG—Consider this remedy for the toothache accompanied by receding and bleeding gums, with ulcers of the mouth. Teeth are loose and eating is painful. The pain is made much worse from salt. The patient will gasp for air while in pain and will want to be fanned. The patient's teeth will hurt every time they are touched by the tongue, and yet the patient will keep touching them with his tongue.

CHAMOMILLA—This is one of our most important remedies for those with toothache. The pain of the toothache is unbearable, worse for cold air and by warm food and drink, especially coffee. The pain is jerking or shooting in nature. The patient is very angry, cannot be satisfied or calmed. He may almost faint with pain. Look for hot, swollen cheeks and red, swollen gums. Often, the patient will have one red cheek with the other quite pale. The pain is worse at night. (Bryonia, Mercurius, Spuphur, Coffea, and, even Belladonna all follow well after Chamomilla.)

CHINA—For the patient with a periodic toothache. This pain is made worse from smoking, from any contact with the tooth. The pain, however, is made better from pressing the teeth firmly together.

COFFEA—The patient is restless and irritable. Pain worse for heat and hot food and drink. Better for applications of ice. The patient will be overwhelmed by pain, frantic. He will tremble in pain. The pain will be worse at night or after the patient has eaten a meal. (Belladonna, Hyoscyamus, or Sulphur follows well.)

DULCAMARA—Consider this remedy for the toothache that comes on in cold and damp weather. Especially in the times of year in which the days are warm and the nights cool. Toothache accompanied by diarrhea. Look especially for profuse salivation. Consider this remedy for cases in which toothache comes on following a cold. (Dulcamara follows Mercurius, Chamomilla, or Belladonna well and completes their actions.)

HEPAR SULPH—This remedy is needed when a tooth is infected as well as aching. The patient's pain will be worse at night, in a warm room, when biting down or pressing the teeth together. The patient's cheeks will be swollen. This remedy often works well for patients who have many mercury fillings and have chronic toothache. (Hepar Sulph follows Mercurius or Belladonna; Silicia follows Hepar Sulph well.)

IGNATIA—Consider this remedy if the toothache pain creates a complete change in the patient's personality. If the previously happy patient becomes angry or wildly moody in his pain state. The patient will weep from his pain. Also for toothache that comes on after emotional upset or from depression. Toothache that comes on in the morning when the patient awakens. The pain is worse from coffee or from smoking tobacco. The patient will say that he feels as if his teeth were broken. (Ignatia follows well after Chamomilla, Pulsatilla, or Nux.)

MERCURIUS—This is the first remedy to consider in cases involving a patient who has spongy gums that bleed very easily, loose teeth, and, especially, very bad breath. Look for the patient's mouth to be filled with saliva, and look for a swollen tongue. The patient will be very thirsty. The pain of the toothache will likely shoot up into the ears. The pain is stinging in nature. The pain worse from both hot and cold. The patient's entire body will be very sensitive to changes in temperature and will be worse from both hot and cold. The toothache will be worse at night, especially after the patient has gone to bed. He will awaken from sleep in terrible pain. Look for a great deal of sweat to accompany the pain. (Mercurius follows well after Belladonna or Dulcamara, and before Hepar Sulph, Sulphur, or Carbo Veg.)

NUX—Consider this remedy for the patient who complains of a sore tooth. Look for the patient to complain of pain in both the tooth and the jaw, although the pain can extend throughout head. The pain is worse in the early morning hours, worse in a warm room, worse for mental labor. It is also worse from contact with anything cold. The patient is irritable, constipated, chilly. (Mercurius or Sulphur follows well.)

PULSATILLA—The patient's emotional picture will be helpful here. Expect the patient to be tearful. The patient will have an earache or a one-sided headache accompanying the toothache. The toothache is better for cold, worse for warm. The patient feels chilly, even in a warm room, but will have a sensation of suffocation in the warm room and may well want to go outside for a walk. The patient will be comforted by motion, especially by taking on a rocking motion, as if sitting in a rocking chair. The patient will want company and attention. The pain will become worse if the patient is left alone. (Pulsatilla precedes or follows Sulphur or Mercurius.)

RHUS TOX—The teeth feel too long and too loose. The patient's gums are swollen and they tend to itch, as well as burn. The patient experiences shooting pains, as if the teeth were being torn out by the roots. The toothache will be worse for cold, damp weather. Or will come on in wet weather. The pain is better for external applications of heat. The patient may want to take a long, hot shower to soothe the pain. Look for the characteristic red tip of the tongue as an indication of the remedy. (Rhus Tox follows Belladonna.)

SEPIA—For the patient who experiences toothache during pregnancy. Or for a toothache that comes on during any time of life at which a woman's hormones are undergoing a great change. Look for the patient to complain of pains going into her ears. They may go along the arms and into the fingers. Look for swelling of the cheeks and glands. Look for constipation or sick headache to accompany toothache. (Sepia follows Belladonna.)

SILICEA—For toothache in which the pain extends into the jawbone. The entire jaw may be swollen. The pain in the jaw is greater than the pain in the tooth. The pain is worse at night. Toothache with a tendency toward abscess. (Silicea follows Mercurius or Hepar Sulph.)

STAPHYSAGRIA—For the patient with overwhelming toothache pain. Toothache from tooth decay. The teeth may be black they are so decayed. Gums will be ulcerated, pale white, and swollen. The gums will feel very tender. The pain is worse in the morning and at night, and after cold food or drinks. Look for a cold sweat on face. Cold hands accompany toothache.

SULPHUR—The teeth feel hollow. The patient's pain extends into upper jaw and into the ears. Teeth feel too long, too loose. The pain is worse each night from the heat of the bed and from cold water. From contact with anything cold. The toothache will become worse every time the patient goes outdoors. Accompanying the toothache, look for the patient to experience burning heat in the head and cold extremities. (Sulphur follows especially well after Aconite or Mercurius.)

ALSO CONSIDER

HYOSCYAMUS—The pain is intolerable, tearing or throbbing in nature. Look for the pain to extend into the patient's cheeks and across lower jaw. Look for spasms of twitching in the patient's fingers, hands, arms, and face along with toothache. Look for pulsing pains from the patient's forehead to jaw. The pain is worse in the morning, worse for cold air. The patient is nervous and excited. His eyes are red and wide open. He looks all around, rather wildly. His face is red and hot to the touch.

PLANTAGO—The pain is worse for cold air, but better from eating. All the teeth feel sensitive—as if they were too long for the mouth and were too exposed. Look for the mouth to be full of saliva. This remains one of our general remedies for toothache. Some practitioners recommend that this remedy be dissolved in water and used as a mouthwash in cases of acute toothache.

GENERAL ACHES AND PAINS
Teeth: Acute Situations—Abscess

This is the bacterial infection of a decaying tooth. Pus has formed, and the tooth is extremely tender, with pain radiating across the jaw, along the side of the nose, or across other teeth. The abscess is a gumboil—a swelling of the gum filled with pus. Fever may accompany the infection. This infection is dangerous and if the boil bursts in the mouth (do not swallow), or if the swelling becomes too great, this may be an appropriate time for the use of an antibiotic. It is certainly a time in which home treatment should be limited only to the amount of time it takes to get into your practitioner's office.

REMEDIES

BELLADONNA—For the patient who experiences abscess with fever. The patient's face, tooth, and gum all feel hot. The face and mouth are both dry. The abscess is red, hard, and painful. The patient will complain of a pain that is throbbing in nature. Look for the pain to come on and to leave suddenly, without warning. Look for the patient's face to be red and hot.

HEPAR SULPH—Think of this remedy first when suppuration, or the formation of pus, is inevitable. An infection is present and the pus is being pushed to the surface. Hepar Sulph will draw the pus into the boil and bring it out of the system. Watch that the patient does not swallow this pus if the abscess bursts.

MERCURIUS—If taken early enough, this remedy will prevent suppuration. It is considered to be the remedy of first choice. Look for swelling of glands, which is keynote to the remedy and will guide you to its use. Also look for the patient to display spongy gums, and for the production of much saliva, for a swollen tongue, and for the patient to have terrible breath. If you become familiar with the smell of the breath of a Mercurius patient, you will come to recognize the remedy by this smell alone. Abscess will be pale in color. Night sweat will accompany the infection.

SILICEA—In this remedy's portrait, the patient's pain is worse for both hot and cold things. The swelling is large and very painful. Discharge from abscess is thin and watery. The abscess is slow to heal. The patient is drained of vital force and is very slow to heal.

GENERAL ACHES AND PAINS
Teeth: Acute Situations—Teething Pains

While this is not a disease state, it can still be a period of time in which the patient is in rather extreme pain. And the fact that the patient is a young child only makes the situation worse. Therefore, I have listed a few remedies that may be of great help as the child cuts his teeth.

REMEDIES

ACONITE—Of great help in cases in which the child is restless in his discomfort. Look for the patient to whine and to cry. He cannot be quieted or comforted. He will not stop thrashing or moving about. He cannot be quieted. The patient will not be able to sleep. He may waken suddenly from sleep due to the pain. Look for the patient to have fever during teething, to have hot, dry skin. He will be very thirsty. Look for diarrhea to accompany teething. The stool will be green or watery. Or look for the opposite to happen and the child to have constipation during teething.

APIS—This patient will also awaken from sleep with pain. He will awaken frequently all through the night. The whole house will be awakened by his teething. The child will scream in pain. Look for the patient to have red spots, like insect stings, all over his body. The patient will yawn often. A green-yellow diarrhea will accompany the teething.

BELLADONNA—The first remedy to consider when the child moans from his pain. He will also awaken from sleep in pain, but he will awaken with his eyes wide open and alert; his eyes will appear wild. The patient stares directly at you. The eyes will be reddened. The pupils will be dilated. Fever accompanies the pain. The patient's head will be red and hot. The patient's gums will look red and swollen. The patient may go into convulsions from the pain.

CALCAREA—A great remedy for teething pains in the child who is slow to develop and is slow to cut his teeth. For teething pains in a child with a large head, or who has trouble holding that head upright. Look for the child to have a sweaty head and for these head sweats to come on during sleep. Look for the patient to have cold, damp feet. Vomiting may accompany teething pains, as might diarrhea. Stool is white and thin. Look for the patient to have a good appetite, even during pain. Look for the patient to have a distended abdomen.

CHAMOMILLA—This is probably the first remedy to think of for the child who is teething. The child will want to be held, will demand to be held, and this may be the only way to him. The patient is very irritable, and very sensitive to his pain. He may rage in his pain. The patient may strike out, throw things. The child awakens from sleep in pain. Even when asleep, he thrashes about in bed. Look for the child to have one red cheek and one pale cheek. Look for twitching of the child's extremites, both when he is sleeping and when he is awake. Diarrhea, smelling of rotten eggs, may accompany teething pains.

COFFEA—The child will be totally sleepless and very excited. He will seem to have a bottomless pit of energy, although the rest of the family will be exhausted. It is as if the patient receives energy from his pain. And yet, in reality, the child is exhausted from lack of sleep. The patient's mood seems to swing wildly: he will laugh one moment and cry the next. The child will be feverish in his pain.

GRAPHITES—Consider this remedy for teething pains that occur in a child whose skin looks unhealthy and/or unclean. Look for raw skin in the bends of the neck and behind the ears. Teething pains accompanied by eruptions of the skin on the head and on the face. Eruptions with a sticky discharge. Constipation will accompany pain.

IGNATIA—The teething pains will be accompanied by hot flashes. Sudden heat, with sudden perspiration. The child will be awakened from sleep by the pain and will literally scream in pain. The patient will tremble in pain. Look for single parts of the body, arms, legs, and head, especially, to jerk and tremble during pain. Watery diarrhea accompanies pain.

IPECAC—An excellent remedy for the child who becomes nauseous during teething. Look for vomiting to accompany pain. Diarrhea may also accompany pain. Stool will have a bright green color, the color of grass.

The child will also have coughing fits during teething. He may cough until he chokes, until he vomits.

MERCURIUS—Called for in cases in which, during teething, the child begins to drool, and his mouth is filled with saliva. Look for the patient to have very red gums, and to have swelling of the gums, tongue, and mouth. The patient will be very much worse at night, especially from the heat of the bed. The patient awakens in pain. Night sweats accompany pain. The patient's bedclothes will be soaking wet from sweat. Diarrhea may accompany teething pains. Look for the patient to have a very strong-smelling urine during teething.

NUX—As is usually the case in this remedy type, the patient will be angry and very irritable, especially if his teething keeps him from sleeping. He will lose his appetite in his pain, but will have increased thirst. Pains tend to come on, or to become worse, in the very early morning. Look for constipation to accompany teething pains.

PODOPHYLLUM—Look for this child to be restless in his sleep and to tend to sleep with his eyes half open. He will grind his teeth in his sleep. The child will roll his head from side to side in pain. Look for diarrhea to accompany the pain. The stool will be watery and very offensive-smelling. The child will also have nausea, and may gag in attempting to vomit. The patient will be worse after eating or drinking. He will also be worse in hot weather.

SILICEA—As with Calcarea, the teething pains in Silicea tend to occur in children who have overly large heads. In this case, large heads with very thin necks. Teething pains in children who have a weak vital force, who seem to have failure to thrive, or always to be ill. Look for the patient to have foul-smelling sweat on his head. Look for a distended abdomen and for that abdomen to be hard to the touch. The patient's gums will be very, very sensitive.

SULPHUR—For the child who experiences itching pains during teething. Itching may be felt all over the patient's body and not just in his gums. The patient's face will be pale. He will be clammy or sweaty. The patient will seem hearty, but may be given to fainting spells accompanying the pain. Look for diarrhea to accompany the teething pain. Gushing diarrhea that comes on early in the morning and drives the patient from his bed to the bathroom. The stool may be bloody or mucus-filled. The passing of the stool may cause discomfort, with burning or itching pains.

General Aches and Pains
Teeth—Acute Situations: Dental Procedures and Surgery

As recovery from dental surgery involves recovery from an incised wound, take a look at the section on wounds and consider the remedies there in addition to these.

Also, in general it is a good idea to remember to try not to swallow any blood that may flow after any dental procedure—always try to spit the blood out. If bleeding continues, apply some gentle pressure on clean gauze for 10 to 15 minutes to stop the flow. After bleeding stops, wash mouth out with a solution of either Aqua Hypericum or Aqua Calendula.

REMEDIES

ARNICA—This is the general remedy to stop swelling and bruising and to promote quick healing. Arnica should be considered for use in the recovery from surgery of any sort. The wise patient would consider using the remedy both before and after dental surgery.

HYPERICUM—This is the first remedy to think of in this situation. It is always of great use after dental operations when there is a good deal of nerve pain. Hypericum and Arnica are often used alternately in the recovery from dental procedures.

PHOSPHORUS—Think of this remedy first when there is a great deal of bleeding and bleeding is hard to stop. Look for the blood to be bright, bright red.

STAPHYSAGRIA—This remedy acts as a follow-up to Hypericum when the Hypericum fails to work. Think especially of this remedy if the patient is overwhelmed by his pain. And if the pain experienced seems far greater than such a situation usually suggests.

General Aches and Pains
Travel Sickness

We all know the general symptoms here: dizziness, vomiting (food, bile, water, mucus), and a general feeling of being better off dead. There are, however, some basic homeopathic remedies that offer hope.

REMEDIES

ARSENICUM—The patient is totally overcome by the illness. He is left helpless by overwhelming nausea. Look for the patient to say that he wishes that he were dead. Symptoms center around nausea accompanied by violent retching. The patient vomits everything that he eats. Drinks very little and must slowly sip what he does manage to drink. The patient will be quite sure that he will die from this ailment.

COCCULUS—A major remedy for travel sickness. The patient feels light-headed, giddy. Nausea begins when patient rises up in bed or to a standing position from sitting. The patient experiences excessive nausea, aggravated by motion of vessel. He is worse from eating or drinking anything at all.

HEPAR SULPH—An excellent remedy to consider for travel sickness that is specific to riding in a car or on a train. From the rocking motion of a land vehicle. The patient will experience a pain in the head as if a nail were being driven into it. Look for the patient's face to be a deep red. The ears may also turn bright red. Look for a spasmodic opening and closing of the eyes.

IPECAC—Travel sickness with constant nausea. No matter what the patient eats or doesn't eat, whether he stands or sits, sleeps or lies awake, he feels incredibly nauseous. Nausea accompanied by copious vomiting. The patient will feel exhausted. He will complain that his stomach feels cold and empty.

NUX—As allopathic as it sounds, it is always a good idea for a patient to take a dose or two of Nux before boarding any vessel—car, boat, plane, or train—on which he thinks that he might become ill. Also very good if the patient becomes sick from traveling. The patient will be dizzy, confused, and will have no appetite. Look for a headache to accompany travel sickness. Also look for patient to be angry, irritable.

PETROLEUM—For nausea, vomiting, and giddiness. Water accumulates in the mouth. The patient will actually feel better for eating during attack, as odd as that may sound. The patient is worse from sitting up or from bright lights. This is a major general remedy for those suffering from this condition.

RHUS TOX—For the patient who experiences severe nausea, with restlessness. Patient feels better for lying down, but feels compelled to move about. May want warm liquids. He may feel better for external warmth as well, such as from taking a hot shower.

ALSO CONSIDER

KREOSOTUM—The patient who experiences nausea, vomiting, and retching that are accompanied by burning pains. The patient will typically be very thirsty. His limbs and extremities will feel chilled. The patient will be restless.

TABACUM—This is another general remedy for travel sickness. It is indicated for the patient who feels weakness, sweating, nausea, and trembling.

GENERAL ACHES AND PAINS
Digestion Upsets—Hiccoughs

Hiccoughs can be the response to eating too quickly, or they can be an emotional response to stress, excitement, or surprise. Homeopathics offer a solution, no matter the cause.

REMEDIES

IGNATIA—For very loud hiccoughs, those that can be heard ringing through the halls. The hiccoughs are spasmodic in nature. They come on quickly and leave just as quickly. This is the first remedy to consider for hiccups that accompany emotional upset.

MERCURIUS—Consider this remedy for cases of hiccoughs that are worse from drinking water.

NUX—This is the remedy of first choice for cases of hiccoughs that come on from eating, especially with overeating and drinking. The hiccoughs may be accompanied by a bitter or sour taste in the mouth. In general, the best, most effective hiccough remedy, excepting those cases that are based in emotional upset.

ALSO CONSIDER

CYCLAMEN—For patients with hiccoughs that either come on or are, in general, associated with breathing distress. The hiccoughs are improved by drinking water.

General Aches and Pains
Digestion Upsets—Bad Breath

While bad breath may be nothing more than the expression of the onions and cheese that you had for lunch, more often than not chronic bad breath is a sign of either tooth decay or digestive disorder.

The following few remedies are to be tried acutely, but a chronic case of bad breath will yield only to the best selected constitutional remedy.

REMEDIES

CARBO VEG—Bad breath from the abuse of mercury, from mercury fillings in the mouth.

NUX—For chronic bad breath in the morning. Bad breath that comes on as the result of overindulging with rich food and drink. Bad breath in alcoholics. Bad breath from drinking coffee.

PULSATILLA—Bad breath occurs both in the morning and at night.

SILICEA—Bad breath from the malnourished. Bad breath in the mornings.

SULPHUR—For chronic bad breath after dinner.

General Aches and Pains
Digestion Upsets—Bad Taste in the Mouth

This is more serious than it sounds. A bad taste in the mouth can be a very helpful symptom in locating a constitutional remedy. For instance, a bitter taste generally means that there are problems with the liver; a foul taste leads to infections of the mouth or throat, a salty taste to chronic lung conditions. Look for an acrid, sour taste in those who have chronic stomach disorders. A loss of taste is a sign of nervous afflictions.

REMEDIES

For a bitter taste in the mouth in the morning, consider: **Bryonia, Calcarea, Carbonica**, and **Mercurius**.

For a sweet taste in the mouth, consider: **Belladonna, Bryonia, Ferrum, Mercurius**, and **Pulsatilla**.

For a sour taste in the mouth, consider: **Calcarea Carbonica, Nux, Phosphoric Acidum**, and **Sulphur**.

For a salty taste in the mouth, consider: **Arsenicum, Carbo Veg, Nux**, and **Phosphoric Acidum**.

For an acrid, biting taste in the mouth, consider: **Arnica, Chamomilla, Mercurius**, and **Pulsatilla**.

For an oily, greasy taste in the mouth, consider: **Silicea**.

For a loss of taste, consider: **Belladonna, Cantharis, Hepar Sulph, Lycopodium, Phosphorus**, and **Veratrum**.

If solid food tastes bitter, consider: **Bryonia, Sulphur**, and **Hepar Sulph**.

If all food and drink tastes bitter, consider: **Bryonia**, and **Pulsatilla**.

If all food tastes sour, consider: **Lycopodium** and **Nux**.

If all food tastes salty, consider: **Arsenicum, Belladonna**, and **Sulphur**.

GENERAL ACHES AND PAINS
Digestion Upsets—Indigestion

From time to time, we all have indigestion, whether from lack of exercise, from stress, or from eating the wrong things. While the following remedies may help, they cannot cure a person of bad habits or poor lifestyle choices. You're on your own there.

This is a section of general remedies for states of indigestion, including flatulence, belching, and vomiting, and the remedies that are most commonly used in the treatment of such things. In the sections that follow, remedies more specific to constipation, diarrhea, and the like will be listed separately.

REMEDY CHECKLIST

For indigestion accompanied by constipation, consider: **Bryonia, Lachesis, Lycopodium, Nux**, or **Sulphur**.

For indigestion accompanied by diarrhea, consider: **Arsencicum, Carbo Veg, China, Mercurius, Pulsatilla, Phosphoric Acid**, or **Veratrum**.

For indigestion associated with a lack of exercise, consider: **Nux, Sepia**, or **Sulphur**.

For indigestion associated with overwork, consider: **Calcarea, Lachesis, Lycopodium, Nux, Pulsatilla**, or **Sulphur**.

For indigestion associated with emotional strain, consider: **Chamomilla, China, Nux, Phosphoric Acid**, or **Staphysagria**.

For indigestion associated with mechanical injury, consider: **Arnica, Bryonia, Rhus Tox**, or **Sulphur**.

For indigestion associated with overeating, consider: **China, Nux**, or **Pulsatilla**.

For indigestion associated with drinking alcohol, consider: **Arsenicum, Carbo Veg, Lachesis, Nux**, or **Sulphur**.

For indigestion from beer, consider: **Arsenicum, Calcarea, Rhus Tox, Sepia**, or **Sulphur**.

For indigestion from coffee, consider: **Ignatia** or **Nux**.

For indigestion from tobacco, consider: **Cocculus, Hepar Sulph, Ignatia, Nux**, or **Staphysagria**.

For indigestion after drinking cold water, consider: **Arsenicum, China, Phosphorus, Pulsatilla**, or **Veratrum**.

For indigestion after drinking milk, consider: **Bryonia, Calcarea, Nux**, or **Sulphur**.

For indigestion after eating bread or other wheat products, consider: **Bryonia, Lycopodium, Mercurius, Nux, Pulsatilla**, or **Sulphur**.

For indigestion after eating meat, consider: **China** or **Sulphur**.

For indigestion after eating fatty foods, consider: **Carbo Veg, China, Pulsatilla**, or **Sulphur**.

For indigestion in children, consider: **Bryonia, Calcarea, Ipecac, Nux**, or **Sulphur**.

For indigestion in the elderly, consider: **Arsenicum, Carbo Veg, China, Nux**, or **Veratrum**.

REMEDIES

ARNICA—For any form of digestive discomfort after a blow to the abdomen. Also for patients with indigestion that leads to a bruised feeling in the stomach. The patient belches a lot, complains of a taste of eggs in the mouth. Look for a sense of fullness in the pit of the stomach. The patient's tongue is coated yellow. He complains of a bitter or putrid taste in his mouth. After eating, the patient has the desire to vomit. He may have bouts of diarrhea.

ARSENICUM—This is an excellent acute remedy for violent digestive disorder that may be brought on from intestinal flu or food poisoning. The patient is restless, although totally depleted. Look for both vomiting and diarrhea, which may occur concurrently. This is the first remedy to consider if the patient is just plain unsure as to which end of the body should be aimed at the toilet first. The patient will be chilled. Will be afraid. Will want someone to take care of him. He may also be very thirsty and will want warm things, but will only sip small amounts at any given time. A leading remedy for any form of indigestion in the elderly.

BRYONIA—This is the first remedy to consider in cases of indigestion in hot or in damp weather and especially in weather patterns that combine hot and wet. Also for patients whose indigestion comes on from drinking cold liquids when they are overheated. Especially when the patient drinks ice cold beer on a hot day and then becomes ill. The patient loathes food; even the smell of food is nauseating. Look for soreness in the region of the patient's stomach. Burping after meals. For everything to taste bitter. The patient will throw up immediately after eating. The indigestion likely will be accompanied by constipation. The stools will be dry and hard. Headache also will likely be a part of the picture. The patient will want to lie still, will be very irritable. (Rhus Tox is often given either before or after Bryonia in cases of indigestion.)

CALCAREA—Perhaps the most important symptom here is that the area around the patient's waist is very sensitive. The patient cannot bear pressure on the waist and must loosen his clothing. He will complain of pressure as if from a weight on the stomach. Or a sour taste in the mouth. Look for vomiting of undigested food. Aversion to meat, to warm foods in general. The patient's feet will likely be both cold and damp. And look for sour-smelling head sweats. The patient's head will be cold and a sick headache may accompany indigestion. The patient will awaken nauseated at 3 A.M. Stools large and hard, and often comprised of only partially digested food. An excellent remedy for patients with acid indigestion. (Calcarea often follows Sulphur in indigestion.)

CARBO VEG—The patient belches and burps often. But this only gives brief relief. The patient will complain of a sensation as if stomach and abdomen will burst from eating and drinking. He will experience pain on the left side, under his ribs. Expect sour belching. Burning in stomach. A bitter taste in the mouth. And a great deal of intestinal gas. This is a good remedy for those who become ill after overeating. The patient feels as if suffocating—wants to be fanned. Nausea is worse in the morning. Digestion is accompanied by heartburn. Also by hiccoughs. (Often follows China in indigestion.)

CHAMOMILLA—For the patient who is experiencing a sensation of bloating that is placed high in abdomen. Sensation as if contents of the stomach were rising up into chest. Aching pain in stomach and under short ribs. Look for a bitter taste in mouth. Vomiting accompanies indigestion. The patient is very impatient, angry.

CHINA—For the patient whose abdomen feels full and tight, as if it had been stuffed. Much gas is passed, but to no relief. The patient experiences aversion to all food and drink. He complains that he continues to taste food long after he has eaten it. He is very tired, must lie down after every meal, as if it takes all the body's energy to digest food. For those who are dyspeptic after a long illness or after losing a good deal of blood.

COCCULUS—A minor remedy for indigestion. Look for the patient to have a sensation of hollowness in his stomach. The stomach feels empty, even after the patient has eaten. He will complain of a sour taste in his mouth. He will feel a strong aversion to anything acidic. The patient's throat will feel dry. Constipation will accompany indigestion. The patient may faint during bouts of indigestion.

GELSEMIUM—For the patient whose stomach and bowels feel empty and weak. His stomach is distended, with pain and nausea. The stomach burns, and the burning pains extend all the way up into the mouth. All symptoms are worse from fright, grief, or bad news, from anticipation of bad events, from test taking or public speaking. This remedy is most often used when dread of future events leads to bouts of indigestion. Diarrhea or vomiting may accompany indigestion.

HEPAR SULPH—As with Carbo Veg, all food disagrees. The patient's stomach becomes painful if he eats any food, no matter how carefully selected or prepared. Yet, the patient will have cravings for acids and for strong flavors. Look for nausea, belching, and intestinal gas—all without taste or smell. The patient's mouth tastes metallic. This is a common remedy for those who have used many different allopathic remedies for indigestion. For those who crave alcohol. Look for constipation to accompany indigestion. The stools are hard and difficult. (Hepar Sulph and Nux, because of the similarity of symptoms, are often used either before or after each other in the treatment of indigestion, especially chronic indigestion.)

IPECAC—This remedy is especially suited to young children who experience indigestion. It is very similar in its symptom picture to Carbo Veg. For cases of indigestion in which the patient feels that his face and extremities are very cold during bouts of indigestion. For indigestion that is accompanied by vomiting or dry retching. The patient will vomit food, drink, and mucus. He will have a sinking sensation in his stomach that warns of each new spell of vomiting.

LACHESIS—For patients with irregular appetites. Sometimes they are very hungry and eat a great deal, other times they are repulsed by food. They tend to crave milk. They also tend to crave alcohol, especially wine. They are highly averse to bread and to other grain products. They will have a sensation of fullness and sluggishness after every meal. Just as a snake must rest after eating in order to digest, the Lachesis must lie down after eating. He feels heavy and weak from eating. Constipation accompanies indigestion. (Works well either before or after Mercurius in indigestion.)

LYCOPODIUM—This is one of our most important remedies for those with indigestion, especially chronic indigestion. The patient's stomach feels full and heavy after every meal. There is a great deal of intestinal gas—just a mouthful of food leads to gas. Stomach feels full up to the throat. The patient will sit down to eat and be very hungry. But, after only a few swallows, he will feel full due to the intestinal gas. Look for the patient to have to unbuckle his pants from the pressure. The patient will experience almost constant fermentation in the stomach, like yeast working. There is much rumbling, especially on the left side of the abdomen. Troubles from eating wheat. Also troubles from milk and other dairy products. No other remedy type craves sugar and other sweet things as much as Lycopodium will, and yet sweets will lead to indigestion. Constipation. Stool is hard and passed with great difficulty. Symptoms worse at 4 P.M. (Works well after Calcarea and before Sulphur.)

MERCURIUS—Pit of the patient's stomach will be very sensitive. When sitting, the patient will feel that the food just eaten feels like a stone in the stomach. Look for a sensation of pressure high in the abdomen. Heartburn accompanies indigestion. The patient has aversion to solid food, to meat, to all warm foods. The patient desires cold things. Expect that the Mercurius patient will have much saliva, accompanied by a salty, metallic taste in his mouth. Diarrhea, involving much straining, accompanies indigestion. Perspiration also accompanies bouts of indigestion.

NUX—Whether for acute or chronic indigestion, Nux is perhaps the single leading candidate for a remedy, especially if the indigestion either is a product of a lack or exercise or comes on from overwork in our modern corporate environment. Also the leading remedy for indigestion that comes on from any form of overindulgence, especially from over-indulging in spicy foods or alcohol. This remedy may also be helpful for those who experience indigestion after becoming very cold. Look for the patient to have a bitter taste in the mouth in the morning. To have much belching. And for the belching to have a sour taste. Food will also taste sour, especially bread and grain products. The patient will not be very hungry, but will crave alcohol, especially beer. The patient's stom-ach region is very sensitive to touch. The patient will have cramps in the stomach, with pressure, worse after any meal. He cannot bear tight clothing. It is keynote of the remedy that the patient will be very irri-table, and will want to be alone. A red face accompanies indigestion. The patient may also have spells of feeling overheated, followed by chills. Constipation will accompany indigestion. Stools large, hard, and passed with great difficulty. Chronic constipation. (Sulphur follows Nux well in indigestion.)

PHOSPHORUS—Should be considered for patients who vomit after every meal. Or who vomit after drinking cold water or other cold liquids. As the liquid warms in the patient's stomach, he becomes nauseous and vomits. The patient will feel terrible burning pains in the stomach. He will crave cold things; he will crave smoked meats. Look for the patient to complain of a sour taste in his mouth and to say that he feels as if his entire system has become acidic.

PULSATILLA—In some ways, this will act on acute cases of indigestion much as Nux will for the chronic. Consider this remedy first if indiges-tion comes on from overeating, especially from eating greasy or very rich food. Look for the patient's tongue to be coated white or yellow, and for there to be a bad taste in his mouth in the morning and evening. There will be much belching after a meal, which will taste like last food eaten. The patient's stomach feels full. And he is made nauseous by fats, pork, pastry, and ice cream. The patient will experience vertigo with indigestion. The patient becomes dizzy when stooping or rising. Dizzy and nauseous in a warm room. Chilly patients, who experience flashes of heat. Diarrhea every night. The stool will be yellow-green in color. The patient will be depressed, even weepy. (Sulphur follows well in indigestion.)

RHUS TOX—Most often used either before or, especially, after Bryonia in the treatment of indigestion. Look for the patient to be very restless, for him to have to keep moving in order to find a comfortable position. The patient's tongue will be very dry. Look for the characteristic red tip on the tongue. The patient will be very thirsty.

SEPIA—For cases of indigestion in which the patient's stomach pulses with pain. For chronic cases of indigestion that involve a great weakness in digestion. Especially for chronic cases in which a sick headache accompanies indigestion. Or for cases in which headache and indigestion alternate in a chronic manner. Look for belching, which tastes sour and bitter. Look for the patient to complain of a sensation of pressure on the stomach. To say that it feels like a stone on the stomach. The stomach feels pressed down upon. The patient's face is yellow. Constipation accompanies indigestion. Stools are knotty and hard, pass with difficulty. It is keynote of the remedy that there is a sensation of a weight in the anus.

SILICEA—The patient awakens with a bitter taste in the mouth in the morning. He experiences nausea that is worse in the morning and after every meal. Even water tastes bad. The patient vomits after drinking water. The patient has no appetite, but has a great thirst. He cannot digest any food. In cases of chronic indigestion of the Silicea type, the patient's system has lost the ability to taken in nutrition from food. The overall vital force is overwhelmed. The patient is emaciated and exhausted. This is a remedy for cases in which indigestion is chronic in nature and develops slowly over a long period of time. Also for cases in that indigestion comes on after any sort of severe disease has weakened the total system. Constipation accompanies indigestion—stool recedes after being partially expelled.

SULPHUR—This is a very general remedy for those who have indigestion. It is also a major remedy for low blood sugar and for the other ailments that arise from that condition. The typical Sulphur indigestion will be deeply related to lifestyle, and to the poor diet and lack of exercise on the part of the patient. This is a remedy to consider for cases involving acid stomach with much belching, much gas. The region of the patient's stomach is very sensitive to touch. The patient feels weak and faint at 11 A.M. and must eat. At that time—indeed, at all times—the patient will desire sugar, salt, and fat. A sensation of burning heat on the top of the head will accompany indigestion. The patient will feel hot and sweaty. He may feel that he cannot breathe after he eats. He is restless. He may experience vertigo with indigestion. He will have a red face. Keynote of the remedy is that the patient will experience early morning diarrhea, which drives the patient out of bed.

ALSO CONSIDER

ANTIMONIUM CRUDUM—For the patient whose discomfort is caused by overloading the stomach. There is a sensation of great fullness in the stomach. This will be accompanied by a great deal of gas. The patient's tongue will have a white coating. Belching brings up the flavor of the last food eaten. Nausea and vomiting. Watery stools, with hard lumps. Patient is thirsty; thirst is worse at night. (Antimonium Crudum is used after Ipecac if Ipecac does not completely cure the case.)

PHOSPHORIC ACID—Indigestion that is combined with either mental or physical depletion. The patient is exhausted, either mentally or physically, and cannot digest his food. Consider this remedy strongly for cases of indigestion—especially chronic indigestion—that comes on from grief or from a loss of love. Or for patients who have lost vital fluids. Weakness from blood loss, or from dehydration from vomiting. (China and Phosphoric Acid both follow each other well in cases of indigestion.)

GENERAL ACHES AND PAINS
Diarrhea

Again, this can be a very broad category and you may well want to check on the remedies listed under the general category of indigestion if none of those listed here seems to fit the case.

While simple acute diarrhea is more unpleasant than it is serious, chronic diarrhea can severely weaken the patient and leave him dangerously dehydrated. Therefore, if the diarrhea does not come under control within 48 hours, be sure to call your health practitioner.

REMEDY CHECKLIST

For diarrhea which is painless, consider: **China, Phosphoric Acid**, or **Secale**.

For diarrhea which is accompanied by griping pain, consider: **Arsenicum, Bryonia, Chamomilla, Colocynth, Puslatilla**, or **Sulphur**.

For diarrhea which is accompanied by vomiting, consider: **Arsenicum, Ipecac, Phosphorus, Rhus Tox**, or **Veratrum**.

For diarrhea after emotional upset, especially fright, consider: **Arsenicum, Chamomilla**, or **Veratrum**.

For diarrhea after excitement or joy, consider: **Aconite, Coffea**, or **Pulsatilla**.

For diarrhea after grief, consider: **Ignatia** or **Phosphoric Acid**.

For diarrhea after anger, consider: **Chamomilla, Colcynthis**, or **Nux**.

For diarrhea in anticipation of future events (fear of tests, public speaking, and the like), consider: **Gelsemium**.

For diarrhea in the autumn or spring—in changeable weather— consider: **Bryonia, Carbo Veg, Dulcamara**, or **Rhus Tox**.

For diarrhea in the summer, consider: **Arsenicum, Bryonia**, or **Mercurius**.

For diarrhea in young children, consider: **Belladonna** or **Hyoscyamus**.

For diarrhea in elderly patients, consider: **Arsenicum, Antimonium Crudum, Opium**, or **Phosphorus**.

For diarrhea in pregnant women, consider: **Nux, Opium**, or **Sepia**.

REMEDIES

ACONITE—Stools are frequent and scanty—watery, slimy. Nausea and sweat before stool. Feeling that you have not finished after passing stool. Vertigo upon rising. Restlessness. Intense thirst. Diarrhea from exposure to dry, cold weather.

APIS—Stools are greenish in color, or yellowish. Slimy mucus. Sensation as if something in the abdomen would break from straining at stool. Tongue is dry and shining red. Little or no thirst. Feet are swollen. Symptoms are worse in the morning.

ARSENICUM—Stools are thick, with dark green mucus, or brown or black and watery. Involuntary stools. Great weakness with diarrhea. Fainting. Exhaustion. Patient is chilly, restless, very thirsty—yet drinks very little. Vomiting after eating or drinking. Worse for eating or drinking anything cold.

BELLADONNA—Stools are thin, green, and covered with mucus that may be white or watery. Stools are small and frequent. Clutching in the abdomen. Pains come on suddenly. Stop suddenly. Patient is sleepy but cannot sleep. Worse at 3 P.M. and worse for sleeping.

BRYONIA—Diarrhea in hot weather, or from drinking cold drinks when overheated. Stools are brown and thin, with undigested foods. Smell like rotten cheese. Nausea and faintness for sitting up. Thirst for large quantities of water, drunk at long intervals. Symptoms worse in the morning, worse for any motion.

CALCAREA—Diarrhea in persons with swollen, distended abdomens, those with good appetites, who are nonetheless emaciated. Chronic poor digestion. Chronic diarrhea, with claylike stools. Profuse sweat on the head when sleeping. Feet are cold and damp. Urination difficult. Urine and stool smell strong and fetid.

CARBO VEG—Stools are light-colored, involuntary. Rotten smell on the person, in his stool. Vital force greatly exhausted. Great amounts of strong-smelling gas. Patient is restless and exhausted. Feels as if he cannot breathe. Must be fanned. Symptoms are worse from 5 until 6 P.M.

CHAMOMILLA—Stools green and watery. Hot stools, smelling of rotten eggs. Bitter taste in mouth, with vomiting. Patient very irritable, impatient. The patient's face has one red cheek and one pale, cold cheek. Symptoms are worse at night.

CHINA—Stools yellowish or whitish, watery. Spastic colon, pain relieved by bending over. Stools can be painless, with undigested food and a great deal of gas. Distention of the abdomen. Body sweats. Patient very thirsty, yet drinks little. Symptoms worse at night, after eating, every other day.

CINA—Look for white stools; for the patient who chronically picks his nose. Restless sleep, with frequent changing of positions. Patient grinds teeth in sleep. Patient troubled with worms.

COLOCYNTHIS—Stools are saffron colored, frothy, or thin. Before stool, there is pain and cramping in the abdomen as if the intestines were being squeezed between stones. Pain is relieved by the patient bending over. Bitter taste in mouth. Symptoms worse for eating anything at all.

DULCAMARA—Stools are yellowish, greenish, and watery. Colic before and during stool. Griping pain in region of the navel. Vomiting of mucus. Symptoms are caused by getting cold and wet, aggravated by cold, wet weather. Skin is dry and hot.

FERRUM—Painless, watery stools made up of undigested food. Bowels feel sore, bruised. Patient has good appetite, but emaciated. Vomiting of food soon after eating. The least emotion or exertion produces a red, flushed face.

GELSEMIUM—Diarrhea from fear, from fright, from grief or bad news. Consider for cases of diarrhea in exhausted or chronically ill patients. Diarrhea with a sudden urge for stool. Stools the color of tea—dark yellow. Desire to be quiet, to rest.

HEPAR SULPH—Painless chronic diarrhea. Stools are light yellow and slimy, with undigested food. Sour-smelling diarrhea. Better for eating. Hot, sour regurgitation of food. Stomach feels full; patient desires to loosen clothing.

IPECAC—Stools fermented. Nausea and colic before and during stool. Vomiting of yellow, jellylike mucus. Pale face, cold extremities. Flatulent colic.

MERCURIUS—Stools are dark green, slimy, frothy, bloody. There is a frequent urge for stool, but stools feels incomplete. Cutting pain in abdomen, with chilliness. Violent thirst for cold drinks. Mouth filled with saliva. Night sweats, especially on the head; forehead cold. Worse at night and in hot weather.

PHOSPHORUS—For those who suffer chronic painless diarrhea, worse in the morning. Stools of undigested food. Stools watery, with little white flakes or lumps in them. Gradual loss of strength from diarrhea. Vomiting of cold drinks and food when they warm in the stomach. Patient is sleepy after eating.

PODOPHYLLUM—Painless diarrhea. Profuse watery stools. Before stool, there is a loud gurgling in the bowels, sounds like water. During stool, patient gags, experiences dry heaves. Cramps in feet, calves, and thighs. Always worse in the morning, at night, and in hot weather. Podophyllum is a good bet for a general diarrhea remedy when the need for stool seems to never end.

PULSATILLA—Stools are greenish yellow like bile. Stool constantly changing. Before stool, rumbling in abdomen, cutting pain in bowels. Diarrhea is worse at night, worse from eating fruit or ice cream. Bitter taste in mouth. The patient is chilly in a warm room, yet craves cool air. Tongue is white coated. Loss of taste. Thirstless.

SULPHUR—Stools are changeable: yellow, brown, green, with or without undigested food. Chronic diarrhea, worse in the morning, drives the patient out of bed. Painless diarrhea. Before stool, however, there may be pain, urging, and colic. Constant heat on the top of the head. Sour or bitter vomiting. Frequent spells of weakness, fainting. Patient is sleepy during the day, wide awake at night.

VERATRUM ALBUM—Stool profuse, watery. Black or green. Severe pain and colic before and during stool. After stool, great weakness and a feeling of emptiness in the stomach. Patient has a cold sweat on the forehead. Violent vomiting of mucus. Intense thirst for cold water. Extreme weakness.

ALSO CONSIDER

ANTIMONIUM CRUDUM—Stools are watery and profuse. Stomach very upset. Cannot digest the simplest foods. Tongue is coated white. Violent vomiting of bitter, slimy mucus. Worse for eating and drinking, especially from overeating.

HYOSCYAMUS—Painless diarrhea, yellow and watery. Involuntary stools. Diarrhea during fever. These patients will be wild, suspicious. They may insist that they have been poisoned.

PHOSPHORIC ACIDUM—Painless diarrhea. Stools are white and watery. Very offensive. Great rumbling in the bowels. The patient is very indifferent to his ailment, wants nothing, and cares about nothing. Profuse sweat at night.

SECALE—Painless diarrhea. Stools are watery brown. Stools are discharged from the body with great force, discharged very rapidly. Patient is very exhausted after stool. Patient vomits without effort, leading to great weakness. Great anxiety. Great sensation of burning in the pit of the stomach. Extreme thirst. Patient has an aversion to heat, cannot bear to be covered up.

GENERAL ACHES AND PAINS
Constipation

You will not get the same sympathy from homeopaths for constipation—or cositiveness, as it is known in the older texts—as you will for diarrhea. Where diarrhea can have many different causes, most of which involve some sort of state in which the patient has come down with some viral infection or eaten tainted foods, constipation is most often seen as a disease related to lifestyle. Usually the patient does not exercise enough or eats an improper diet. Therefore, most practitioners faced with a patient who is constipated will likely look first at lifestyle changes before considering homeopathic remedies.

I include here, however, a few of the most commonly used remedies for constipation for use with the acute case.

REMEDY CHECKLIST

For constipation in those who are too sedentary in their lifestyle, consider: **Bryonia, Lycopodium, Nux, Phosphorus, Platina**, or **Sulphur**.

For constipation in pregnant women, consider: **Nux, Opium**, or **Sepia**.

For constipation in the elderly, consider: **Antimonium Crudum, Opium**, or **Phosphorus**.

For those who are chronically beset with constipation, consider: **Bryonia, Lachesis, Lycopodium, Nux, Sepia**, or **Sulphur**.

REMEDIES

APIS—A good remedy for acute constipation. The patient will complain of a pain in his forehead that may extend into his eyeballs, which accompanies the constipation. He will feel that the region around the waist is very tender and will not want it touched in any way. The abdomen is so tender that the patient will feel that something within would literally dbreak if he made the effort that would be necessary to pass a stool. So he does not want to struggle to pass a stool. He does not want to even try.

BELLADONNA—For acute cases in which the patient feels a throbbing sensation in his head that accompanies the constipation. The patient will complain of a rush of blood into his head, or of throbbing headache. His face will be flushed red. When moving the head downward, and especially when stooping, the patient will feel as if he were about to faint.

BRYONIA—One of our most important remedies for those who are constipated, especially for those who are suffering chronic constipation. The patient may lose all appetite, but he will be very thirsty and will, from time to time, drink great amounts of water. He will not want to move, as any form of movement increases his pain. Terrible headaches are likely to accompany the constipation. The patient will feel that his head will literally split open from the pain. Look for the patient to have dry lips and a dry mouth during constipation. The patient will belch often and may vomit up whatever food he does eat. The stools will be small, hard, and dry. He may seem to have been burnt. The patient will be irritable and will want to be left alone.

CALCAREA—The odd keynote that the patient will feel better when he is constipated than he will at any other time. For patients with constipation due to lack of exercise and poor diet. The Calcarea patient will be drawn to the foods that he cannot digest. He will also, especially in childhood, eat things that are not even food: chalk, paste, dirt, and the like. Constipation accompanied by head sweats. The head will be chilled and the sweat will smell sour. The feet, too, will be cold and damp. The stools will be large and hard and partially composed of undigested foods. The patient will be moody and depressed after passing stools.

CARBO VEG—A remedy to consider for patients with chronic constipation, usually due to lack of exercise. The patient will usually be overweight and out of shape. He will often have trouble breathing and will need to be fanned in order to feel that he is taking in enough air. The patient will feel exhausted, debilitated by his constipation. Look for constipation to be accompanied by hemorrhoids or by rheumatic pains.

CAUSTICUM—The keynote here is that the patient will experience a great deal of soreness in his anus. He will complain of pain and soreness in the rectum and anus especially when walking. The patient has a frequent but unsuccessful desire for passing stool. The patient will be anxious and very restless. Look for his face to take on a bright red coloring. Stool will be small and soft and very hard to pass.

GRAPHITES—This is a remedy especially for those with chronic constipation, who seem naturally given to constipation. The patient will have skin that looks very unhealthy. He will seem to lack the ability to fully digest and metabolize food. His skin will itch when he is constipated. The stools will be hard and knotty. Often the lumps passed will be strung together on ropes of mucus. This is a remedy to keep in mind any time a patient passes a large quantity of mucus with the stool.

IGNATIA—These patients will be very anxious in their state of constipation. They will be moody and, in turns, angry and very depressed. They are very anxious to pass a stool. They feel that there is total inactivity in their system. This is an excellent acute constipation remedy, especially for cases in which constipation has come on while traveling or after catching a cold. For constipation when accompanied by hemorrhoids. After these patients pass stool, there will be a sharp and violent pain that moves upward from the anus.

LACHESIS—This is perhaps the first remedy to consider in cases in which constipation has come on as a part of an acute disease state. Especially consider in cases of stubborn constipation that comes on during a fever.

LYCOPODIUM—One of our most important remedies for patients with any sort of digestive troubles, chronic or acute. In acute constipation, look for it to accompany respiratory infections of all sorts. In chronic conditions, consider Lycopodium for cases of stubborn constipation that involve poor diet, especially for those who are allergic to certain foods, which cause constipation. Most especially for those allergic to wheat and to dairy products. The patient will likely display the other characteristics of Lycopodium. Look for the patient to have a great deal of intestinal gas, especially just after eating. And listen for the sound of loud gurgling in their bowels. These patients may be very hungry, but just a few bites of food seem to fill them up, as they swell with gas. Look for them to have to unbutton the top of their pants to get relief. Also look for the other keynote of Lycopodium, which is an aggravation of all conditions at 4 P.M. Since Lycopodium, like Sulphur, speaks to those with low blood sugar, expect this aggravation daily in the late afternoon. They will feel better after 8 P.M. (Sulphur's aggravation is in the late morning, at 11 A.M.) The stools will be very hard and passed only with the greatest difficulty.

NUX—There is no better remedy to consider for stubborn constipation in businessmen than Nux. Chronic constipation in those who work with their minds, and not with their bodies. Constipation also from overuse of alcohol and from eating a diet of spicy foods. Look for hemorrhoids to accompany constipation. These patients will make frequent but ineffectual efforts to pass stools. They may complain of a sensation that their anus were closed tight. They will feel a fullness in the head. A headache, like a nail being driven into the forehead, may accompany the constipation. The patient will be very sensitive in the region of the abdomen; he will not be able to bear any touch, or tight clothing, around the area of the waist. The patient will be irritable when constipated. This is also an excellent remedy for constipation during pregnancy, if the characteristic personality traits are present. The stool will be large and hard, and passed only with great suffering.

PHOSPHORUS—This is an excellent remedy to keep in mind in cases in which diarrhea and constipation chronically alternate, especially when those cases occur in older patients. The patient will have a great deal of belching that accompanies the constipation. He will belch a great deal after each meal. He will also become very sleepy after eating, especially after he has eaten dinner. The stool will be long and thin and hard, like a dog's.

PULSATILLA—The symptoms will often resemble Nux, but the behavior of the patient will be your guide. Both Pulsatilla and Nux will have constipation as a result of eating the wrong things. Nux will want spicy foods and alcohol; Pulsatilla will want greasy foods, rich foods. Afterward, these patients will become silent as nausea sets in. Look for patients to be weepy in their constipation. To want others to pity and care for them. This is another remedy to keep in mind for cases that alternate diarrhea and constipation.

SEPIA—Consider this remedy when a sick headache accompanies constipation. The patient will complain of a pressing down feeling in the abdomen. Also of a weight or a lump in the anus. He may also complain of flashes of heat in his body. This is an excellent remedy to consider for constipation in pregnant women. The stools will be hard and knotty and may contain mucus. They are passed with a terrible cutting pain.

SILICEA—Consider this remedy especially for children who have constipation. The patient's stomach will be distended and hard to the touch. The patient will complain of a sour taste in the mouth. Heartburn will accompany constipation. Swollen glands may also accompany constipation. In Silicea cases, it may seem that the patient's system simply lacks the strength to pass the stool.

SULPHUR—One of our greatest remedies for constipation and any other form of digestive disorder. The disorder here is usually functional; it is caused by the lifestyle of the patient. Chronic constipation in those who will not exercise, or who exercise without discipline and regularity. And in those who eat an unhealthy diet. Sulphurs are the typical junk-food junkies. They crave salt, grease, and sweet things. They love sodas and candy and baked goods. Pizza and hamburgers and fries will be their favorite foods. And, like Calcarea, they seem drawn to these things, all the while they are aware that they are the worst things that they could possibly eat. The patient will often feel faint while trying to pass stool. He will complain of hot sweat while straining to pass stool. Often, the first effort will be so painful and difficult that the patient will not want to try again. The stools will be hard and lumpy and mixed with mucus. After passing a stool, the patient will complain of burning pains in the rectum and anus.

VERATRUM—This is the first remedy to think of for constipation in infants. Especially when it is a chronic problem. It will seem as if the patient's system were totally paralyzed. The patient will pass stool only with much straining and forcing. Look for the patient to have a cold sweat all over the body, but especially on the forehead when attempting to pass stool. The stool will be large and very hard.

ALSO CONSIDER

NITRIC ACID—For cases of constipation that are totally painless. This is another remedy that is especially recommended for cases of constipation in the elderly. The passing of stool becomes irregular, rather than stopped. The patient will usually complain that his urine is especially strong-smelling during this bout of constipation. He may also say that he feels as if there were a band being drawn tight around his head. The stools will be hard and dry and few and far between.

OPIUM—This is the first remedy to think of for those who have taken many allopathic medicines, for either diarrhea or constipation, and now find that their system is totally out of whack. Often, the patient will experience days of chronic diarrhea, followed by days and days of constipation, during which they will not even have the desire for a stool. Constipation will be accompanied by a loss of appetite. The constipation may come on after a deep fright or shock. The stools will consist of small, hard black balls.

GENERAL ACHES AND PAINS
Heartburn

While this ailment in general is related to and covered under the topic "Indigestion," I have here listed some of the most common remedies for this condition and the related idea of "sour stomach" in a simple checklist form.

By "heartburn" I mean the burning sensation in the stomach that often rises up into the throat, causing an inclination to vomit and a general feeling of nausea and anxiety. I also include that sensation called "water brash" in the older texts, which consists of either the rising of bitter or acidic fluid into the back of the mouth, or the coughing up of watery fluid.

REMEDY CHECKLIST

For cases of heartburn, consider: **China, Nux, Phosphoric Acid, Pulsatilla, Sepia**, or **Sulphur**.

For cases of water brash, consider: **Arsenicum, Calcarea, Carbo Veg, Lycopodium, Nux, Phosphorus, Sepia**, or **Sulphur.**

For vomiting up of acid, consider: Calcarea, Chamomilla, China, Nux, Phosphorus, or **Sulphur**.

For vomiting up of food, consider: **Arnica, Bryonia, Carbo Veg, Nux, Phosphorus, Pulsatilla**, or **Sulphur**.

For belching, consider: **Arnica, Bryonia, Carbo Veg, Nux, Pulsatilla, Rhus Tox**, or **Sulphur**.

REMEDIES

CARBO VEG—The leading remedy for cases that involve water brash, especially when it occurs at night. The patient will complain both of a burning sensation in the stomach and of belching that brings a sour taste into the patient's mouth. Carbo Veg is especially helpful for cases of heartburn after the patient has been drinking too much and indulged in too many parties.

CHINA—To be considered particularly for chronic cases of heartburn. When the patient experiences heartburn after each and every meal. The patient will experience a sensation of fullness after every meal, as well as a sensation of pressure in the region of the stomach. There will be increased saliva in the patient's mouth, and the patient will suffer from empty retching spasms after eating.

NUX—Will often speak to the sensation of water brash or heartburn after the patient drinks alcohol. Also, stomach upset after eating foods that are too spicy. The patient will be irritable. The region of the stomach will be very sensitive and the patient will want nothing to touch him in the area of the waist. He will have a bitter taste in his mouth and a sensation of pressure in the abdomen. Constipation often accompanies this heartburn.

PHOSPHORUS—A great general remedy for heartburn, especially when it is accompanied by the rising of acid fluids in the back of the throat. The patient may also gulp up watery fluids. Also for those patients who experience a sour regurgitation of food after eating. Nausea may come on after cold fluids have heated in the patient's stomach. The patient may also be very sleepy after eating, especially after eating supper.

PULSATILLA—The patient will belch and then will taste the flavor of the food that he has been eating. For the patient who says that his food is "repeating" on him. Also for vomiting of acid fluids, or the rising of acid fluids into the back of the mouth. The patient will feel that his stomach is empty, even if he has just eaten.

SEPIA—For the patient who experiences water brash after he has been eating or drinking. He doesn't need to have had any solid food to feel the churning in his stomach. The patient will also experience burning pains in his stomach. This remedy is especially suggested for women who experience heartburn during pregnancy.

General Aches and Pains
Colic

Colic as a term can be applied to almost any pains in the abdomen. Most often, however, it is used to describe pains in the colon or large intestine. Characteristically, colic pains are crampy, gripping, twisting, and severe. With the pain may come symptoms such as diarrhea, vomiting, belching, and perspiration.

Our older texts tell us of three types of colic. *Bilious colic* is typified by a severe gripping pain in the abdomen that is, at first, made better by pressure but later is very sensitive to touch. Vomiting may accompany this form of colic, as might a distension of the abdomen. The patient will experience coldness in the extremities and the skin will have a yellow tone.

Flatulent colic involves both belching and the passing of intestinal gas; neither brings relief. Here, too, the abdomen tends to become very distended and may be stretched like a drum. The patient will have a great deal of pressure pain.

Finally, there is what used to be known as *painter's colic,* the onset of which is usually a feeling of exhaustion, which is followed by a sensation of pain that wanders all throughout the region of the abdomen. The lower limbs feel heavy and yet the patient will be restless because of the discomfort. Often, the patient will have to bend forward in order to relieve the discomfort.

REMEDY CHECKLIST

For cases of bilious colic, consider: **Bryonia, Colocynthis, Chamomilla**, or **Nux**.

For cases of flatulent colic, consider: **Carbo Veg, China, Cocculus, Lycopodium, Pulsatilla**, or **Sulphur**.

For cases of painter's colic, consider: **Belladonna, Mag Phos**, or **Platina**.

For colic that is accompanied by chronic constipation, consider: **Nux** or **Opium**.

For colic that is accompanied by hemorrhoids, consider: **Carbo Veg, Colocynthis, Lachesis, Nux, Pulsatilla**, or **Sulphur**.

For colic that is accompanied by indigestion, consider: **Belladonna, Bryonia, Carbo Veg, China, Nux**, or **Pulsatilla**.

For colic that comes on after mechanical injury, consider: **Arnica, Bryonia, Carbo Veg, Lachesis**, or **Rhus Tox**.

For colic that comes on after exposure to cold, damp weather, consider: **Bryonia, Pulsatilla**, or **Rhus Tox**.

For colic that comes on after taknig a chill, consider: **Aconite, Chamomilla, Colocynthis, Mercurius**, or **Nux**.

For colic during pregnancy, consider: **Arnica, Bryonia, Chamomilla, Pulsatilla**, or **Sepia**.

For "menstrual colic" (PMS), consider: **Cocculus, Coffea, Mag Phos, Pulsatilla**, or **Veratrum**.

For colic in children, consider: **Aconite, Belladonna, Chamomilla, Cina, Coffea**, or **Sulphur**.

REMEDIES

ACONITE—For inflammatory colic that involves the bladder. For bouts of colic that come on suddenly. The patient will also experience difficult and scanty urination. The abdomen is very sensitive, with cutting pains in the belly. The pain can be so severe that the patient cries out with great anxiety and fear.

ARNICA—The first remedy to think of when cramping in the abdomen comes on after physical injury. Also for colic during pregnancy. The patient will feel a fullness in the stomach, as if he has eaten too much. There will be a sensation of pressure that extends to the spine and up into the chest. The pressure will be worse after the patient eats or drinks and he is very much worse from being touched. The patient will not want to be touched and will often insist that there is nothing wrong with him although he is in obvious pain. The pain is made better from any discharge, especially from urination or diarrhea.

BELLADONNA—The patient will suddenly feel as if something is clawing at the area of his abdomen from the inside. Look for a protrusion in the transverse colon. The patient will clutch the abdomen in pain. The discomfort will center in the area of the navel. Look for the external pressure and bending over double to relieve the pain. It is keynote of Belladonna that pains come and go suddenly. In the case of colic, the attack is like a bolt of lightning. (Mercurius, Lachesis, and Hyoscyamus follow Belladonna in cases of colic.)

BRYONIA—The patient will complain of a sensation of fullness and pressure in the region of the abdomen that comes on after eating. He will experience stitching pains in the bowels. Bryonia is specific to colic that comes on, accompanied by diarrhea, in the summer, or from having cold things to eat or drink after becoming overheated. Also colic from drinking milk.

CARBO VEG—Cramping with a sensation of fullness in the abdomen, which feels as if it will burst. The patient will feel intestinal gas trapped in the abdomen. The patient passes much gas with only brief relief. Gas has a terrible odor. Constant downward pressure in the abdomen. Keynote here is audible rumbling in the bowels. The pain will be worse from 4 until 6 P.M.

CHAMOMILLA—Cramping with terrible flatulence. Look for the patient's abdomen to be distended like a drum. There will be continual pains in the abdomen, without a moment's peace. Cramps will be accompanied by the sensation that the bowels are rolled up in a ball. The patient will be furious while he is in pain. This remedy is to be especially considered for cases of colic in which the patient drinks coffee daily. This is also a leading remedy for cases of colic in children. Especially when the pain comes on late at night, toward sunrise.

CHINA—For cases of colic that involve flatulence with thirst. The patient will experience violent cutting pains around the navel that will be relieved by bending over double. The abdomen feels full and tight as if it had been stuffed, as if it would burst. Colic from eating fruit or drinking beer. From any mistake in diet. The pain will be worse at night. Worse also after the patient has experienced any other severe illness or blood loss.

COCCULUS—This is a major remedy for flatulent colic. Look for the patient to experience spasms of the stomach with a gripping sensation. Contractions of the abdomen with downward and outward pressure. Belching relieves the pain. The patient's abdomen is distended and feels as if it is full of sharp stones. The patient will complain of a feeling of fullness in addition to the pain. He may have trouble breathing.

COFFEA—For patients who experience laborlike pains in their abdomen. The patient complains of a sensation as if the bowels were being cut to pieces. The patient cries aloud and grinds his teeth in pain. Their whole body is too sensitive to be touched. A sensation of coldness in the limbs will accompany colic. The patient may also experience a sensation of suffocation. He will be in despair over his condition.

COLOCYNTHIS—Colic that consists of violent cutting, constrictive or spasmodic pains. The patient feels as if the whole abdomen is being squeezed between stones. Relief only comes from bending over double.

Pain comes on after feeling of indignation or anger. Also especially indicated for cases of colic that are accompanied by diarrhea. It is keynote of this remedy picture that the pain is spasmodic in nature and that it extends into the patient's throat. The patient will literally moan in pain. Cramping may also extend into patient's limbs. The patient will be very restless. This is the closest thing we have to a general colic remedy.

IPECAC—Consider this remedy for the patient who is experiencing a horrid pain that is accompanied by a sick feeling in the stomach. The pain centers on the navel region. The patient is worse from any motion, better from rest. The patient experiences constant nausea and vomits easily. Vomiting makes patient weakened, inclined to sleep.

LYCOPODIUM—Consider for cases of colic that are accompanied by flatulence. The patient belches without relief. Passes much intestinal gas without relief. There is a sensation as if the abdomen would burst from pressure. The patient must open his pants or loosen any clothing around the waist in order to get some relief. He will become hysterical if anyone attempts to touch the area of his waist, often even if he is not, at that moment, in pain.

MAGNESIA PHOSPHORICA—For cases of colic, or for any cramping that is made better by the application of heat to the site of the cramp, and by rubbing that area of the body. Especially indicated for patients who experience flatulent colic. The patient must bend over double to receive some slight relief. The patient will be made better by belching.

MERCURIUS—In this remedy picture, the pit of stomach is very sensitive. The patient's pains are accompanied by chilliness and shuddering. Pain in the area of the liver is common. The patient will be unable to lie on his right side because of the pain. Coughing or sneezing brings on a terrible pain in the chest. There will be a frequent urge to pass a stool— which consists of slimy diarrhea. Look for a cold, clammy sweat on the patient's thighs and legs. Look also for the patient's urine to be dark-colored, or even to contain blood.

NUX—Cramps in the stomach, with upward pressure. The patient will experience cutting and pinching pains that accompany a desire to vomit or belch. He may be very nauseous. He may feel dizzy, or have shortness of breath. There is pressure as if there were a stone in the stomach. The patient experiences a frequent urge to stool, without result. The patient will be angry, irritable. He may complain of a sense of fullness or tenderness under his ribs. The area of the liver may be very sensitive. The patient may complain of throbbing pains in the liver. This is the first remedy to consider in cases of colic with chronic liver troubles.

PODOPHYLLUM—Especially suggested in cases of colic in which the patient experiences pain in the area of the liver or the gall bladder. The liver will feel swollen and very sensitive. Look for the patient to constantly rub the area of the liver to get relief. The patient will awaken with a headache, will have a headache all morning. Look for his tongue to be coated white and for him to complain of a foul taste in his mouth. The patient will have frequent stools. The stool will be chalklike and very offensive smelling. Nausea and vomiting may accompany the colic.

PULSATILLA—Colic that is accompanied by a bitter taste in the patient's mouth, and when the patient is made worse for any food and drink. Aching, drawing pains in the pit of the stomach. The patient belches a good bit, and tastes food last eaten. The patient has frequent loose stools, and the stools are changeable. He may experience either constipation or diarrhea. The patient is made worse by eating greasy or fatty food. He is also made worse by being in an overly warm room.

SEPIA—Especially indicated for colic in pregnant women. These patients will complain that it feels as if their intestines were "turning over" inside them. There are spasmodic pains. The pains are worse after any motion. Look for a distended and swollen abdomen. Patients will complain of a sensation of pressure and of a bearing-down sensation. Look for a rumbling in the bowels after the patient eats. Either diarrhea or constipation may accompany colic.

VALERIANA—Should be considered for cases of colic in hysterical patients. Consider especially in cases in which the subject is emotionally sensitive or high strung, and the apparently well-chosen remedies have failed. The patient will complain of cramps that come on immediately after eating or after going to bed at night. Spasmodic pains all throughout the abdomen. The patient's abdomen is bloated as well. Look for the patient to have convulsive movements of the diaphragm as well.

VERATRUM—Consider for cases of colic in which the patient experiences knifelike pain here and there, all around the abdomen. The patient's abdomen feels as if cut with knives. For cases of colic with nausea and vomiting. Look for the patient to have a great thirst for cold drinks in large quantities. The patient will be filled with anxiety and despair. He will complain of feelings of great weakness during bouts of colic. A cold sweat, especially on the forehead, will accompany colic. (Veratrum and Coffea follow each other especially well in cases of PMS.)

ALSO CONSIDER

HYOSCYAMUS—Colic that is typified by spasmodic gripping pain. The patient will cry from the pain. He may also vomit. Look for a hardness and swelling in the region of the abdomen. This area is very sensitive, although the patient will most often allow it to be touched. The patient will complain of a headache that accompanies the colic.

PLATINA—For cases of colic that come on after anger or fear, or cases in which the colic pains alternate with the emotions of anger and/or fear. The emotional distress will disappear just as the physical pain begins, and vice versa. The patient will complain of a pressure in his abdomen that comes on after he eats anything. The sensation of the pain will be contracting in nature, as if a shoe were laced up too tight. The patient will also experience a pain that is bearing down in nature. He will weep while in physical pain.

GENERAL ACHES AND PAINS
Hemorrhoids

Hemorrhoids are enlargements of the veins that run along the rectum. The enlarged veins form lumps which can be located either inside or outside the the anus. They are sensitive and/or painful to touch and may become inflamed, causing terrible itching and burning whenever the patient passes a stool.

REMEDIES

ACONITE—A leading remedy for hemorrhoids that bleed. The patient will complain of stinging pains and of a sensation of pressure in his anus. The pain will make the patient very restless, and he will have great difficulty staying still. The patient's skin will be, in general, hot and dry.

APIS—Consider this remedy for cases in which the hemorrhoids burn like fire, or sting like the sting of a bee. The pain will be made better by any application of cold water. The patient will complain of a sensation of sensitivity in his abdomen. He will feel that something inside him will break if he puts forth the effort to pass a stool. Constipation will accompany hemorrhoids.

ARSENICUM—For hemorrhoids that are more painful at night. Especially after midnight. The burning pains will keep the patient from sleeping. During the day, the patient will complain that a stinging pain comes on when he walks. And yet, the patient will be restless and will want to pace about the room in pain.

BELLADONA—A major remedy for hemorrhoids that bleed. The area of the anus is very sensitive. The pain comes on any time the hemorrhoids are touched in any way. The pain of the hemorrhoids extends up into the back. The patient will want to lie still in order to limit the pain. Pains will come on suddenly and leave just as suddenly. The patient will be sleepy, but will not be able to sleep.

CALCAREA—For hemorrhoids that protrude from the anus and bleed a good bit. There will be an almost constant pricking pain in the anus that will drive the patient into a frenzy. He will not be able to keep still. The area is particularly painful after the patient passes a stool. Cold sweat on the patient's feet accompanies the hemorrhoids.

CARBO VEG—For very swollen hemorrhoids that protrude from the anus. For hemorrhoids that bleed a great deal. They may also ooze mucus. The area of the anux emits a terrible odor. The patient experiences a tickling, itching, and burning sensation in the anus. The patient passes stools that are foul, loose, and bloody.

CAUSTICUM—The patient will have trouble passing stool depending on the size and location of the hemorrhoids. The patient will have stinging and burning pain that is so severe that he will be unable to walk due to the pain. A sensation of pressure in the abdomen accompanies the hemorrhoids.

GRAPHITES—The remedy to consider when the area of the anus is cracked and swollen with hemorrhoids. The patient has the sensation of burning and itching in the anus. This is the remedy of first choice for those who have hemorrhoids accompanied by chronic constipation.

IGNATIA—Consider for cases involving hemorrhoids in which the pain shoots way up into the rectum. The pain extends all the way up into the pelvis. The patient will experience both bleeding and burning pains, both of which will be worse if the stool that is passed is loose. The patient will have an empty feeling in the stomach.

NUX—An especially good remedy for those with bleeding hemorrhoids. The patient will experience a flow of pale blood after passing each stool. Hemorrhoids with tearing pains that move up into the patient's lower back. The patient will have constipation as well as hemorrhoids. The patient will feel a frequent ineffectual desire for stool. Consider this remedy especially for those who have constipation and hemorrhoids after the misuse of drugs of any sort, or from drinking alcohol.

PULSATILLA—Consider this remedy for cases of hemorrhoids in which a sensation of pressure in the anus is the outstanding symptom. The anus will feel sore, although there may well be itching and burning pains as well. The patient may have constipation as well as hemorrhoids. He will awaken with a bad taste in his mouth every morning.

RHUS TOX—Consider this remedy for cases in which the burning and itching of the hemorrhoids is relieved by motion. The patient will keep moving to a new position in order to find relief. The pain will be worse if the patient becomes wet, or during damp weather. Also from over-lifting or overstraining on the part of the patient.

SEPIA—For bleeding hemorrhoids that protrude outward when the patient passes a stool. The patient will experience a sensation of heat, burning, and swelling in the anus. The patient will complain of a sensation of oozing in the anus. He will have the sense of a weight or a lump lodged in the anus that is not relieved by passing a stool.

SULPHUR—A leading remedy for bleeding hemorrhoids. The patient will have constant urges to pass a stool. This urge continues even after the patient has just passed a stool. Stools will be thin and bloody. The patient will experience stinging and burning pains in the anus. He will have a great deal of itching in the anus and throughout the body. The anus will be very sore as well, especially if the patient passes a firm stool. The patient will feel heat all throughout his body. He may experience hot sweat all over his body, especially on his head. The patient will experience aggravation in the morning and may be driven out of bed by the need to pass a stool, which begins the itching and burning for the day.

GENERAL ACHES AND PAINS
Skin Conditions: Rash

This general category indicates any circumscribed redness of the skin, or any eruption of redness or spots that is—and this is important—generally unaccompanied by fever or by any other symptoms that could be considered constitutional. Rashes come in various types and from various causes—dietary, mostly—but all general rashes will respond to the correctly chosen remedy.

REMEDIES

ACONITE—Children especially will get rashes that respond to Aconite. The rash will usually appear after the child has been outside playing in a cold wind. The child becomes overheated in play and does not realize that he is beginning to feel chilly. The child comes indoors, is suddenly chilly. The affected area will be bright red. Fever can sometimes accompany the rash. The patient will be anxious, restless.

BRYONIA—Consider Bryonia especially for rashes that come out in a patient who is bedridden or one who does not move around enough. Also used for heat rash, and for general rashes that come out in hot weather.

CHAMOMILLA—The leading remedy for cases that involve red rashes on the cheeks and on the forehead. This is the first remedy to consider for the typical rashes in infants that come out during nursing and dentition. The child is impatient and even angry with rash.

DULCAMARA—This remedy responds to rashes that break out in red spots that look as if they were flea bites. The rash is worse during changes in the weather, from hot to cold and during times of the year that have hot days and cold nights. Rashes in the spring and autumn.

IPECAC—Consider this remedy for itching of the skin that is accompanied by nausea. The rash is not clearly defined on the skin, appears and disappears suddenly, and is followed by nausea and vomiting.

MERCURIUS—The rash here will tend to bleed after being scratched. The rash is very itchy. Look for the patient's skin to have pustules and/or running sores, with itching and burning. The sensation of itch is much worse at night. The skin will look raw.

PULSATILLA—Rash after eating heavy or greasy foods. Rashes that itch violently when you are in bed. Rash will look like measles. Patient is weepy, clingy. Patient and itching worse for closed, warm room, better in open air.

SULPHUR—For a red rash all over the body. Rash will sting and itch. Body has hot sweat with rash. Pimply eruptions filled with pus. Also dry and unhealthy skin. Whole skin red. Patient is very thirsty.

GENERAL ACHES AND PAINS
Skin Conditions: Itching

Usually severe itching or itching that continues for some time will be an indication of a chronic condition. It certainly makes for a very unhappy patient. Here we are talking about cases in which there is no rash on the skin, no strong redness or marking of any kind, just maddening itching. An alcohol bath of the affected parts will often help with the itching. If it does not, consider the following remedies.

REMEDIES

ARSENICUM—Consider this remedy for a sensation of itch that accompanies dry skin. The patient's skin is very dry, even parchmentlike. The patient's skin both burns and itches. This is the first remedy to think of for cases of chronic itching in elderly people. The patient is chilly, worried about his health.

IGNATIA—For itching that is worse when the patient gets into bed. The itch feels like flea bites. When the itch is scratched, it moves to another part of the body, only to begin again.

MERCURIUS—Itching is worse at night, and worse from the warmth of the bed. Dry, rashlike eruptions. The keynote here is that the skin bleeds when it is scratched.

NUX—Itching begins upon undressing and extends over the whole body. The itch may center on the area of the rectum. The patient will be very irritable during the itch. Muscular twitches and spasms may accompany the itch.

PULSATILLA—Consider this remedy first for cases that combine biting with itching here and there on the body. The itching and burning moves from place to place on the body. The movement of the itch has no rhyme or reason. The itching feels like ants on the skin. Itching begins when the patient gets warm in bed.

RHUS TOX—Itching is accompanied by intense burning. Itching extends over the whole body, particularly on the hairy parts of the body. Often the skin feels shrunken during itching. The itch will be made better by taking a shower, and by applications that are hot and moist. The patient will be restless and will have to change positions often in order to get comfortable.

SULPHUR—Itching with tingling, also with burning that comes on after scratching. The body is sore from scratching. The itching sensation will be made much worse by heat, especially the heat of the bed. The patient's skin will be hot and sweaty. This is the first remedy to think of for itch, especially for chronic itch.

GENERAL ACHES AND PAINS
Skin Conditions: Abscesses

An abscess is a collection of pus, of what the classical homeopaths loved to call "purulent matter." It may be either acute or chronic in nature.

Acute abscess begins with the usual signs of inflammation, such as heat, redness, swelling, and throbbing pain. Then the pus begins to form. Often such abscesses come on after fevers.

Chronic abscesses are more subtle in their formation. They are generally the result of a low-level infection, which is itself a chronic condition. They may appear very slowly, internally or externally, and are a gathering of the toxins in the system. As such, they should be taken quite seriously.

I include here the abscesses called "felons" or "whitlows" that are particular favorites of mine. I used to get them all the time and they really hurt. These are infections of the fingertips, usually next to the nail. They can swell up like balloons and can last for weeks. People who, like me, do a lot of typing tend to get them from the pressure of the fingers on the keys.

REMEDIES

ACONITE—Consider this remedy when a tumor has formed and that tumor is swollen, red, and shining. The patient will complain of cutting, violent pain. The area of the infection burns, as if it had been burnt by fire. The patient is very nervous. The patient, desperate in the pain, insists that "something must be done!" Great fear, great excitement. Look for the patient to experience aggravations in the evening and at night.

APIS—This remedy is especially good for felons. For cases that involve burning and stinging pains when the patient feels like he's been stung by a bee. Cold water relieves the pain. (Consider this remedy especially for abscesses that come forth after using the remedy Sulphur.)

ARSENICUM—For cases of abscess. When the patient's whole system is weakened by the infection. Look for a violent burning of the affected part. The abscess burns like fire. The patient is very restless and tosses about. The patient is very thirsty, but drinks very little. Look for aggravations during periods of rest. The patient better for motion. Look for aggravations after midnight.

BELLADONNA—Consider this remedy for cases of abscess when the tumor is very swollen and feels very hard to the touch. The patient will complain of congestive or pressing pains. He says that the abscess throbs or stings. Pains appear suddenly and disappear just as suddenly. The swelling also has a hot, dry sensation. The patient will be worse daily at 3 P.M. Look for a throbbing headache to accompany infection. This is also a remedy for patients with felons.

BRYONIA—This remedy is very good in the early part of abscess. Especially in cases in which the swollen part feels heavy. The area of the swelling is hard to the touch. The tumor alternates in color, and can be very red or very pale. The patient complains of stitching pains that are aggravated by the slightest motion. Wants to stay very still. Look for constipation, with hard dry stools to accompany the abscess.

HEPAR SULPH—For abscesses in which the infection has formed and must now burst. It is too late for the body to reabsorb the infection. The patient experiences throbbing pains. The period of pain is often preceded by chill. Hepar Sulph is suitable for chronic abscesses as well. Also suitable for felons and whitlows. The remedy will cause felons to burst and heal faster.

LACHESIS—If the pus has formed already, Lachesis will expel it externally from the body. For abscesses with purple color, great swelling; abscesses formed from the introduction of poison into the system. The purple color and the swelling are keynote of the remedy, as is the fact that the area of the infection will swell greatly if scratched.

MERCURIUS—If taken in time, this remedy will cause the system to reabsorb the abscess and keep it from having to burst. Consider this remedy first in all cases that involve glandular abscesses. Also for abscesses that are not yet inflamed, or for cases of abscess that involve intense, shining redness and stinging pains. Look for the pain to extend into the joints. Consider this remedy as well for felons and whitlows that hurt into the bone of the finger.

PHOSPHORUS—Consider this remedy for the early stages of infection only. Phosphorus prevents the formation of pus. The remedy also guards against scars in the healing process.

PULSATILLA—Consider for abscesses that bleed easily and that are accompanied by stinging and cutting pains. Consider especially for cases of abscesses that are accompanied by itching. Look for the patient to produce copious pus that is yellowish green in color. This is also the leading remedy for abscesses that come on after other infections. The patient will be tearful and will want a lot of attention.

RHUS TOX—Consider this remedy especially for underarm abscesses. The patient complains of stinging and gnawing pains. The abscess is painful to the touch. Look for a discharge of bloody pus. The pain is worse for rest, better for motion.

SILICEA—When the abscess must burst, or in chronic cases in which the discharge has become thin, watery, fetid. Consider this remedy especially for felons and whitlows on the fingertips. This is the most important remedy to consider for any abscess that is especially slow to heal. Think of Silicea when the patient's entire vital force is threatened by the infection.

SULPHUR—This is the remedy to think of in chronic cases in which there is a good deal of discharge of matter. When there is a chronic tendency to return to disease. Especially for persons who are troubled by boils. For lean, stoop-shouldered persons. For chronic cases in which the patient's skin, no matter how often he washes, looks unhealthy and smells foul.

GENERAL ACHES AND PAINS
Skin Conditions: Boils (Furuncles)

A boil—or as the old texts would call it, a "furunclus growth"—is a hard, round, and inflamed tumor that will ultimately burst and release its discharge. The matter will start out mixed with blood and afterward will be just pus. When the growth bursts, it will reveal a small, grayish, fibrous mass called the core. This particular abscess will not heal until the core is expelled.

A "blind boil" does not completely form and does not burst, but becomes a particularly nasty chronic infection. Some people just seem more likely to get these than do others. No one knows why.

Aren't you glad you're studying homeopathy?

REMEDIES

ACONITE—Consider this when the boil is highly inflamed and will be accompanied by fever and by great restlessness on the part of the patient. Look for the patient to complain that the abscess burns as if from hot coals.

ARNICA—This remedy is very good for blood boils. For tumors of dark color, with dull, sore pain as if from a bruise. This is the first remedy to consider in cases involving small, painful boils that reappear in the same spot, one after another. For single boils that appear anywhere on the body.

BELLADONNA—Consider especially for cases of boils that have a fiery red appearance. Look for the boil to feel hot and dry to the touch. Look for the patient to complain of a throbbing pain. This remedy is specific for swollen glands under the arms and in the groin.

HEPAR SULPH—Think of this remedy if the boil has become infected to the point that it must burst. The patient will complain of throbbing pains that are preceded by a sensation of chilliness.

MERCURIUS—Consider this remedy if the boil is inflamed and hard and very painful. When the boil matures slowly. Look for the patient to experience profuse sweating that brings no relief.

SULPHUR—This is the first remedy to consider in cases of chronic boils. Especially for boils in patients who have dry, scaly skin. Or in patients who have skin that appears unhealthy.

GENERAL ACHES AND PAINS
Skin Conditions: Sores/Ulcers

These are basic injuries and come in several types. Among them are:

The *simple ulcer*. This is the result of some superficial injury, such as a bruise, burn, or abscess. This form of ulcer will heal itself in a matter of a very few days if the patient is constitutionally strong.

The *irritable ulcer*. This sore is hot, tender, and subject to gnawing pain. The edges are sore and ragged, and the skin is red and inflamed. The ulcer may contain greenish or reddish matter, which is acrid and excoriates the surrounding skin. This type of ulcer will usually form on the lower limbs and is usually linked to a poor diet.

The *indolent ulcer*. This is the most common form of a sore, and also the most difficult to heal. The surface is flat and has a gray crust to it. The sore is very tenacious. The edges are raised, thick, white, and have no sensation of pain on touching. The discharge is thin and scanty. The ulcer lasts a long time. These ulcers are most common in persons who live in filthy surroundings, again with poor diets.

REMEDIES

ARSENICUM—Consider this remedy for patients with ulcers that bleed easily and are very painful. The site of the sore burns as if from fire. The edges of the ulcer are hard and turned outward. The discharge is thin and offensive, bloody or blackish. Also the remedy for old ulcers that won't heal and for ulcers in the elderly.

BELLADONNA—Consider if the ulcer is very sore and has a burning sensation when it is touched. The patient's skin will be both dry and hot. Consider Belladonna especially if a black crust of blood forms on the ulcer.

CARBO VEG—Consider in cases of patients with ulcers that bleed readily and have a putrid smell to them. The patient will complain of burning pains.

GRAPHITES—For ulcers on patients with chronically unhealthy skin. Consider especially when every little injury to the skin causes suppuration. This is the first remedy to think of for cases of ulcers that have fetid pus, and itching and stinging pains. The discharge is thick and glutinous.

HEPAR SULPH—For ulcers that itch and have gnawing pain. The sore will tend to throb at night. Consider this remedy for patients with ulcers that bleed even when tightly wrapped up. The discharge has a sour smell to it, like old cheese.

LACHESIS—Consider for flat ulcers of various sizes, scattered all over the body. Ulcers that are very sensitive to touch. That may have itching pain. Consider especially for cases involving uneven ulcers, especially sores that form on lower limbs. Around the ulcer will be many small pimples on a purple skin. The skin around the sore will swell if scratched.

LYCOPODIUM—Consider this remedy for cases involving hard, red, and shining ulcers with upturned edges. The ulcers will look like craters.

MERCURIUS—This is the leading remedy for deep ulcers and for ulcers that spread quickly. Look for them to bleed easily. The ulcers will be very sensitive to touch, and even the lightest touch will cause the patient severe pain. Typically, the sore has a reddish look like raw beef. The edges of the ulcer are raised. This is the most important remedy for syphilitic ulcers.

SILICEA—Think of this remedy first for cases of old ulcers. Ulcers that will not heal. Ulcers occurring in unclean patients. And especially for ulcers in patients who have become debilitated. Consider this remedy for ulcers with rough edges, like calluses. Look for the skin around the sore to be enlarged and blue-red in color. Look for the discharge thick and discolored. It may also be bloody.

SULPHUR—Think of this remedy first for cases of ulcers that occur on patients with dry, scaly skin. Sulphur is to be thought of especially for ulcers that are slow to heal, and for irritable ulcers that bleed easily and that have raised and swollen edges. Look for the discharge to be thin and watery. Look for it also to be somewhat fetid. Look for the patient most commonly to complain of pricking pains, although there may be no pain at all associated with the ulcer.

ALSO CONSIDER

NITRIC ACID—This is the first remedy to think of for cases of bleeding ulcers that occur in association with stinging pain. Look for patients to say that they feel as if there are splinters in the skin. The discharge from the ulcer will be bloody. This is a common remedy for use in ulcers occurring in elderly patients.

GENERAL ACHES AND PAINS
Skin Conditions: Warts

Warts are fungal growths that chiefly grow on hands, especially the fingers, and the face. An application of Aqua Thuja or Thuja ointment is the usual topical application for this condition, and such a treatment can be undertaken before the following remedies are considered.

REMEDIES

CALCAREA—Consider this remedy especially for warts occurring on the sides of the fingers.

CAUSTICUM—For patients with fleshy and seedy warts. Consider this remedy especially for elderly patients and most especially for patients with warts on the face. This is the first remedy to think of for those with warts on the nose like those associated with Halloween witches.

DULCAMARA—Think of this remedy for those with warts on the back of fingers. These warts appear on delicate skin that is sensitive to cold.

THUJA—Whether used topically or internally, Thuja is perhaps the leading remedy for warts of all sorts on all parts of the body. Thuja should always be considered first in cases that involve genital warts.

ALSO CONSIDER

ANTIMONIUM CRUDUM—This is the remedy to think of first for warts that are flat, hard, and brittle.

GENERAL ACHES AND PAINS
Skin Conditions: Shingles (Herpes Zoster)

Shingles are a row or belt of inflamed sores that appear on the skin, extending around the body or over the shoulders. The rash burns, itches, and stings and may be accompanied by a fever. While these sores are not dangerous, they should be considered a constitutional situation and the remedies listed below are here as a stopgap until you can get into a homeopathic practitioner's office.

REMEDIES

ACONITE—Consider Aconite if the patient is sleepless, feverish, and very excited. The patient will be very restless. He will complain of a burning sensation on the skin. Look for the skin to be red and hot.

MERCURIUS—This remedy picture calls for an eruption that extends from the back around the abdomen like a girdle. The sores are moist and form dark scabs. The sores burn when touched. The condition will be worse at night. Especially worse when the patient is in bed.

PULSATILLA—Consider this remedy for shingles that are associated with gastric troubles, those that come on from a poor diet of overly rich food, and especially after the patient has been eating pork. Look for the eruption to be worse at night when the patient is in bed. Look for the patient to be mild and tearful. It is keynote of the remedy picture that the patient does not want to be alone.

RHUS TOX—Here we have a shingles rash that looks like poison ivy. It appears in patches, and burns and itches violently. Look for the patient to say that his skin feels shrunken. Look for sharp pains in affected parts; the patient will say that he feels as if his skin had been pricked by needles. This is the first remedy to think of if the shingles come on after the patient has gotten wet in the rain, or if the rash comes on after any exposure to cold damp.

SULPHUR—Consider this remedy in cases of pus-filled rash. That rash will be terribly itchy. The itch will be aggravated by any application of heat, and especially from the heat of the bed. Look for the rash to form yellow and brown crusts. The patient is in general troubled by old sores and chronic skin conditions.

GENERAL ACHES AND PAINS
Skin Conditions: Poison Ivy and Oak

For those who are highly allergic to poison ivy, this rash represents a major ailment and must be treated as a constitutional condition, but for most of us, poison ivy just represents one of the painful realities of summer.

Remember that if you are trying to prevent a poison ivy outbreak, you should go high with your potency (choose the remedy that matches the patient's usual outbreak symptoms). But if you are treating an existing poison ivy rash, you must stay very low in potency—not over 12C, usually—or you will risk spreading that rash all over that poor patient's body.

REMEDIES

BELLADONNA—If the face is the part of the body affected by the rash, give in low potency every two or three hours. The face will be dark red and hot. The patient will want quiet. He will be driven crazy by his symptoms and will want to lie down in a cool, dark place. He will especially be aggravated by noise.

BRYONIA—The patient here will want to be very still. Any movement of any sort will aggravate all his symptoms. Because of this, although he is thirsty, the patient will drink seldom but will drink a great deal at one time. The patient wants cold water, cold applications. He may be very angry. As a classical general poison ivy remedy, bathe the parts of the body affected in warm water and give Bryonia every three hours.

RHUS TOX—This remedy is made from the leaves of poison ivy and is therefore the most commonly used homeopathic remedy for poison ivy. For those who are highly allergic, it is important to take a high-potency dose a month or so before poison ivy season to help ward off the rash. If a patient already has the rash, however, you must never give Rhus in high potency—that will cause the rash to spread like wildfire until it covers the whole body. Give the Rhus in a very low potency—6c or below—to help contain the rash. For Rhus to be the correct remedy, the patient must want to take a hot shower to stop the rash from itching.

ALSO CONSIDER

ANACARDIUM—This will stop the rash only if it is used immediately upon coming in contact with the poison ivy. Look for the patient to have a reduction of all his senses during the rash. There will be a good deal of swelling, along with the itching. The itch will be accompanied by anger and irritablity. The patient will want to rub his rash. The itch is much worse from warm applications, especially warm water. Classical home-opaths also suggest that the infected part be soaked in milk.

SANGUINARIA—Works for poison ivy that is worse for a hot shower and better for a cold shower. Consider this remedy especially for poison ivy early in the season, poison ivy rash in the spring. The rash appears as red, blotchy eruptions that occur in round spots. The patient will be better in darkness. He is worse from any heat, from any motion. He does not want to be touched. Pain in the head may accompany the rash. The pain will be described as a bolt of lightning.

GENERAL ACHES AND PAINS
Skin Conditions: Dandruff

This is the most superficial condition we treat. It is characterized by irregular patches of thin scales on the scalp that are removed by brushing or combing the hair. After the scales have been brushed away they are quickly replaced by more. Dandruff does not form crusts. It is not contagious.

To fight dandruff, keep the scalp clean, the head cool, and the diet healthy. The following remedies may have a positive impact.

REMEDIES

CALCAREA—One of our major remedies for those whose digestive tract is not functioning very well. Look for the patient to be fair, fat, and flabby. The patient's head will have a tendency to feel cold. And the patient's head will sweat as well, especially at night.

GRAPHITES—Consider this remedy for cases of dandruff that are usually accompanied by a feeling of intoxication. The patient will complain of a sensation of burning on the top of his head.

LYCOPODIUM—This remedy is for dandruff accompanied by early balding. Consider this remedy also for cases of dandruff in patients with prematurely graying hair. Also for cases of dandruff in those with chronic indigestion, with intestinal gas. The patient may say that his scalp itches as if covered by fleas.

SEPIA—Consider this remedy especially for cases that combine dandruff and ringworm. This is also a good general remedy for all cases of dandruff, especially in women. The patient's scalp is dry and itchy. The scalp may also be sweaty and burning.

SULPHUR—The first remedy to consider in all cases. In general, you are looking for a patient with dry, scaly skin and scalp. This is indicated in patients with unhealthy skin. The patient's scalp itches, then burns after he scratches it. This is our most important remedy for cases of chronic dandruff, especially in messy patients.

COMMON AILMENTS
Colds and Flus and Fevers

Everyone gets a cold from time to time, and it can actually be a very good thing—a cleansing experience for your body, and an excuse to rest your body, mind, and spirit. But be sure that what you have is truly a cold and not something deeper.

For instance, if you have just begun a constitutional treatment, it is quite common to get a cold. And this cold should not be treated; it is part of the uncovering of the chronic condition. In this case, you simply have to have that cold.

Also if you have been on a constitutional remedy for some time and that remedy is working and you are getting better and if in that case you get a cold, you are far better off having that cold than you are in treating it acutely.

If, however, that cold (or any other acute illness, for that matter) is becoming a real health issue for you, then you must put aside your constitutional remedy before treating the condition acutely. This, of course, means that you must contact your practitioner and make him aware and a part of all you are doing.

Take acute remedies for colds and flus as needed. For the most part, a moderate 30C potency will do nicely.

The trick is what you do after the cold has gone. Most people want to just jump back on their constitutional remedy. But what you must do is wait and see if the symptoms for that remedy return. The cold may have been the initial manifestation of a new constitutional remedy appearing, and you may not need to return to that old remedy at all. So, when the cold ends, do nothing until there is something to do.

As to other treatments for colds, there's rest and rest and rest—not only for your sake, but for everyone else's. Not another soul in the world wants your cold, so stay home, rest, and keep it to yourself. Ginger tea, hot baths, and vitamin C will all help in your recovery.

REMEDIES

ACONITE—Will only help with a cold if you take it in time, and that usually means in the first 12 hours of the infection. Here the cold has come on usually from exposure to dry, cold wind. The cold comes on with a great deal of sneezing. The patient is suddenly very chilly, although his face is burning hot. There is a shallow, dry cough with tickling in the throat. The patient is very restless.

ALLIUM CEPA—Think of the onion from which the remedy is made. The eyes are tearing; the nose is running. The tears from the eyes are bland; the mucus (which is clear) from the nose burns the skin around the nose. For those colds with the red crust forming under the nose. Upper lips also irritated. Symptoms are worse in warm rooms, better in the open air. The sore throat is of a tickling nature. The cough is dry and causes enough pain to the patient that he will grab his throat when he coughs. Usually, there is little or no fever.

ARSENICUM—Another chilly patient, one who wants to go to bed and get cozy. The patient sneezes a good deal and has a good deal of mucus flowing, and it is very thin, clear, and watery. Eyes tear, and the tears are burning. There is a loss of taste in the mouth and the mouth is very dry. Patient is very thirsty, usually for warm things, especially tea with lemon. Look for the patient to sip his drinks. Overall, patient is much improved from heat, but if headache accompanies cold, patient will want cold applications or cold air on head. Patient is restless, unless very sick, in which case he will lie in bed and not want to move at all, as if giving up. In addition to these symptoms, Arsenicum is the remedy of choice for flus in which you have both vomiting and diarrhea. Patient is nauseous above all else and seems to be losing all his vital force to the illness.

BELLADONNA—Usually comes on very quickly, like Aconite. Like Aconite, cold will usually be accompanied by fever. Skin will be hot and dry. Cold begins with fever and sore throat. Voice hoarse. Throbbing headache, worse for any motion. Ulcers in mouth and nose. Dry cough—coughing may be painful enough to make the patient cry. Patient alternates between hot and cold. Sleepy but cannot sleep.

BRYONIA—The nose feels stopped up, but there is no flow of mucus. Lips will be dry and cracked. Dry cough; cough hurts down in the stomach. Cough is worse from drinking liquids. Commonly used as a flu remedy; look for body aches and pains as well as cold symptoms. Patient very thirsty. Constipated. Stool is very hard, as if burnt. Patient is very irritable, wants to stay very still. Often wants to be left alone.

CAMPHORA—Very good at the beginning stages of a cold. Look for the patient to feel very chilly, and there is a great deal of sneezing. The nose is very stopped up—that is the usual first symptom. No great flow of mucus. Headache in the front of the head, sore throat in the front of the throat.

CARBO VEG—Cold with headache. Head feels as if it is pulsing with each heartbeat. Eyes burning and tearing. Nose feels stopped up, especially at night. Mucus flows more during the day. Voice hoarse. Chest feels raw. The patient will often feel that he cannot breathe, will want to have a fan on, have air moving.

CHAMOMILLA—Here there is a great deal of discharge from the nose. Discharge is acrid, burning. Look for the traditional sign of Chamomilla: The patient will have one red and hot cheek; the other will be pale and cold. Rattling mucus in the chest. Hoarseness and loose cough. Cough worse at night. Worse during sleep. The patient will be very irritable, often will be very demanding but will be unsure what he wants. Patient may want to be held or rocked.

DULCAMARA—Best for colds that come on from exposure to cold, damp weather, or that come on from a change in the weather. All symptoms are aggravated by changes in the weather or by becoming cold or wet. Patient is better from moving about, worse from lying still.

EUPHRASIA—The symptoms are the opposite of Allium Cepa. Here the eyes are tearing and the nose is running, but the tears cause the eyes to burn and become red; the clear mucus from the nose is bland. Symptoms are worse in open air, worse from lying down. Usually there is a loose cough; the cough is made better from eating. All symptoms are worse in the daytime.

EUPATORIUM—When used as a flu remedy, look for the patient to seem similar to the Bryonia patient. However, here the body aches are deep; the pain seems to be in the bones themselves. Shivers will go up and down the spine. Aching from head to toe. It is painful to move. Worse for any change in temperature, change in weather.

FERRUM PHOS—Very useful in the first stages of a cough/cold/flu. The initial symptoms may resemble Belladonna, but the patient is not as ill. General fever remedy. Patient will not be sluggish, as in Belladonna, but will be mentally alert. Look for the face to have red patches on the cheeks.

GELSEMIUM—Also will take cold from changes in weather, but illness will not be as severe as in Dulcamara. Gelsemium colds can be very slow to come on. Patient will feel dizzy, weak, and tired for a number of days before cold begins. Cold usually begins as a sore throat with pain on swallowing that extends into the ear. The keynote symptom is fever without thirst. Patient is very content to lie still and rest.

HEPAR SULPH—Cold with infection. Look for the glands in the neck to be swollen. Cold with sore throat that has the sensation of a stick caught in the throat. Loose cough that chokes the patient. Mucus may be clear or greenish.

IPECAC—Cold with an aching pain over the eyes. Much discharge, with stoppage of the nose and loss of smell. Loose cough, with rattling in the chest. No relief from coughing. Nausea accompanies the cold, and the patient will usually vomit mucus. Breathing labored, as if patient had asthma.

KALI BI—A remedy that is usually used to clear out the last stage of a cold. Acutely, it is also the remedy to think of first for sinus headache. Look for the mucus in the cold to be green and ropy. It is thick and tends to be long and stringy. It may be so thick that it cannot be blown out of the nose. It may form crusts or mucus plugs in the nose. The discharge may have an offensive smell. There is also thick postnasal drip and a constant clearing of the throat. Pain at the root of the nose. Pain in the frontal sinuses.

LACHESIS—Look for profuse discharges in Lachesis. Eyes tear and nose runs. But mouth is very dry. Patient may say that he tastes pepper or that the mouth burns as if he had eaten food with too much pepper. Dry cough that hurts in the chest. Patient is very protective of his throat—may cover throat with a loose scarf. Will let nothing touch his throat. Will cough if you touch his throat. Feels as if he is suffocating. Look for the darting of the tongue from the dry mouth. Patient will be able to swallow solid food more easily than liquids. Patient worse in the afternoon and worse for sleeping.

MERCURIUS—Here we have some sort of infection present. Sinus headache with the cold. Swelling of glands in neck. Eyes burn from profuse tears. Pain in teeth and jaws. Look for a swollen tongue (you will see teeth marks on the sides) and profuse salivation. Patient drools on pillow while sleeping. Usually, patient will have bad breath. Inflamed tonsils with the cold. Short, dry cough, worse at night. Night sweats that bring no relief. Patient better for warmth and warm room. Worse, however, from being too hot or too cold.

NATRUM MUR—An excellent general cold remedy. Cold will begin as sneezing fits and loss of sense of smell. The patient speaks with a nasal voice. The mucus will be clear and thick, like raw egg white. Total loss of smell, much sneezing. Much postnasal drip. Lips tend to be dry and cracked, particularly in the corners. Cold sores are common. Loss of appetite. Patient feels depressed but does not want to be fussed over.

NUX—For colds that are slow coming and slow leaving. Patient starts to get ill by becoming chilly. Feels cold inside, cannot get warm. Patient cold with fever. Look for frontal headache with cold. Nose has a great deal of discharge during the day, stopped up completely at night. Dry cough, makes headache much worse. Patient is very irritable and cannot be pleased. If you feel like shoving the food tray through a slot in the door and running, give him Nux. Cold with constipation. Symptoms worse in the morning.

PHOSPHORUS—Colds here tend to begin in the throat and move quickly to the chest. Not a usual head cold remedy. Cough may be dry or loose. It may be croupy in nature. It may be very deep and the cough may cause a great deal of chest pain. The patient is thirsty for cold things, wants ice cream and other cold foods. Patient may become nauseous, may vomit when food or drink warms in the stomach. Usually the patient will lose his voice during the cold. Coughing may bring up mucus, may bring up blood. Patient is worse for lying on left side. Feels tightness in chest. Cough is worse for cold air, for laughing or talking. The patient wants attention, wants company. Does not want to be left alone.

PULSATILLA—Usually used at the end of a cold. Look for the characteristic yellow-green discharges. Mucus will have a fluffy, cloudlike quality. Thick. Loss of taste and smell. Cold with toothache. Patient craves fresh air, cannot bear a warm room. May feel chilly, however, even in that warm room. Symptoms are worse toward evening. Look for the Pulsatilla personality to emerge—patient wants to be taken care of, may whine for attention. May feel very sorry for himself. May want to be held and rocked.

SEPIA—The nose is swollen and inflamed. Nostrils are sore, ulcerated. Obstruction of the very slight mucus flow. Loss of smell. Pain in the back and shoulders often accompanies the cold. Neck feels stiff. Cough is worse in the morning, often violent enough to lead to dry heaves. Stomach feels very empty, but patient is not hungry.

SULPHUR—Mucus flows by the gallon, clear and watery. Complete loss of taste and smell. Patient does not usually feel that sick. May want to just lie in bed and watch soap operas. Will usually crave very salty things that he can taste—potato chips feel good in the throat. Coldness in the extremities, cannot bear to have feet under the covers, so they go in and out of covers all day and night. Cold often accompanied by morning diarrhea, which will drive the patient out of bed in the morning.

COMMON AILMENTS
Sore Throat and Laryngitis

It may well be hard to tell the difference between the occasions on which this list of remedies is needed, as opposed to those for colds and flus. In fact, many remedies appear on both lists. And, as many colds begin with sore throats, if one can learn to quickly treat that problem, the deeper illness may be avoided.

REMEDIES

ACONITE—Here again we think of Aconite first for a sore throat that comes on quickly, most especially if that sore throat begins after exposure to cold, dry wind. Look for the throat to look red and swollen and for the patient to feel chilled, even though there may be a fever. Patient's face may be red as well.

APIS—Think of the general Apis picture and apply it to a sore throat. The throat is red and swollen; it feels stung and burning. The throat is made worse by drinking warm things, and is better for drinking very cold things. The throat is dry, the patient is thirsty. The throat may look to be shiny as well as red. In Aconite, the throat looks swollen. In Apis, it feels swollen as well. The patient will say that the throat hurts whether or not he swallows. The patient will not allow anything around his throat.

ARSENICUM—Will usually begin on the right side and move left, or be more painful on the right side. Here the throat is made better by warm drinks, worse by cold. The patient will be chilly, fussy, restless. Nasal flow will be clear and watery.

BELLADONNA—The problem here is usually tonsillitis, but it may be useful in other sore throats as well. The pain comes on quickly. The tonsils and throat will be bright red. Very red. The pain is burning in character, and the patient swallows constantly, even though it hurts for him to swallow. He may have trouble swallowing food or water. He wants lemons or oranges. Look for a fever with the sore throat.

CARBO VEG—Especially indicated for patients with long-lasting hoarseness that is worse morning and evening. Speaking at all weakens the voice, hurts the throat. Carbo Veg is especially useful for sore throat, hoarseness, and cough following measles.

CAUSTICUM—For a hoarse and rough throat that is accompanied by a hoarse voice. The condition is worse in the morning. This is a very good remedy for obstinate cases, especially with pain in the chest as well as the throat. Usually an emotionally related remedy. Patient loses voice when shouting about causes that excite him, or loses voice in order not to be able to speak up.

CHAMOMILLA—For sore throats that come on when you go out into cold air while perspiring. Stinging and burning pains in the throat. There is a sensation that you should be able to cough something up from the throat and then you will feel better. Often the remedy for children's sore throats, especially when the child is cross.

FERRUM PHOS—Again, this remedy is thought of usually for cases of tonsillitis. The pain does not come on as quickly as in Belladonna nor is the situation as severe. The pain, however, will usually still be accompanied by a fever, and hoarseness is common. This is also a remedy for people who lose their voices a good deal from overuse. Especially from singing, and especially when cold drinks make the throat feel better.

GELSEMIUM—Consider this remedy in cases in which the patient's voice is very weak. Look for a loss of voice due to nervousness, especially fear of public speaking. Look for the patient to suffer raspy pain in throat, paralysis of the glottis. Look for difficulty in swallowing. The throat feels ulcerated, burnt. Great exhaustion in the patient is common.

HEPAR SULPH—The pain feels as if there were a stick caught in the throat. As with Aconite, the pain begins usually after the patient is exposed to cold air. The sore throat will ache into the ears, especially on swallowing. Pain is better for hot drinks. Hepar patients will not want to be touched.

IGNATIA—Like Lachesis, people with these sore throats will be better for swallowing solid food, worse for swallowing liquids. Here you have the sensation of "a lump in the throat." And since this is a medicine for strong emotion, look for the pain to have an emotional origin. Usually there will be a loss of voice here, also, from not having said something that it was important to speak up about. Patient sighs.

LACHESIS—Everyone knows that Lachesis is made from snake venom, and so it goes to follow that the throat, a snakelike part of our being, will be most vulnerable in a Lachesis state. The pain is usually on the left side, or begins on the left and moves to the right. Look for the left side of the throat to be more swollen or deep red-purple in color. Pain is worse for swallowing liquids, especially warm liquids, better for swallowing solids. Throat is overly sensitive to touch. Nothing can cover the throat and no one can touch it.

LYCOPODIUM—Pain begins on the right and moves left, or throat is more painful on the right. Pain is better for warm drinks, worse for cold. There is often a sensation of a plug in the throat. Pain worse in late afternoon. Patient especially weary at that time. Look for the patient to be too tired to have you in the room, but to want you to stay in the house.

MERCURIUS—Here we have some sort of infection present. Usually it is not simple sore throat, but rather a situation in which a cold has settled into the throat. Therefore, Mercurius is not a remedy for a new throat condition, but rather to be considered when a throat continues to be sore for a period of time. Look for swollen glands under the jaw. Look for a swollen tongue and for a great deal of saliva. The pain is raw, the throat is constricted. Tonsils will be swollen.

NUX—Consider this remedy for the patient who experiences scraping pains in throat. Who exhibits hoarseness or loss of voice. Usually accompanied by constipation. Patient is chilly, angry. Look for postnasal drip. Nostrils clogged. This sore throat is slow coming on, slow to build, and slow to leave.

PHOSPHORUS—A great remedy for losing your voice from overuse. "Preacher's throat." Think of it in terms of having given over too much of yourself, and now you are exhausted. You lose your voice because you have nothing left to say. The throat demands cold drinks, ice, ice cream. Patient may become nauseous as these things warm in the stomach. Patient wants to be made to laugh, even if that makes the throat hurt worse. Look for tightness of chest.

RHUS TOX—A great remedy for those who lose their voices often due to overuse. Pain is worse on initial swallowing, better for continued swallowing. Worse for cold and better for warm drinks. The patient will, in general, feel better from warmth, especially the damp warmth of a hot shower.

SULPHUR—Think of this remedy as a general tonic for the throat. The pain is better from cold drinks, worse from warm in any form. Patient feels hot, sweaty. Pain is better for salt and for eating salty things. The patient will want to eat potato chips—things that are both greasy and salty. The pain in the throat is burning in character.

ALSO CONSIDER

WYETHIA—The throat pain isn't the worst thing here—the itching on the roof of the mouth is. The itching stimulates coughing and the coughing makes the throat hurt worse than ever. Also for use with loss of voice from overuse—the throat is dry and hot, there is difficulty in swallowing.

COMMON AILMENTS
Coughs

There are just a few basic cough remedies, although getting to be able to tell the difference among them just by the sound of a cough takes a lot of practice. So try to use the cough as just one of several symptoms and you'll have a much higher success rate.

REMEDIES

ANTIMONIUM TARTARICUM—This is the remedy for a deep cough, one that is moving or has turned into bronchitis. Listen for rattling in the chest and a chest full of mucus. The symptoms come on very slowly, and the cold, which may have been a mild ailment in and of itself, has moved deeper and become a more serious situation. The patient will cough and cough and will be unable to bring up any of the abundant mucus that is inside. The patient may be too weak to expectorate the mucus. In general, the patient is short of breath. Consider Antimonium to be the remedy for a drowning man, and give it when the patient is drowning in his own phlegm.

DROSERA—This is a remedy for dry, spasmodic, and croupy coughs. Here the cough sounds like a dog barking. Listen for the ringing sound to the cough. The patient's larynx is inflamed and irritated. Like Spongia, there is a constriction in the throat, a tickling in the throat. The cough may be croupy in the throat or deeper in the chest. Sometimes the patient may insist that the cough is coming from the abdomen. Spasms of coughing appear after midnight and may cause vomiting. Look for the patient to have to support his chest and/or stomach from the coughing fit.

IPECAC—A cough that is moving toward bronchitis. Illness comes on swiftly, moving from a simple head cold down into the chest in just a day or two. The cough is damp and very deep. Listen for a rattling sound in the chest when the patient coughs. There will be a great deal of mucus in the chest. The cough can be accompanied by choking and suffocation. The patient may have a hard time breathing. Coughs can be accompanied by vomiting. Patient will often be nauseated along with the cough. Coughing fits may end in vomiting. Patient is worse in a warm room. Look for a stuffy nose that bleeds easily. Patient is needy, but often doesn't know just what he needs.

RUMEX—Made from yellowdock, Rumex heals coughs that are dry and shallow. These coughs are set off by a tickle in the throat or in the pit of the throat just above the breastbone. The keynote symptom is that the patient will keep the covers up over his mouth as he breathes in order to warm the air before breathing it in, as cool air triggers a coughing fit. Another keynote symptom of Rumex is that the patient feels that it is taking all his strength of body and mind to keep from coughing. So the patient will breathe as shallowly as possible and as slowly as possible. The patient does not want to talk, because it will make him cough. Doesn't even want to be spoken to. The cough is worse before midnight and when lying down. Touching the throat will bring on a coughing fit.

SPONGIA—The easiest remedy to tell by sound alone. Listen for a harsh cough that sounds like a dog barking or a saw cutting through wood. While Aconite and Hepar Sulph will both also have croupy coughs, neither will have the jarring surprise quality of Spongia. The cough has a rasp to it. Spongia patients will be awakened by the sound of their own cough, usually before midnight. Like Lachesis, the Spongia patient will feel a constriction and suffocation in the throat. He is worse for talking, for cold things, and for overexcitement.

COMMON AILMENTS
Whooping Cough

Whooping cough is a disease of childhood. It most commonly strikes in children age fourteen and under. The condition generally has two stages. In the first, the patient will have a bad cold, with runny nose and sneezing as well as fever. Most notably, the patient will have a cough that is both irritating and painful. The patient may have some trouble breathing.

At the second stage of the ailment, the fever subsides and the cough increases. Whooping cough is so named because of the sound of the cough itself. The cough is spasmodic and convulsive. During the spasms of cough, look for the patient's face to be flushed and for the patient to cough up a good deal of mucus and even some blood. The patient's breathing difficulties greatly increase during these bouts of coughing.

It is all but impossible to tell the difference between the first stage of this illness and a typical cold. Therefore, the remedies listed under the general category of cold are those that should be considered. Those listed here are remedies for the second stage of the illness, once the whooping has begun.

REMEDIES

ACONITE—Should be considered if the cough has a whistling sound to it. The patient has been sick with a cold for a few days, and the coughing comes on and the coughing is very dry, with the characteristic whistling sound. The patient will have hot, dry skin. He will complain of a burning sensation in his windpipe. Look for the patient to hold his throat when coughing due to the pain. Because of its nature as a very brief-acting remedy, Aconite will seldom clear the symptoms of the case, but it will bring about improvement. Another well-selected follow-up remedy will usually be needed to totally clear the case.

ANTIMONIUM TARTARTICUM—Should be considered as a remedy in cases in which the patient seems to be drowning in his own mucus. In cases in which there is a rattling in the lungs. The patient will be unable to take a deep breath without coughing. The patient will be very sleepy and very thirsty. He will be in a state of total exhaustion. Vomiting may accompany the bouts of coughing. Diarrhea may also accompany the cough.

ARNICA—Not a common remedy for this illness, but one with a clear keynote. Arnica is indicated when the patient begins to cry after he has been coughing or begins to cough after he has been crying. The patient's left cheek will be red and swollen. Look for the patient's head to be hot, but his body cold. The patient will feel bruised all over his body. It is common for the patient's nose to bleed from the coughing.

ARSENICUM—A remedy suggested by suffocative fits of coughing. The cough is dry in nature. The patient will stop urinating, or urinate very little, during the illness. Look for the patient's complexion to take on a waxy and pale tone. The skin will feel cool. The patient feels completely exhausted in his illness. He is chilly as well and will want to be covered up and to be in a warm room. The patient will be worse at night, especially after midnight.

BELLADONNA—Should be considered if the patient cannot bear light, noise, or any sort of motion. The patient will complain of a throbbing or congestive headache that accompanies the cough. A nosebleed commonly accompanies the cough. The patient will be burning up with fever. He will be very thirsty. He will be exhausted by his illness, and yet will be thrashing about. He will often be delirious with his fever. (Bryonia often follows Belladonna in whooping cough.)

BRYONIA—The remedy picture will be similar to Belladonna, although the fever stage of the illness may have passed. The keynote of the remedy is present here: the patient will be much worse from any form of motion, even the motion necessary to coughing itself will cause great discomfort. The patient will feel as if he is suffocating from his coughing fits. The patient is likely to cough much more in the evening and at night. He will cough up brownish-colored mucus. The fits of coughing are likely to come on after the patient eats and drinks. The coughing may induce the patient to vomit all that he has eaten. Look for the patient's lips to be dry and cracked.

CARBO VEG—A major remedy for those with whooping cough, at both the first and second stage. Carbo Veg works best if it is given just as the patient's cough first takes on the whooping sound. The patient will complain of a terrible sore throat that is worse when he swallows. He will, in general, be worse in the evening. He will also be worse during damp or cold weather, or upon becoming cold or wet—similar to Dulcamara. Look for the patient to complain of pain shooting into his head and chest whenever he coughs.

CHAMOMILLA—Indicated when all of the usual symptoms common to the remedy are in place. Look for the patient to have one cheek that is red and hot, the other cold and pale. Look for the patient to demand to be carried all through the illness. The patient will be angry in his pain and may even strike out in anger. The patient will have a warm sweat on his head. Diarrhea, smelling of rotten eggs, may accompany the cough.

CINA—For cases of whooping cough that also exhibit the characteristic symptoms of worms. Look for the patient to pick his nose and to complain of itching of the anus and pains in his abdomen. Keynote of the remedy is that the patient will becomes stiff during bouts of coughing. The entire body will become rigid. After the coughing and the stiffness have ended, expect to hear a gurgling sound that descends from the patient's throat to his stomach. The patient may cough up mucus, blood, or both. The cough will be aggravated by any motion, especially by laughing or talking.

DROSERA—A good general remedy for whooping cough. Consider this remedy when there is actually a whooping sound to the patient's cough. Look for violent fits of coughing, fits that wrack the patient's entire body. The patient may or may not have fever, but look for a hot perspiration to cover his body at night. The patient may alternate between heat and chill but will be thirsty during the stage of heat. He may vomit up whatever he eats. The patient will feel better from motion. He will want to keep moving around.

DULCAMARA—Indicated for whooping cough that is characterized by a loose, moist cough. Look for the patient to cough up a good amount of mucus that is thin and clear. The remedy is especially indicated by a case of whooping cough that has been brought on by exposure to cold and damp. It is also indicated in cases of the illness that occur in the autumn or spring, at the times of year in which we have warm days and cold nights.

IPECAC—Indicated in cases of whooping cough in which the patient becomes stiff as a board during fits of coughing. It is also keynote of the remedy that the patient will become blue in the face from coughing. The patient's chest will sound as if it is filled with mucus, and yet none is coughed up. The cough will bring on a gagging reflex. The patient may vomit from coughing.

MERCURIUS—The first remedy to consider if the patient coughs up blood. The patient may also bleed from the nose during fits of coughing. The patient will be worse at night. The patient will cough all night and not at all during the day, or cough all day and not at all during the night. This remedy is especially indicated if the patient has two bouts of coughing and a period of perfect rest and calm before the onset of two more closely linked bouts of coughing. Look for night sweats when the patient is sleeping.

PHOSPHORUS—An excellent remedy for whooping cough, especially if the first stage of the illness appears to be a simple cold that moves very quickly to the throat and chest, all but bypassing the nose. The patient will complain of burning pains in the throat and chest. He may have to hold his throat when he coughs in order to control the pain. The patient will be very thirsty for cold drinks, but may vomit those up just as soon as they become warm in the stomach. The patient will be worse at twilight, worse if left alone.

PULSATILLA—Indicated in cases in which there is a great deal of mucus being coughed up from the first onset of coughing. The patient will also vomit mucus, food, or both. Diarrhea may accompany the coughing, especially at night. The patient will feel chilly, even in a warm room, and yet may also feel that he cannot breathe in a warm room. Although chilly, he may feel better outside. The patient may also have vertigo upon rising.

VERATRUM—Indicated in cases of whooping cough in which the patient is greatly weakened by his condition. The patient's pulse will be very quick, but weak. He will have a low fever that is constant. The patient will have a cold sweat on his face. He will be unable to lift his head. The patient will not want to move or speak. He will no longer seem to care whether he gets better or not. The whole body may be covered in a red, prickly rash. (Veratrum follows Drosera well in whooping cough.)

COMMON AILMENTS
Bronchitis

This inflammation of the lining membrane of the bronchial tubes can be an offshoot of a cold or flu and can be acute or chronic.

In acute bronchitis, the illness is characterized by chilliness, hoarseness, tickling in the windpipe, difficulty in breathing, frequent cough, expectoration that begins with scanty mucus and grows to a copious flow that may be blood-streaked. As the illness worsens, breathing difficulty increases, along with a sensation of tightness in the chest. The cough becomes painful. Breathing has a rattling or wheezing sound. The body may become covered in a cold and clammy sweat. Both young children and the elderly have a tendency to acute bronchitis.

In its chronic state, bronchitis represents an ongoing weakness of the system. Every cold or other inflammation can bring a return of the disease. As the chronic condition worsens, hoarseness of the voice can become permanent, as can the cough and the difficulty in breathing.

REMEDIES

ACONITE—Only of use in acute attacks. Look for the patient to experience chill with fever, to have dry, hot skin. The patient is very restless. He will suffer from a short, dry cough, with constant irritation in the larynx. The patient will be filled with great fear and anxiety. The patient is nervous and afraid that he will die. Aconite is especially suggested by illness that comes on after exposure to cold, dry winds.

ANTIMONIUM TARTARICUM—Consider this remedy for the condition of a large mass of mucus in the bronchia. The patient can breathe only with the greatest difficulty. Patient seems to be drowning in his own mucus. When the patient coughs, it seems as if much would be expectorated, but nothing comes up. Look for the patient to exhibit both nausea and vomiting, with much mucus being vomited up. The patient will complain that his chest feels heavy. The patient is exhausted.

APIS—Consider this remedy when the patient's chest is sore and feels stung and/or bruised. The patient will have a tendency to cough, especially after lying down or sleeping. A clear, stringy phlegm arises from the patient's throat. Look for frequent hawking.

ARSENICUM—For the patient with a dry, hacking cough. With soreness in the chest, which feels raw. Also look for the patient to exhibit moist cough, difficult breathing, and blood-streaked expectoration. The patient must sit up to breathe. He will have a great thirst but will drink only a little at a time. The patient's behavior combines restlessness and exhaustion. He has a deep fear of death, and is worse when alone. Consider this remedy especially in cases of bronchitis in the elderly.

BELLADONNA—Face is flushed and the eyes are red. The patient's head feels pressurized. He will complain of a throbbing headache, as if his head would split. Look for the characteristic hot skin, which will tend to be sweaty. Look for the patient to exhibit a spasmodic cough. Cough is so constant that it does not leave time to breathe. Patient may cry after every coughing spell. The patient is very sleepy but cannot sleep. Patient jumps during sleep.

BRYONIA—For when the patient's breathing is difficult and shallow. The patient must sit up to breathe but does not want to move. He lies there trying to breathe without moving. His chest feels tight. The patient complains of a dry cough with stitching pains in the chest. There is a violent cough in the morning, with expectoration of a large amount of mucus. When coughing, patient feels as if his head and chest would fly to pieces.

CARBO VEG—Bronchitis with obstinate hoarseness, particularly in the evening. Severe burning in the chest, as if packed with hot coals. Look for the patient to exhibit a violent cough, with a characteristic discharge of yellow pus. The patient complains of stitching pains between the shoulders. Patient cannot breathe, craves air, wants to be fanned in order to breathe.

CAUSTICUM—Consider this remedy if the patient's throat is rough or hoarse. Especially in the morning. Look for the patient to exhibit a short, hacking cough, with roughness in the throat. Patient feels pain over the hip when coughing. Involuntary emission of urine from coughing. The cough worse in morning. Look for a loss of voice, especially in the morning.

CHAMOMILLA—Hoarseness and cough, with rattling of mucus in the trachea. The place from which the mucus was removed feels painful. The patient has a scraping cough, with tickling in larynx, which is worse at night, and especially worse during sleep. One cheek of the patient's face is red, the other pale. Patient is very impatient, irritable, rude.

HEPAR SULPH—Dry cough, with roughness in the throat. Rattling, choking cough that is worse after midnight. Look for the patient to be hoarse, and to wheeze when breathing. The patient will feel that there is a danger of suffocation when he is lying down. Consider this remedy especially in cases of acute bronchitis that come on from exposure to cold dry wind. The patient's throat feels as if a stick were caught in it.

IPECAC—Consider this remedy for cases involving the rattling of mucus in the bronchial tubes. The patient has bouts of suffocating cough. He has great difficulty breathing. The chest is full of phlegm. But coughing does not bring up mucus. Look for the patient to exhibit much nausea and vomiting with the cough. Patient vomits mucus.

KALI BI—Helpful in cases involving burning pains in the trachea and the bronchia. The patient will exhibit cough, with expectoration of green stringy mass. The keynote to the use of this remedy is the quality of the mucus itself; it must be ropy or stringy and green and firm or hard.

LACHESIS—Consider when the patient's voice is hoarse and feeble. And yet, he will want to keep on talking. The patient will complain of a sensation of constriction of the throat. He will exhibit a short, hacking cough, caused by a tingling in the throat. Look for difficult expectoration of yellow mucus. The patient's throat is painful when touched, and the patient can bear nothing around the throat. Pressure on throat brings on violent coughing. Patient is worse for sleeping and in the afternoon.

MERCURIUS—For a sore throat with violent cough, particularly at night. Look for the patient to feel as if his head and chest would burst. Patient feels hot, then cold, then hot again. The cough typically is worse from lying on the right side. Look for swollen glands—glands swollen throughout the body. The patient exhibits much sweat, which brings no relief.

NUX—Consider this remedy when the patient's larynx feels rough, scraped. The rough throat causes coughing, causes the patient to try to clear his throat. He will repeatedly, constantly, try to clear his throat. Look for a dry cough, from midnight until sunrise. Cough with head-ache, as if there were a nail being driven into the skull. The patient's nose is stopped up. Look for fever in a chilly patient. Patient feels cold with the slightest movement of air. He is worse at 4 A.M. Consider this remedy for cases of bronchitis accompanied by constipation. Bronchitis in those who use too much allopathic medicine, especially cold medicines.

PHOSPHORUS—For cases of bronchitis that involve a total loss of voice. The patient cannot talk because larynx is too painful. He will complain of tightness in the chest. Cough, with expectoration of pale red or rust-colored mucus. The cough is severe and exhausting. The patient dreads the cough and trying not to cough. He may hold his throat to keep from coughing. The patient will complain of a sensation of weakness in the abdomen. The cough is worse when the patient is lying on the left side.

PULSATILLA—For bronchitis with dryness in the patient's throat. Look for the patient to exhibit a dry cough at night that is worse when the patient is sitting up in bed. The patient exhibits a loose cough, with expectoration of yellow mucus. The patient will be chilly, even in a warm room. He will have hot, dry skin. The patient has no thirst, even during fever. Patient is tearful.

RHUS TOX—For a cough brought on by a sensation of tickling under the breast bone. The cough is worse from laughing or from talking. The cough will be accompanied by rheumatic pains in the bones that are worse when the patient is at rest, and better from gentle motion. The patient is worse at night, especially after midnight.

SPONGIA—Consider this remedy for cases involving a dry larynx, with a hoarse, hollow, wheezing cough. The cough is worse at night. Cough that sounds like sawing wood. The patient's voice gives out midsentence.

SULPHUR—Consider this remedy for cases of hoarseness and loss of voice. The patient will complain of a sensation as if there were something crawling through the inside of the throat. The patient has a loose cough, with expectoration of thick mucus. Look for him to complain of soreness in the chest. He will exhibit stitches in chest that extend to the back. The patient will especially complain of pain in the left side. Look for frequent fainting spells. Also for a constant rattling in the chest. This is the single best remedy for chronic cases of bronchitis.

VERATRUM ALBUM—Consider this remedy for the patient who exhibits a dry, hollow cough, as if it came up from the lower part of the chest or from the abdomen. Look for a rattling of mucus in the chest that cannot be coughed free. The cough may be accompanied by vomiting, diarrhea, and great exhaustion. The patient's face will be covered with a cold sweat.

COMMON AILMENTS
Pneumonia

Pneumonia is, of course, a rather serious condition—one that is beyond the scope of simple home treatment. It is an inflammation of the lungs that usually begins with chills, which are soon followed by a high fever.

The patient's pulse will be very quick and full. The patient typically will have trouble breathing and will complain of a sticking pain in the chest. Cough will usually be a central issue in the case, and the patient will usually try to avoid coughing because of the pain it causes. The cough is usually dry at first, later becoming loose. The patient will usually cough up large amounts of mucus. Over time, this expectoration will usually take on a red or rusty color and may be blood-streaked. Other indications of pneumonia are rapid and shallow breathing, headache, thirst, and general restlessness.

The first sign of recovery from pneumonia is usually to be found in the skin. When the patient's skin begins to assume a natural moisture and temperature, things are moving in the right direction. By the time the patient begins to cough up large amounts of mucus, the danger is usually past.

Pneumonia is especially serious in the young and the old, but it is a condition that should be treated by a professional practioner. The remedies listed here should be used as a stopgap until a visit to a medical professional can be arranged.

REMEDIES

ACONITE—This remedy is very helpful in the beginning stages of pneumonia. The symptoms are the usual portrait of the remedy. The patient is restless and fearful, and cannot be calmed or comforted. The patient will be particularly afraid that he will die. The patient will exhibit a high fever; his face will be red, hot, and dry. Look for a full and bounding pulse. The patient will feel shortness of breath. He will be very, very thirsty, especially during fever. The patient complains of a sticking pain in his chest. Vertigo will accompany the illness; the patient will become dizzy if he attempts to sit up in bed.

ANTIMONIUM TARTARTICUM—Suggested in cases in which the patient seems to be drowning, in which there is a rattling sound in the patient's chest. The patient will exhibit short, difficult, and oppressed breathing. His lungs seem to be filled with mucus; it rattles in his chest, but none is brought up by coughing. The cough will be loose in nature, however. The patient will say that his lungs feel paralyzed. The patient will say that it feels as if the inside of his chest were lined in velvet. The patient will also have a great deal of nausea. He may vomit, or strain to vomit, in order to bring up mucus.

ARSENICUM—This is a remedy suggested by a patient who is both restless and exhausted. These are chilly patients who will want to be warmed, want to be in a warm place. They will crave warm drinks, which they will sip a little at a time. They will complain of burning pains in the chest and of a sensation of heat in the chest. Their skin will be clammy. Their arms and legs, and especially their feet, will be very cold. The patient will be worse at night, especially after midnight. This remedy is particularly called for in elderly patients and in those whose vital force is depleted by their illness.

BELLADONNA—For cases of pneumonia that include a congestion of the head and a throbbing headache. The patient will have a wild look in his eyes; he will be frantic in his pain. He may be delirious in his high fever. The patient may try to escape or may physically strike the person attending him. His face will be bright or dark red and very, very hot. The patient will exhibit a high fever that is sudden in its onset and leaves suddenly as well. The patient expectorates mucus that is blood-streaked. He is very thirsty. Look for the patient to have a cracked tongue and lips. The patient is very sleepy, yet cannot sleep. He starts suddenly in his sleep. The patient is worse at 3 P.M.

BRYONIA—Here the patient has a fever that is less violent than in other remedy pictures. A moderate fever. The patient has a cough and expectorates a mucus that is reddish or brownish in color. The patient will complain of shooting or stitching pains in his sides or chest. The patient's pain is worse from any motion, even from the motion of coughing. Even the motion involved in breathing increases the pain. The patient breathes in a shallow manner. The patient will say that he feels as if his lungs would not expand if he were to try to take a deep breath. The patient will be constipated and will pass stools that are hard and dry, as if they were burnt.

CARBO VEG—Considered a remedy for the later stages of pneumonia. The patient is completely exhausted. He is very weak. He will especially complain of a sensation of weakness in his chest. The patient will experience coughing fits, during which he will cough up mucus that is brownish in color. His face will be very pale. His pulse will be very weak. The patient's extremities will be cold. He will feel that he cannot breathe and will want to be fanned. He will have an easier time breathing cold air.

CHINA—This remedy is especially indicated in cases of pneumonia in which the patient has lost a good deal of blood or other body fluids. It can also be indicated in cases in which the patient has received a blow or other mechanical injury, such as a fall. Whatever the cause, the patient will complain of pressure in his chest. He will feel stitching pains in his sides. The patient will also complain of heart palpitations that come on after fits of coughing. In severe cases, the patient may experience palpitations from trying to breathe. Look for the patient to have a tongue that is coated yellow. Look for him to have a quick pulse. The China patient has a vital force that is depleted. He is all but defeated by his illness.

LYCOPODIUM—Suggested especially in patients who are given to chronic conditions of the lungs. Look for the patient to cough up a mixture of mucus and pus. Look for the patient to have cheeks that are red in bright circles as if makeup had been applied. The patient will have trouble breathing. Fanlike motions of the nose as the patient attempts to breathe are characteristic of the remedy type. The patient will be fearful, will not want to be alone, and yet will be too weak to have others near. He will be comforted by the sounds of others moving through the home. The patient will be much worse between 4 and 8 P.M.

MERCURIUS—Usually characterized by a pain that moves through the chest from back to front. The patient will say that they he has a stitching pain that begins in the back under the shoulder blade and moves through from back to front. The patient will have trouble breathing. His cough will begin dry, but become loose. The patient will cough up bloody mucus. There will be great tenderness in the area of the patient's liver. The patient will be worse at night. He will be covered with sweat, especially at night, which offers no relief.

PHOSPHORUS—One of our most important remedies in pneumonia. Think of Phosphorus for violent cases of pneumonia, for cases in which the patient feels as if his chest were too small, as if it were constricted. Stitching pains in the patient's chest will be greatly aggravated by coughing or even by breathing. The patient will have to hold himself when he coughs to help control the pain. He may hold his throat or press against his chest or back. The patient's cough will be dry. He will ultimately cough up or choke up mucus that is rusty-colored. Pneumonia that resonds to Phosphorus usually involves a large part of the lung, which makes the patient very weak. He will want to sleep a good deal of the time. He will be very thirsty for cold things, but these cold liquids may make the patient nauseous, or even cause him to vomit, when they are warmed in the patient's stomach. The patient will be worse at sunset.

RHUS TOX—Suggested in cases of pneumonia in which the patient is very restless, especially late in the evening. The patient will feel that he has to keep moving in order to be comfortable and in order to breathe. The patient may be delirious and may thrash about. The patient will exhibit a terrible cough that seems as if it would tear something from the patient's chest. The patient will be better from heat, and much worse from becoming cold or wet or during damp, cold weather.

SULPHUR—Consider this remedy particularly in cases in which the pneumonia tends to recur. In which the patient seems to be getting better, only to get worse again. The patient will feel as if the lungs were paralyzed. He will experience fainting spells and periods of great weakness. Worse in the late morning, usually around 11 A.M., at which time the patient will feel dizzy and weak. He will also, from time to time, experience flashes of heat throughout his body, and especially in his chest. He will also feel heat in his head, especially at the top of his head. The patient will have a coughing fit if he tries to breathe too deeply. Look for the patient to feel that he must have open air in order to breathe. He will open doors and windows in order to breathe.

ALSO CONSIDER

PHOSPHORIC ACID—The remedy to keep in mind as often being the final remedy needed in the treatment of pneumonia. The remedy is indicated if, after the danger of pneumonia has passed, the patient remains totally exhausted. This exhaustion will be accompanied by diarrhea. A dose or two of Phosphoric Acid will often bring the patient back to full health.

COMMON AILMENTS
Croup

If you are a parent who has experienced croup, you already know that most of the time it seems so much worse than it really is. Your child seems so sick and you feel so helpless. Actually, it is often pretty easy to deal with homeopathically.

Croup is the inflammation of the mucous membrane that lines the larynx and windpipe. By far the most common type of croup is classically called "false" croup. Here the symptoms come on suddenly, usually in the middle of the night, after your apparently healthy child has gone to sleep. A few hours later, the whole house is awakened by the child's noisy breathing—wheezing, mostly—and dry, loud cough. It sounds worse than it is.

What is dangerous is the "true" croup, which can come on as a common cold—far more slowly than in "false" croup. Here, the cold just seems to get worse. In a matter of hours, the pulse accelerates, the skin grows very hot, and the child begins to have trouble breathing. The cough is dry, hoarse, and croupy-sounding. As the child becomes more ill, the cough gets shrill. Symptoms are worse through the night but better in the morning. The danger here is of exhaustion and suffocation, as the symptoms get better and worse but do not pass. This is definitely a case for a medical professional and not for someone playing "guess the remedy."

REMEDIES

ACONITE—Should be considered as the most important remedy for the first stage of croup. The patient will have a high fever. Look for his skin to be dry, hot, and red. The patient will have great emotional and physical restlessness. Look for the child to cry over the pain of the sore throat. Look for the patient to exhibit loud breathing while exhaling. Yet he is quiet while breathing in. Each exhalation ends with a hoarse, hacking cough.

ANTIMONIUM TARTARTICUM—For advanced stages of croup. Consider this remedy when the patient's breathing threatens to stop altogether. When the breathing sounds as if it is clogged by mucus, but none can be coughed up. When it seem as if patient is drowning. The patient's respiration will be shrill, hoarse, short, and whistling. The patient's chest expands with great difficulty. The head is thrown back in order for the patient to breathe. Look for the patient's forehead to be covered with a cold sweat. The whole body may be covered with sweat.

BELLADONNA—This is a remedy to think of for cases of croup that come on suddenly, and in which the pains leave just as suddenly. A great heat of the head—a high fever with red face—is typical here. The patient's eyes are also very red. The area of the larynx is very sore and when throat is touched, the child feels as if he will suffocate. Look for a bright red throat internally. Look for a dry, barking cough. Look for a spasmodic cough. The child can only breathe in short, shallow breaths. The child is very sleepy but cannot sleep.

CALCAREA—Croup in a child with a pale flabby body. The patient's scalp is very sweaty. On breathing in, the child makes noises that are hoarse, loud, and difficult. Child cries out in pain. Consider this remedy in cases of croup in which the child is exhausted and yet is worse after sleeping. This is also an important remedy to consider in cases in which croup chronically occurs again and again.

CHAMOMILLA—Look for a good deal of mucus here, especially in the windpipe. Look for the patient to have a dry short cough, especially at night. This cough will be present even while the child is sleeping. The child will be very angry and will want to be carried all the time. The child will scream and react violently any time he is put down. Look for one red cheek, with the other cheek pale—that is keynote of the remedy.

HEPAR SULPH—Consider this remedy in cases in which the patient exhibits a loose, rattling, and choking cough, and for cases in which the patient's air passages seem to be clogged with mucus. Look for the child to exhibit violent fits of coughing that make him suffocate or vomit. The child cannot bear to be uncovered, coughs wildly if any part of the body is uncovered. Profuse sweat and great drowsiness are common.

KALI BI—Remedy for "true" croup. The disease comes on gradually, at first with just a cold, then there is a loud hoarse cough as well. As the disease progresses, the difficulty of breathing increases, and the air traveling through the trachea sounds as if it were passing through a metallic tube. Tonsils and larynx are red and swollen. The child's throat looks as if it were covered in a newly grown membrane. Look for the child's head to be inclined backward to aid breathing, with violent wheezing and rattling in the trachea.

LACHESIS—Consider this remedy for advanced cases in which it seems the lungs will become paralyzed. The patient's larynx is very painful. The child cannot bear for the throat to be touched. Look for a suffocating cough. Child is worse for sleeping, tosses and moans in sleep. The child will also have trouble swallowing liquids but will have a much easier time swallowing solid food.

PHOSPHORUS—Consider this remedy first when the child's voice is too hoarse for him to speak. When it is simply too painful to talk. The child's whole body trembles from the cough. The patient's chest is constricted. The patient may complain of the sensation of an iron bar drawn tight across the chest. Look for shortness of breath, although the breath has a normal sound to it. This is a good remedy for children who are chronically given to croup. It may also be used to follow and complete the actions of other remedies when croup has a tendency to reappear.

SPONGIA—For simple "false" croup. This is one of our most important general cough remedies. The patient's cough has a crowing, barking, or wheezing sound to it. His respiration is slow, loud, or wheezing. Often it can even sound as if the patient is sawing wood. The patient will also be prone to fits of suffocation. The patient can only breathe when the head is bent backward. The patient's cough, which is dry in nature, is made worse by the action of breathing.

COMMON AILMENTS
Inflammations of the Eye

This is a general category that relates to any form of inflammation or infection of the eye or any of its parts. Characteristic symptoms include: pain, redness in the eyeball or in some other part, sensitivity to light, and a general sense of irritation. This inflammation may also be accompanied by headache.

The following are the remedies that most often speak to a general irritation or inflammation of the eye. In the sections that follow, remedies for more specific eye conditions are listed. It should be noted as well that today several companies have produced eyedrops containing homeopathic remedies. While I am in no way a fan of combination remedies in general, I do want to suggest that these drops, used acutely, can be of wonderful help when a patient is in crisis. And these drops can be an excellent topical alternative in the treatment of acute inflammations.

REMEDIES

ACONITE—For conditions of the eye that are accompanied by fever, in which the skin is red, hot, and dry. For conditions that come on suddenly. The patient will be nearly frantic in his pain. He will not be able to be comforted or calmed. He walks the floor in pain. Look for the patient to have a full and quick pulse. Look for the affected areas to be red, hot, and swollen. Look for the patient to complain of throbbing pains, and for his cheeks to be flushed. The affected eye will have aching pains, and the pains will be worse from any motion of the eye. Look for a copious flow of tears from the eye, but the patient will say that the eye feels dry and irritated. The patient will not be able to bear any form of light. The patient will likely be very thirsty.

APIS—For any condition in which the eyelids are swollen and inflamed.

Look for the eyelids to be so swollen that they are turned inside out. The patient will complain of a stinging pain, as if the eye had been stung by a bee. The white of the eye will be red, swollen, and shiny. Look for the eye to tear easily and often. Discharges from the eye will tend to be watery. The eye will feel better from cold applications. The patient will also be better from cold things, cold drinks especially.

ARNICA—Should be considered for any case of irritation to the eye that is brought on by mechanical injury. The patient will complain that his eye is sore, that it feels bruised. For more information on conditions brought on by mechanical injury, turn to the section of this guide called "Injuries to the Eye," which is listed under "Wounds."

BELLADONNA—Strongly indicated in situations in which the white of the eye is very red and inflamed, and the patient is completely intolerant of light. (This is the leading remedy for snow blindness.) The patient will also be very sensitive to noise. He will be in a state of nervous exhaustion. Look for either a copious flow of tears or for the eye to be completely dry. The eye will ache deep inside and the entire area around the eye will ache as well. The pain will be throbbing in nature. The pain will be increased by any motion of the eye. A violent headache may accompany the eye pain. The headache will be throbbing and congestive in nature. The patient may complain that he sees either black spots or sparks of color before his eyes. (Belladonna follows Aconite for almost any inflammation of the eye. It also works well both before and after Mercurius or Hepar Sulph.)

BRYONIA—Should be considered for long-lasting redness of the eyes. The patient's eyelids will be swollen, and the patient will complain that he has pain in his eyes any time the eyes are opened. The patient will want to lie very still and very quietly with eyes closed. The patient will want to be left alone and will become very angry if he feels that he is being bothered. The pain will be worse in the night. (Bryonia follows Pulsatilla well in inflammations of the eye.)

CALCAREA—Should be considered in cases that involve swelling and redness of the eyelids. When the eyes are glued together every night. The patient will complain of stinging pains. These pains will be made much worse by any form of light, especially firelight. Even the light of a candle will cause the patient much pain. This is a remedy to consider in cases of chronic inflammation of the eyes. In which the patient wants to spend all his time indoors in darkness. And especially in cases of inflammation in which the glands are also swollen.

EUPHRASIA—The keynote feature of this remedy is the copious flow of tears from the eyes. The eyes water all the time. The patient will complain of a pain, not only in the eyes, but extending upward into the forehead. The pain will be pressing in nature. The pain will be worse in the morning. The patient will also likely exhibit a cough. The cough will be loose in nature. Look for the patient's nose to run as much as his eyes. The flow from the nose is bland. (Eupharasia follows Belladonna well in inflammations of the eye. It is also the first remedy to consider if Belladonna fails to work.)

IGNATIA—Should be considered for the patient who complains of pressure pains in his eyes. The eyes will not be very red, or very inflamed, but the patient will still be very sensitive to light. Look for a copious discharge from the eye to be matched by a copious nasal discharge. The patient's pain will be worse in the afternoon and in the evening. Look for the patient to be very emotional, to be very moody. To weep easily.

LYCOPODIUM—Should be considered in inflammations that begin in the right eye and move to the left. Especially if the patient complains of a sensation of sand in the eyes. And if a sediment like sand is also present in the patient's urine. Consider this remedy in cases of eye inflammation in patients, especially in children, who are given to many colds and upper respiratory ailments of all sort. Consider also in cases in which the inflammation is accompanied by constipation and intestional gas. The patient's abdomen will be bloated and swollen with gas. The patient will be worse from 4 until 8 P.M.

MERCURIUS—Suggested by any violent inflammation and/or redness of the eyes. The patient will complain of cutting pains in the eyes, and of the sensation of glass in the eyes. He will be very sensitive to light and to temperature. The patient will become too hot and too cold in alternation, will have very little tolerance for changes in temperature. Consider this remedy if pustules form in the eye or on the lids or in the margin of the lids. Consider the remedy also if the regular symptom portrait is present: night sweats, which do not improve the patient's state; swollen glands; an increase in the flow of saliva; and terrible breath coming out of the patient's mouth.

NUX—Should be considered when eyes are bloodshot. This is the first remedy to think of in cases of bloodshot eyes. The patient will say that he feels as if his eyes were filled with sand or glass. The corners of the eyelids will be very red and itchy. The patient's eyes will water a good deal and these tears will irritate the eyes. The eyes will also itch. The eye pain will be accompanied by a stuffed-up nose. The patient will dread the light of the morning on first opening his eyes. An early morning headache is also very common, as is a coated tongue.

PULSATILLA—A very effective remedy for many different types of inflammation. The patient may complain of burning, cutting, or tearing pains in his eyes. These pains will be worse if the patient is in a warm, closed room. He will feel better in open air, even if he is chilly—even in that warm room he will usually be chilly. The patient's eyes will be very sensitive to light. This is a good remedy to remember in chronic inflammations of the eyes, especially for inflammations that lead to discharges from the eyes that are yellow-green in color. And in cases that involve itching of the eyes more than anything else. The eyes will look puffy and swollen. The pain will be worse in the afternoon and in the evening. The patient will want a great deal of attention and likely will be weepy and clingy.

SPIGELIA—Consider this remedy when the patient's eyes feel achy. When the patient complains of a pain that is boring in nature. That bores deep into the eye. The patient will say that his eye feels too large for his head. The pain that the patient experiences will return at the same time every day. This pain may be utterly unbearable.

SULPHUR—This is an excellent remedy for general inflammations of the eyes, especially those that appear and reappear from time to time. Consider this strongly for any inflammations that occur after any suppression of a rash or any other skin condition by allopathic drugs. Consider this remedy for any inflammation that might be the result of allopathic suppression of any sort. The picture matches the general portrait of Sulphur: these patients will experience flashes of heat in the affected part and throughout their whole body; they may be covered in a hot sweat; they will be thirsty and sluggish; they may feel faint or exhausted in their pain state. Their eyes will feel hot and burning and itchy. The itch will be increased by any form of heat or warmth and will be better in open air. The pain will be worse in the late morning, especially at 11 A.M.

COMMON AILMENTS
Conjunctivitis

Conjunctivitis is an inflammation specific to the conjunctiva, the thin transparent lining that covers the surface of the eye and the inside of the eyelids. This inflammation can be caused by an infection or by an allergic reaction, although conjunctivitis is most common during the time in which the patient has a cold. The patient only has to sneeze and then wipe his nose and then touch his eye to spread the virus to the eye. Because most of us have learned in adulthood—by repeated experience, if nothing else—not to rub our eyes after we blow our noses, this is for the most part an illness of childhood. We grew up calling this condition "pinkeye," and the symptoms are what you remember: red bloodshot eyes, swollen lids, yellow or green secretions from the eye, the lids glued together in the morning, and itching and irritation in the eye.

REMEDIES

ACONITE—Consider this remedy when the eye inflammation is accompanied by fever, when the patient's skin is dry and hot. Look for the eye to be intensely red and swollen. Look for the patient to complain of a good deal of acute pain. The patient's eyes will have a great intolerance to light. The patient may also complain that his eye feels dry. As is typical to this remedy, look for the patient to have a good deal of fear, anxiety, and to be both physically and emotionally restless. Look for flushed cheeks to accompany inflammation. (Pulsatilla often follows Aconite well in cases of conjunctivitis.)

APIS—Consider this remedy when the patient's eyelids are swollen. They may be so swollen that they turn inside out. The patient's eyelashes fall out. Look for the patient to complain of burning and stinging pains. The pain will be like that of a bee sting. Look for a great deal of tearing of the eyes. The patient's whole eye itself may be swollen. The eye will be bloodshot. The area of the swelling will be not only red, but shiny.

ARSENICUM—Consider this remedy for cases of inflammation of the conjunctiva with dark red color. The patient will complain of burning pains. The patient's eye literally feels as if it were on fire. Look for swelling of the eyelids. You may also find ulcers on the cornea. The patient's eyelids will be glued together every night. The patient will be in great pain and anxiety and he will be both physically and emotionally restless. The patient will not want to be alone. He will display the characteristic intense thirst of the remedy—drinks little, but often.

BELLADONNA—For the patient who displays a great intolerance to light and/or noise. The patient's eye is very red, with a discharge of hot, salt tears. Either that or there will be a great dryness of the eye. The patient's eyelids will be red and swollen. They stick together easily and may bleed when they are pulled apart. The edges of the eyelids may turn outward. Look for the patient to complain of sharp pains all around the eyes, pains that extend into the head. A feeling of congestion in the head and a throbbing headache will accompany the inflammation. Pains appear suddenly, and leave suddenly. The patient may also experience double vision.

CALCAREA—Look for swelling and redness of eyelids, which glue themselves together nightly. The patient's eye will have a red, hard swelling and a copious secretion of swelling. The patient complains of stinging pains that are worse from any form of glare. The eye pain will be worse if the patient looks at any firelight, even a candle. He will also complain of burning pains after he has been reading. The patient will have a strong desire to remain in the darkness. Glandular swellings in the neck, eruptions on the scalp. Look for ulcers on the patient's cornea.

COLOCYNTHIS—Should be considered as a remedy for cases that involve violent pains in the eyes that extend all the way back to the back of the head. The patient will complain as well of a violent pain that cuts up into his forehead. The pain will also extend down into the nose. The pain will increase if the patient stoops or is lying down on his back. Vomiting may accompany eye pain. (Colocynthis follows Aconite or Belladonna well in eye pain and inflammation.)

EUPHRASIA—Consider this remedy in cases in which the eyelids are red and swollen and the margins of the eyes are ulcerated. The patient will complain of a terrible itching of the eyes during the daytime. The pain will be worse from any sort of light. Look for a profuse flow of both tears and mucus. The patient will complain of a terrible headache, which accompanies the inflammation. The patient will also feel heat inside his head. The patient's eyelids will be glued together every morning. (Euphrasia may be followed by Nux if the patient is made worse in open air, or by Pulsatilla if the patient is better in open air.)

HEPAR SULPH—Consider this remedy when the upper lid is the one that is glued down. The upper lid is also swollen and aching. The patient will complain that the upper lid feels bruised. The lid will be very swollen and very painful if touched. The patient's eyes will be very sensitive to light. The patient's eyelids may go into spasms if the patient is exposed to light. He may also spasm every morning. (Hepar Sulph may follow Aconite, Belladonna, or Mercurius in cases of conjunctivitis.)

LYCOPODIUM—As with other remedy pictures, here, too, you will find the gluing of the eyelids at night. Also look for the burning pains in the patient's eyes. But, keynote to this remedy is that the patient will complain of a sensation as if there were sand in the eyes. This will be combined with another keynote: red sediment like sand in the urine. Constipation accompanies inflammation. The inflammation usually begins in the right eye and may spread from there to the left eye.

MERCURIUS—Consider this remedy for cases of violent inflammation and redness of the eye. The patient will complain of cutting and burning pains. The eye will have excessive sensitivity to glare, to any firelight, or to any light at all. Look for pustules to form around the eyes and on the margins of the lids. The patient will have trouble opening his eyes, not just from the fact that they are glued together, but also from the ulcers and pustules that have painfully formed. Along with this, look for other symptoms that are typical of the Mercurius type: swollen glands in the neck; a swollen tongue; and an overabundance of saliva. The patient will also be sweaty as well, and will have terrible breath.

PULSATILLA—This is the major remedy to consider for conjunctivitis that accompanies a common cold. In fact, for any eye inflammation following a common cold. Often the inflammation will spread to both eyes. Typically, the patient's eye secretions are yellow or green. The patient's eyes are glued together nightly. The patient's eyes will both burn and itch, and the patient will very much want to rub them. The itching and burning will be worse in the afternoon and evening. The itching and burning will also be worse when the patient is in a warm, closed room. This is true although the patient may be chilly, even when in a warm room. Expect the patient to be very needy. May also be weepy.

SULPHUR—This remedy is typically called for in cases involving itching and burning in the eyes and eyelids. The patient will be made worse by moving or by any exposure to light. As with Lycopodium, the patient will feel as if there were sand in the eyes. Look for specks and ulcers on the patient's cornea. The patient will also experience flashes of heat in the eyes. The patient will feel weak while he is in pain. He may experience fainting spells. Look for the patient to complain of a burning sensation on top of the head. The itching and burning will be worse at night when the patient is in bed. Think of this remedy for stubborn conjunctivitis, when it reoccurs with every cold.

COMMON AILMENTS
Styes in the Eyes

Styes are small boils that form on the eyelid. They are infections that most often form at the root of an eyelash. It certainly can be a painful event, often coupled with fever, but styes are not serious illnesses and will clear up on their own in about seven days.

REMEDIES

GRAPHITES—An excellent general remedy for styes. It is often used both topically (as Aqua Graphites, with the potentized remedy dissolved in pure water) and internally in the treatment of those with this condition. The patient's eyelids will be red and swollen. Look for dryness of the eyelids.

HEPAR SULPH—Consider this remedy when styes appear often. Also think of Hepar Sulph when styes leave hard spots behind. When there are biting and burning pains in the corners of the eye, where dry pus forms. Even in acute cases, think of this remedy when pus is present.

LYCOPODIUM—Consider this remedy for styes occurring in the right eye. The eye itself may have an internal sensation of being too large for its socket. The eyelids will typically be red and somewhat swollen. Styes commonly occur where the external lid meets the internal canthus.

MERCURIUS—The situation is similar to that of Hepar Sulph, but a more generalized infection is present, of which the stye is only a part. Look for the general indications of the remedy, with a swollen tongue, a great deal of saliva, swollen glands, and night sweats.

PULSATILLA—This remedy should be given in the early stages of the ailment, as the boil is forming. If taken early enough, the remedy will nearly always disperse the stye. Pulsatilla is especially adapted to styes on the upper lids.

STAPHYSAGRIA—Consider this remedy when the stye tends to appear again and again. Give the patient Staphysagria once or twice a week until all styes have disappeared. Often the patient will complain of extreme discomfort from the stye, far more than should be associated with the ailment.

COMMON AILMENTS
Earaches in General

This again is a general category. In it I list the remedies that most commonly relate to the broad category of earache. Earaches can have many different causes, from exposure to cold and damp weather to a buildup of wax in the ear. An earache may also be caused by a sinus infection, a throat infection, or even simple tooth pain. Or the pain may be the result of an actual infection of the ear. This infection may be of the outer ear (you can be sure of this cause by pulling on the earlobe; if this increases pain it is an outer-ear infection), or, perhaps most commonly, there may be an infection of the middle ear, which often occurs as an aftermath to a cold. The inner ear may also be the site of the infection. If this is the case, we have a more dangerous event, one that not only is extremely painful but that also might have long-range impact on the patient's health and well-being and professional treatment is required.

But an earache often occurs when there is no perceptible inflammation present. And for no obvious reason. Then we do what we always do in homeopathy—we treat the patient by matching the totality of the symptoms to the remedy that best mimics those symptoms. In the case of earache, the pain is often very severe, with a cutting, digging, burrowing, tearing, shooting, or throbbing character.

REMEDY CHECKLIST

For a sensation of sorness, consider: **Graphites, Lachesis, Mercurius**, or **Sulphur**.

For a sensation of itching, consider: **Lycopodium, Pulsatilla**, or **Sulphur**.

If the ear swells, consider: **Lycopodium, Pulsatilla, Sepia**, or **Sulphur**.

REMEDIES

ACONITE—Consider this remedy first in cases of acute earache that is caused by exposure to cold wind. When the earache comes on suddenly, especially after the patient has come into a warm house after being out in the cold, dry wind. Also consider this remedy for earaches that come on after a sudden stoppage of a chronic discharge from the ear. That the stopping of the discharge is sudden and that the discharge has been flowing for some time are both very important. Look for the other parts of the Aconite picture to be present as well. Look for the patient to be anxious, fearful, both emotionally and physically restless. A sudden high fever may accompany earache. The patient will be thirsty. He will be fearful.

Note: Aconite is the most important remedy to consider in cases in which the eardrum has burst due to infection or mechanical injury. While the eardrum will heal itself, this remedy will treat the pain and panic that accompanies the rupture.

ARNICA—An excellent remedy to consider in the treatment of the patient with earache. Consider this remedy especially in cases in which the patient's earache is worse whenever the patient is touched. He will not want to be touched and may withdraw from even the most tender touch. He may insist that nothing is wrong with him and that he wants to be left alone. Also consider if the earache is worse from noise. The patient will complain of stinging pains that are located both in and behind the ears. The patient will typically have a hot head and a cold body. He will also typically complain of a sensation of heat in the internal ear.

BELLADONNA—Consider this remedy for a sudden, throbbing earache that is made worse from warmth. The patient will complain of boring or shooting pains. The pain will be accompanied by a sensation of roaring and humming in the ears. The patient will have a great sensitivity to noise. He may also be very sensitive to light. The patient will typically complain of pain in the head and the eyes at the same time. He will have a feeling of congestion and heat in the head. A sudden, high fever may accompany the earache. Look for the skin to be red, hot, and dry.

CHAMOMILLA—This is one of our most important remedies for earaches in children. Consider this remedy for earaches that are bad enough to cause the child to scream in pain. The child will be inconsolable in his pain. He will want to be carried, and is only calm and quiet when he is being carried. In adults, this remedy should be considered in cases of severe earache, most especially when the patient is made very irritable by the pain. The patient will complain loudly about acute shooting pains, as if a knife had been thrust into the ear. Chamomilla earaches, typically, are accompanied by a cold, or are the result of suppressed perspiration. The pain typically is made worse from open air and is worse at night.

DULCAMARA—Consider this remedy if the earache pains are worse at night, especially when the patient is at rest. These earaches especially come on during autumn and spring, the seasons of the year when the days are hot and the evenings cold. The patient will be worse from every change in the weather from warm to cold. This is the first remedy to think of if the earache is accompanied by nausea.

HEPAR SULPH—Consider this remedy for a throbbing earache, which is soothed by warmth. The patient will complain of a roaring or throbbing in his ear. This remedy should especially be considered for the earache that accompanies a cold and sore throat, especially if that sore throat seems to hurt into the ear. The patient will complain that his ear hurts every time he blows his nose. Look for the glands under the patient's neck to be swollen. (Hepar Sulph often follows Belladonna in cases of earache.)

MERCURIUS—This is a major remedy for earaches that are caused by the presence of an infection. (See the next section.) If you know the Mercurius picture, you may treat with the correct remedy at the onset of the infection and save the patient a good deal of suffering. The earache begins as suppuration is imminent. The pain is intense. The patient will complain of a tearing or pricking pain. It is keynote of the remedy that this pain will extend into the cheeks. That is very important, as are the other parts of the symptom picture: look for the patient to sweat a good deal, without the sweat bringing any relief; look for the patient to be worse at night and worse during any form of damp or rainy weather. The patient's tongue will be swollen, as will the glands under the neck. Look for the patient to have foul breath and an abundance of saliva.

NUX—This is an excellent remedy to consider for earache, especially if the patient is very angry or irritable when he is in pain. The patient will be cold; he will not be able to bear the movement of any air, especially any air on his ear. The patient will complain that his ear pain moves upward into his forehead. He may also report that the pain moves into his temples. The patient may even say that the pain of the earache extends into all the bones of his face. The pain will be stinging in nature. The pain will be worse in the morning. (Nux is an excellent follow-up to Chamomilla in cases of earache.)

PULSATILLA—The patient's behavior is very helpful here. Pulsatilla is indicated as a remedy when the patient is very needy, very emotional. Especially if the patient is clingy or weepy. He will complain of a sensation of pressure behind the eardrum. Also of darting pains in the ears. He will report that his ear feels stopped up. He will report a sensation as if something were about to be pressed out of the ear. Externally, the ear feels hot, is red and swollen. The patient will be made better for rocking and for being in fresh air. This remedy is suitable to persons who are tearful in their pain, who are chilly but worse in a warm, closed room. (*Note*: As this remedy type is typically improved by motion, especially rocking motion, and by being outdoors, this is the remedy suggested when in the dead of winter you bundle your screaming baby up to rush to the doctor's office, only to find that the baby falls into a peaceful sleep during the drive. The baby is now in open air and being rocked and the pain lessens and the patient improves. A dose of Pulsatilla usually is indicated by such a case.) Pulsatilla is perhaps our single most important remedy for cases of simple earache.

SPIGELIA—Consider this remedy first when the patient complains of an earache that feel like a nail is sticking in the ear. The pain is severe and may drive the patient into a frenzy. The patient will report that the aching pain extends into the cheekbones.

COMMON AILMENTS
Ear Infections: Inflammations of the External Ear

An inflammation of the external ear can affect any area in front of the eardrum, including the external ear itself and the canal that leads into the eardrum. Certainly a condition of swelling and redness of the outer ear has much in common with the ailment mumps, and it is strongly suggested that the reader consider the remedies in that section as well.

An inflammation of the external ear will almost always involve redness and swelling of the area. There may or may not be an actual infection involved. It may be difficult at times to determine whether the inflammation has more to do with the internal or external ear. Remember to give the external ear a gentle tug. If this action greatly increases the pain, consider the remedies listed here. In acute cases, the situation pretty much narrows down to three remedies. If there is no sign of pus or any discharge, the choice is between Belladonna and Aconite. If discharge is present, then Mercurius is almost always the indicated choice. In cases in which the external ear is chronically inflamed, Graphites is the usual remedy.

REMEDIES

ACONITE—Consider this remedy for cases of acute infection in which the patient complains of sharp or shooting pains. These pains come on suddenly and the patient will be frantic in his pain. Especially for inflammations that come on after the patient has been in contact with cold, dry winds.

BELLADONNA—Consider this remedy when the ear and the face are all swollen, red, hot, and dry. The patient will be frantic, but exhausted. The swelling and heat come on quickly. A high fever may accompany the infection. The patient will be exhausted, will want to rest in a cool, dark place. The patient will be worse from light and worse from noise. This is a good remedy for any sort of general infection in the area of the external ear. Belladonna is the remedy to think of if Aconite fails in its action.)

GRAPHITES—Think of this remedy first for cases of chronic inflammation of the outer ear, especially when there is no apparent infection present. Itching will be the major symptom of the inflammation. This is the first remedy to consider when you have a patient with these chronic inflammations and the patient is slow to heal and has dirty, unhealthy-looking skin.

MERCURIUS—This is perhaps our most important remedy for this condition. Consider Mercurius in cases of external ear infection in which pus is being produced. Look especially for swelling of the glands in the patient's neck. This is always the first remedy to think of in inflammations of the ear—internal or external—in which pus has formed.

COMMON AILMENTS
Ear Infections: Inflammations of the Internal Ear

An inflammation of the internal ear affects the area behind the eardrum. This is a very painful condition that typically involves redness and swelling of both the external and the internal ear. The pain will most often be burning, stitching, beating, or itching in nature. The pain may extend deep into the ear or may spread into the bones of the face and head. The patient may also experience nausea and vomiting and coldness of the extremities.

REMEDIES

ACONITE—For cases of sudden ear pain that is usually brought on by exposure to cold air. Look for the patient to be very restless and filled with anxiety. The patient's ear will look bright red and swollen, both inside and out, and will feel hot to the touch. The inner parts of the ear will be inflamed. The patient will complain of pain that is beating in nature. Look for the patient to have a great sensitivity to noise.

BELLADONNA—Again, think of this remedy's keynote of sudden onset of pain and you have the leading indicator. Also look for the patient to have a hot face and fever that has also come on suddenly. Look for the patient to also have a great sensitivity to touch. His sense of sight and hearing will also be affected. He will not be able to bear light or sound. Look for the patient to have glazed, staring eyes. His pain will be deep-seated and throbbing in nature, as if the ear would be pushed out of the head. The patient will be exhausted and will want to rest in a cool, dark, quiet place. But he will be unable to sleep. The patient will suddenly start as if in fright just as he is drifting off to sleep.

HEPAR SULPH—The other remedy, along with Mercurius, to think of first in cases of ear inflammation in which pus is present. In this case, examination will show that the eardrum is red and swollen. Typically, there will also be a buildup of pus in the middle ear. The pus is thick and yellow-green in color. The patient may have a great deal of pain accompanying the inflammation, or he may have no pain at all. If there is pain, look for the patient to become angry with his pain. Look for the patient to feel warm, even if there is no fever present, and to crave open air. Look for the pain to be worse at night, and worse when the patient is in a warm room. The Hepar Sulph inflammation usually comes on at the end of a cold, when the patient is already fairly weak and crabby. The inflammation only exaggerates what is already in place.

LYCOPODIUM—An excellent choice for a remedy for ear inflammation and infections that occur in the right ear or in which the right ear is more painful than the left. The patient will have a good deal in common with the Chamomilla patient. He will be angry and impatient in his pain. He can be very demanding and even abusive while the pain persists. The patient will typically be afraid of the dark and afraid of being left alone, although he will not want others in the room with him. He will want to hear the sounds of the family in the other rooms of the house, but he will want to be left in peace. The pain will be worse from 4 until 8 A.M.

Lycopodium is especialy useful as a remedy in the early stages of inflammation.

MERCURIUS—This remedy is indicated if the ear pains are much worse at night and are of a beating and tearing nature. The patient will complain of a buzzing in the ears. Look for a discharge of bloody pus from the affected ear. The patient will have profuse sweating of the head, but the sweating will give no relief. The patient will have no tolerance for changes in temperature. He will become very hot and very cold easily. Look for night sweats to accompany the inflammation. Look for swollen glands in the neck and, perhaps, a swollen tongue as well. The patient will have offensive breath and will have increased salivation in his mouth.

PULSATILLA—The keynote symptom of this remedy is the presence of a pressure pain behind the patient's eardrum. This is an excellent remedy to consider in cases of inflammation of the external and internal ear. Often, the pain will be accompanied by terrible itching. Also by hardness of hearing. The patient will complain of darting pains in ear. This remedy is especially indicated in cases that also involve a discharge of pus from ears, especially after measles. The remedy is suitable to the chilly patient, especially for the patient who is chilly even in a warm room, and yet is better in open air. The Pulsatilla patient is weepy and wants to be taken care of. The pains improve when the patient is rocked.

SILICEA—An important remedy for the child who is chronically given to ear infections. This Silicea patient, like the Pulsatilla, will be rather needy and will want a great deal of attention. But the Silicea patient will not be as loving or as clingy as the Pulsatilla. These patients are indeed weepy and whimpering, but they want help with their pain, instead of just attention. This is also the child who is allergic to everything, who always seems to be underweight and sick, and who seems to have earache after earache, no matter what the parents do about it.

COMMON AILMENTS
Drainage from Ears

This is a common disease of childhood, especially as a result of chronic ear infections. This discharge is sometimes offensive and is a source of great annoyance to patients and parents alike. Often this drainage will take place after a bout of measles or a high fever.

REMEDY CHECKLIST

For drainage of bloody matter, consider: **Lachesis, Mercurius**, or **Pulsatilla**.

For drainage of mucus, consider: **Belladonna, Calcarea, Mercurius, Pulsatilla**, or **Sulphur**.

For drainage of pus, consider: **Calcarea, Hepar Sulph, Mercurius**, or **Pulsatilla**.

If the drainage is very offensive, consider: **Hepar Sulph, Lycopodium, Mercurius, Pulsatilla**, or **Sulphur**.

If the drainage occurs after measles, consider: **Pulsatilla** or **Sulphur**.

If the drainage occurs after a high fever, consider: **Belladonna, Hepar Sulph**, or **Mercurius**.

REMEDIES

ARSENICUM—For cases in which the drainage is accompanied by a burning sensation. This discharge often extremely offensive, although it tends to be thin. There will usually be a great deal of discharge. Roaring in the ears and hardness of hearing accompany discharge.

BELLADONNA—Consider this remedy especially in cases of drainage after high fevers. The drainage will usually be accompanied by a swelling of the glands in the neck, which are made sore from touch. The patient will complain of a humming and roaring in the ears, with hardness of hearing.

CALCAREA—This is especially suited to overweight patients with sluggish digestion. In children, look for delayed milestones. The remedy will speak to those with chronic discharge from the ears. This discharge is of offensive pus, mostly from the right ear. Look for the patient to have a swollen abdomen and a good appetite. The glands in the patient's neck will be swollen. The patient will likely have cold, damp feet and head sweats. Consider this remedy for pale, fair patients—especially children—with soft, flabby muscles.

HEPAR SULPH—Consider this remedy for cases of discharge of fetid pus from the ears. The patient will also complain of a whizzing and throbbing in the ears. The patient may also be hard of hearing during the discharge. This remedy is especially helpful for drainage at the end of a bad cold.

LYCOPODIUM—For cases involving purulent discharge and difficult hearing. This remedy is most called for and most suitable after a bout of high fever. Right ear has dominant symptoms. (Lycopodium often follows Belladonna or Aconite, after those remedies have cleared the initial inflammation.)

MERCURIUS—Think of this remedy first in cases involving truly offensive discharge, which is accompanied by ulceration on or behind the external ear. The patient will complain of hardness of hearing, that his ears feel obstructed. Look for splotchy eruptions on the face and/or pustules on the lower limbs.

PULSATILLA—Look for a discharge of mucus or thick pus from the ears. The pus is yellow or green in color. The discharge will be accompanied by hardness of hearing. The patient will say that his ears feel stopped up. He will complain of tearing or stitching pains in the ears. This remedy is especially suited to those who are tearful, mild persons who do not want to be alone. Pulsatilla is especially useful in cases of discharge after a bout of measles.

SILICEA—Think of this remedy first for cases of stoppage of the ears in which the ears are closed at times, open at others, with a loud crackling sound in the ears when they are open. Look for a discharge of pus from the ears and for the external ear to be swollen. Look for scabs to form behind the ear. This is an excellent remedy to keep in mind for cases of children who have chronic discharge from the ear. Especially in thin, weak, and whiny children.

SULPHUR—Think of this remedy first in cases of offensive discharge that is mostly from the left ear. Look for eruptions behind the ear at the time of discharge. The patient will complain more of itching than of pain. The affected area will bleed after the patient scratches it. This is the first remedy to consider in cases of ear discharge after the suppression of some eruptive disease or after the drying up of old sores.

COMMON AILMENTS
Deafness Following Inflammation of the Ear

Since this category strongly follows earache or the categories of inflammation and discharge, I offer a quick checklist of remedies. Refer to the listings under the previous categories of ailments of the ear. These remedies are for temporary, not possible long-term, deafness, in which case a professional must be consulted.

REMEDY CHECKLIST

For sudden deafness that lasts only for a short time, consider: **Gelsemium**.

For deafness that is accompanied by discharge from the ears, consider: **Calcarea, Mercurius, Pulsatilla**, or **Sulphur**.

For deafness that is accompanied by a congestion of the head, consider: **Belladonna, Nux, Silicea**, or **Sulphur**.

For deafness with a sensation that the ear is filled with water, consider: **Graphites** or **Sulphur**.

For deafness in which the noises in the ears are so loud that the patient cannot hear anything else, consider: **Hepar Sulph**.

For deafness in which all sounds seem to echo or vibrate, consider: **Mercurius**.

For deafness after a high fever, consider: **Belladonna** or **Hepar Sulph**.

For deafness after measles, consider: **Carbo Veg** or **Pulsatilla**.

For deafness that is caused by a buildup of earwax, consider: **Carbo Veg, Causticum, Graphites**, or **Lachesis**.

COMMON AILMENTS
Noises in the Ears

Noises such as roaring, buzzing, or ringing may accompany the earache or any inflammation or drainage of the ear, as well as any common cold. Consider the following checklist as a part of putting together the complete picture of the symptoms.

REMEDY CHECKLIST

For the patient who is, in general, sensitive to sounds, and who hears a noise in the ears, consider: **Aconite, Belladonna**, or **Sulphur**.

For a roaring in the ears, consider: **Aconite**.

For a humming in the ears, consider: **Belladonna**.

For a hissing sound in the ears, consider: **China**.

If the noise is worse in damp weather, consider: **Carbo Veg**.

If the noise is worse in dry or hot conditions, consider: **Sulphur**.

If the noise is worse in the morning, consider: **Nux**.

If the noise is worse at night, consider: **Pulsatilla**.

For noises in the ears of patients who sweat, consider: **Mercurius**.

For noises in the ears of patients who don't sweat, consider: **Chamomilla**.

COMMON AILMENTS
Measles

For the first few days, measles can look just like a cold. But come the fourth or fifth day, the eruption makes an appearance, first on the face, then on the neck, chest, and abdomen and, finally, on the extremities.

The measles look like small irregularly shaped red spots. After two more days, the measles will be at their height and will begin to disappear in the same order in which they appeared. Accompanying the rash will be swelling and inflammation of the glands in the neck, as well as weakness of the eyes and discharge from the nose and ears.

REMEDIES

ACONITE—Must be taken at the very beginning of the illness, when the skin first becomes very dry and hot. The patient will have a sudden high fever. The rash associated with measles may not have even appeared as yet. But the patient's eyes will be red, watery, and very sensitive to light. He will have a dry and hacking cough that accompanies the illness. Patient is very irritable, anxious, and restless. He will be very afraid in his illness and may even predict the hour of his death. He will not be able to relax or be comforted. The patient will be very thirsty. Look for headache and vertigo to accompany the fever.

APIS—In this remedy picture, the patient's skin is swollen and covered with hot, red eruptions. The rash will resemble bee stings—they will be red, hot and swollen. The patient will complain of a cough, and a soreness of the chest, the quality of which he will describe as feeling as if he were bruised. The patient's chest feels constricted. The patient will not be able to bear being in a warm room. He will be better from cool applications and cool drinks. His urine will be very yellow. Look for the patient to have diarrhea in the morning, with greenish yellow stool.

ARSENICUM—The rash here is accompanied by burning and dryness and itching of the skin. Eruptions appears and disappears suddenly. The patient's face is very bloated, and the lips are dry and parched. The patient has great anxiety and is very restless. The patient craves liquids, usually craves cold water, but drinks little. He is worse at midnight. The patient will be chilly and will want to be bundled up to stay warm. He will want to be in a warm room, although the patient may want to have cool air on his face if a headache has accompanied the fever.

BELLADONNA—The giveaway here is the bright red appearance of the patient's throat and tongue. The patient has difficulty swallowing. His face is red and hot, with a throbbing headache. A feeling of congestion in the head accompanies the outbreak. The patient will have a sudden high fever. His skin is bright or dark red. The patient will complain that his back feels as if it will break. Look for a dry spasmodic cough. The patient will be always drowsy, but is restless in sleep.

BRYONIA—Consider this remedy when the eruption is imperfectly developed. When the rash is very slow to appear. The patient will complain of congestion of the chest, of shooting pains that are increased by deep breathing. He will complain of a dry and painful cough. Sitting up in bed causes nausea and faintness. The patient will be very thirsty for vast amounts of water. The patient will have a headache, which is worse from coughing. As is keynote of the remedy, the patient will be made worse from any motion. Even motion of the eyes will cause the headache to worsen. The patient will be irritable and will want to be left alone. Constipation may accompany the measles.

COFFEA—Consider this remedy when the patient's skin is dry and hot at night. When the patient is very sensitive and cannot bear to be touched. The patient will be very wired, very excitable. He will be extremely wakeful. He will not even want to try to go to sleep. Look for a dry, hacking cough, with constant tickling in the patient's throat.

IPECAC—Consider this remedy if the measles are slow in making an appearance. Especially if the patient complains of a a feeling of constriction in the chest. The patient will be driven crazy by a tickling cough. Look for a rattling of phlegm in the patient's chest. The patient will display much nausea and vomiting. He will complain of a constant sense of nausea. He will be unable to eat and even the smell of food will cause nausea. The smell of tobacco will be especially troubling.

MERCURIUS—As always in this remedy picture, the glands in the patient's throat will be swollen. The patient will have great difficulty swallowing. He will complain of a sore throat and ulceration or swelling of the tonsils may accompany the measles. Look for the patient to produce profuse saliva. Especially at night. The patient's pillow will be wet from drool. The patient will have bad breath. He will experience a great sensitivity in the pit of the stomach. He will have night sweats, which will not relieve the fever. Look for the patient to experience bouts of green and slimy diarrhea.

PHOSPHORUS—Consider this remedy when the lungs are involved. The patient will complain of a tightness in his chest. Look for a violent exhausting cough, which produces rust-colored expectoration. The patient will complain of sticking pains in his chest, which are aggravated by talking, coughing, or breathing. Look for the patient to experience hoarseness, with loss of voice. The patient will be very thirsty for cold liquids, which once warmed by the stomach may be vomited up.

PULSATILLA—Useful when illness is still at the stage of a cold. In fact, Pulsatilla is useful before, during, and after a bout of measles. It is perhaps our most important remedy for this condition. Look for the patient's eyes to be red, watery, and sensitive to light. Look for a thick yellow or yellow-green discharge from the nose. The patient's mouth will be very dry. And yet, the patient will be thirstless, even during a fever. The measles rash will be slow to appear. Look for the patient to have a loose cough, which brings up more thick yellow mucus. Look for the patient to have nightly diarrhea, in which no two stools are alike. The patient craves cool air, although he will be chilly, even in a warm room.

SULPHUR—A useful remedy once the rash has appeared. The rash is slow in forming. The patient is irritable. Look for the patient to have a high temperature. For the patient to be both hot and sweaty. The patient will complain of a sensation of heat on the top of his head. The patient will be very thirsty for cold liquids and will drink a good deal. Look for the patient to have a dry, hacking cough. The rash itself will be bright red or purple in color.

COMMON AILMENTS
Mumps

Mumps is an inflammation of the parotid or large salivary glands, which are located under the lower jaw. In the early stages of the illness, the patient feels sluggish and low-spirited and complains of pains in the limbs, loss of appetite, chills, fever, and headache. Within a few days, one or both glands will begin to swell, becoming both hard to the touch and painful. The swelling will increase for four or five days, and then will begin to disappear. Sometimes the whole neck will be involved, and in that case, there is great difficulty in moving the jaw to chew or swallow food.

REMEDIES

ACONITE—Only an effective remedy if it used in the very early part of the illness. Likely before the diagnosis of mumps can be made. A high fever begins suddenly. And suddenly the patient is very sick. The patient is chilly, anxious, fearful. He is very thirsty in his fever stage. Patient is very restless. He will not be able to rest or be comforted.

BELLADONNA—Look for bright or dark redness of face and eyes as your indicator. Also look for bright red swelling of the patient's glands, especially on the right side. Expect the sudden disappearance of the swelling as well. All the patient's aches and pains are accompanied by a throbbing headache and a sense of congestion in the head. He may experience delirium during fever. He may complain of seeing sparks of light in front of his eyes. The patient will be very sensitive to noise and light. He will want to rest in a dark, cool place. He will be very sleepy, but he cannot sleep.

CARBO VEG—Consider this remedy when the fever is slow to come on and slow to build. The keynote symptom is that the swollen glands become very hard and swelling lasts a very long time. Too long a time. And then the illness moves from the glands to the stomach, where the patient experiences a burning pressure. He also complains of a sensitivity in the throat. Even simple foods disagree. The patient experiences much belching of sour and rancid food. He will feel as if he cannot breathe. He will want moving air to help him breathe.

MERCURIUS—Here the disease begins as a cold and then builds to a fever. In the fever stage, heat alternates with chills. The patient will be very sensitive to changes in temperature and always seems to be either too hot or too cold. During the heat stage, look for the patient's body to be covered in sweat, which does not relieve his symptoms. Look for a hard swelling of the glands in the neck, with stiffness in the jaw and difficulty swallowing. The patient produces profuse saliva and has very offensive breath. Look for diarrhea of dark green slimy stools. The patient will say that it feels as if he has never finished passing all of the stool, that there is always some left to pass. Everything is worse at night and in damp or rainy weather.

PHYTOLACCA—This is a very small remedy for mumps, but may prove useful. In this remedy picture, the glands are swollen very hard, as if they were small stones. That is keynote to this remedy and must be strongly considered in its use. The patient complains that his pain extends into the ears on swallowing.

PULSATILLA—Consider this remedy especially if the inflammation moves to the female breast or the male testicles. If the patient complains of vertigo, especially when rising from a sitting position, or in a warm, closed room. The patient is chilly, but worse for a warm, closed room. He wants open air. He will want to be rocked. Children will want their mothers to rock them. Adults will sit in a rocking motion at the edge of their bed. Look for the patient to have a thickly coated tongue, accompanied by a very bad taste in the mouth. The patient will be tearful, will not want to be alone. He will be worse in the evening.

RHUS TOX—Consider this remedy when there is a great deal of body and joint pain accompanying the mumps. The pain travels to all the limbs. The patient will complain of stiffness and lameness in all his limbs. This pain is worst on first motion after rest. The patient will want to keep moving in order to stay pain free. He will be restless at all times, trying to find a comfortable position. He is restless at night as well, and must toss and turn to find a comfortable position. Look for a dark red swelling of the left side of the jaw. Look for the patient to be worse from getting wet or from damp, cold weather. Look for the patient to feel better from applications of heat.

ALSO CONSIDER

HYOSCYAMUS—For when the patient is in a delirium. He will have a red face. Look for the patient to have a wild, startled look on his face. The patient will complain of throbbing pains in his head and jaw. Look especially for twitching and jerking of the patient's limbs. He will thrash about. The patient combines delirium with great nervous excitability. Giddiness, with stupefaction. He may strike out at his caretaker. He may be very suspicious. He may even insist that he is being poisoned.

COMMON AILMENTS
Chicken Pox

Chicken pox is one of the most common of childhood ailments. I've never had it, so stay away from me if you even *think* you might have it. Chicken pox in childhood will run its course rapidly and is usually not at all dangerous. The fever is usually low, and the blisters, which form on the skin and are filled with milky fluid, appear irregularly on any part or all over the entire body. At the end of three or four days, the pustules dry up and fall off, sometimes leaving a small scar. In adults, however, the illness can be far worse, with high fever, pustules covering the whole body and the possibility of long-lasting effects.

REMEDIES

ACONITE—If the chicken pox come on suddenly, and with a high fever. This remedy, in fact, will be useful only during the onset of the disease, or at the stage of fever. It is a useful remedy if the patient complains of a sense of congestion in the head and/or lungs. The patient will complain of headache. He will be very thirsty. The patient will be emotionally and physically restless and anxious. A nosebleed may accompany the chief complaint.

ANTIMONIUM TARTARICUM—Very helpful if the blisters are large and the patient—especially if the patient is a child—whines and will not be left alone. The patient may feel a congestion in the chest and may have some trouble breathing. The patient may have an audible rattling of mucus in his lungs.

BELLADONNA—Look for the patient to have fever, red face, congestive headache, and a sore throat. He will mostly complain of a congestion of the head. A throbbing headache may accompany the outbreak. Most obvious, however, will the fact that the patient, while very sleepy, will have trouble sleeping, will have a troubled and restless sleep.

MERCURIUS—Consider this remedy toward the end of the patient's illness. Mercurius is helpful if, when the patient's fever goes down and the spots begin to heal, some seem to become infected. Or if there seems to be a general infection present. Also a good chicken pox remedy when the glands under the neck swell, or when the tongue swells. The patient's fever will be high and the patient will sweat a good deal, but without relief.

PULSATILLA—Helps especially if the symptoms of a cold are dominant over the symptoms of the chicken pox. Also the pox will be slow to appear. But the patient will be driven totally and completely crazy by the itching. The itch will be worse in a warm room. The patient, in general, will be worse in a warm or closed room, although he will be chilly. And the patient will have watery eyes and nightly diarrhea. The patient will be clingy and weepy and will want a great deal of attention.

RHUS TOX—This is an excellent remedy for the patient with chicken pox. Look for the rash to be accompanied by fever; look for the patient to be very restless. The pox will be like poison ivy, bright red and very itchy. The patient will want to scratch and scratch. He will be driven crazy by the itch and will have to change positions constantly in order to get comfortable. He may walk the floor in his discomfort and be unable to rest at all. The itch may be made better by heat, especially by the heat of a long, hot shower. The patient will complain of a sensation as if his skin has shrunken on his body, as if his skin is too tight. The patient will be worse from cold and damp. Look for the characteristic red tip of the patient's tongue as an indication of the remedy.

SULPHUR—While this remedy picture has the traditional combination of rash with fever, it has the unique symptom that the patient will be very hungry and thirsty throughout his illness. The patient will drink a great deal, and will, unlike most patients, retain his appetite. He will crave salty and greasy things. He will want potato chips, french fries, or pizza. He will have the sensation of great heat on the top of the head and a hot sweat may cover the entire body. The patient will suffer from itching, and the itching will be made worse from any form of heat, especially from the heat of the bed. He will kick off the covers in order to sleep. The patient will be better from being in the open air.

ACUTE ASPECTS OF CHRONIC COMPLAINTS
Sinusitis

Sinusitis is a general term for any inflammation of the mucous membranes of the sinuses. Usually it is brought on as an aftermath of another viral or bacterial infection, such as a cold. Symptoms include a blocked nose, nasal, speech, and perhaps a frontal headache. The pain may also extend into the patient's jaw.

REMEDIES

BELLADONNA—Consider this remedy for cases of sinus pressure or infection that come on suddenly. The sinus infection will be accompanied by a fever that also comes on suddenly. The patient's face will be red, hot, and dry. Sinusitis may also be accompanied by nosebleed. The patient will complain of pressure in the frontal sinuses. He may also feel a heat and congestion throughout the head. The patient will be very sensitive to noise and to light. He will want to rest in a cool, dark place.

The patient may want to sleep, but his symptoms will be aggravated when he lies down.

CALCAREA—This is an excellent remedy to consider in cases in which there is chronic nasal blockage and sinus pressure. Look for the patient to have ulcerated nostrils. Look for a chronically diminished sense of smell. The patient will complain of a gnawing pain at the root of the nose. Look for a nasal discharge of thick, fetid pus. This remedy should especially be considered in cases of sinusitis in overweight patients, in patients who have chronic digestive problems. The patient will often feel quite sluggish while his nose is blocked. He will have a cold sweat on his head and especially on his feet. The patient's feet will be both cold and wet. This is a chilly patient with a chronically blocked nose and with chronic sinus pressure or infection.

HEPAR SULPH—When this remedy is called for, there is a true infection present. Look for the patient to discharge yellow mucus. The patient's face will be very tender and sensitive. The sinus pressure and, indeed, the patient in general will be better from applications of heat. The patient is chilly and irritable. This sinus infection has a great deal of sneezing accompanying it. It may be brought on from contact with cold, dry air. Look for the glands in the patient's neck to be swollen. Look for the patient to also complain of a sore throat, of drainage down the throat. The patient will say that he feels as if there were something caught in his throat. He will typically feel as if there were a stick caught in his throat.

KALI BI—The first remedy to think of in any case involving sinus infection, especially an acute sinus infection. Look for the patient to discharge stringy mucus that will be green, knotted, and tough. The patient will complain of a feeling of blockage and congestion on either side of the nose. Only one side of the nose at a time will be affected, although the affected side may alternate frequently. He will also complain of pressure at the root of the nose. It is especially keynote of this remedy that the patient will be able to identify the specific spot of the pain, and that spot will be small. This is also an excellent remedy to consider in cases of sinus headache, especially chronic sinus headache, that matches the pattern of specific small spots of pain. Also think of this remedy when the mucus does not flow, but when the pressure and pain are consistent with the type. When the mucus does not flow, there typically will be a violent sinus headache.

LACHESIS—Consider this remedy in cases that involve a chronic nasal discharge of both mucus and blood. Lachesis is especially indicated if the blood is dark in color. The patient will complain that the inside of his nose is painful. The patient's face will be flushed a dark red purplish color. Look for the sinus symptoms to either begin or to be dominant on the left side. Look for a sore throat to accompany sinus pain. The patient will have difficulty swallowing liquids, but will be able to swallow solids. Look for all symptoms to be made worse by the patient sleeping.

MERCURIUS—This is a remedy for those patients who are experiencing a true infection in their body. Look for the patient to discharge a greenish pus through the nose. And look for the patient's nose to bleed every time he blows it. Look especially for a swelling of the nasal bones and of the patient's tongue. The sinusitis may be accompanied by a swelling of the glands in the patient's neck. Look for a terrible odor to come from the patient's nose and mouth. Look for an increase in saliva from the patient's mouth.

NUX—A remedy that can be helpful to those with chronic sinus problems. Especially for those patients who experience sinus blockage and pressure accompanied by chronic constipation. Consider Nux first for cases of "snuffles," or chronic blockage in which the patient has to struggle to take in any air through his nose. The patient will make a "snuffling" sound as he attempts to breathe. The patient will be chilly, and will feel worse from the movement of any air. He will crave alcohol and spicy foods, which, for a moment at least, will make his nose run and give him a short-term solution. The Nux patient will be angry and irritable. Even though his nose is blocked, the Nux patient will be very sensitive to smells. The smell of perfumes, of flowers, will be especially difficult for the Nux to bear and may make the patient feel faint.

PULSATILLA—An excellent remedy for chronic sinus infection or for simple sinutitis that accompanies a cold. Look for the patient to complain of sinus pressure and pain above the eyes. He will complain that his nose is constantly stuffed up, especially if the patient is in a warm, closed room. The patient may be chilly, but his sinus symptoms will be improved by open air. Look for a discharge of yellow mucus, mucus that may come forth in a large, thick cloud. The patient may complain that he experiences pain in the frontal sinuses as well, especially on the right side of his face. The pain may extend into the bones of the face, especially on the right side of the face. The patient will experience rapid and almost contradictory shifting of pain from one part to another. The patient will be weepy in his pain.

SILICEA—Consider this remedy for cases of chronic sinus blockage and pressure. Especially consider this remedy for cases of sinusitis in thin and

depleted patients, patients with a chronic tendency toward upper res-
peratory infections of all sorts, and in patients with many allergies, especially food allergies. The patient will experience deep pain in the
frontal sinuses and the bones of the face, and often the jaw as well. He
will also complain that his nasal discharge irritates the skin around the
nose. But it is particularly keynote of the remedy type that the tip of the
patient's nose will be chronically itchy, which will drive the patient
crazy. The patient will also likely lose his sense of smell altogether.

ALSO CONSIDER

BAPTISTA—Consider this small remedy when there is a thick mucus discharge from the patient's nose. This will be accompanied by a severe
drawing pain along the nose. The patient will also complain of a dull
pain between his eyes. The patient will complain of a beating or pulsating
headache. He will say that he feels lightheaded, or that his head feels too
heavy. Look for the patient's face, especially his cheeks, to be red hot.

PHOSPHORIC ACID—Indicated in cases of sinusitis in which there is a
bloody discharge of pus from the patient's nose. Look for the patient to
bore his fingers into his nose in an attempt to clear his sinuses. Look for
a terrible smell to come from the patient's nose. The patient will complain of a buzzing in his head. He will say that his head feels heavy. He
may complain of a headache that is made worse from any motion of the
head. The patient will be exhausted and may feel intoxicated by his pain.

ACUTE ASPECTS OF CHRONIC COMPLAINTS
Seasonal Allergies and Acute Allergic Response

First, it is important to note that, of all the homeopathic treatments possible, those for allergies and those for headache are probably the most
difficult. There are many, many remedies to consider and may different
symptoms possible. (See the sections of this guide entitled "Sinusitis" and
"Colds and Flus and Fevers" in order to review a complete list of remedies.
Any remedy for a cold may be a potential remedy for allergies and all
should be considered, especially Euphrasia and Allium Cepa. Remember,
homeopathically speaking, it doesn't matter whether the symptoms are
caused by a virus or by exposure to an environment to which the

patient is sensitive. It is only important that we match the symptoms to the appropriate remedy.)

To make things even more difficult, allergies and allergic reactions of any kind are not truly ever acute situations. They must be dealt with constitutionally. I include the following remedies as stopgap measures to be used only until a visit to medical professional is possible.

REMEDIES

APIS—This remedy is perhaps the best single remedy for acute allergic response, especially for any allergic reaction that brings about a shock response. Most especially think of this remedy for the shock that can result from a beesting. But Apis is also excellent in cases of allergies to foods such as peanut butter. Keynote to the remedy is red swelling of the affected parts. Look for the area of the swelling to shine. It will feel hot to the touch. This is true even in cases of allergic reactions to foods. A part of the patient's body, most often the eyelids or the throat, will swell and sting and feel very hot. The patient will want cold applications. He will be very anxious. Apis is also an excellent remedy for seasonal or chronic allergies that follow the same pattern of symptoms. The rims of the patient's eyes will be red and inflamed. He will be very thirsty for cold water.

ARSENICUM—Consider this remedy when the patient is completely worn out by his allergies. And yet, the patient will be fussy, irritable, and restless. He will not want to be alone. The patient will be much better from warmth. Look for the patient to complain of burning pains, especially in his eyes and nose. The patient blows his nose often, but with little result. The patient's mucus is thin and watery. Look for the allergic symptoms to be worse on the right side. The patient will be thirsty, either for cold or for hot things, and is likely to want lemon. He will drink only small amounts of liquid at any one time. Consider this remedy especially for allergies that return at precisely the same time every year.

DULCAMARA—Consider this remedy for the patient whose allergic symptoms alternate between a stuffy and a constantly running nose. Expect the patient to be constantly sneezing. Look for his eyes to be swollen and watering. Look for the patient to be made worse by being out of doors or in damp weather. Hy will be especially worse from smelling newly mown grass, which will be the last thing that the patient smells for several days. Consider this remedy especially for patients whose allergies are worst in spring or fall when days are warm and nights are cool.

GELSEMIUM—The keynote here is sneezing without stopping. The patient sneezes and sneezes and sneezes. His eyes are heavy and puffy, and water constantly. The patient's eyes will be sensitive to light. Patient is listless, feels dizzy and exhausted. Look for a coating of the tongue, especially a yellow coating. The patient's lips will be dry. The patient will complain of a burning sensation in his mouth that extends into his throat and stomach. Look for the patient to complain of a sensation of congestion in the lower part of his chest. This is an excellent remedy to consider in cases of long-term low-grade allergy in which the patient is never incapacitated, but always uncomfortable.

NATRUM MUR—As it is perhaps *the* remedy for patients with colds, especially at the beginning of a cold, it is also perhaps our most important remedy for patients who have chronic allergies. Think of this remedy first in allergies, especially spring allergies, that resemble a simple cold. The patient will have a discharge that is thick and clear, like raw egg white. He will have a total loss of smell and taste. His nose will be totally blocked, although it flows freely. He will sneeze a good bit and his eyes will tear during the sneezing. The patient will complain that his nose feels dry, although it is flowing. Consider this remedy first in cases of allergies that begin with sneezing alone. This is also the first remedy to think of in cases of acute allergies that come on when the patient visits the seashore, or for chronic allergies that are made worse from a visit to the seashore. The allergies will be worse during the daytime and the patient will be worse outside, especially in the sunshine. The patient will be very thirsty for cold water.

SABADILLA—The very portrait of hay fever makes up the symptoms of Sabadilla. The patient sneezes constantly—ten, twelve sneezes at one time. This is keynote of the type: they cannot stop sneezing. The patient's nose will run freely, and the discharge will be a clear, thin liquid. The patient's eyes water constantly. His throat feels hot. The patient will be very, very thirsty. Thirsty most especially for cold water, but the patient will drink virtually anything and in great amounts. The patient's whole body will be covered in a hot sweat during a bout of hay fever. This is the first remedy to think of in cases of seasonal allergy or long-lasting allergies that are associated with heat and sweat.

SILICEA—Again, consider this in chronic cases of allergy that are typified by a stuffed-up nose, especially when the patient is worse upon waking in the morning. The patient will complain that his sinuses are painful.

And this pain may extend into the bones of the face. This is the best remedy to consider in cases of allergies in patients who are chronically depleted, and chronically given to colds, flus, and other infections and inflammations. In the patient who is slow to heal. An excellent remedy for patients who are allergic to dust. Who have both allergies and asthma. Look for a general chilliness on the part of the patient. A general weakness. Look for a total loss of the sense of smell to accompany the allergies. Look for the discharge from the patient's nose to irritate the skin around the nose.

ALSO CONSIDER

ARSENICUM IOD—It is keynote for this remedy type to have a thick, honey-colored discharge from the nose. This is the second stage of the patient's allergies. In the first stage, the patient will sneeze and sneeze. After three or four days of sneezing, the honey-colored flow will begin. The patient will complain of sore nostrils and of a burning sensation in his nostrils. The patient's eyes and ears will also burn. The patient will complain of burning and pressure in his ears, and of a constant tearing of the eyes, which also burn. The patient will be much worse from any form of heat, from both applications of heat and being in a warm environment. Look for the patient to have dry skin. Look for a burning throat to accompany the allergies.

ARUNDO—This is a general hay fever remedy. In fact, almost the only use of this remedy is in cases of patients who have hay fever. Consider this remedy most usually for cases in which the symptoms come on early in the allergy season. The symptoms usually will begin with a tickle in the patient's nose. With sneezing, but no mucus flow. The patient will complain that the roof of his mouth and his ears are both itchy. The patient will have a burning in his mouth. He will have a total loss of smell once the discharge begins. The patient will also experience burning and itching in his hands and feet. His feet will be hot, sweaty, and itchy.

KALI IODATUM—This is an excellent remedy for either acute or chronic allergies. The patient will have a constant nasal discharge. This discharge, while it is watery in appearance, will burn the patient's nostrils. The patient will complain of a sensation of rawness inside his nose. The patient's eyes and throat will feel raw and inflamed as well. The patient's sneezing attacks will be worse in the morning, just after awakening.

SANGUINARIA—A somewhat small remedy, but important to cases of chronic allergies. Think of Sanguinaria for cases in which the patient's nasal membranes are both dry and congested. And in which there is a discharge of watery mucus that is accompanied by burning pains. When the patient is without discharge, look for crusts to form that will bleed if detached. The patient will complain both of the discharge and of postnasal drip, which nearly maddens the patient. He will also complain of a dry throat that has burning pains, and of soreness in the area of the tonsils, especially the right tonsil. Look for the patient's tongue to be swollen and ulcerated, especially on the right side. The patient will also experience a tickling cough. This is also an important remedy for those with nasal polyps.

WYETHIA—Again, this remedy is suggested by patients whose symptoms come on very early in the season. And this remedy is especially suited to patients who have fall allergies only. The major symptom here is itchy palate. Although the patient will have a full range of symptoms, it is the itchy palate that drives him crazy. He will also have a sensation of swelling and burning in his throat. He will have to constantly clear his throat. He will have a constant need to swallow, but will have trouble swallowing. The patient will say that his mouth feels scalded. He will complain of a dry, hacking cough and of a sensation of weight that extends from his throat to his stomach. The patient will be worse in the late morning, especially at about 11 A.M. During that time, the patient will feel a chill and will be very thirsty when chilled.

ACUTE ASPECTS OF CHRONIC COMPLAINTS
Acute Asthma

Asthma is certainly a chronic condition, usually hereditary, and considered by many homeopaths to require miasmic treatment—treatment designed to reconcile a genetic predisposition to the condition. As with the other illnesses in this section, I include asthma not to encourage home treatment, but to give an indication of the constitutional types requiring treatment for asthma. Often the presence of this type of chronic disorder will lead a homeopath to a specific remedy or group of remedies. Chronic asthma must be professionally treated.

The symptoms of asthma center around a difficulty in breathing, which is typically worse at night. There is a sense of tightness or constriction in the chest and a desire for fresh air, although the patient will usually be unable to bear fresh air. Breathing with wheezing. Face flushed and bloated. Dry cough, later with expectoration. Spasmodic coughs. Attacks can last three or four hours and usually subside slowly. Attacks can come on frequently or may not reappear for months or even years. Attacks can be caused by breathing in dust or fumes, or from emotional states.

REMEDIES

ACONITE—For acute attacks and for attacks that occur suddenly. Look for shortness of breath, especially when sleeping. The patient cannot take a deep breath. Look for a spasmodic, choking cough, with a sensation of constriction of the patient's windpipe. Look for the patient to be in a state of great fear, restlessness, and anxiety. Patient will fear death, and will predict the day and time of his death. (Aconite is considered to be the acute remedy for a condition of asthma for which Sulphur is the chronic remedy.)

ANTIMONIUM TARTARICUM—Consider this remedy first in cases of asthma in which the patient sounds as if he were drowning. For cases in which there is an obvious rattling sound in the patient's chest. It is key-note of this remedy that the patient will have anxious breathing. Look for a sensation of weight or of oppression of the chest. Consider this remedy when breathing seems all but impossible. The patient must sit up to breathe. When the patient breathes, it seems as if his bronchial tubes were filled with mucus, but none appears when the patient coughs.

ARSENICUM—For cases of shortness of breath and attacks of suffocation, especially after midnight. The patient will feel great anguish and fear, great restlessness. Look especially for fear of death. The patient cannot lie down because of feeling of suffocation. Patient feels chilly, wants to be in a warm room. He may want cold air on face, but only on face, will want the rest of the body covered. This remedy is especially important to cases of asthma in the elderly, or in persons of a chronically weakened condition. Look for extreme thirst usually for warm things, but also for cold, but patient only sips a little liquid at at time.

BELLADONNA—For cases of asthma that comes on in wild attacks, usually occurring in the afternoon or early evening. The patient will complain of a sensation of dust in the lungs. Patient feels better for holding his breath, better for bending the head backward. The patient's face and eyes are red during attack; his skin is hot, red, and dry. Look for a dry, spasmodic cough, occurring especially at night. Patient is sleepy, but cannot sleep. This is perhaps our most important remedy for asthma in very young patients.

BRYONIA—The patient wants to stay very still, does not want to move at all, as the least exertion makes the patient worse. Look for the patient to have frequent bouts of dry cough. Also look for that frequent cough to move a good deal of mucus. The patient will complain of stitches in the chest. The patient may feel a sensation as if his ribs were broken. The patient's pain will be worse on breathing in. Breathing in causes coughing. Sitting up causes nausea. Look for chronic constipation with hard, dry stools to accompany asthma.

CHAMOMILLA—Consider this remedy first if the patient's breath feels trapped in his throat. Hoarseness accompanies asthma. The patient will suffer from a cough, and this will be accompanied by a rattling of mucus in the patient's windpipe. Look for hot sweat on the patient's forehead. Look for the patient to have one cheek red, the other pale. Patient is very irritable, rude. This is an especially useful remedy for patients who are children. Look for that child to want to be carried all the time. And to become very angry if he is put down.

CHINA—Consider this remedy first for cases of asthma that come on in suffocative fits from mucus in windpipe. This remedy is especially indicated when the attack comes on when patient is in bed at night. The patient's breathing will be very difficult. His breathing pattern will be a labored and slow inhalation, with quick exhalation. Look for an expectoration of clear mucus. The asthma will be worse at night. Worse for drinking. And look for the condition to alternate days, to be better every other day.

IPECACUANHA—Indicated in cases of spasmodic asthma. Asthma that is accompanied by violent contractions of the throat and chest. Look for the patient to have a sudden, spasmodic pain in his chest that forces him into a pattern of short breathing. The patient will have to pant in order to breathe at all. Look for the patient to have a rattling noise in the area of the bronchial tubes on breathing in. Suffocation threatens from the terrible constriction. The patient will be much worse from any form of any motion. It is keynote to this remedy that nausea accompanies asthma. That the patient has a feeling of emptiness in his stomach. That vomiting may accompany the asthma. Consider this remedy for cases of asthma that comes on from fright or anger.

NUX—Should be considered for cases of asthma in which the patient feels a spasmodic constriction in the lower part of their chest. In which the patient complains that even loose clothing is too tight and constrictive. The patient will have a short, dry cough. The patient may sometimes cough up a bit of blood. The patient will complain of the terrible congestion in his chest. He will be made better by lying on his back. The patient will want to lie still, and only occasionally will turn over or sit up. Nux is especially suggested by cases of chronic asthma in alcoholics, or those who use drugs. Also for asthma in angry or irritable people.

PHOSPHORUS—Indicated for the patient who displays very loud breathing during asthma. The patient will pant in his struggle to breathe. Look for a spasmodic constriction of the chest. The patient coughs constantly and the cough exhausts the patient. There will only be slight expectoration, which is usually thin and watery. Look for the asthma to be accompanied by a complete loss of voice. The patient will complain of a sensation of weakness and emptiness in his abdomen. Of a terrible burning in his throat. He will be very thirsty for cold water. Asthma will be accompanied by long, hard, narrow stools that are very difficult to pass. Asthma in thin, slender patients. Think of this remedy first for asthma in children who are very thin and sensitive.

PUSLATILLA—An excellent remedy to consider for cases in which asthma is caused by the inhalation of smoke or vapors. The patient will feel as if he is choking before the asthma attack begins. This is also an excellent general remedy for cases of asthma in children. Especially in weepy or clingy children. The patient will be worse at night and worse from lying down. Although he will be chilly, the patient will be worse in a warm room and better in open air. He will be thirstless. He will be worse from lying down and better from walking. Look for an expectoration that contains much yellow or yellow-green mucus, and that may contain blood as well. The patient will complain of a sensation of pressure in his chest.

SPONGIA—This is truly an acute asthma remedy. Look for difficult respiration, as if the throat were cut off by a plug. Look especially for the patient to wheeze when breathing. Or the patient's breathing may be very slow and deep, as if each breath would be his last. Difficult breathing will be accompanied by a rush of heat and blood to the patient's head. Look for the patient to awaken in fright from sleep. The patient will especially fear suffocation during sleep. Look for the patient to display a hoarse, hollow, wheezing cough.

SULPHUR—Look for the attack to come on during sleep. The patient will be worse after sunset. Worse every night. Look for the patient to complain of a feeling of tightness in his chest. Also of a feeling of dust in the lungs. Look for the patient to have a dry cough that is accompanied by hoarseness, or by a loose cough that is itself accompanied by soreness.

The patient may cough up white mucus, or the expectoration may be bloody. Look for the patient to complain of a feeling of pressure in his chest. The patient will feel weak and may faint. The patient will complain of a constant feeling of heat on the top of his head. Consider this remedy for cases of asthma attacks that are caused by the patient breathing in any type of smoke, including cigarette smoke.

VERATRUM—Consider this remedy for attacks of asthma that occur during cold, damp weather. Also for attacks that often occur very early in the morning. The patient will be filled with anguish and fear. The patient will feel as if he is about to suffocate. Look for the asthma attacks to be accompanied by oppressive pains around the patient's heart. Look for the patient's nose, ears, and lower extremities to feel cold. It is keynote of this remedy that the patient will have a cold sweat on his forehead. Also for the patient to be utterly exhausted. Look for the asthma to be accompanied by diarrhea, which will further exhaust the patient.

ACUTE ASPECTS OF CHRONIC COMPLAINTS
Rheumatism

There is not an actual medical diagnosis for the term *rheumatism*. It is, rather, a general condition in which a person feels worse in cold damp weather, with multiple aches and pains. It may progress into the condition of rheumatoid arthritis (always a chronic condition to be treated by a professional), and may also be a sign of food allergies, candida infection, or a genetic tendency toward a number of illnesses.

Therefore, this category is an important one. It should be used in conjunction with other illness categories and will be especially helpful with those listed under "Strains and Sprains."

REMEDIES

ACONITE—The key to the remedy picture is the sudden appearance of sharp pains. The pain will be worse in cold, dry weather. The patient will be both emotionally and physically restless. Look for red swelling in affected part, which will be very sensitive to touch and to motion. Look for a sudden, high fever to accompany the pain. The patient will complain of stitching pains in chest, which will make breathing difficult. Look also for retention of urine, and for the patient to experience the same stitching pains in his kidneys. Aconite would be considered an acute remedy for rheumatism—Sulphur is most often considered to be the remedy that speaks to the same conditions that have been made chronic.

ARNICA—Another acute remedy for rheumatism. The thing that will be keynote is the hard, red, and shining swelling of affected part of the body. And everything will seem too hard to the patient. Every chair, every bed. Like the Princess and the Pea, the patient will feel every little disruption on a physical surface. And so the patient will not be able to become comfortable, will not find a comfortable place to be or a comfortable postion to be in. The patient will experience lameness. He will complain that he feels as if the affected areas of his body were sprained or bruised. If any mention is made of treatment, the patient will insist that he is fine and that he needs nothing. The Arnica patient is afraid to be touched. This is important in identifying them. They panic if they think that they will be touched. (Arnica is often followed by Rhus Tox in cases of rheumatism.)

ARSENICUM—Here we will see a picture of a patient with burning, stinging, tearing pains. And with pale or white swelling of the affected parts. All the patient's pain will be relieved by application of warmth. The patient will want to be made warm, will want to be "cozy." Look for a profuse sweat, which relieves the pain, but leaves the patient very weak. The patient will be on a roller coaster of internal temperature; look for the patient to have frequent chills, alternating with sensation of heat. These are restless patient—look for them to be constantly moving the affected limbs. It is keynote of the type that they display an extreme thirst—especially for warm liquids—but that they drink little at any given time.

BELLADONNA—Another acute remedy for rheumatism. The keynote of this remedy is the characteristic appearance of affected joints. Look for red, shining, and swollen joints. The patient will complain of a cutting pain that extends deep into his bones. And of darting pains in his joints. These pains will come on suddenly, and also leave quite suddenly. The affected areas will also have the combined sensations of congestion and heat. The patient may experience a sudden fever as well, with dry, hot skin, thirst, and a throbbing headache. The patient will be drowsy, sleepy, but cannot sleep. Every time the patient begins to fall asleep, he will be startled awake by sudden pain. Look for an aggravation at 3 P.M. The patient will also be aggravated by motion or touch.

BRYONIA—Another major remedy. The aches and pains associated with this remedy type are worse in cold, dry weather. The pains are worse especially from any motion, but also from touch. The pains will be made better from pressure, from lying on a hard floor. The Bryonia patient will be very irritable. He will be disinclined to speak or to answer any questions. He will become angry if you try to get him to move. Look for stiffness, with swelling and a faint redness to the inflamed part. Look for dry, hot skin, or a good deal of sweat that is of an acrid nature. The patient will complain of a bitter taste in mouth; he will say that he feels as if his mouth had been burnt. (Bryonia follows both Aconite and Belladonna well for cases of rheumatism.)

CALCAREA—Consider this remedy for chronic cases of rheumatism. Few remedy types are as sensitive to cold, and especially to the combination of cold and damp, as is the Calcarea. The patient's joints will be swollen, and the patient's aches and pains will be worse with every change in the weather. Especially when the weather is getting colder. The patient may have aches and pains from Thanksgiving till Easter. The patient will have cold, damp feet, as if he were wearing wet socks. Also look for head sweats. The patient's head will be very chilly. And yet, it will be sweaty as well, especially when the patient sleeps. Consider this remedy strongly for the overweight, middle-aged patient who is out of shape, exhausted, and disinclined to exercise.

CAUSTICUM—This is a major remedy for patients with rheumatic pains. It is especially helpful to those with chronic neck and shoulder pain. Look for pain in the jaw and neck. Causticum is considered the most important remedy for those suffering from TMJ (transmandibular joint disease) or chronic pain in the jaw. It is also the remedy most associated with carpal tunnel syndrome, for the pains in the wrist that chronically begin with repetitive movement of the hands and wrists, such as in typing. This is also an excellent remedy to consider for those who suffer muscle spasms. The patient's pains will be relieved by warm, wet weather. This is very helpful in the selection of this remedy, as most other rheumatics are worse in wet weather. The patient will still, however, experience discomfort from the change in the weather. Look for great weakness and lameness in the patient's lower limbs. The pain will be worse in the evening, and from exposure to cold.

CHAMOMILLA—This is another excellent acute remedy. Look for the patient to complain of a tearing pain, one that is accompanied by a sensation of numbness in the affected part. The pain is continuous and gets worse at night, which causes the patient to attempt sleep only with much tossing and turning. The Chamomilla patients are furious in their pain. They can become verbally abusive. They can even throw things in their anger. Look for the patient to be covered in hot sweat, especially on the patient's head. Look for redness of one cheek, paleness of the other. The patient may complain that the pain moves upward into the head, ears, and even the teeth.

DULCAMARA—This is a remedy to consider strongly for both acute and chronic cases of rheumatic pain that are deeply tied in to weather. Look for the patient to experience both pain and stiffness that will be made much worse in cold, damp weather. The patient will be so sensitive that he will even be worse from moving from a warm to a cold place. Especially consider this remedy for those patients who suffer pain during the times of year in which the days are hot and the nights cold. Also the times of year in which there are wild changes in weather. Rheumatism in the autumn and the spring. Look for the affected parts of the patient's body to feel bruised. The pains associated with this remedy type are mostly in the back, and the joints of the arms and legs. The pains will often come on when the patient is sleeping.

IGNATIA—An unexpected but excellent remedy to consider for cases of chronic rheumatism. Consider this remedy when the patient insists that his pain has the sensation that the skin had been ripped apart from the bone. The patient will have to continually change his position, toss about, in order to achieve any level of comfort. Look for the patient to have trouble sleeping, or to have only a very light and brief sleep, due to his pain. The patient will complain of a jerking in his limbs as he begins to fall asleep. He will have pain in the calf muscles. He will have pain in his soles. The pain will be worse at night. The patient will feel better while eating and just afterward, especially just after breakfast.

LACHESIS—This is a remedy to consider for chronic rheumatic conditions. A keynote of this remedy is swelling, especially the swelling of the index finger and wrist joint. The patient will also complain of stinging pains in the knees, with swelling. Left-sided symptoms are worse. The affected areas will also be discolored, will take on a reddish purple color. Look for the patient to have profuse sweating, but the sweating brings no relief from the pain. The patient will be worse from sleeping. All the pains will increase after sleep.

LYCOPODIUM—Consider this remedy for chronic cases in which the pain symptoms are worse on the right side. The patient will complain of drawing and tearing pains. The patient's pains will be worse in the late afternoon, and worse again at night. It is keynote of this remedy that there will be a painful rigidity to muscles and joints, which is accompanied by a sensation of numbness. The patient will be chilly and the affected parts will be especially chilly. This is a major remedy for chronic rheumatism, especially in old people. The patient's urine will be dark in color, will have a sediment of red sand. The pains will be accompanied by constipation, flatulence, and sour belching.

MERCURIUS—Consider this remedy for the patient with aches and pains that are worse at night. The patient will be worse from any change in the weather. But, more important, the patient will also be worse if moved outside a narrow temperature comfort range. What changes in weather are to other patients, changes in temperature are to the Mercurius. These patients become hot and cold very easily, and they move into pain with these temperature changes. Also, the patient experiences uncomfortable sweats, especially at night. These sweats bring about no relief. The pain will be worse when the patient is in bed, and in the late night, toward morning. Look for a puffy swelling of affected parts that is a light pink color. The pain will be accompanied by green slimy diarrhea. (Lachesis often follows Mercurius in cases of rheumatism.)

NUX—Consider this remedy especially for cases in which the patient's pains are in the back, loins, chest, or joints. The pain may center in the area between the shoulder blades. The affected areas will be colored with a pale swelling. Spasms are keynote to this remedy; all affected parts will experience jerking pains that are aggravated by touch or motion. Also by a twitching in the muscles. The affected areas of the body will also experience numbness. The patient will have a storng aversion to open air and great sensitivity to cold. He will feel heat in affected parts that is mixed with a general sensation of chilliness, especially when the patient is moving about. The patient will also be very sensitive to noise and to smells. Certain smells may make the patient feel faint. If the patient can be made to sweat, either from motion or by contact with moist or dry heat, the sweat relieves the patient's pain. Chronic constipation accompanies the rheumatism. Chronic irritability is keynote to the remedy. This is one of our most important remedies for chronic rheumatic pains.

PHOSPHORUS—Consider this remedy for rheumatic pain that sets in when the patient becomes cold. The patient will complain of a sense of lameness of the affected parts. Of weakness in his lower limbs. This will be accompanied by a sensation of weakness and emptiness in the abdomen. Look for the patient to belch large quantities of wind after eating. Look for the patient to have difficulty with stools as well—for long, narrow, hard stools that are very difficult to expel. While Phosphorus does not speak to a wide range of specific rheumatic pains, it is a very important remedy of the type, in that the Phosphorus patient is considered a "human barometer." No other remedy type, with the possible exception of Rhus Tox, is so sensitive to changes in the weather. The Phosphorus will be made much worse from changes from warm and dry to cold and damp. He will be especially worse when storms approach. He may be sensitive enough to sense storms days before they appear. The Phosphorus may experience emotional, as well as physical, aggravations from changes in the weather. In addition to rheumatic pains, the Phosphorus will typically have headaches during weather change. This is an important acute and chronic remedy.

PHYTOLACCA—Consider this remedy for chronic rheumatism. Dullness is the key here. The patient will complain of dull, heavy, and aching pains, especially in damp weather. These pains will be rather low grade, but will be constant, and therefore maddening. The pain will be worse on the right side of the body. The pain will be worse from pressure and from any motion. The patient may complain that a headache accompanies his pain. The pain will be in the forehead and will also be a dull ache. Look for the patient's urine to be dark red and to leave a deep red stain.

PULSATILLA—This is one of our most important remedies for those with chronic rheumatic pains. It is keynote here that these pains constantly move and shift location throughout the patient's body, seemingly without rhyme or reason. The patient will complain of a sensation of numbness; he may even complain of a sensation of paralysis. There will be a puffiness to the affected parts. Warm, stuffy rooms make everything worse, even though this is a chilly patient. The patient's pains will be relieved by exposure to cool, open air. The patient will also be better for comfort, touch. The patient's digestion will also be upset. The patient will experience a bad taste in the mouth every morning.

RHUS TOX—This is perhaps the first remedy to think of in general cases of acute or chronic rheumatism. No other remedy so speaks to the rheumatic aches and pains as does Rhus Tox. Consider this remedy for patient who experiences aching and stiffness of joints, especially in cold, damp weather. The patient will be made worse from too much rest and is especially worse on first motion, but will be made better by gentle sustained motion. Therefore, the patient is restless and is always seeking relief and rest. These patients will say that they have to get "warmed up," that they have to get their joints moving before they will feel better. When they are in great pain, they may not be willing to sit down or to stop moving at all because they know their distress will increase if they stop. But they will also be made worse by overdoing, by moving too much, which also aggravates their condition. Look for a characteristic swelling and redness of affected parts. The patient may say that he feels as if his skin had shrunk, that it is too tight on his body. The patient's pains are drawing and burning in nature; the patient may feel as if the affected parts of the body had been sprained. Look for the patient to have the characteristic red tip on his tongue as a guide to the remedy. The Rhus Tox patient will be worse from any change in the weather and is especially bad on rainy, cold days. His aches and pains will be improved by heat, especially by damp heat in a hot shower. That will help his aches and pains and relax the shrunken sensation in the skin as well.

RUTA—This is a great remedy to remember for patients with pain in their joints, especially for pains in the knees. This remedy is also specific to the area of the hips as well. The patients' pain will be in their tendons, rather than their muscles. Look for any ascending motion to be difficult. It is especially difficult for any Ruta patient to rise up out of a chair or a car seat. The pain will extend from the small of the patient's back down into his legs. The patient may also complain of a sensation of stiffness in his wrists and hands that extends into his fingers. Also of pains in the feet and ankles. He will say that he feels as if his muscles and tendons were shortened and had shrunk.

SULPHUR—This is perhaps our most important remedy to consider in cases of chronic rheumatism. But it should not be discounted in cases of acute rheumatism, either. More important, think of this remedy when a patient suddenly has rheumatic pains and, although the case seems acute, the pains linger on and on. The patient will complain of tearing, stitching, or dull, aching pains. The pains will be worse on the left side of the patient's body. The patient's hands will tremble. He will have hot, sweaty hands. He may have pains all throughout his arms and hands. Also, look for stiffness of the knees and ankles that keeps the patient from walking totally erect. Consider this remedy for the patient with rheumatic pain in the left shoulder. This patient's walk will be stoop-shouldered. He will also have a constant sensation of heat on the top of his head. His whole body may be covered in hot sweat. The patient will complain of frequent spells of weakness, or of fainting spells. He will be worse from any form of heat, especially the heat of the bed. (Sulphur is a remedy that follows many others well in cases of rheumatism. It especially follows Aconite, Belladonna, Bryonia, Mercurius, or Pulsatilla.)

THUJA—Suggests another remedy type that is very sensitive to changes in the weather. The Thuja patient will experience pulsating pain, as if there were an infection under the skin. He will also complain that the affected parts feel cold and weak. The patient will be made worse from resting and will especially be worse from the heat of the bed. It is keynote of this type that the patient will complain that his limbs feel as if they were made of wood or of glass. As if he were fragile and would easily break. Look for the hands to be affected, for the tips of the patient's fingers to be swollen and red. The patient will say that his hands feel dead. This is a remedy that has much twitching. Look for muscular twitching, weakness, and trembling all throughout the body. The patient will complain of a pain in his heels. He will be worse from cold, worse at night, and worse from cold, damp air.

VERATRUM—Should be considered in cases in which nausea accompanies the rheumatic pain. In cases in which the patient is covered in a cold sweat during his pain. The patient will say that his pain has a bruised quality. That he feels very weak and is trembling. The patient will, however, be better from motion. He will feel better especially when he walks. The patient will say that his pain comes on in electric flashes. He will complain especially of pain and cramping in the calves. He will say that his arms feel swollen and cold. He will feel that the muscles in his arms are paralyzed. The patient will be made worse from cold and will be better from warmth. He will be worse at night.

ALSO CONSIDER

COLCHICUM—For cases of rheumatism in which there is moderate swelling that is accompanied by pale redness of the affected parts. The patient's pains are burning in nature. The patient is chilly, even when sitting by a fireplace. He will also experience flashes of heat throughout his body, especially in the affected parts. Look for the pain to move to the area of the heart: the patient will feel stitches of pain in his chest. He will have heart palpitations as well. Look for profuse sweat. The patient's urine will be dark and scanty. Consider this remedy for patients who have a sharp pain in the left arm. Who complain of tearing pains in the limbs in warm weather and stinging pains in cold weather. The patient will have a sensation of pins and needles in his wrist and hand. The rheumatic pains shift from joint to joint. The pain is worse at night. A tingling accompanies the rheumatic pains.

RHODODENDRON—This is a small remedy, but it can be very important for cases of rheumatic pain. Consider this remedy for patients with aches and pains in muscles and ligaments. These pains will be worse from rain, especially from thunderstorms, and worse in cold weather. The patient will be worse before the storm begins. He will also be afraid of the storm. He may feel an aching in his temples at the approach of a storm. All the joints will ache, especially those in the patient's big toe. The pains will be worse on the right side of the patient's body. Look for the patient also to experience pain in his neck and shoulders, which may extend into his arms. The pain is worse when the patient is at rest. It is an odd keynote of this remedy that the patient will not be able to sleep unless his legs are crossed.

SABINA—Consider this remedy for cases of chronic rheumatism. For cases in which the patient cannot bear a hot room. He will have to have the windows open. The patient feels better only when he is in cold air or in cool rooms. The patient will complain of pain in all his joints. Also of shooting pains in his heels that move throughout the feet and up the leg. He will feel pain in the front of his thighs. Look for the affected areas to be red and shining and swollen. The patient will be worse from any motion and from any form of heat.

ACUTE ASPECTS OF CHRONIC COMPLAINTS
Headache

Any sort of pain occurring in any part of the head can be termed a headache. It is usually not to be considered a simple acute disturbance, but is, rather, symptomatic of an underlying general disease. Some headaches have to do with chronic sinus complaints, some are gastric, some menstrual, some nervous, and some rheumatic. Therefore, as with allergy, the remedies listed here are to be used only as a temporary solution. If headaches reoccur, it is a clear sign that you should get in touch with a professional homeopath, and someone with chronic headaches should be under professional care.

REMEDY CHECKLIST

For a headache that comes on from a mechanical injury, consider: **Aconite, Arnica**, or **Belladonna**.

For headaches that are accompanied by a congestion in the head, consider: **Aconite, Belladonna, Bryonia, Nux**, or **Pulsatilla**.

For headaches that accompany colds or other respiratory infections, consider: **Aconite, Chamomilla, Mercurius, Nux**, or **Sulphur**.

For headaches that accompany rheumatic pains, consider: **Bryonia, Chamomilla, China, Ipecac, Pulsatilla**, or **Nux**.

For the headache that comes on from a change in weather, consider: **Chamomilla, Nux**, or **Phosphorus**.

For a headache that comes on from being overheated, consider: **Aconite, Belladonna**, or **Bryonia**.

For a headache that comes on from lack of sleep, consider: **Carbo Veg, Cocculus, Lachesis, Nux**, or **Pulsatilla**.

For a headache from overwork, consider: **Lachesis, Lycopodium, Natrum Mur, Nux, Silicea**, or **Sulphur**.

For a headache that is accompanied by nausea or gastric distress, consider: **Antimonium Crudum, Bryonia, Iris, Nux, Pulsatilla**, or **Veratrum**.

For a headache that is accompanied by constipation consider: **Bryonia, Lycopodium, Nux, Pulsatilla, Sepia, Silicea**, or **Sulphur**.

For a headache that comes on after drinking coffee, consider: **Chamomilla, Ignatia**, or **Nux**.

For a headache from drinking alcohol, consider: **Arsenicum, Lachesis**, or **Nux**.

For the nervous headache, or for chronic headaches in nervous patients, consider: **Aconite, Arsenicum, Belladonna, Coffea, Colocynthis, Ignatia, Pulsatilla, Sepia**, or **Veratrum**.

For a headache from grief, consider: **Ignatia** or **Staphysagria**.

For a headache from anger, consider: **Chamomilla** or **Nux**.

REMEDIES

ACONITE—Consider this remedy for a violent, stupefying headache, especially on that is accompanied by a feeling of heaviness in the forehead. The patient will complain of a sensation as if his brain were pressing on the forehead from the inside. He will have vertigo when rising from a sitting position. The pain may be accompanied by bitter, bilious vomiting, by great anguish, and by great emotional and physical restlessness on the part of the patient and a fear of death. The Aconite headache comes on suddenly. A slowly forming headache counterindicates the remedy. Patient cries out, says he cannot bear the pain.

ARNICA—Here we would usually first think of a headache as being from a bruise or blow to the head. But Arnica is a helpful general headache remedy. Consider this remedy when the patient says that his head hurts over his eyes. For stitching pains in the forehead that are made worse by stooping. When the patient's head and face are hot, but the rest of the body is cool. Sore stomach often will accompany the headache. Look for much belching, which the patient says tastes like spoiled eggs. Look for nausea and vomiting that is worse after eating or drinking.

ARSENICUM—A major remedy for a periodic headache, one that recurs in a specific pattern of days or weeks. (Also think of Belladonna for this kind of headache.) There is a feeling of a great weight in the head, most often in the forehead. The patient complains of beating pains in the forehead. Vomiting will usually accompany this sick headache. Violent vomiting, especially after eating or drinking. Patient is very thirsty, but only takes small sips of liquid. Patient is restless, fearful—especially fears death. Pains worse when patient rests, better when in motion. Pain is better for cold applications or cold air on the head. The patient feels chilly, however, and wants to keep the rest of the body warm.

BELLADONNA—Consider this remedy for the classic sick headache. When the patient's whole head feels as if it would burst. When there is a feeling of a congestion of blood in the head, with throbbing pains, especially in the forehead. Extreme sensitivity to light makes the patient close his eyes. Boring pains, with headache on the right side of the head. Vertigo, with a loss of sight. Nausea, some vomiting of bile, mucus, or food. The patient cannot bear light or noise. (This is also true of Aconite or Cocculus.) Headache worse at 3 P.M. The patient's face is flushed.

BRYONIA—Consider this remedy when the patient's head aches on first waking in the morning. (Consider also Calcarea Carbonica or Nux.) Especially for chronic headaches that come on the first thing in the morning. The head aches as if it would split open. Patient is aggravated by any motion, even the motion of the eyes. Patient wants to stay perfectly still. Patient becomes sick or faint from sitting up. Lips are parched, dry, and cracked. Constipation may accompany headache, with hard, dry stools, as if burnt. Patient is very irritable.

CALCAREA—An important remedy for those who suffer chronic headaches. Dull, oppressive pains in the forehead are most common in the Calcarea headache. Chronic headache that dulls the intellect. The patient forgets what he was saying, what he was thinking. He seems confused when he has a headache. Throbbing headache in the morning, continuing the whole day. Feeling of coldness in the head. Feet cold, as if the patient were wearing wet socks on his feet. Vertigo when going up stairs. Headache improves at night.

CHAMOMILLA—This is an important remedy for those who suffer sinus headaches. Headaches from drinking coffee. Heads aches on one side only. Headache extends into jaw. Acute shooting pain in the forehead. One cheek is red and the other pale. (This may also be true for Aconite or Nux.) The patient is overly sensitive to his pain; the patient will actually become almost giddy. He will be very impatient, very irritable.

CHINA—Consider this remedy for the headache that comes on from blocked sinuses. The patient will complain of a pressure in his forehead as if it would burst. The brain feels sore, bruised. Worse from any mental exertion. (Also consider Nux or Sulphur for this.) The patient will have a ringing in his ears, and fainting may accompany headache. Keynote for this remedy is that the patient has a headache every other day.

COCCULUS—Sick headache that comes on from traveling by car or boat, etc. Throbbing headache that is worse in the evening. Patient is worse from talking, laughing, noise, or any bright light. Patient feels better while sitting up. Travel sickness with vertigo.

COFFEA—For a headache during which the patient is very excitable. Very sensitive, especially to light and noise. Headache as if a nail were being driven into the head. Headache will be much worse from noise, especially from music. Headache worse in open air. Head feels too small. Headache with insomnia.

IGNATIA—Headache in forehead, with boring pains. Headache better from lying down. Pain as if a nail were being driven through the side of the head. Headache as if an object were being pressed down hard on the brain. Patient emotionally upset, may be filled with suppressed grief. Headache with an empty feeling in the pit of the stomach. Headache accompanied by constipation.

IPECAC—Most pronounced symptom of headache is nausea and vomiting. (Veratrum is the other remedy that shares this symptom.) Headache feels as if the brain and skull were bruised all the way down to the root of the tongue. Stooping causes vomiting. Headache accompanied by diarrhea, with green stools.

KALI BI—The remedy for a sinus headache, or for a headache during the last stages of a cold when the sinuses are blocked and the head feels pressurized. Throbbing headache in the forehead, usually worst over the left eye. Characteristic of Kali Bi headaches is that they affect only one small part of the head. Patient will point and say, "It hurts right here." Headache worse from eating. Feeling of weight on top of the head. Vision is dimmed. Vertigo from looking up.

LACHESIS—The most important thing about this headache is that it tends to induce sleepiness. Nausea with headache. Throbbing pain in temples. (Also consider Aconite, Arnica, or Belladonna for patients with this symptom.) Headache begins upon waking in the morning. Patient cannot bear anything tight around the waist. Pale face with headache. Vertigo with headache. Throat very sensitive to touch. Headache worse from sleeping.

LYCOPODIUM—Think of this for chronic headaches, especially for chronic right-sided headache pain. Also for periodic headache, usually beginning or aggravated at 4 P.M. Headache may come on daily, or in a specific pattern of days or weeks. Headache feels as if temples are being nailed together. Headache with dizziness, with intestinal gas. Patient is irritable and chilly during headache.

NATRUM MUR—Throbbing headache. Chronic migraine headaches that are worse in the daytime, better at night. Headache caused by the sun. Warmth and motion make headache pain worse. Sinuses feel congested, nose stopped. Headache may be preceded by tingling in lips, nose, or tongue. Think of this headache especially for pain that moves with the sun, that grows worse as the sun moves up in the sky and fades as the sun fades over the horizon. This is also a remedy for headaches from overstudying. The patient's eyes may tear during the headache.

NUX—Consider this remedy especially for the patient who has a tendency toward gastric headaches. For the headaches associated with hangovers. Headache with sour, bitter vomiting. Sensation as if the skull were too big. Sensation as if the skull would split from the pain. Stupefying headache, especially in the morning, aggravated from mental exertion. (Calcarea and Sulphur both share this symptom.) Headache follows chronic constipation. Constipation with large stools, frequent urging. Patient tends to be chilly, irritable. The irritability is so strong a symptom that its absence counterindicates the remedy.

PULSATILLA—Consider this for the headache that is connected to dietary troubles, especially for the headache from eating rich or greasy foods. (Also consider Ipecac or Nux.) Headache worse toward evening. Patient craves cool, fresh air, cannot bear a closed, warm room. Patient is chilly, even in a warm room. The patient will have a bad taste in his mouth every morning.

RUTA—This is an excellent remedy for the eyestrain headache, usually beginning by reading in too dim a light or by doing close work, such as sewing. The headache will have a pressing and/or bursting quality. Headache from becoming overfatigued. Headache may be accompanied with lower back or hip pain.

SEPIA—Consider this remedy for headache pain in forehead and/or temples. This headache will be accompanied by violent pain. Also by nausea, with a feeling of emptiness in the stomach. The patient's face will appear yellow, especially across the nose. Headache with constipation, with hard, knotty stool. The patient's urine will be strong smelling and will contain claylike sediment. Patient is angry, and cries—especially when he considers his pain.

SILICEA—Think of this remedy for chronic headache with pain in forehead. Tearing pains, usually worse on one side, with pain traveling through the eyes. Pains worse from any mental exertion, from stooping, talking, or from cold air. Pain better in a warm room. Headache with constipation. Stools recede after being partially passed.

SULPHUR—Pains are usually in the forehead and temples. Pain has a pressing or burning sensation. There is a feeling of constant heat on the top of the head. The headache may also be accompanied by a hot sweat over the patient's whole body. His hands will be hot and sweaty. Headache with diarrhea. Diarrhea may drive the patient out of bed in the morning. Fainting spells with headache. Periodic headache that may share that same dull throbbing quality of a Calcarea headache.

THUJA—Consider this remedy for the headache that occurs over one eye. The pain will have a boring quality. This is a classic sick headache. The pain will be relieved by pressure. The patient may press against his forehead, or press his forehead hard against a wall. Also for headaches that press into the frontal sinuses. (Thuja often follows Belladonna in cases of sick headache.)

VERATRUM—Consider this for the nervous headache. For when a high-strung patient is given to frequent headaches. These have violent pains that are unbearable for the patient. Cold perspiration all over the body accompanies the headache. Patient feels weak, faint. Headache with vomiting, with exhausting diarrhea. Patient has great thirst for cold drinks.

ALSO CONSIDER

ANTIMONIUM CRUDUM—Another remedy to consider, along with Bryonia, Nux, or Pulsatilla, for the headache that comes on accompanied by an aversion to food. The patient will be very nauseous and will not be able to stand even the smell of food. The patient will be worse from any ascending motion, especially from going up stairs. He will feel better in open air.

IRIS—This is perhaps our most important remedy for the migraine that is accompanied by nausea. The headache is also accompanied with blurring of the patient's vision, or blurred vision may precede headache. The patient feels that his scalp is tight. Vomiting and deep nausea accompany sick headache. Headache tends to be right-sided. Pain is improved by motion.

PHOSPHORIC ACID—This remedy is specific to the headache in which the pain is on the top of the patient's head, as if his brain were being crushed. Headache after long-term grief. Also consider for headaches after long-term illness, which has left the patient very weak. Headache with pain in the region of the liver. Sensation as if the stomach were being pushed up and down. Headache may be accompanied by painless diarrhea.

SANGUINARIA—Consider this remedy for the headache that is worse in the morning. This is a remedy for the patient with a right-sided headache. Headache begins at the back of the head and travels forward. Pain can extend into the right shoulder. Headache pain is worse during the day and improves as evening comes on.

ACUTE ASPECTS OF CHRONIC COMPLAINTS
Fever

While the basic remedies for fever have been listed previously in the category "Colds and Flus and Fevers," I wanted to consider more carefully this very important symptom. Like headache and allergy, fevers can reveal a good deal about our overall constitutional health. Therefore, consider the following remedies for fever and their constitutional implications.

In general, fever can be said to have three features: heat, cold, and the sweat. The sensation of cold usually begins with a feeling of exhaustion. The patient may also feel pains in the back of the head or in the legs, and may stretch and yawn a good deal. Coldness usually begins in the extremities and moves throughout the body. Coldness may be extreme enough to cause chattering of the teeth. The cold stage may last from just a few minutes to two or three hours.

The sensation of heat usually begins just as the chill ends. The face flushes, the skin becomes hot, the pulse races. Look for a dry tongue and mouth, much thirst, headache, and restlessness. The hot stage can last up to eight hours in an acute situation; in a constitutional situation it can last much longer.

The sweating stage, when the fever "breaks," ends the cycle. The fever has burned out the toxins in the system and recovery begins, except in constitutional situations, in which the cycle may begin again.

You will find, however, that some fevers will have only hot stages, some only cold, and some will have no sweat involved at all. And the balance of the stages will differ from case to case, person to person. So, in selecting the right remedy, we are going to balace the three features of fever and place them once again within the context of the whole person.

REMEDIES

ACONITE—Violent chill, followed quickly by heat, especially on the head and face. Cough during fever. Shortness of breath. Of great use in the first stage of fever—chills from a cold, dry wind. Violent thirst. In bilious fevers, everything tastes bitter, except water. Pain in stomach after eating or drinking. Pressure in the region of the liver. Throbbing headache, worse for any motion. And yet, patient is restless and wants to move about.

ANTIMONIUM TARTARICUM—Fever with nausea and vomiting, with a sinking sensation in the stomach. Patient feels that he will not survive. General weakness in the whole system. Patient is very ill. Profuse cold sweat. Pulse is rapid and very weak. Great drowsiness, although patient may resist sleep in the fear that he will never awaken.

APIS—Chills at 4 P.M., like Lycopodium. Patient is worse in a warm room. Becomes chilly at the slightest motion, with great heat on hands and face. Sweat alternates with dry skin. Pain on the left side, under the lower ribs. With high fever, patient may slip into unconsciousness and delirium. Unable to talk. Tongue is cracked, ulcerated. Mouth and throat very dry. Great difficulty swallowing. Soreness in the pit of the stomach and the abdomen. Fevers with constipation. Also diarrhea of stools with mucus and blood. Great weakness. Cannot bear light or noise.

ARNICA—For fevers in the patient who is in an apathetic condition. Patient is indifferent to his condition. Tongue dry, with a brown streak down the middle. Patient is confused, forgets words when speaking. Falls asleep in the middle of a sentence. Patient feels sore and bruised, constantly changes position in bed. Feels that the bed is too hard. Fever with involuntary urination.

ARSENICUM—Illness begins with headache, yawning, and stretching. With general discomfort. Chill and heat are intermingled rather than separate states. With fever there is great anguish. Internal chilliness with external heat. During fever, great fear, great anguish, fear of death. Great restlessness. After fever, great exhaustion. Face is pale, shrunken. Cold sweat on forehead. Constant licking of the lips. Tongue dry. Violent thirst, but drinks only a little at a time.

BELLADONNA—High fevers that are quick in coming on. Slight chill with much fever or vice versa. Some parts of the body are hot while others are cold. Face is flushed and bloated. The skin is red. The eyes are sparkling, pupils dilated. Throbbing headache accompanies fever. Patient cannot bear noise or light. Patient is delirious, with a wild expression on the face. Wants to bite, strike out. Patient is sleepy and cannot sleep, or jumps and starts in the night. Choking sensation in the throat. Tongue is red, cracked. Tenderness in the abdomen; the slightest jarring or movement is painful.

BRYONIA—Face is red and burning. Swollen. Chill predominates. Lips are dry and cracked. Tongue is coated with a thick, white fur. Oppressive headache. Pain as if the head would split from the slightest motion. Delirium day and night. Violent, dry cough that causes stitching pain in the region of the liver. Constant desire to sleep, with sleeplessness and tossing about. Patient does not want to be moved or touched. Dryness of mouth, usually with the desire to drink great amounts of liquid. Does not drink often, but drinks a great amount when thirsty. Cannot sit up due to nausea and faintness. Soreness in the stomach. Constipation accompanies fever, with hard, dry stools.

CALCAREA—Chronic fevers. Thirst during a chill. Chills alternating with heat. External coldness with internal heat. Hardness of hearing accompanies fever. Feet feel damp, as if the patient is wearing wet socks. Patient very weak. Vertigo. Shortness of breath, especially on going up stairs. Diarrhea containing undigested food. Palpitations of the heart with fever. Rapid pulse, much anxiety. Fever with chronic dry cough.

CARBO VEG—Irregular attacks without pattern. Often begins with sweat, shortness of breath, and then chill. Attacks are preceded by toothache and pains in limbs. The patient is thirsty, but only during chill. Vertigo. Eyes are dull and sunken. Cannot bear light. Redness of face and sick stomach during heat stage. Extremities are cold and covered in cold sweat. Eating or drinking causes fullness of stomach, sensation as if abdomen would burst. Diarrhea, brown and bloody. Patient wants to be fanned in order to breathe.

CHAMOMILLA—Little chill, great heat and sweat. Much thirst with heat. Face is red, with one cheek red and one pale. Patient is angry, rude. Hot sweat on face and head. Pain in the abdomen accompanies fever. Frequent pale urination. Fever may be accompanied by vomiting. Stools green, watery, and slimy.

CINA—Before fever, the patient vomits, feels great hunger. Thirst with chill and heat. The face is pale through all stages of fever. Nose tickles. Patient is restless at night. Look for dilatation of the pupils. Look for a perfectly clean tongue.

FERRUM PHOS—The keynote here is that there is no keynote. This is the general acute fever remedy. The fevers generally come on rather quickly, and without warning. The patient is thirsty during the chill stage. Look for swelling of the face, especially around the eyes. Patient may have stomach upsets with fever, may vomit all food eaten before it is digested. Any exertion flushes the face. Patient is exhausted with fever.

GELSEMIUM—Chill tends to come on in the evening and begins in the hands and feet. When fever comes, patient becomes anxious and is restless, although exhausted. Vertigo. Intoxication with fever. Patient is sensitive to light and noise. Gelsemium is a wonderful preventative remedy for fevers and flus. Good for both acute and chronic conditions. Here the fever is not too high, the patient is not very ill, but the illness lingers. Fevers with Southern flu. Fevers in chronic fatigue syndrome.

IGNATIA—Thirst with chills. External heat follows and brings with it internal shuddering. Chill can be relieved by external heat. Fever with red rash covering the whole body. Very little sweat. Sweat usually only on the face. Headache and pain in pit of the stomach accompany the fever.

IPECAC—More chills than heat. Or much heat and little coldness. Fever comes on with yawing, and a collection of saliva in the mouth. Chill is increased by external heat. Patient is not thirsty during the cold stage, but very thirsty with heat. Fever accompanied and almost overridden by nausea and vomiting.

LACHESIS—Look for the characteristic dry, red tongue, which is cracked at the tip. Tip of the tongue may bleed. Delirium is very common and patient talks a good deal in delirium. Patient cannot bear to have anything touch his throat. Trouble swallowing liquids, can swallow solids more easily. Fever tends to come on in the afternoon, chill dominates over fever. Chattering of teeth. Sore chest. Violent headache. Patient is worse for sleeping.

LYCOPODIUM—Fever begins at 4 P.M. and ends at 8 P.M. Face is yellow.

Tongue is dry and black, or covered with thick mucus. Must breathe with the mouth open. Look for fanning of the nostrils as patient tries to breathe. Patient uses the wrong words when trying to express ideas. Constant sense of fullness in the stomach and abdomen. Feels as if he would burst. Fever accompanied by intestinal gas. Obstinate constipation. Red sandlike sediment in urine. Patient is fearful. Does not want to be alone. Patient is irritable.

MERCURIUS—In the early stages, the patient may not be aware that he is sick. He doesn't complain of any symptoms, but feels very weak and wants to go to bed. Face is yellow. Tongue is coated with yellow fur. Breath is very bad. Look for ulcers on lips, gums, and cheeks. Bitter, sour, or sweetish taste in mouth. Look for a great deal of saliva. Look for a swollen tongue. Tongue may be so swollen that it has teeth marks running along both sides. Region of the stomach is sore to touch. Stinging pains in area of the liver. Diarrhea with dark green stools. Dark urine. All symptoms are worse at night or during rainy weather.

NATRUM MUR—Chill comes on at 10 A.M. with great thirst. Patient wants cold water and drinks much and often. Violent headache with fever. Dry tongue. Corners of the mouth are ulcerated. Patient will usually have sore throat with fever, craves salt, and says that it makes his throat feel better.

NUX—First remedy to think of for simple fevers in angry patients. Fever may be very slow to come on. Starts with chill. When chilly, the patient becomes more angry. Cannot be made warm. Fever with headache that feels as if a nail were being driven into the head. Bitter taste in the mouth. Belching, which is also bitter. Fever may be accompanied by vomiting, constipation. Constrictive cramplike pains in abdomen. Sleeplessness at 3 A.M. Aggravations in the morning.

PHOSPHORUS—The patient must breathe through an open mouth. Deep fevers with blackened lips and tongue. Mild delirium. Thirst for very cold drinks; wants only cold food, like ice cream. The patient vomits cold food and drink as soon as it warms in the stomach. Painless diarrhea that is very watery. Abdomen is very empty-feeling. Patient is very weak. Patient does not want to be alone.

PULSATILLA—Fever with melancholy. Patient is disgusted by everything. Patient becomes dizzy on rising from sitting. Headache, with beating pain in the head, worse from stooping, from being in a warm room, in the evening. Tongue is coated yellow. All mucus is yellow. Putrid taste in mouth. Vomiting mucus. Nausea, no desire for food. Nightly diarrhea, especially from fatty foods. Fever without thirst. Symptoms are very changeable; the patient feels well one hour, worse the next. All symptoms worse toward evening.

RHUS TOX—Face is red and swollen. Blue circles around the eyes. Lips take on a brownish color and are very dry. Tongue is dry, red, smooth, or red only at the tip in a patch the shape of a triangle. Patient talks to himself. Ears are stopped up; patient loses the sense of hearing. Fever with dry, troublesome cough, especially during the chill stage. Severe pains in the limbs, worse for rest. Diarrhea, involuntary stools. Patient is very exhausted, especially from diarrhea. Lower limbs are very weak, may be drawn up to body. Red rash may cover the whole body. Patient is worse at night, especially at midnight.

SEPIA—General cold feeling, with pressure over the temples and eyes, begins the attack. Great coldness of the hands, with a sensation as if the fingers were dead. During the fever, vertigo, even incoherence. Sweat over the whole body, accompanied by anxiety and by a dry throat. Total absence of thirst.

SULPHUR—To be used in fevers when the best selected remedies have little or no effect. For chronic fevers of unknown origin. Patient is burning hot on the top of his head, with cold extremities. Tongue is dry and brown. Patient is very thirsty. Patient sleeps during the day and is sleepless during the night. Patient is mentally sluggish. Look for early morning diarrhea that may drive the patient out of bed. Spells of weakness, faintness.

VERATRUM—Patient has yellow or blue face. Face is cold and covered with cold sweat. Lips are dry, brown, and cracked. Look for violent trembling, and cramps of the feet, hands, and legs. Fever is accompanied by violent vomiting. Intense thirst for cold drinks. Excessive weakness, pulse almost absent. Cramps in limbs, with cold sweat.

ALSO CONSIDER

ANTIMONIUM CRUDUM—Fever with gastric disturbances. Look for a white-coated tongue. Patient is very sad. Feels depleted. Cold stage dominates fever. Great desire to sleep. Fever without thirst, as with Pulsatilla.

BAPTISTA—Face is dark red with fever. A dull headache accompanies heat, with confusion of ideas. The patient's head feels as if it were in scattered pieces. Tongue is coated brown, is dry, especially in the center. Bad breath. Diarrhea accompanies fever. Sweat, urine, and stool are all offensive.

CHINA—Fever preceded by nausea, headache, hunger, palpitations. Thirst comes on before chill and again during sweating stage. Chills alternate with heat. Skin is cold and blue. Ringing in the ears, with dizziness and a feeling as if the head were enlarged. Pain in the region of the liver and spleen, especially when patient bends or coughs. Yellow skin.

HYOSCYAMUS—Face is swollen and red. Tongue is red, dry, and cracked. Lips look like scorched leather. Fever very high. Delirium with fury. Loss of consciousness. Loss of ability to speak coherently. Muttering. Patient picks at bedclothes. Great restlessness. Patient jumps out of bed, tries to escape. Eyes are wild—red and sparkling, rolling of the eyes. Twitching of limbs, twitching of tendons. Patient is convinced that you are trying to poison him. May refuse all remedies.

NITRIC ACID—For very serious fevers. The patient is very weak. Fever with very loose bowels—green, slimy diarrhea. Stools accompanied by severe pain. Hemorrhage from the bowels. Abdomen is very sensitive. Urine is very offensive, like horse urine. Pulse is irregular. For fevers that occur again and again in chronic fatigue syndrome.

OPIUM—Face is swollen and purple with fever. Patient has trouble breathing, and breathing may sound like wheezing. Patient cannot stay awake. Comalike sleep. Delirious talking with the eyes wide open. Pulse is labored and slow. Retention of urine. Involuntary stool while in stupor.

PHOSPHORIC ACID—Patient is greatly weakened by illness and has become indifferent to his condition. The patient does not want to talk—it takes too much energy to talk. Answers questions very slowly. Tongue is dry and cracked. The patient stares at things, mutters. Great rumbling in the bowels with watery diarrhea. Cold sweat on face and hands, and on the region of the stomach. Pulse is weak and intermittent.

STRAMONIUM—High fever, with loss of consciousness and involuntary movements of the limbs. Ceaseless talking. Patient is very earnest. Constant jerking of the head on the pillow. Desire to escape. Tongue is yellow-brown. Tongue is dry. Lips are sore and cracked. Mouth is very dry, but there is not desire for water. Look for black diarrhea.

Materia Medica

Introduction

THE STUDY OF materia medica is the very heart of the practice of homeopathy. A serious student can come to grasp the complex philosophy of homeopathy, but if he is unable to recognize the remedies "on the hoof" in the living human being, the practitioner will never have more to offer than platitudes. And when you are yourself lying sick in bed, or worse still, when a loved one is lying there looking up at you, it is only by the study of materia medica, the study of the remedies themselves as they reveal themselves in their "remedy portraits," that you will know how to be of any real help.

Therefore, it is important that we take some time to consider the remedies themselves. I have here listed the most basic and commonly used remedies and have attempted to give an overview of their uses. As you read through this section, please remember that any materia medica study is only as good as the insights of its teacher. While I have attempted to put together as well rounded a look as possible of each of these remedies, it is only my point of view of these remedies. It is important for all serious students of homeopathy to inspect several materia medicas, in order to get as much information from as many sources as possible.

In selecting the remedies included, and in creating the portraits of those remedies, I have used the framework of acute treatments, listing the remedies that I think should be in every household, the remedies that are most basic and most important to most families. I do this to help bridge the gap between philosophical and hands-on experience.

Now, a few notes about how this section is put together. You will find that under the listing of each remedy, the first section is called "Remedy Source." Here I have given the history that the substance has had before it became a homeopathic remedy. In some instances, the healing action of the substance is the same as the action of the remedy. In some cases it is not. Please be careful not to confuse the substance with the remedy.

I also give the history of the remedy, who created it, who proved it, and in what year if, at all possible. When important, I will also give the names of other remedies that are a part of the same "families," as with the Rhus or Kali remedies. All of this is listed just to give you a background on the remedy, how it is put together, and the history of its use.

Next you will find the section called "Situations That Suggest . . ." Here I list the major clinical uses for each remedy. I do this with some hesitation, because I never want a reader to begin to think of Rhus Tox as a remedy for poison ivy but always as a possible remedy for a person who is suffering from poison ivy. Indeed, there are several other likely remedies for that specific condition.

But I think that it is important to look at the wide range (or, in some cases, the narrow range) of symptoms that a particular remedy can cover. This is one way that we can actually avoid the trap of thinking of Rhus Tox as a "poison ivy remedy." If we look at the huge range of ailments that Rhus Tox can speak to, we can only come away with more respect for this wonderful remedy.

So take a look at these clinical uses, but be aware that all of the remedies listed here will transcend any or all of these uses. Don't think, for instance, if Sulphur is not specifically listed as having "Colds" under its clinical uses that it can never be the appropriate remedy for a person with a cold. Use this section as a tool and not as the final reality.

The next section is called "Remedy Portrait." Here I attempt to give you an overall look at the remedy and how the patient who needs this remedy is likely to look and act. In some cases, how he may feel or smell. In that so many of the remedies listed here are both acute and constitutional remedies, I have stressed their acute uses. Certainly there is much more to be said about each remedy, and especially about the remedies that may be considered our most important, like Sulphur or Natrum Mur, but the goal here is to create a starting point for education, and not to be the last word about these remedies.

Next, I've gathered together the keynotes for each remedy. Keynotes are the symptoms that are particularly associated with a remedy. We should, of course, never select a remedy based solely on the keynotes, but we must always look to the totality of the symptoms and match that to the totality of the Remedy Portrait.

The next two sections will be very helpful in selecting a remedy. These have to do with what makes the patient or his specific symptoms feel better or feel worse. The sections are called "Aggravations" and "Ameliorations." Use these as you use the keynotes to help refine your understanding of the remedies and their selection.

Next is the section entitled "Dosage and Potency." In this, I give the general guideline in the use of specific remedies. Some work better in higher potencies, some in lower. Again, this is not meant to be a final word on any specific remedy, but is, rather, a general guideline. So, if the remedy called for says it works best in 30C, and you only have 12C, don't panic. Use the 12C and it will at least do some good until you get your hands on 30C. Or it may do the whole job itself.

But if a remedy has a specific warning about using too high a potency and you are about to take a 1M, you might want to think again about taking that remedy in that potency. You might want to go out and get a 30C. So don't get caught up in the trap of worrying about potency or dosage, but do pay attention to them.

It is especially important that you pay attention to dosage, since the true power of homeopathy is usually expressed in the dosage. And the rule of thumb is always the same: give the remedy until improvement begins; then stop. So, if you see some changes with the first dose, if the patient is improved in general energy, even if every specific symptom is not improved, leave it alone. Give the remedy again only if you have to—only if the case begins to decline and the patient begins to grow worse. Remember that more cases are ruined by giving too many doses than by any other way.

If you give too high a potency, you are likely to bring about an aggravation of the entire condition. And, if a patient is very weak, this can be a bad thing. If the patient has a cold or a rash, he may become more uncomfortable and may get a bit angry with you, but he will get well all the same. But if the patient is very weak, if he is elderly, or if he has had a good many allopathic treatments (and who, these days, has not?), then you really are better off, all in all, by starting with a lower potency and building up to a higher potency if you feel you have to.

So use the information in this section as a guideline. Note that some remedies will take repetition well, and with some remedies you should even expect to give more than one dose. Other remedies work best in a single dose, and still others, in high potencies, even demand it. Use this section as a guideline before giving any remedy.

The final section listed under each remedy is called "Relationships." Here I have given you what information I could about what remedies may be considered complements to the one being considered. These complements are remedies whose actions are in harmony with the remedy at hand. This does not mean that I am telling you to use more than one remedy at a time, or that I am even trying to predict what other remedies you will have to use in a given situation. Instead, I am giving you information as to what remedy or remedies seem to naturally come after the one at hand in the majority of situations. Or what remedies tend to be used before this one. Or what remedies almost always tend to be used after this one. And, in some cases, I list what remedies should never be used just before or after a specific remedy, in that their actions are antagonistic to one another.

Again, this does not replace your need to take the case and research the case. The method of homeopathic treatment is still the same as always. You have to look at the totality of the symptoms and watch as the patients shift when the first remedy has been given.

Part of mastering homeopathy has to do with knowing when to go from the first remedy to the other, as well as with the selection of the second remedy. Both of these are hard skills to master. Both take a good deal of time and dedication. Because of this reality, and because we are dealing with acute situations that, in many cases, will actually be fairly simple to figure out, I have given you, where possible, the general flow of the case. This does not mean that in the situation at hand, Symphytum will be needed to follow Arnica and complete its action in the case of a broken leg. It just means that in many cases, in the majority of cases, it will be true. So again use this section as a guide and not as the final word.

I have gathered together sixty remedies here, trying to select the same remedies that are contained in most home kits. Are they the best and only remedies that I could have selected? Probably not. But they are useful remedies all of them.

Note: While homeopathic remedies are often gender-linked in their constitutional use—men will often need remedies such as Lycopodium or Nux, while women require remedies like Pulsatilla or Sepia—there is no such link when the remedies are used in acute situations. For simplicity's sake, therefore all patients are referred to in the masculine singular unless the specifics of the case demanded otherwise.

Materia Medica: Remedies

1. ACONITUM NAPELLUS

Remedy Source: Vegetable Remedy. Aconite is created from the roots and stems of the plant *Aconitum napellus,* which is also known as wolfsbane and monkshood. The plant is native to Europe, and must be gathered in the flowering stage in order to be made into the remedy Aconite. It was first created as a homeopathic remedy by Hahnemann in 1805.

Situations That Suggest Aconite: Shock. Also angina, arrhythmia, headache, injury and trauma, Neuralgia, vertigo. Also upper respiratory infections, colds and flu, conjunctivitis, croup, otitis media, pneumonia, tonsillitis. Also panic attacks.

Remedy Portrait: Aconite is among the most "restless" remedies. A historic homeopath named Nash lists Aconite, along with Rhus Tox and Arsenicum, in his "restless trio." So, the Aconite patient will be very restless and he will not be able to be quieted. Look for the Aconite patient to pace the floor, or, if he is forced to lie down, to thrash about. Because of this general restlessness, the Aconite patient will be startled very easily. He is easily frightened, especially by noises or from a change in his symptoms. And the Aconite patient's symptoms will appear and change suddenly as well. In the same way, almost everything about this person will suggest haste. He will do everything in a hurry, everything in a panic. Because of this, he may seem somewhat careless or accident prone.

Speed is, indeed, the keynote of the remedy. All the symptoms of the remedy type come on quickly. They often will come on if the patient is exposed to a cold, dry wind, which chills him and brings on illness. This is the first remedy to think of for colds and flus that come on very suddenly after the patient has been outside on a cold day.

As a matter of fact, an onset of symptoms that is slow, even if those symptoms themselves match those of Aconite, will counterindicate the remedy. The illness has to travel like a freight train for this remedy to be of help. And Aconite, since it is such a speedy remedy, will also only be of help in the first few hours of any illness. Once that illness has moved beyond its initial, shocking stage and has begun to define itself more fully, Aconite will be of little or no use.

The Aconite's patient's symptoms will seem to overwhelm him, and will especially seem to overwhelm or distort his senses. Sight, smell, and, especially hearing will become distorted and may even disappear altogether. In that Aconite disorders hearing, it is a major remedy for patients with noises or ringing in their ears. The Aconite patient will be especially sensitive to sound and to sight. He will be startled easily by strange or sudden sounds and will have a strong sensitivity to light.

The Aconite patient's pain tends to be numbing in nature, with tingling and pricking sensations also being very common. The patient's muscles, especially the leg muscles, will become very relaxed, and every attempt to move will become difficult and painful. Because of this, Aconite is a major remedy for sciatica when the symptoms of that condition match the general sudden pattern of Aconite.

Aconite is a remedy common to inflammatory diseases of all sorts and can be very useful in cases of tonsillitis, laryngitis, bronchitis, pneumonia, and ear infection, all of which come on during or are worse during cold, dry weather or exposure to cold wind. It is also the first remedy to consider in conditions like toothache that follow the Aconite pattern of quick onset in which the pain is unbearable. Aconite, surprisingly, can be a helpful remedy in cases of chronic ailments as long as the patient's symptoms follow the general remedy portrait.

Aconite is one of the first remedies that we consider for all cases of fever. The Aconite fever, of course, comes on quickly, most often after the patient has been exposed to cold, dry winds. These fevers are characterized by a red face, or a face that alternates between red and pale. The patient's skin will be dry and hot. He will have a great thirst for large quantities of cold water. His whole body will seem burning hot. The patient will be restless but will refuse to lie still or to rest.

But we must not overlook the emotional symptoms of the Aconite patient, as they are very important to the understanding of this remedy type. The patient is frantic and filled with fear. Look especially for a fear of death. The patient will also commonly predict the time of his death. Fear, like the pain in Aconite, will be worse at night. Aconite patients will have the irrational fear of having their hair cut. Some will even seem afraid of having their hair touched. Look for ailments to come on after fear and anger, or from hearing shocking news.

As a shock remedy, Aconite is often used in alternation with Arnica. In cases in which the patient has received both physical injury and shock, the two remedies, depending upon the potency on hand, may have to be repeated in alternation as frequently as every five minutes.

The color red is also common in Aconite. The face will be red with fever. The ears will be red during the onset of the illness. All blood will be bright red in color.

The general modalities of the remedy find the Aconite patient worse at night; worse for lying on the painful side; worse on rising; and worse for music, which most Aconites cannot bear to hear. The patient is better in the open air, which he often feels he can breathe although unable to get heated air into the lungs. He often feel betters after sweating.

Keynotes: Aconite is a remedy of particular importance to young people, and to the diseases of young persons that come on quickly; illnesses from exposure to dry, cold air, especially north or west winds.

Also look for, as Hahnemann wrote, "anguish of mind and body." Look for restlessness. Notice that the patient's fears concerning his own illness cannot be quieted.

Look for the skin to be hot and dry. And note that, as Allen tells us, "Aconite should never be given simply to control the fever, never alternated with other drugs for that purpose. If it be a case requiring Aconite no other drug is needed; Aconite will cure the case."

Aggravations: Evening and night. Also aggravations from the pains of the illness—for instance, the patient will not be able to tolerate the pain, no matter how intense or mild it may be. Aggravations from a warm room; from lying on the painful side of the body; from rising up in bed. Also from breathing in and from listening to music.

Ameliorations: Ironically, the Aconite who has been made ill from exposure to cold air will also be ameliorated by open air. The patient is also improved by sitting quietly and by perspiring.

Dosage and Potency: The remedy is most commonly given in low potencies of 12C or 30C for most acute conditions. Higher potencies may be needed for conditions that involve an acute fear of death. In that one dose of this remedy usually will not hold longer than six hours, Aconite is repeated often in acute illness.

Note that conditions that seem to fit the Aconite portrait but fail to yield to the remedy, or become long-lasting in nature, may yield to the remedy Sulphur, which is considered to be the constitutional equal to Aconite. Sulphur is often given both before and after Aconite in inflammatory illness.

Relationships: Aconite is complementary to both Arnica and Coffea. Its actions work best in concert with Sulphur, as noted above. Aconite is also followed well by Arsenicum, Belladonna, Bryonia, and Pulsatilla.

2. ALLIUM CEPA

Remedy Source: Vegetable Remedy. The remedy is made from the common onion, belonging to the Natural Order of Liliaceae. This common food product is found all over the planet.

The remedy is made from the fresh red bulb of the vegetable. The remedy Allium Cepa was created by Constantine Hering in 1847.

Situations That Suggest Allium Cepa: Allergies of all sorts. Hay Fever. Seasonal allergies. Colds. Coughs. Inner-ear infections. Upper-respiratory infections. Headaches. Sore throat.

Remedy Portrait: Think of how your body reacts when you slice an onion and you will have the usual portrait of Allium Cepa. Your eyes will run, as will your nose. Moisture seems to run from every part of your face. There is profuse watery discharge. Look for the patient to have to stuff tissues into the nose to stop the flow.

With Allium Cepa colds and allergies, the water coming from the eyes is bland—that is, it does not burn or itch the eyes. They tear and tear, and the flow is very watery. The discharge from the nose, however, causes irritation. The skin around the nostrils is red and sore and often cracked. These are the colds in which the nose becomes so sore that you do not want to blow it.

Allium Cepa is so effective when dealing with allergies that we have to be a little careful when using it. The remedy will help with allergies in up to a third of all cases for at least that season. However, seasonal allergies are never truly acute situations, and a remedy that is deeper acting and more specific to the case is usually called for in order to clear the allergies away for all time. If we are to use the Band-Aid approach with Allium Cepa, we will find that although the allergies will grow better for one season in the next the remedy will be of much less help. We are warned that using this acute remedy for a constitutional situation can ultimately suppress the allergies into a deeper condition like asthma.

But this aside, the wise use of this remedy when the symptoms match the remedy's action will be a great blessing to all involved, as Allium Cepa is perhaps our most important acute remedy for persons with colds.

It is interesting to note that those needing this remedy will usually reveal themselves by the fact that they crave onions. They will refuse to eat cucumbers.

Allium Cepa is helpful with headaches, especially headaches that accompany colds or allergies.

The patient will tend to also have symptoms involving the eyes. The eyes will burn, will ache, will feel as if they were tearing from smoke. The patient will want to rub his eyes.

The throat also presents symptoms. The patient will have laryngitis. This loss of voice may or may not accompany a cold or allergies. The throat will also be sore, and the pain will be made much worse by coughing. The patient will have to grasp his throat and hold it still when he coughs, because the coughing makes him feel that he is going to tear his throat open.

Keynotes: Sore and *raw* are the two words that best sum up the pains of Allium Cepa. In some cases, the patient's whole body will feel raw during his cold.

The allergies in Allium Cepa tend to come on every year in August. The remedy is also very useful for spring allergies, especially those that come on after damp weather, or from northeasterly winds. These allergies cause discharges from the nose that burn both the nose and the upper lip. The nose drips so much that drops of watery discharge will drop off the tip of the nose.

Aggravations: There is a general aggravation from being in a warm room. Aggravation also from getting wet.

The Allium Cepa patient who has a headache will find that the headache is made worse by closing his eyes.

The patient is worse when having to sit still.

The patient's allergies tend to be worse in the late afternoon. The patient, however, will have a general aggravation in the evening.

The patient will also be worse for eating salad, which he will not be able to digest well. The same is true for peaches.

Ameliorations: There is a general amelioration when the patient is outside in the open air. Even if the allergies are made worse by being outside, the patient will want to be outside.

The patient is better for moving about. He will want to go outside and walk.

Dosage and Potency: This is a light, quick-acting acute remedy. A dose will last from a single day to a week. The lower potencies are most commonly used. The potency 30C is most common for the treatment of colds. Higher potencies work best in single doses, although the lower potencies may be repeated as needed. Allium Cepa in general does not take repetition too well, and should be repeated with reservations.

Relationships: Allium Cepa is complementary to both Phosphorus and Pulsatilla. In cases of allergy that have been helped by Allium Cepa, Phosphorus should be considered a constitutional remedy.

3. ANTIMONIUM TARTARICUM

Remedy Source: Mineral Remedy. This is one of the oldest medicinal substances known to mankind. Antimonium is taken from antimony, one of the basic alchemical substances. The ancient name is "tartar emetic," as it is a remedy taken from the compound of antimony and potash. The resulting chemical salt causes nausea and distressed breathing.

This is a remedy created by Hahnemann. It was later reproven by Hencke.

Situations That Suggest Antimonium: Influenza. Bronchitis. Pneumonia. Whooping cough. Respiratory infections of all sorts. Also chicken pox, digestive distress, vomiting. Also general muscle pain, lumbago, rheumatism.

Remedy Portrait: Antimonium Tartaricum is often considered the drowning man's remedy. Think of the death rattle in the chest, the final gasps for air as the drowning man who has been beached tries in vain to remove the liquid from his lungs. So, too, with the Antimonium patient. He cannot take a deep breath. He rattles with a wet cough and strangled respiration. He coughs and hacks to remove the phlegm from his system, but as hard as he tries, he cannot cough up the mucus.

In general, the Antimonium patient will be totally exhausted. He will want to lie still. He will want to sleep most of the time. You will find that all the patient wants to do is sleep, and yet he does not seem to recover strength from sleeping. Vertigo will accompany or alternate with this sense of sleepiness. Vertigo will come on if the patient attempts to rise.

The Antimonium patient will likely want to be held as well. Children needing this remedy will want to be carried. Adults will want you to sit at the top of the bed and cradle their head in your arms. The patient will not, however, want to be fussed with. He refuses to have his pulse taken and refuses to take his medicine.

The patient's face will be pale and covered in a cold sweat. Look for the eyes to appear sunken. Look for the patient to flap his nostrils in attempting to breathe. Listen for the rattling sound of his breathing.

Accompanying these symptoms you will most usually find nausea. The patient will be too nauseous to eat and will refuse food—except perhaps for apples, which are often craved by those needing Antimonium Tartaricum. Acidic fruits in general may be craved. The patient will be averse to milk and dairy foods, will be worse in his digestive distress if forced to drink milk. The patient has no thirst.

Keynotes: The most important keynote is the concept of suffocation. The patient will have shortness of breath. He will not be able to take a deep breath. He will have to sit up in order to breathe or to cough. Coughing and gasping for air (as with whooping cough) accompany each other in this remedy.

Central to the remedy also is the rattling of mucus in the chest with little expectoration. There is a great deal of mucus present, but, no matter how the patient coughs and hacks, he can't get any out.

A lack of reaction is also keynote to the remedy. The patient will want to rest and sleep and will still become weaker. You will sit by his side and want to speak to him in a loud voice in order to get a reaction. You will feel the need to cheer him on, to shout, "Come on, you can do it."

The cold sweat on the face is also keynote, as is the patient's thirstless condition. Also look for trembling, for trembling of the whole body but especially of the hands and of the head.

Also keynote to this remedy is a sense of weight. The patient will feel as if a heavy weight has been placed upon him, especially upon his chest. Also the patient will seem almost to be deadweight, as he will seem heavier than usual. This is especially true of the patient's head, which will seem too heavy for him to lift.

Finally, although this is a chilly remedy, and the patient will likely feel cold all the time, he will be worse from warmth. He does not want to be covered. He does not want to be bundled up in warm clothing.

Aggravations: The patient is worse from warmth. Worse in a warm room or from warm covers or warm clothing.

The patient will also be worse in cold or wet weather. Look for the patient's condition to worsen when the weather changes to rain, especially in spring.

The patient will be worse also from lying down in bed at night. Breathing and expectoration are much worse from lying down.

The patient will be worse from any motion or movement; worse from touch; worse from any strong emotion, especially anger, which aggravates the cough.

The patient is, in general, worse at night. Look for dramatic aggravations in the middle of the night, Especially at 4 A.M. Cough, however, will be worse at either 4 A.M. or 4 P.M.

Ameliorations: The patient feels best when he reclines but has many pillows behind him so that he is in nearly a sitting position. He is also better when lying on the right side.

The patient will be better in the cool, open air.

He will be especially improved if he can manage to cough up some mucus.

Dosage and Potency: This is not a good remedy to use in a low potency. Below 30C, Antimonium Tartaricum has been shown to create powerful aggravations. The remedy will have to be repeated as needed, but make sure to stop treatment when improvement begins.

One dose of Antimonium Tartaricum can hold for up to two weeks.

Relationships: It should come as no surprise that Antimonium Tartaricum is complementary to Ipecac, which also follows this remedy quite well in cases involving respiratory and digestive distress.

Carbo Veg, Silicea, and Sulphur all also follow this remedy well and complete its healing action.

4. APIS MELLIFICA

Remedy Source: Animal Remedy. Apis is created from the venom of the honeybee. And, because it is much harder to extract venom from a bee than it is to milk a cow, none of the methods by which the remedy is made are very pleasant for the bee.

The remedy was created in 1852 by Dr. Fredrick Humphries.

Situations That Suggest Apis: Allergies (especially to bee stings). Also: acute asthma, arthritis, herpes, headache, shingles. Also sore throat, colds and flus, fevers, pneumonia, chicken pox. Apis may also be useful for ovarian cysts, endometriosis, miscarriage, urinary incontinence.

Remedy Portrait: Just think about the sensation of a bee sting and you are thinking about the symptoms that we associate with the remedy Apis. When you get stung, you are likely to find the area of the sting swollen, red, and hot. You will feel a burning pain in the area of the sting. This is the picture of the patient who needs Apis. He is experiencing burning pains in some area of his body. Those pains are linked to swelling and the swollen area is red and somewhat shiny. It doesn't matter where in the body the symptoms occur and it doesn't matter what caused them. The presence of these remedies suggests the remedy Apis. (It is easy to get a little confused between the aches and pains that suggest the remedy Arsenicum and those that speak to Apis. Both will have redness, and both will have burning pains. But with Apis these pains will be better from applications of cold. Arsenicum will need warm applications in order to feel better. Remember this and it is easy to tell the two apart.) So for ailments, from infections to arthritis, these are the symptoms that will guide the use of the remedy. It will be particularly useful in the home as a remedy for those with sore throats, for the patient who complains of burning in the throat, and if the throat itself looks red and glossy, and—this is important—if there is swelling present. The patient will be very thirsty for cold water, which will improve the pain in the throat. It all adds up to Apis.

Look for the Apis patient's personality to follow the physical symptoms. Because of the swelling and the heat, the patient will often feel that a portion of the body or that the whole body itself will burst. Like a bee, he may seem overly intense and to be "busy as a bee." He will want to keep moving. The patient will hurry about, driven by his pain. He may also want to keep talking, in spite of his pain. And he will talk and issue orders.

Apis patients are not angry patients, like Nux or Bryonia, nor are they particularly fussy like Arsenicum, but they will not suffer fools gladly. Apis patients will seem as if it is all that they can do to maintain an even keel. They will be too busy concentrating on their pain to put up with much from you, so they may appear somewhat short-tempered and irritable, but they will not strike out like Chamomilla patients will. They will, however, demand the things that they think that they need in order to get well. Therefore, they will demand cold drinks when they are thirsty and will become very aggressive if their needs are not met.

This same symptom portrait will be in place for Apis patients who are having troubles with allergies, especially for those who are experiencing an acute allergic response. Think of this remedy first for those who go into shock as an allergic response. Of course, this is especially true for those who are allergic to bee stings, but it is also very true in cases of food allergies, those that create the Apis picture: swelling, redness, burning pains, and patients who are demanding. Most commonly, the swelling in cases of food allergies will take place around the patient's eyes. Apis is also a major remedy for hives, and for allergic reaction to puncture wounds.

As an acute remedy, Apis is often used for punctures. Remember that for the homeopath any insect bite is considered a puncture wound—just as if that wound had been made from the patient stepping on a nail. The Apis puncture wound will have the typical symptoms of Apis: it will be red and swollen, and will feel hot. (This will make it easy to tell Apis apart from Ledum, which is another of our great remedies for puncture wounds. The Ledum patient will have a wound that feels cold and the Apis patient will have a wound that feels hot. Both will, however, want to put cold things on the wound.) The patient will want to put cold things on the wound in order to soothe it. In fact, this desire for cold, from cold applications on wounds to cold water for a sore throat, is so common a symptom of Apis that if the patient does not want cold, it is likely not an Apis situation.

Another strong indicator of the remedy has to do with sides of the body. Apis is a right-sided remedy. This means that symptoms most often will begin on the right and move toward the left; either that, or the symptoms will be worse on the right side of the patient's body. In any case, the patient's symptoms will also migrate. They will move suddenly from one part of the body to another, apparently without rhyme or reason. (Apis is one of our most important remedies for pains that migrate. Pulsatilla is the other remedy that most often includes this picture.)

Apis is also a remedy to be strongly indicated by the presence of a rash that is bright red, and is better from cold applications. The patient will be worse from warm applications. It is also an important remedy for cases of measles in which the symptoms match the remedy portrait.

This is also an important remedy for sore throats. These can be dangerous because they involve tremendous swelling. The patient's throat can swell up so much that it will keep him from swallowing any solids, and he may have a good deal of difficulty with liquids too. The patient may even begin to choke from the swelling. While it is most common for the patient to crave cold water, it can happen that the Apis patient will have no thirst at all. Consider the remedy if the other symptoms of Apis match. Typically the pains associated with the sore throat will extend into the patient's ears on swallowing. The patient's tonsils may be swollen and red, and Apis should be kept in mind for cases of tonsillitis as well.

Apis should also be considered in cases that involve any inflammation of the eye, most especially when these inflammations include enlarged blood vessels and swelling of the eyelids. The patient will complain that his eyes burn and sting. The patient will feel both pain in the eyes and a decrease in the quality of vision if he looks at any flame, from a fireplace to candlelight. The patient also is worse when looking at anything that is white, and when moving the eyes from right to left.

Apis is also a useful remedy in many cases of joint pain. The pain may be caused by arthritis or by injury to the joint. Look for swelling of the joint. The joint will be worse for heat and better for cold. The pain is stinging in nature. Note that the heat of the joint is internal and the joint does not feel hot to the touch. If the joint feels hot to the touch, consider the remedy Belladonna instead of Apis.

Certainly Apis is the first remedy to consider in cases of bee sting, especially for those who are allergic to these stings. In cases of anaphylaxis, Apis is the first remedy to consider.

The symptom picture of this remedy includes a general aggravation of all symptoms at 3 P.M., at which time the patient may experience fever with chills. If the patient becomes thirsty at all, it is most usual at 3 P.M., during this period of chill.

The patient is worse in the heat and especially in a stuffy room. The patient is also worse for the heat of the bed. This is a patient, like a Sulphur patient, who kicks off the covers and wants to be left uncovered.

Warmth in general is the greatest aggravation for the Apis person; even the heat of a warm room will cause all the symptoms to get worse. The patient cannot bear a stuffy room. Even the mental symptoms will be worse for a stuffy room. The Apis patient will be better from cold in nearly any form: from a cold bath; from being uncovered; and from being outside in the cool open air.

The patient will also feel worse if he is made to lie down but will feel better when sitting up erect. He will usually want to move around and feels better afterward. This especially true for exercise in the open air. The Apis patient is also made worse from being touched, from any pressure, especially on swollen parts of the body.

Keynotes: The pains of Apis are characterized as being "burning, stinging, and sore" in nature. Look for the pains to suddenly migrate from one part of the body to another. Look for swelling of the area under the eyes; also swelling of the hands and feet, which will look puffy.

Look for the affected areas of the body to be red, swollen, and shiny. Look for the heat of fever to alternate with chill. Look for the patient to complain of a sensation of heat in the affected area. This heat will be internal in nature.

Aggravations: The Apis patient will awaken in aggravation, as will the Lachesis patient. He is worse from sleeping, and even worse for just lying down.

He feels much worse in closed, warm rooms. A hot room will be intolerable, as will hot applications. The Apis patient will also be worse from the warmth of the bed.

The patient is also made worse by getting wet. However, he will feel better by washing individual parts of the body (usually the face) with cold water.

The critical time of day for the Apis patient is late afternoon, usually around 3 P.M. He is also worse for pressure and will not want to be touched.

Ameliorations: The Apis patient will feel better from cold water, both by drinking it and bathing in it. He will want a cold bath, or a cold washcloth on the head.

Apis patients are also better for slight exertions, and should not be forced to remain lying down at all times. They will seek to change positions frequently, both when sitting and when lying down. They like to sit upright.

They are also improved by uncovering themselves. They will kick off their bed covers and will loosen their clothing. They are greatly improved by cool, open air.

Dosage and Potency: Apis may be used successfully in all potencies, although the 30C and 200C potencies are most common. Potencies of 1M and above should be considered in cases of severe acute allergy attack and in cases of shock reaction to bee stings.

The remedy bears repetition well and should be used as needed.

Relationships: Apis is a complementary remedy to Natrum Mur, which may be considered the constitutional equivalent for the remedy. It is also complementary in action to Pulsatilla and to Arsenicum.

It should be noted, however, that Rhus Tox is inimical to Apis and the two remedies should never be used back to back.

5. ARNICA MONTANA

Remedy Source: Vegetable Remedy. Arnica was used as an herbal remedy for centuries until it became a part of the homeopathic pharmacy. It is known that the Roman legion carried Arnica with them when they went into battle to use to help the wounded of both sides recover. Also, the Germans historically have been known to say that Arnica plants, commonly found on mountaintops, grow just where they are needed to help tend injuries from falling, tripping, skiing, and so on. Arnica, as an herbal remedy, is used both as a poultice and brewed as a tea.

The whole plant is used in the preparation of the remedy, with the roots, leaves, and flowers collected for potentization at the flowering-stage. As a homeopathic remedy, Arnica was created by Hahnemann.

Situations That Suggest Arnica: Physical trauma, blows and bruises, head injuries, concussion, arthritis after physical trauma, rheumatism, nosebleed, vertigo, strains and sprains, pains associated with childbirth, post-surgical pain, dental procedures. A very valuable remedy for the period of home recovery after heart attack or stroke.

Also influenza, pneumonia, gastritis, headaches, eczema and boils, nightmares, and emotional trauma.

Remedy Portrait: If there is one remedy that is universally suggested as the best starting point for homeopathic treatment, it is Arnica. This is true because the situations in which Arnica is useful seem simple enough to identify. It is also true because this remedy seems almost miraculous in its action. You only have to ask a homeopath to tell you about the first time he used Arnica to set his eyes aglow as he starts to relate three or four hours' worth of true-life adventures in homeopathy.

Arnica is a wonderful acute remedy. It speaks to so many of the aches and pains and blows and bruises to which we are all victim. It is also an important constitutional remedy as well. In fact, Arnica has so many uses that, at times, one might be tempted to throw out the other remedies and just give everyone Arnica.

When we think of Arnica, we think first and foremost of physical trauma. This is the first remedy to think of in situations in which there has been a blow to the body. Whether that means that your child has fallen from the swing set, or you have tripped on the stairs, or another loved one has been mugged, Arnica is the remedy of first choice.

But we want to avoid the allopathic mindset here. While the picture of Arnica extends to nearly all mechanical injuries, we have to be sure that the patient in his total symptom picture matches the remedy's symptom picture. When we think about Arnica, we do not just think about the patient who has a bruise—there are probably a good ten or twelve remedies for those with bruises—we think about the patient who is in the Arnica state.

The first part of this is shock. Arnica is the first-choice remedy for those who are in shock. Think of the patient as being on a seven-second delay. You ask him a question, and you see that he is a little disconnected from what happened. He is not quite sure of his own state of health.

The Arnica patient is commonly known to insist that he is fine and that he needs no help. Kent tells us that the Arnica patient will send the doctor home, assuring him that he is fine. There is a form of denial in Arnica, denial of the patient's own condition. You may be puzzled by the patient, therefore. He has received an injury, but says that he is well. How can you know whether to treat him or not?

A way to tell if the patient needs Arnica or not is by gently attempting to touch the injury. The Arnica person is terrified of being touched, and is terrified by even the idea of pain. Kent says, "You will see the old grandfather sit off in a corner of the room, and, if he sees little Johnny running toward him, he will say, 'Oh, do keep away.' Give him a dose of Arnica and he will let Johnny run all over him."

Another keynote to the remedy has to do with body temperature. The Arnica patient's head will be very hot and his body will feel very cold. All the patient's extremities especially will be very cold. And it is a keynote symptom of Arnica that the tip of the patient's nose will feel very cold after injury.

Look for the patient to say that he feels bruised. The sensation of the pain will be bruising, even if the situation at hand does not have to do with physical trauma. For instance, headaches that can be helped by a dose of Arnica have the same bruising pain as would a head injury.

The Arnica patient will be in a state of extreme sensitivity. Look for the patient to complain that he cannot get into a comfortable position, that his chair or bed is too hard, that everything is too hard. To get the idea, think of the Princess in Hans Christian Andersen's story "The Princess and the Pea." Like that royal daughter, the Arnica person will find that, if you put one uncooked pea at the bottom of a pile of twenty mattresses, he will not be able to sleep because the mattress is just too hard. Like the princess, the Arnica person is too sensitive to touch. The touch of a human hand, or to the touch of a mattress, a chair, or even clothing, can likewise be too hard to bear.

Of particular sensitivity for the Arnica person is the region of the abdomen. The pelvis and uterus are particularly sensitive. Pregnant women who feel the movement of the fetus, which makes them feel sore and bruised, find great comfort in Arnica. It is also useful in cases of abdominal gas and bloating.

Arnica is also very helpful for cases of sprains, and/or general injuries, bruises, and shocks, particularly for injuries to joints. A sprained ankle, for instance, can be almost miraculously cured just with Arnica, a dose of which may allow the patient to put his full weight back on the ankle instantly.

Arnica can also be used to prevent pain. It is always a good idea to take a dose before visiting your dentist. Arnica used after dental procedures and surgery will also aid in the quick healing of that physical trauma. And, as Arnica is also a very useful remedy for situations in which the patient has overexerted himself, it is a useful remedy to take when returning to aerobics class after an absence of several years. In fact, the middle-aged among us who are trying to get back in shape once more after a decade of ignoring our physical condition need to keep Arnica on hand to deal with the traumas that we are likely to face—emotional and physical—as we work our way back to a physical peak.

Arnica is also an important remedy for use when a patient is home, recovering from either a heart attack or stroke, most especially in situations in which the left side of the body has some paralysis, with a full and strong pulse, and in which the patient sighs often and mutters quietly. Look for this patient to have a red face.

Arnica may be taken orally or used topically, and most health food stores will sell the remedy both ways. If all you have is the pellet form, you can simply dissolve the remedy in water and apply the remedy topically to the injured part of the body, giving the remedy orally at the same time. But please make note that Arnica should never be used topically on any injury that involves broken skin. While Arnica will do no lasting harm, it will hurt like hell. In fact, those who make this mistake once will never make it again. Instead, the remedy Calendula can be very helpful topically for injuries that involve broken skin—scratches, scrapes, cuts, and the like—but Arnica will only work on blows, bruises, sprains, and other injuries in which the skin is whole and healthy, although in either case the remedy may be taken internally to speed healing.

Keynotes: The patient needing Arnica is in shock. Therefore, look for him to insist that he is fine. Look for the patient to also be a little slow in answering, as if he is on a seven-second delay.

Look for the patient to feel sore, lame, and bruised. The patient will feel like he has been beaten. The whole body will be oversensitive.

Look for a hot head and a cold body, or a hot head and cold hands and/or feet.

Look for the patient to feel that the surface upon which he is lying is too hard, that everything is too hard. The patient will therefore keep moving or changing position in search of a soft place.

Aggravations: The patient will feel worse after too much rest, will feel worse if the surface lain upon seems too hard. He will feel worse when lying on one side too long, worse from any touch.

The patient will also be worse from wine, and from cold and damp.

The patient will be worse from blowing his nose.

Ameliorations: The patient is made better by cold, open air. He is also improved by uncovering his body and from changing positions when sitting or lying. He is also better when lying down with his head hung low.

Dosage and Potency: Arnica is given in all potencies, from the low-potency topical rub to the highest dilutions. It is considered that 30C, 200C, and 1M are the most common potencies for acute circumstances. The higher potencies are most often used in cases of old injuries that have never healed. The topical rubs are helpful in simple aches, pains, and strains.

In recent injury, the remedy may be repeated as needed, and the potency may be increased until improvement begins. Old injuries respond best to single doses of Arnica.

Relationships: Consider using Arnica with Aconite, Veratrum, Hepar Sulph, Hypericum (with which it works especially well), Ruta, and Bellis. Arnica also is often used with Rhus Tox, and Rhus often completes the healing action begun by Arnica.

6. ARSENICUM ALBUM

Remedy Source: Mineral Remedy. The substance arsenic was for a very long time an important part of the allopathic pharmacy. The remedy Arsenicum Album was created, not just from arsenic alone, but from a chemical compound of arsenic and oxygen. It was created as a homeopathic remedy by Samuel Hahnemann and was one of his first and most important discoveries.

Situations That Suggest Arsenicum: Mental disorders: anxiety, neurosis, obsessive behavior, compulsive behavior, depression, panic attacks; allergy: shingles, seasonal allergies, hay fever, food allergies, environmental allergies; respiratory infections of all sorts: bronchitis, influenza, pneumonia, pharyngitis, isophagitis, colds. Also fever, chronic fatigue; digestive disorders: colitis, food poisoning, irritable bowel, chronic diarrhea; insomnia.

Remedy Portrait: The Arsenicum patient is pretty easy to spot. Despite the fact that that patient might be suffering from any number of ailments, the common thread to these ailments is fear. The Arsenicum patient is afraid. He is afraid that he will die from his illness, whatever it is and however mild an illness it might be. He is afraid of death, and most particularly that death is near at hand. And he is afraid to be alone. It is an important feature of this remedy picture that the Arsenicum patient will actually grow sicker and his symptoms will increase if he is left alone.

Another important aspect of this remedy picture is that the patient will be worse around midnight, particularly during the hours from midnight until 2 A.M. Not only will the Arsenicum patient be most afraid at this time, and most unwilling to be left alone, but he will also have an increase in his physical pain. Even an Arsenicum patient who has fallen asleep in the earlier part of the night might awaken at midnight. He will feel sure that he is going to die. He will also feel sure that there is a stranger in the house, that someone has come to rob him, that someone has come to harm him. The Arsenicum that awakens at midnight might be awake for the rest of the night, as he keeps watch over his house and his health.

The Arsenicum patient is among our most depleted patients. His vital force is depleted. In fact, it may be all but exhausted. And yet, Arsenicum patients are restless patients. (They are among Nash's "restless trio" of Arsenicum, Rhus Tox, and Aconite.) Arsenicum patients will not just go and lie down. In fact, they may be afraid do so, because in their minds, they would by lying down to die. (When they are very ill and very depleted, however, Arsenicums will go and lie down, and will cover themselves up with many blankets and then they will lie perfectly still. This is a sign of deep illness in Arsenicums. It is not a good thing.) Instead, Arsenicums will fuss. In fact, they are among our fussiest patients. They go to bed, and settle in for a moment until they decide that they want some tea. They make their tea and go back to bed, after doing the dishes, only to stop to straighten a picture on a wall. And on and on. In and out of bed, fussing with their blankets and bedclothes. They may not even be aware that they are doing this, that they are constantly fussing, but they keep on, exhausting themselves even further as they refuse to just relax.

The Arsenicum patient is also a very chilly patient. He feels cold down deep inside. He will want to be warmed and be comforted. He may use the word *cozy* in describing his goal. This patient knows that if he just can get warm, all will be well. And the Arsenicum can get warm. This is one of the ways that you can tell him apart from the Nux Vomica patient, who is also cold but who can never get warm. The Arsenicum, if he is in a warm room—which he craves—and huddled under enough blankets, will begin to get warm. And it will be as if he begins to melt. As he grows warm, he becomes calmer, softer, and easier to deal with. It is one of the important tricks in dealing with the Arsenicum patient. Help him to get warm and he will let you leave for a few minutes.

The exception to this rule is the Arsenicum's head. Often, especially during a headache, the Arsenicum will want his head uncovered and exposed to cold, fresh air. So here is the picture of the Arsenicum patient: a person wrapped up warmly in blankets, sitting in a comfortable chair by a window that has been cracked open so that fresh air will blow on his face. If you are in that picture, sitting nearby, keeping company and standing guard, then we have the closest thing to happiness that is possible for the Arsenicum patient.

Think of this remedy for all sorts of common ailments, especially upper-respiratory illnesses. Think of Arsenicum for the patient whose cold begins on the right side and moves left—Arsenicum is a right-sided remedy—also for the patient whose cold is worse on the right side of the body and whose throat hurts worse on the right than it does on the left. Also consider Arsenicum for the patient who has an earache on the right side, or whose head hurts on the right side.

And look for the Arsenicum patient with an upper-respiratory ailment to complain of burning pains. An Arsenicum patient will always experience burning sensations in the affected parts of his body. And yet, these pains, like all the aches and pains in the Arsenicum patient, will be relieved by warm applications and by the patient becoming warm. Arsenicum belongs to Nash's "burn trio," along with Phosphorus and Sulphur. These three remedies are known for their burning pains. Among them, only Arsenicum has burning pain that is relieved by warmth.

During the cold or flu, look for the patient to have a good deal of nasal discharge and for that discharge to be thin and watery. This will also be true in cases of hay fever that are treated by Arsenicum. The discharge may burn the skin around the nose. The nose may also bleed during this discharge. The patient will say that his nose feels stopped up. He sneezes and sneezes, but it brings no relief. The nasal symptoms will be worse when the patient is in the open air, and better when he is in a warm room.

The patient's eyes will also tear profusely and those tears will burn as well. Look for the patient's eyes to be red-rimmed. You will often see swelling around the eyes as well. The patient's eyes will be light-sensitive. The patient may also say that he feels as if he has glass or some other sharp object in his eyes.

Just looking at the patient's face will give you some indication of the remedy. The Arsenicum patient will have a face that is pale or yellow in color. It may appear a bit swollen. The skin of the face will feel cold, and it may be covered by a cold sweat. The patient's mouth will be dry. His tongue will be dry and clean and red or blue in color. The patient will complain of a metallic taste in the mouth.

The patient may also have swelling in his throat, which will also take on a red or blue color. He will have difficulty in swallowing, especially in swallowing solid food. He will, however, be very thirsty. Arsenicum is one of our thirstiest remedies. The patient is most usually thirsty for warm things; in fact, he especially likes tea with lemon—anything with lemon, actually. The Arsenicum patient may also want cold liquids, so the temperature of his desired drink is not a solid clue to the remedy. The clue is the manner in which he drinks. The Arsenicum, thirsty as he is, will only sip his drink. He will only drink a little at a time, but he will drink frequently.

The Arsenicum patient usually will not want to eat, however. Arsenicum is one of our most important remedies for cases of intestinal flu and food poisoning. Either way, the Arsenicum patient will be nauseous. He will not be able to bear either the sight or the smell of food, and he will be made worse by eating. The only items that he may want are coffee and other acidic beverages. Consider this remedy in cases of heartburn in which the patient brings up acid and bitter tastes from his stomach. Consider it also for cases of indigestion that are caused by the patient eating ice cream. Also for indigestion brought on by vinegar, ice water, or tobacco. The indigestion can also be brought on by the patient eating fruit, especially watery fruits like melon.

This is a remedy to consider in cases of diarrhea and also cases of vomiting, but most especially in cases where the two are combined. Think of Arsenicum for flus in which the patient does not know which end of his body to aim at the toilet first.

In either case, the patient will complain of burning pains in the abdomen, a terrible colic. He will say that it feels as if he has live coals in his intestines. The patient's abdomen will be enlarged and swollen. The area of the patient's liver may be swollen and sensitive to touch as well. The pain in the region of the abdomen will be increased each time the patient coughs.

In cases of diarrhea, the stool will be very dark and may be bloody as well. The diarrhea will usually be accompanied by, or preceded by, a chill that centers in the area of the abdomen. After the stool, the body will be as cold as ice. All bouts of diarrhea will weaken the patient.

The patient's vomit, too, will usually contain some blood. It, too, will be dark-colored and may also contain green mucus. The patient will vomit up anything that he eats.

Look for the Arsenicum patient to experience heart palpitations. He will also feel as if he is going to faint. This patient will not want to lie down, as he will be afraid that he will suffocate if he lies down. Consider this remedy as well for any condition in which the patient has trouble breathing, fears suffocation, and cannot lie down. This patient will also complain of a burning sensation in the chest and, possibly, in his lungs. Consider this remedy for cases of asthma that match the symptom picture, especially for asthma patients who are worse after midnight.

Also consider Arsenicum for patients with rheumatic pains, especially when these pains are accompanied by trembling, twitching, and muscle spasms. The Arsenicum patient will feel weak. He will feel that the muscles in his limbs are weak. He will have cramps, especially in his calves. He will suffer all sorts of sciatic pains, especially burning pains. Look for the patient's feet to be swollen.

Finally, think of Arsenicum in cases of fever—for high fevers that exhaust the patient, for high fevers that alternate with cold sweats. These fevers will be worse after midnight. The patient will be restless from the fever and may thrash about. He may be delirious from his fever. The Arsenicum patient will also have disturbed sleep—he will dream dreams that upset him and are filled with worrying things and terrible images.

The Arsenicum will have to have his head raised in order to sleep without fear of suffocation. He will stack up his pillows in order to sleep.

Keynotes: Look for the patient to be depressed, anxious, and irritable. Look for a fear of death, and look for the patient to be sure that his present condition, no matter how mild it may be, will lead to his death. He will be emotionally anxious but will be too weak to move.

Look for burning pains. The affected parts of the body will feel as if they are on fire, and yet the patient is made worse for cold things, and wants warm drinks and applications.

Look for difficulty in breathing; for asthmatic breathing. Look for difficulty with digestion and elimination. Look for emaciation and exhaustion.

Aggravations: From night, especially midnight. Typical aggravation takes place from 1 until 2 A.M., although it can also occur at 1 to 2 P.M.

From cold, from cold food or drink, from cold applications, from cold air, from cold bathing.

Also from wet weather. From dampness in any form. By being at the seashore.

From lying on the painful side. From lying down with the head low. Also from movement. The patient is exhausted and is made worse by any exertion, especially from ascending stairs.

Ameliorations: From warmth. From warm food and drink. From warm rooms and warm bathing. From the warmth of bed. (*Note*: The headache of an Arsenicum is improved by cold applications and air.)

From company. The Arsenicum feels better in every way when he has people near him, especially if he is receiving a lot of attention.

From using many pillows. The Arsenicum will want his head supported and lifted up high. He will feel better after sleeping with pillows.

Dosage and Potency: It is important not to use this remedy in high potency for those with a weakened vital force. Therefore, it is used in low potencies of up to 30C for most conditions. High potencies are very useful in cases in which the characteristic fears dominate the portrait.

Arsenicum is repeated often in acute situations. In a crisis, it may be repeated as often as every fifteen minutes until improvement begins. In general circumstances, however, one dose of Arsenicum may be said to hold for up to thirty days.

Relationships: Arsenicum is one of our most important polycrests, and is therefore to be used both before and after nearly every other remedy in our homeopathic pharmacy. There are no remedies inimical to Arsenicum. Phosphorus, however, is particularly complementary to the remedy, as are Carbo Veg and Apis.

7. BELLADONNA

Remedy Source: Vegetable Remedy. Belladonna is taken from a plant that for many years has been used as an herbal medicine, Deadly Nightshade. As the name implies, the plant is indeed poisonous. Eating the plant creates symptoms similar to those that the remedy removes: high fever, fears, throbbing pain, and rage. It is interesting to note that the plant itself, like those who are treated by the remedy taken from it, is very sensitive to sunshine and prefers to grow in the shade.

The remedy is created from the whole plant, picked at the flowering stage. The remedy was created by Hahnemann.

Situations That Suggest Belladonna: Fever, migraine, convulsions. Also constipation, hemorrhoids, influenza, low back pain, sinusitis, tonsillitis, vertigo. Also Ménière's disease and otitis media. Consider for hallucinations, delirium, mania. Also sunburn, sciatica.

Remedy Portrait: The term *belladonna* means "beautiful woman," and refers to the wild look in the eyes that Belladonna produces. In the patient needing Belladonna, the homeopathic remedy, you will see an intensity that is lacking in the rest of us. The eyes seem deeper, larger, and wilder than human eyes.

In home use, we often equate Belladonna with fever. And, indeed, this remedy is a great blessing to the parent whose child has suddenly spiked a high fever. The patient's eyes are wild, the skin is dark or bright red, and it is very hot and dry to the touch. This is the most common picture of the remedy, and it will apply to fevers of all sorts, including sunburns, that come on quickly and leave the patient in a state of confusion or exhaustion.

But Belladonna is useful for many other different situations, making it one of our most important acute remedies. The two keynotes of the remedy have to do with speed and with intensity. Perhaps no other remedy, with the exception of Aconite, moves with the speed of Belladonna. All pains associated with the remedy come on suddenly and leave just as suddenly, and without warning. And all ailments associated with the remedy attack violently as well. The onset of an ailment that is suited to treatment by Belladonna will be a stunning thing: it is sudden, unpredictable, and wildly violent.

Thus, it is a good remedy for use in children's ailments, when the child reacts with heat, flushed skin, glaring eyes, and hypersensitivity of all senses.

The Belladonna response to the illness is that the patient will want to rest in a cool, dark, and quiet place. All the senses have been shoved up a notch by his pain. He will be especially sensitive to light and to noise and cannot bear either. In fact, his discomfort is such that he cannot bear using any of his senses. More than anything else the patient will want to sleep, but he will be unable to sleep. The pains of Belladonna are all associated with congestion and with throbbing. The patient is beset with throbbing pains that are driving him crazy and he cannot sleep. He will lie down and try to rest, but every time he dozes off, he will be startled into an awakened state. The patient will be startled by any sound, any light, or any motion. He will by startled by the throbbing pulse in his own body. The Belladonna patient is exhausted but cannot sleep.

Consider this remedy in any ailment that combines heat and dryness. The patient's skin will be very hot but it will stay dry. The patient's head especially will always stay dry. In the same way, no matter how high the patient's fever, there will be no thirst. Look for the patient, however, to complain that his feet are cold, no matter how hot the rest of his body may be.

The patient's skin will be red as well as hot, although this red color may alternate with pale, pale skin. The skin will be swollen as well, and also very sensitive to the touch. The patient will be startled unless touched very carefully.

Obiously, this is a good remedy to think of in cases of colds and flus that are accompanied by fever. It is also an excellent remedy to keep in mind for ailments that accompany or follow colds or flus. Remember this remedy for cases of conjunctivitis, for instance, in which the patient's eyes feel congested and have throbbing pain. This pain will become worse if the patient lies down. The eyes will be dry, and they will be very sensitive to light. The patient may see sparks of light in front of his eyes.

This is also an excellent remedy to consider for patients with pain in the external or middle ear, most especially if this pain is accompanied by swollen glands in the neck. The patient's hearing will be very acute. The patient may also hear his own voice echoing in his ear.

This is also a remedy for patients with nosebleed, especially for nose-bleeds that accompany fevers or colds. The bleeding will begin and end suddenly. The nose will be red and swollen. Other keynotes of the remedy will also be present: a throbbing sensation in the face and especially in the nose; a red skintone and heat accompanying the bleeding; and a sensation of a sudden rush of blood to the head preceding and accompanying the bleeding.

This sensation of congestion is very important to the remedy type. The patient will feel a sudden rush of blood to the affected area of the body. This sensation of congestion will be accompanied by throbbing. Most pains of any sort will be throbbing in nature.

Think of Belladonna in cases of sore throat and tonsillitis in which the tonsils are red and swollen and the patient's throat feels constricted, cases in which the patient has trouble swallowing. The pain will be made worse if the patient drinks any liquids. He will complain of scraping pains in his throat and will report that his throat feels dry.

The Belladonna patient will have a distended and hot abdomen as well. The whole area of the abdomen will be tender and swollen and must be touched with great care. The patient will complain of pains in the left side of the abdomen and of a cutting pain that moves across the region. The pain will be worse from any violent, quick motion, such as sneezing or coughing, and especially from touch. Even the touch of clothing will cause pain.

This is also a remedy to consider in cases of body aches and pains, rheumatic pains. These pains will be shooting in nature. The patient's limbs may jerk suddenly. He will complain of a sensation of coldness in his extremities. Look for the patient's joints to be red, swollen, and hot. Look for the patient's pains to shoot from the joints all along the limbs. As always, these pains will both appear and disappear suddenly and without warning.

Consider Belladonna for the patient with palpitations. The palpitations will be violent and sudden. They will reverberate into the patient's head. The patient will say that he feels as if his heart were too large. The patient's pulse will be rapid but weak.

Also consider this remedy for the patient who has vertigo. The patient will feel that he is falling either to the left side or backward. The vertigo will be accompanied by palpitations, or by a throbbing heat in the head. The vertigo will be worse when the patient rises from stooping.

This is, of course, an excellent remedy to consider for those with head-ache—if the headache is accompanied by a sense of congestion and by throbbing pains. The headache will be centered in the forehead but may extend to the back of the head or to the temples. The headache is worse from light, from sound, from motion, and from touch. The patient to rest in a semi-erect posture. He will not want to lie down flat. The pain will be improved by pressure. The headache may accompany a stopping up of the patient's nose. In that case, the headache will cease if the nose begins to flow. The headache will usually be worse on the right side. Think of this remedy for headaches that come on with colds or allergies, although our classic texts also note that this is the remedy for headaches that come on from having your hair cut.

Keynotes: Symptoms appear suddenly. Suddenness runs all through the remedy. Look for the patient to move his eyes quickly, looking from side to side, looking all around the room.

Redness is also common; particularly the head and face will become red. The skin will give off heat. The skin is dry.

This is a congestive remedy. Look for the patient to feel a flushing and a rush of blood to the affected area. The headaches, particularly, are congestive in nature. The headache will be accompanied by a red face.

Aggravations: There are many aggravations for Belladonnas. They are aggravated both by heat and by cold. Aggravated by cold wind, by any draft. Also by heat and by summer weather. Aggravation by the sun is quite common. Belladonna cannot bear strong light, particularly sunlight.

They are made worse by motion and by touch. They do not want even the slightest touch.

They are also sensitive to pain. They cry out in pain. They are made worse by lying on the painful side of the body.

They are worse at 3 P.M.; worse also at night, especially after midnight.

They are also worse from looking down, from bending their head forward. They are worse from stooping.

Ameliorations: They feel better from resting, especially from resting in a dark room. They are better in darkness in general.

They are better from standing or sitting upright, and are made worse by lying down. Patients will want to stay on their feet. Often, they will be unable to sit still because they are driven to move about by their pain.

They are better in a warm room, but will insist that it be neither too hot nor too cold. They feel better when their head is covered.

Dosage and Potency: Most often, Belladonna will be used in either the 30C or 200C potency, although it can be used in higher potencies quite effectively. In that the patient is so reactive to his pain, we often will want to give a 1M or higher potency from the very beginning, but remember that this strong yin or yang reaction to pain is common to the type and quite often the 30C will do the trick, even in cases of high fever. In fact, it has been my experience with the remedy that the lower potencies are actually more effective for most inflammatory conditions.

This is a short-acting remedy, and its benefits often hold for as little as a day. Therefore, be prepared to give more than one dose of the remedy, carefully watching not to give it before it is again needed.

Relationships: Belladonna is a complementary remedy to Calcarea Carbonica, which often is used to finish the cure that Belladonna has begun. The two remedies work well either before or after each other.

In that Belladonna's ailments come on suddenly, it is also used successfully with Aconite. But in this case, Aconite should be given before Belladonna and does not follow it well. Arsenicum, Sulphur, Lachesis, Nux Vomica, and Rhus Tox all follow Belladonna well and can complete the healing action begun by the remedy.

Dulcamara is a remedy that does not blend well with Belladonna's actions. The two remedies should not be used back to back.

8. BELLIS PERENNIS

Remedy Source: Vegetable Remedy. The remedy is created from the daisy. The mother tincture is created from the whole plant.

Burnett gives us our best look at the remedy and its uses.

Situations That Suggest Bellis: Physical fatigue, physical trauma, bruises, injuries in the spinal area. Also tumors, boils, and acne. Also headache, especially from injury; sleeplessness. Also rheumatic aches and pains. The pains associated with pregnancy and childbirth.

Remedy Portrait: This remedy is perhaps best thought of in terms of Arnica, in that it seems to have an action that is most similar to that remedy, but Bellis is deeper acting than is Arnica and is able to bring about healing in situations in which Arnica fails to act.

Think of Bellis in cases involving any sprain, bruise, or laceration that has generally weakened the patient. Most especially think of Bellis in cases in which Arnica has already been given, and has failed to work. (*Note*: Bellis is not the remedy of first choice—nor is Arnica—in cases in which an old bruise has failed to be reabsorbed by the body. In that case, think first of Calcarea Carbonica.)

Like Arnica, Bellis is also an excellent remedy for boils as well as for other growths, such as soft tumors, that appear on the skin. It has even be known to be effective in cases of malignant tumors.

Bellis, like Arnica, is also an excellent recovery remedy. It can be used in the period following childbirth to end pain and speed recovery. It can also be used before and during childbirth for the same reason, but here Arnica is the more common and, often, more effective choice during this time frame. (The keynote here is that if the woman cannot walk during pregnancy due to pain, the first remedy of choice is Bellis, otherwise, Arnica.)

In the same way, Bellis is an effective remedy—again, as is Arnica—during postsurgical recovery, greatly speeding healing and also reducing pain.

It is also a wonderful remedy for abscesses, wherever they might appear in the body, and for boils, which will both burn and itch. Bellis can also be used as a remedy for those with varicose veins, when the legs feel bruised and sore, from the pain. Bellis should also be thought of in cases that involve acne and eczema, when the condition of the skin is red and dry with blistering.

This is another general rheumatism remedy. It is considered to be the remedy of "old laborers," in that the pains appear over years of work and overwork. The Bellis rheumatic is the person who has used his body for hard labor over a period of years and now feels pain in the joints and muscles both. The limbs have a bruised feeling and are both cold and stiff. Often the patient will complain of a sensation of a band wrapped around a joint.

The pulse in Bellis is irregular. The rhythms will be off. Again, as with Arnica, this is a general heart remedy, to be considered in cases involving angina.

The patient will, in general, have a desire to move, to use his body, not in the restless manner of a Rhus, but in the manner of a person who is used to being strong and able and cannot bear to find himself weakened or in pain. Bellis patients will be somewhat slow mentally, as if they are having a hard time grasping any concept, but they will want to use their minds, as they do their bodies, and will tend to be somewhat keyed up over their own slowness. They are aware that their mind is sluggish and this upsets them.

Finally, but perhaps most important, this is a remedy that excels in situations involving trauma to tissues. It is also for deep muscle pain and for the sensation of soreness and bruising. The sensation of pain also seems to run along the nerves, as with Hypericum. The pain here is improved by applications of cold water. Bellis is a wonderful remedy for injuries that involve swelling. It is a remedy specific to the area of the pelvis and is extremely helpful in injuries to the pelvis. It is for this reason that it is such a help in the recovery from childbirth.

Keynotes: As with Arnica, the sensation of soreness or of having been bruised (whether or not that is actually the case) is keynote to the remedy Bellis. It is also important to note that the aches and pains here are improved by cold applications, which will often help separate the action of this remedy from that of Rhus Tox, which it can closely resemble.

Also keynote is the remedy's action in the area of the pelvis. Therefore, it is the remedy of first choice for trauma in that area, from accident, attack, surgery, or childbirth. For this reason, Bellis should also be considered an excellent remedy for injury to the coccyx, and for any fall that injures the pelvis.

Look for the patient to awaken at 3 A.M. and not to be able to sleep again until 5 A.M. Expect dreams of anger, and expect the patient to be excitable over his condition. The greater the pain, the more excitable the patient.

Finally, it is keynote of this remedy that illness comes on from taking cold drinks when the patient is overheated. While this is a solid general indicator for the remedy, it is also a great fun fact that Bellis is the remedy of choice for ice cream headaches.

Aggravations: The patient will be worse from warmth, worse from any application of heat, worse from a hot shower or bath. He will feel worse especially when he becomes cold after a hot bath.

Like Arnica, the Bellis patient is also worse from any touch. He will not want to be touched and will become very excited and animated if you are about to touch his wound.

Bellis patients are worse before storms and will, in their rheumatic complaints, often be able to predict the approach of a storm by their "trick knee" or other painful joint. They are especially bad when the storm also involves a cold wind.

They do not wish to remain totally still and are worse if immobilized. If at all possible, the patient should be allowed some sort of mobility. They are worse when lying on their left side.

Ameliorations: The Bellis patient will feel better, as will the Rhus Tox, from continuous, gentle motion.

He will also feel better if he himself is allowed to place gentle pressure on the painful areas of his body. For instance, the Bellis patient with a headache will be discovered pressing on his head, or pressing his head against the wall.

Bellis patients are also better for a cool environment and from cool applications to the body.

They are also improved by eating. They tend to have an insatiable hunger and will crave exotic and spicy foods.

Dosage and Potency: Bellis is most often used in the 30C potency, which suits all of its activities. It is also often used topically in the mother tincture.

It bears repetition well and may be repeated as needed.

Relationships: Obviously, the remedy most related to Bellis is Arnica. And Bellis is often used in follow-up to Arnica in situations in which Arnica has failed to complete the case.

Bellis is also used with Hypericum, Calendula, and Staphysagria in recovery from trauma and postsurgical recovery. Although it is seldom mentioned in homeopathic literature, Bellis is also a remedy that complements Ignatia in the treatment of grief and emotional pain. Like Arnica, it may be given in a single high-potency dose to clear away the ill effects of traumatic news or circumstances.

9. BRYONIA ALBA

Remedy Source: Vegetable Remedy. Bryonia is created from wild hops. The mother tincture is made from the roots of the plant, which must be picked just before the first flowering.

Bryonia was created by Samuel Hahnemann.

Situations That Suggest Bryonia: Consider for influenza, bronchitis, pneumonia, cough. Consider strongly for constipation, diarrhea, gastritis. Also toothache, nosebleed, headache, migraines, coma, vertigo. Also rheumatoid arthritis, physical trauma, tendonitis, connective tissue disease, low back pain, sciatica, bursitis.

Remedy Portrait: The Bryonia patient has been called the "Bryonia bear." And the patient has earned this name. When you disturb a Bryonia at rest, it is as if you had disturbed a bear in hibernation. You will regret it. Bryonia patients want to lie very still. They do not want to move at all. In fact, a patient with a Bryonia headache may find that it hurts even to move the eyes. Therefore, the Bryonia will want to lie down and be left alone. The motion of looking at another person, of having to talk, especially to answer questions about his case, just makes all his aches and pains worse. And that makes him very angry.

Bryonia patients are angry and irritable. You may confuse them with Nux patients, in that both are far better left on their own if they are sleeping. If it can be avoided at all, neither should be awakened when sleeping. Both of these patients will be constipated—perhaps chronically constipated. But the differences in the ways in which they display their symptoms will help the homeopath to tell them apart.

Bryonia patients will experience dryness in all mucous membranes. These will be thirsty patients, but because of the pain that they associate with movement of any sort, look for Bryonias to drink infrequently. And, when they do, look for them to drink great amounts of water.

These patients are also very concerned with work. In this way, they are similar to Calcarea and to Nux, both of whom will talk on and on about all the things they should be doing, all the reasons why they should get up out of bed and go to work. Bryonia patients will certainly do this as well. They may even try to get up from bed and go to work, but they will be unable to do so. The aggravation that they feel from any motion will put a stop to their desire for work, as will their overwhelming sense of vertigo.

Always consider Bryonia in cases involving vertigo. The patient will experience vertigo, usually accompanied by nausea, upon getting up. These patients will feel faint, and feel confused when they rise.

Bryonia is a remedy for patients with headache. Patients will complain that they feel as if there is a hammer inside their head that is slamming against their brain. The headache may begin in any part of the head, but the pain will center in the occiput, the back of the head. Bryonia may also be considered a remedy for the traditional sinus headache that is characterized by pain in the forehead and pressure and congestion in the frontal sinuses. In all cases of headache, the Bryonia patient will be worse from motion of any sort, even from moving the eyeballs.

Bryonia is a major remedy for those with flu, for the body aches and pains associated with influenza. Again, these pains will be made worse by any motion. Patients will suffer abdomal distress as well. They will feel tenderness and swelling in the region of the liver. They will complain of tenderness in the walls of their abdomen. Patients will complain of burning pains all through the region and the pains will be made worse by motion or any form of pressure.

Consider Bryonia for any ailment that is accompanied by stubborn constipation. In the Bryonia case, again, as with the Nux case, constipation will accompany nearly any other set of symptoms. The patient's stool will be brown, thick and dry, as if it were burnt. It may also be bloody.

The Bryonia patient will likely experience nausea as well. The patient's stomach will be sensitive to touch and to pressure. The patient will be made worse by eating. He will complain after he eats that it feels as if there is a stone in his stomach.

The patient's throat will be dry and constricted, similar to the conditions found in the Belladonna's throat. He will feel that anything he swallows will get stuck in his throat due to its extreme dryness. Look for the patient to have mucus in the throat, tough mucus that is very difficult for the patient to move. He has to cough hard to bring up the mucus, and the motion of coughing brings on pain.

The patient will experience discomfort throughout the throat and respiratory system. Bryonia patients are bothered by a dry, hacking cough that gives them no peace. They will have to sit up to stop coughing and will experience vertigo when they sit up.

As the Bryonia patient is thirsty but has to wait a long time until he can finally move to drink, he is also in great need of a deep breath. The Bryonia will breathe as shallowly as possible so as to keep from feeling pain, but he actually craves being able to take a deep breath. He will feel that he must expand his lungs fully. And so, from time to time, the Bryonia patient will take a long, deep breath that, while it soothes his need to breathe, will cause him physical agony.

Because of this aggravation from motion, and because of the pain and pressure in the chest that is unique to this remedy, Bryonia should be considered the remedy of first choice in cases of cracked or broken ribs.

It should also be considered in cases in which the patient's knees are stiff and painful; also in cases of rheumatic pains, especially sciatica, in which the patient feels stitching and tearing pains in the affected parts.

The patient complains of stiffness and pain in the small of the back, which extends down the legs. The patient's feet will be swollen and hot. The left leg will be in constant motion during the pain. The patient's left arm may also be in motion.

Look for the Bryonia patient's skin to take on a yellow color. His skin will be pale, his hair will be greasy. Look for the affected areas of the body to become swollen and tender.

Bryonia is a remedy for ailments that come on in hot weather. Consider it for any abdominal pain or colic that comes on when the patient becomes overheated in the summer and then eats or drinks something cold. Consider it for all cases of summer diarrhea. Look for the stool in this case to be brown and bloody. Look for the diarrhea to be worse in the morning, and worse if the patient moves.

Also consider this remedy for nosebleeds in the summer; these also will be worse in the morning. Often, the Bryonia nosebleed will relieve the patient's headache. Consider this remedy for any nosebleed that is accompanied by swelling in the tip of the patient's nose, especially when the nose itself is tender to the touch.

In general, the Bryonia patient will always be worse from motion, and worse from coming into a warm room. His pulse will be full, hard, and quick. The patient will have external chilliness but will have a sensation of internal heat. He will be given to sweating, especially during fever.

Bryonia patients are sleepy patients. They will want to be left alone to lie still and rest. It is best for everyone that they be allowed to do so.

Keynotes: The major guiding symptom of this remedy type is that Bryonias do not want to move. They demand absolute rest and will become very angry if they are told that they need to move. Bryonias many even experience pain from the movement of the eye.

This need for rest will be on the emotional as well as the physical level. They tend to want to be left alone in silence. They will not want to answer questions or make decisions.

Look for them also to experience an amelioration of symptoms when lying on their painful side. They will want to put weight and/or pressure on their painful spots.

Look for Bryonia patients to be very thirsty. They will drink a great deal of water at one time and then will not drink again for many hours.

Aggravations: Motion, of any sort, no matter how gentle. Think of this as the remedy for persons with cracked ribs. If you have any idea of how painful those are, you will understand. Every motion, every touch brings on agony.

Bryonia patients are particularly worse from any ascending motion. They are worse from sitting up—which will cause them to feel either faint or sick or both. The motion of changing from the lying position to the sitting position is very difficult.

Because of their trouble with motion in general, anything that jostles them causes pain: coughing, sneezing, and swallowing can be particularly difficult. In that they are also made worse by fasting, the swallowing issue can be particularly tricky.

They are also made worse from closing their eyes, and from sleeping. Given this, it is to be expected that morning would be the worst time of day for Bryonias.

They are also worse from warmth and cannot bear the thought of a too-warm room. Their symptoms are worse in summer.

Ameliorations: Bryonia patients are better when lying on the painful side and when putting their weight on the painful area of their body.

They are better for quiet, for rest, and better in a darkened room.

They are better for cool things: cool temperatures, cool open air, and cool food and drink.

They feel much better when they belch.

Dosage and Potency: All potencies are used. Lower potencies, 30C most commonly, are used for simple flus and other inflammatory conditions. Chronic digestive ailments often call for higher potencies.

This remedy is short-acting and often calls for repetition. Clarke tells us that one dose usually lasts from seven to twenty-one days.

Relationships: Bryonia and Rhus Tox work well together and often complete each other's actions in acute situations. Aluminia, a remedy that also speaks to chronic digestive disorders, particularly constipation, also works well with Bryonia.

Calcarea Carbonica does not work well with Bryonia and the two should not be used in conjunction with each other.

Bryonia is often used before or after Nux Vomica, which also speaks to digestive troubles. Carbo Veg and Sulph should also be considered in cases that have been improved but not cured by Bryonia.

10. CALCAREA CARBONICA

Remedy Source: Mineral Remedy. Calcarea Carbonica is taken from calcium carbonate, derived from the middle layers of oyster shells.

It was created by Hahnemann.

Situations That Suggest Calcarea: Digestive disorders and malnutrition; heartburn; constipation; functional disorders and immune dysfunctions: chronic fatigue, environmental poisonings, night sweats; allergies: rhinitis, food allergies, sinusitis, acute asthma; respiratory disorders and inflammations: colds, flu, bronchitis, otitis media, pharyngitis; PMS; connective tissue disorders: low back pain, sciatica, rheumatoid pain, and rheumatoid arthritis; skin diseases: acne, eczema, rash; anxiety and related disorders: phobia, depression.

Remedy Portrait: If there is a homeopathic remedy that can be considered a general tonic, it is Calcarea. As the remedy is taken from the calcium that builds the bones in our bodies, it is a particularly benign remedy, one that works simply and wonderfully well. But, given all this, we must still make certain that we use this remedy, as well as any other homeopathic remedy, only when it is called for, and only when the symptoms of this remedy match those that the patient is already experiencing.

The constitutional Calcarea is an overweight, somewhat slow patient. He is slow in body and in mind. And this theme will carry over to those who need the remedy on an acute level as well. Look for this patient to feel a weight, not only in the head but in the mind as well. He will complain of a weight in the head, and may even say that he is having trouble holding his head up, in supporting it on his neck. In the same way, the patient will feel as if his mind is being weighted down as well. This patient will feel as if he is not thinking clearly, or functioning mentally at his best.

Look for Calcareas to be apprehensive patients. They may feel that they are losing their mind. The fact that they cannot think clearly will bother them a great deal. They may feel that they have no time to be ill, that there is work that they should be doing. Like Bryonias, Calcareas may talk about work a great deal, and may seem to alternate between feeling that they are shirking on their work responsibilities and a sense of relief that because they are sick they don't have to work at all.

Often, Calcarea patients will have become sick in the first place because of overwork. In the acute case, Calcareas may have gotten a cold or flu due to overwork. They do not sleep enough and feel constantly over-whelmed by their responsibilities. If they continue the pattern and move into more of a constitutional state, look for Calcarea patients to have one bout of acute illness after another, to always be a bit ill.

When Calcareas become ill, when they can use this illness as a reason to not work, they will often become totally averse to work or to any form of mental exercise. They will want to operate on a very simple level. They will want to watch television and read magazines. Any sort of mental exertion will cause palpitations and anxiety. Suddenly they will complain that their head is becoming very hot.

The head is the site of many of the Calcarea symptoms. Except for the moments of mental exertion, the patient will have a cold head. His whole body, in fact, will tend to be chilly. The right side of the patient's head especially will be cold. The patient's scalp will itch as well, and it will sweat. It is keynote of this remedy that the patient's head will be covered with sweat, especially during sleep. The patient will awaken with a wet pillow.

Digestive symptoms will also be pronounced. Look for the patient to have a strong aversion to meat but to crave eggs. (The Silicea patient will also crave eggs—it is one of the many symptoms that the two remedies have in common—but the Calcarea will digest these eggs well and will be very happy that he ate them. The Silicea will become sick after eating the eggs.) The Calcarea may also crave a variety of things that would not be considered food—look for them to eat chalk, paste, pencils, even dirt. He will also want to eat salty things. And he will also crave sweets of all sorts.

Calcareas are patients with good appetites, except for the times in which they feel totally exhausted. Then they may lose their desire to eat alto-gether.

Calcareas will tend to have frequent heartburn. Look for them to belch and burp a good bit. They will have a sensation of pressure in their stom-ach. They will have a sour taste in their mouth. Look for the region of the patient's stomach to swell, to form into a rounded dome. Patients will feel cramps throughout their abdomen. These cramps will be worse from pressure and from drinking cold water.

Calcareas will crave cold water. It does not sit well with them but they want it badly. They will also tend to like cool or cold foods. Hot foods will nauseate them. Calcarea patients are made worse by eating. They will go into an aggravtion of symptoms while they are still eating.

This swelling of the stomach is an important symptom. In fact, look for

Calcareas to have swelling throughout their body. Look for patients to have swelling of the upper lip, also swelling at the root of the nose, and swelling of all affected parts of the body.

Consider this remedy for patients whose faces have become very pale. They will have dark rings around their eyes. Look for swollen glands in their necks that are also tender, and look for these glands to stay a bit swollen for a long time.

Calcareas are sensitive patients. They are sensitive to light, and sensitive to their environment. They get chilly very easily. They will become sicker if they stay chilly. These patients need to be warm. Their feet will be especially vulnerable to cold. Look for Calcarea patients to have cold, wet feet. Their feet may sweat so much that their socks become wet as well. Calcareas must keep their feet warm and dry, and if they can do this one thing, they will feel much better.

The Calcarea will always feel worse in cold weather, and especially in cold, wet weather. Rheumatic pains of all sorts are common in the Calcarea who has become wet. Look for all sorts of illnesses after exposure to cold and wet weather. Look for the patient to have pain between his shoulder blades and a sensation of pain and weakness in the lower back. The patient will complain of cramps in the calves. He will also complain of knee pain, and especially he will feel as if his knees will give out from under him when he climbs stairs. He will complain of a sensation of weakness in all his extremities. He will say that his feet feel cold and dead, especially at night when he is in bed. He will also complain of a weakness in the ankles, as if they, too, will give out from under him. Calcarea is a remedy to be strongly considered in cases in which old sprains, and even old bruises, will not heal but just keep getting a little better and then a little worse.

This is the tonic aspect of the remedy. Consider Calcarea for the patient who seems unable to totally kick any acute ailment, who never seems to be quite well again. This will especially be true for the patient who seems to take on the ailment again after becoming cold and wet, or who becomes ill again every winter.

Calcarea is a remedy for the patient who has diarrhea or constipation, and especially for the patient in whom both alternate and in whose system the conditions seem to be becoming chronic. The patient will feel swelling and pressure in the abdomen. He will be unable to bear any sort of tight clothing in the stomach area. And he will feel exhausted by his digestive upset. It is keynote of this remedy, however, that the patient will feel both better and happier, however, when he is constipated. During diarrhea, the patient will literally tremble with exhaustion.

Calcarea speaks to a wide range of respiratory ailments. Consider this remedy for patients who experience an ongoing tickling cough; also for those who have a condition of hoarseness that is painless. The cough and hoarseness will be worse in the morning. Look for these patients to only bring up mucus in the daytime, although they cough all day and night. Patients will have a sensation of suffocation. Their breathing will be worse when they climb stairs or undergo any form of ascent. Calcarea patients, even though they are chilly and vulnerable to cold, will want to breathe cold, fresh air.

Keynotes: Calcarea patients are chilly, sweaty, exhausted patients. They want to be warm, especially their feet, which are so often cold and clammy that classic homeopathic texts will say that they "feel like they are wearing wet socks." Their head may be hot, although many Calcareas have cold heads as well; but their head will be sweaty, Especially at night, when the pillow will be wet from their head sweat.

Calcareas feel exhausted, totally drained. They often have trouble breathing, and feel as if they cannot get enough air into their lungs, and this terrifies the patient.

Calcarea patients also are most often constipated. And they feel better when they are constipated.

Look for them to act a bit needy, to want attention, and to want to watch movies on the VCR when they are sick. They will want to cry at sad romantic movies and will feel better for crying. They will want to be taken care of, to have special meals made. They will not want to eat meat but will crave eggs. They tend to crave milk products as well when they are sick.

Aggravations: Calcarea patients are at their worst during the period just before they fall asleep. They are also worse from stretching, or from lifting anything with any weight to it.

They are worse after eating, and worse in the morning, when they feel their most exhausted.

They are worse for getting cold and worse from washing with cold water. They are much worse from getting wet, especially if their feet get wet or cold.

They are worse for any mental exertion; worse from having to tend to the needs of others.

Ameliorations: Calcareas are greatly improved in dry weather. They feel better when warm, and after sleeping.

Dosage and Potency: In acute situations, the lower potencies, especially from 6C to 30C, work well. The potencies of 1M and above are used only in constitutional treatments.

Calcarea does not repeat well if you stay with the same potency. It is better used in single doses of one potency and the potency then changed if the remedy needs repeating.

Relationships: As part of one of the most basic triads of remedies, Calcarea follows Sulphur well and precedes Lycopodium well. The order of these three remedies is important. Calcarea does not follow Lycopodium well, nor should it be given just before Sulphur.

Calcarea is complementary in action to both Rhus Tox and Belladonna. It both precedes and follows these remedies well, and any may complete the healing action of the other remedies.

Nux Vomica also follows Calcarea quite well in cases in which depletion is pronounced, such as cases of chronic fatigue syndrome.

Nitric Acid, while similar in action to Nux Vomica, does not relate well with Calcarea and should be given neither directly before nor after the remedy.

11. CALENDULA OFFICINALIS

Remedy Source: *Vegetable Remedy*. This remedy is created from the leaves and flowers of the marigold.

Situations That Suggest Calendula: Wounds, abrasions, cuts, scrapes. Also recovery after surgery, infected wounds, burns, sores, most especially infected sores of all kinds.

Remedy Portrait: The remedy Calendula is one of the first homeopathics that most of us discover. It is part of every homeopathic kit in the form of a salve that may be applied to almost every injury, certainly to every form of cut or scrape. It is a natural antiseptic as well as an astringent, and therefore it is one of our most important acute remedies. But Calendula is certainly far more than just an ointment; it has been potentized at every level, and is very useful both topically and orally.

Think of Calendula first when you are dealing with a patient who has any form of lacerated wound. It is especially important if the wound has become infected or is in danger of becoming infected. In such a case, Calendula will not only promote healing of the injury, but will heal the accompanying infection. Consider using Calendula both topically and internally, with the salve applied topically to the wound and a 30C dilution of the remedy taken internally at the same time. Calendula may also be used in combination with Hypericum and/or Arnica in emergency situations. While this is not good homeopathy, in that it breaks the Law of Simplex, I have seen enough clinical situations to know that it might well be necessary to bring the patient into healing. If the skin is not broken, one might decide to use the Arnica topically while taking the Calendula internally. Or the Calendula may be used topically while the Arnica is taken internally.

The remedies Calendula and Hypericum have a special affinity. Both promote healing to injuries, especially to lacerations. Hypericum is the remedy of choice in cases of nerve pain, in cases in which the patient will experience a pain that shoots all along a nerve. Calendula is a remedy for the general promotion of healing and the forestalling of infection. Therefore, in the case of a severe laceration, such as might be caused by a gunshot wound, both of these remedies will likely be called into play. Since the Calendula salve is very low potency in most cases, the patient may well need a stronger homeopathic dilution. Therefore, the remedy may need to be taken internally in a higher potency, or Aqua Calendula may need to be created by dissolving the potency pellet in pure water. Hypericum and Calendula may need to be alternated in the treatment of a patient with a severe laceration.

Calendula is also a very important remedy for stopping bleeding, and is therefore very useful for healing any sort of cut or incision. It is also an important remedy to use after dental surgery. In the case of dental surgery, the patient may swish Aqua Calendula around in his mouth to promote healing and soothe pain. In this situation, Calendula may again be used in alternation with Arnica, and the Arnica may be given in a high-potency pellet to bring about healing.

Note that I personally prefer to use Aqua Calendula instead of using the remedy in the form of a petroleum salve, or in its tincture form in an alcohol-based liquid. I find that it works best by simply dissolving the pellets in water and using this liquid both topically and internally. This method also give you the ability to select the potency of the remedy that is best for the situation at hand and does not force you to use the potency of the salve only.

Also note that while the salve is very gentle and soothing for scrapes, it should never be used for burns because the petroleum jelly base will seal the pain of the burn in and will increase pain and slow the healing process. For burns, Aqua Calendula again is the best bet. The alcohol-based liquid should never be used for conditions of dry skin or eczema; the alcohol itself will further dry the skin. Aqua Calendula is once more the best option for these conditions.

Calendula may also be of great comfort in patients with all sorts of joint pain. It should also be considered for patients with any sort of arthritis pain. The salve, liquid, and water-base may all be used very effectively and may allow the patient to avoid the use of topical cortisone, which itself can be highly suppressive and toxic to the whole system.

Look for the Calendula patients, who are likely to be in great pain, to be very irritable. They are usually easily frightened and very nervous, although some may be so overcome in their vital force that they become disconnected from reality, and appear sleepy. They tend to be very chilly from their pain, and, as they move into chill, they become very worried; they are sure that something terrible is about to happen. In that they are already wounded, it is important that persons needing this remedy place their fears not in the recent past or the present but in the future, as if something bad is about to happen.

In general, Calendula patients are in need of reassurance and will be improved with attention and with the reassurance that things will be all right. They are worse for cold, and need to be kept warm and to be soothed.

Keynotes: Calendula is keynote in cases of physical trauma, often in which there is a breaking of the skin. Allen tell us, "Calendula is almost specific for clean, surgical cuts of lacerated wounds, to prevent excessive suppuration." By that he means that the use of the remedy will not only promote healing but will also prevent the onset of infection of the wound.

The patient is in shock, is exhausted—possibly from loss of blood.

Aggravations and Ameliorations: There are no set aggravations or ameliorations for Calendula, in that, unlike the other remedies listed here, it is purely an acute remedy. Therefore, its use, unlike that of other remedies, is largely determined by the situation itself, by the nature of the trauma, and not by the behavior of the patient. Any wound may be treated internally and externally by Calendula.

Dosage and Potency: While Calendula is most often available in the form of a topical salve, it is also available in potencies of homeopathic tablets. And it may be used topically in addition to its internal use. All potencies are available and all are used.

Calendula is a short-acting remedy and will need to be repeated during recovery.

Relationships: Calendula is most similar in its action to Hypericum in that both speak to the pain of injuries to parts of the body that are rich in nerve endings. Both tend to feel pain as running along those nerves. Therefore Calendula is often used topically, while Hypericum is taken internally. It may be used in exactly the same manner in combination with Arnica or Bellis in cases involving physical trauma or postsurgical recovery.

Calendula is also very helpful when used topically while Hepar Sulph is taken internally. These remedies are combined in their actions when a wound has become infected and the patient's vital force is threatened.

12. CAMPHORA

Remedy Source: Vegetable Remedy. The remedy Camphora is taken from the gum of the *Laurus camphora*. From this, the remedy is made into a mother tincture and potentized.

Situations That Suggest Camphora: Ill effects of allopathic or homeopathic medicines. Also influenza with chills, fever with chills, pneumonia, measles. Also diarrhea with cramps. Also arthritis. Also sunstroke, headache, fainting, chronic fatigue syndrome, insomnia.

Remedy Portrait: Think of those television commercials for toothpaste in which the people brush their teeth and then suck air into their mouths and cry out, "It's so fresh!" and you have the idea of this remedy. Every achy part of the body is minty fresh—that is, it is chilled to the bone, as if you rubbed it with that toothpaste and blew on it. (And, yes, it is keynote of the remedy that the patient's breath will be, if not so minty fresh, at least cold.) So the patient is in pain and is icy cold in his painful state, and yet the Camphora patient will not allow you to cover him. He will even want to be covered, to be warmed in concept, but will be unable to bear the actual warmth of covering.

The Camphora patient is in a state of collapse. His strength is all but gone. And it is keynote of this remedy that, in this state, the patient must concentrate upon his pain in order to keep it under control. Camphora patients are actually improved by thinking of their pain.

The pains that run through this remedy also are most commonly throbbing in nature. Look especially for a throbbing headache to accompany other ailments. This headache will be placed in the occiput, the back of the head. Look for the patient to pull his head to one side, left or right, during this headache.

The patient will feel as if he is about to be consumed by his pain, that it will actually swallow him whole. He will feel as though his whole life will become this pain. But if the Camphora patient actually thinks about the pain and its specific location and quality, it will disappear, and so the patient will tend to be all but silent. He will not argue or complain; instead he will spend his time and energy concentrating on his pain. But Camphora patients do not want to be left alone. They fear being alone. They fear that if they are alone, they will lose the battle and disappear into their pain. For this reason, you may find that the Camphora patient will want some slight physical contact. They may want to hold your hand, or grip your arm, while they are in pain. This gives them an anchor for their concentration and a method of controlling the pain.

Their senses will be distorted by their pain, especially their senses of smell and taste. Their nose will be cold to the touch. It will be blocked. Look for nosebleeds, persistent nosebleeds. The patient will feel very cold during the nosebleed. Smells will bother the patient greatly. Any form of smoke, especially tobacco smoke, will greatly aggravate the patient.

Food will taste strange, bitter—especially meat, which will tend to make the patient nauseous with its strange bitter taste. The patient will be very thirsty, however.

In the home, the major use of the remedy Camphora, however, is as an antidote. It, along with Nux Vomica, is considered to be the universal antidote for both homeopathic and allopathic medicines. It is used to antidote the ill effects of medicines that are causing harmful aggravations to the patient. For this reason, if for no other, it belongs in every home kit. Check the Appendix, "On Antidoting Specific Remedies," for the names of the remedies that are antidoted by Camphora.

Aggravations: Camphora patients will be worse from any cold air, any drafts. They are worse from any bad news, any strong emotions. They are worse when they do not receive any attention.

The worst moment of the day for them occurs when they are just falling asleep. At this moment, they lose their ability to concentrate upon, and therefore control, their pain and it comes raging back at them, preventing sleep. Some Camphora patients will actually be driven to tears by the pain that comes on at the moment of sleep. Because of this syndrome, all will have great difficulties in getting to sleep. This sometimes sets in motion chronic patterns of insomnia that will remain even after the pain has ended.

Ameliorations: Camphora patients are better when thinking about their pains.

They feel better from drinking cold water.

They feel better for bodily discharges, especially sweat.

Dosage and Potency: Camphora may be given in any potency, from the lowest to the highest. The lower potencies, up to 30C, may be repeated as needed, but the higher potencies should be given in a single dose.

Relationships: Camphora is considered the antidote to all vegetable-based remedies. It is further considered to be the general antidote for food poisonings involving any form of vegetation. It is, therefore, the remedy of first choice in cases involving the ingestion of poison mushrooms. While Camphora is not antidoted by coffee, tea, or lemonade, beverages that are common antidotes of homeopathics, those sensitive to coffee's actions should avoid it during treatment with this remedy.

Camphora is antidoted by the remedies Phosphorus and Dulcamara.

13. CARBO VEGETABILIS

Remedy Source: Vegetable Remedy. As charcoal had been used as a substance in the treatment of indigestion, Samuel Hahnemann created the remedy Carbo Veg from vegetable charcoal. Specifically, he burned beechwood. The wood was heated until it was red and then ground into milk sugar until it had become fine enough to dilute in water.

Situations That Suggest Carbo Veg: Acute asthma, chronic fatigue syndrome, failure to recover from illness, fainting and states of collapse, recovery after surgery, comas. Also headaches, pneumonia, eczema.

Remedy Portrait: Carbo Veg is an excellent remedy to know when a patient is failing to recover from illness. Look for the person to feel that he has never been well since some past illness. For instance, he will have asthma that it is said came on after a bout of measles or from some period of life during which he drank heavily. The person's general health has broken at some point and he hasn't recovered since.

Illnesses also come on from poor diet, especially from too much salt in the diet. They are also brought on by eating spoiled foods and by food poisoning caused by bad meat or fish; also from consuming fatty foods.

Look for the patient to look broken down. He will have bad skin color. The face will be pale, and yellowish or grayish. The face will also be puffy. The head will be cold and will display a cold sweat, especially on the forehead. Gums will bleed easily. It is keynote of the remedy type that the Carbo Veg patient has cold breath.

This is a common remedy for nosebleeds, specifically for those who have nosebleeds day after day. Look for the patient's face to grow very pale before the nosebleed begins. This is a fairly general keynote of the remedy: the patient's face gets pale before the onset of symptoms.

Look for the patient to crave foods that are sure to disagree with him. He wants alcohol. He wants sugar. He wants salt.

As with Sulphur, this is a remedy for those who cannot digest even the simplest foods. Look for an excessive accumulation of gas in the intestines. The patient will feel, as with Lycopodium, that his stomach is very full, even if just a little food has actually been eaten.

The patient will be relieved by belching. This is so pronounced a reaction that he often will drink carbonated beverages to induce eructation. The patient is also gassy and very flatulent, especially in the evening and especially when lying down. This is a remedy for bloated people, and for people who are suffering from both bloating and indigestion.

This is a wonderful remedy for those who become ill after eating too rich a meal. Look for them to want to loosen their clothing around the waist. Carbo Veg patients want no tight clothing on their body.

Look for them also to want to constantly be fanned. They will feel as if there is not enough air in all the world for them to breathe. Although they tend to be a bit chilly, Carbo Veg patients will want air moving on them, especially on their face. They will run the fan or the air conditioning.

Patients will feel that they cannot breathe. They will be worse when lying down and will want to sit up in bed in order to breathe. This sensation of lack of breath will be improved by belching.

Because of these symptoms, Carbo Veg is a major remedy to consider in cases of pneumonia; also for asthma and emphysema; also for bronchitis, if it follows the general pattern of the remedy portrait.

This is also a major remedy for anemia if it again follows the general pattern.

Keynotes: It is keynote of this remedy that the patient wants to be fanned. He wants moving air in order to help him breathe. Lachesis is another remedy that likes moving air, but Lachesis wants the air to move from the opposite side of the room. He does not want too much stirring of the air. Carbo Veg wants that fan right on his face, because he fears that he will not be able to breathe any other way.

It is also keynote that the patient will crave the things that he cannot tolerate. This is true in terms of food as well as in terms of lifestyle choices. This is a person whose health has been broken, and who does nothing to improve this situation. He will neither change his diet nor begin even the mildest exercise program to improve his overall health.

It is also keynote that the Carbo Veg cannot take pressure. This is true on both a physical and emotional level. The simple pressure of a hat on the head will give such a patient a headache. In the same way, the simple pressure of a mate asking the patient to try to exercise or work will start him off on an asthma attack. These are people who are exhausted and in whom an acute situation is in the process of becoming a chronic condition.

Aggravations: From pressure of any sort. From being asked to sing or read aloud. From any exertion, mental or physical.

The patient is also aggravated by all but the simplest foods. Aggravated by butter, pork, and any other fatty food. By alcohol, by sugar, by salt—all of which he will crave.

The patient's aggravated by tight clothing, especially clothing that is tight around the waist.

The patient is worse in warm and damp weather, worse from any change in weather. He is worse from lying down. He is also worse from becoming overheated, worse when near an open fire, and worse in hot air.

The Carbo Veg patient, although exhausted, is easily angered. And he is made worse by his anger, which exhausts him.

Ameliorations: The patient is better when being fanned. Belching and flatulent discharges make him feel better.

The patient will fear the dark and in general be worse at night. He will better during the day and better from light in general.

Dosage and Potency: Low potencies are suggested for cases of simple indigestion or lingering exhaustion. Potency 30C is most common in these cases. Higher potencies are called for in constitutional cases.

Carbo Veg may be repeated as needed in low potencies. Higher potencies—1M and above—are best if used in a single dose.

This is a slow-acting and a long-acting remedy. Clarke tells us that one dose will work for up to sixty days. This is not a remedy in which we look for immediate dramatic changes, but rather for a slow gathering of strength as the patient recovers from his ailments.

Relationships: Carbo Veg works well with other remedies of depleted patients—Nux Vomica, Lycopodium, and Phosphoric Acid. It also acts as a good follow-up to Aconite, and, in stubborn cases of asthma, should be considered with Arsenicum Album.

14. CAUSTICUM

Remedy Source: Mineral Remedy. Like the Kali family of remedies, Causticum is a potassium-based remedy. In this case, the remedy is taken from a mixture of lime and bisulfate of potash. The mixture is dissolved in alcohol, from which the mother tincture is then made.

The remedy was created by Hahnemann.

Situations That Suggest Causticum: Burns. Also ailments involving the voice: stammering, loss of voice, laryngitis, paralysis of the tongue, Also bronchitis, cough and cold, whooping cough; ear ailments: Ménière's disease. Also goiter. Also headache. Also hemorrhoids, constipation. Also rheumatism, arthritis, sciatica, neuralgia, carpal tunnel syndrome, muscle aches and pains, hip pain, back pain, neck pain, tendon pain. Also warts, boils, acne, eczema, herpes.

Remedy Portrait: I have to be upfront in stating that in many people's minds, the Causticum patient is the picture of the old Halloween witch. This is true because we tend to think of Causticum first in cases involving warts on the face, especially warts on the end of the nose.

But there is also a more subtle reason why Causticums are equated with witches. Like Phosphorus and Rhus Tox patients, Causticum patients are deeply tied to the planet, especially to changes in the weather. They are weather witches, in that they can often predict when the weather is about to change by their body's aches and pains.

And, like the Phosphorus type, the Causticum will seem a bit psychic, as if he can tell what people are thinking. But, where Phosphorus will be able to do this one-on-one, Causticum seems to be able to read the underbelly of society. He seems able to sniff out exactly where the culture has chosen to bury its bodies.

Causticum is, in its constitutional form—which is all that we have been discussing up to this point—a political animal. Causticum types seek justice. They seek revenge.

Most Causticum types will move into jobs that have some depth and meaning, at least to them. They make great investigative journalists. They are wonderful researchers. Even those who hold average jobs will volunteer their time in the evenings to good causes. Our not-for-profit organizations are filled with Causticums who are doing their good work.

But, as Phosphorus, whom Causticum can resemble, will always put the individual in front of the pack, and will always seek to end the suffering of the person who is in front of him right now, Causticum puts the cause in front of the need of the individual. How did Spock put it in that *Star Trek* movie? "The needs of the many outweigh the needs of the one." Something like that. Very Causticum.

For this reason, you will find that Phosphorus and Causticum just don't mix. They will work together in these community groups, but their ultimate goals just won't blend. Also, the serious Causticum just won't get Phosphorus' jokes. It is interesting to note that while physically, the two remedies have the same sort of rheumatic aches and pains, Phosphorus will feel much worse for the change from dry to wet weather, while Causticum improves when the dampness begins. So while their issues are very similar, their approach is opposite.

Even in acute situations, look for the ailments in Causticum to come on from grief. This is a remedy type that we tend to enter slowly. Again, as with other remedies like Nux and Calcarea, we wear ourselves down into the Causticum type. It is not usually a remedy associated with sudden infections and the like—of the Aconite or Belladonna type—but, instead, even the acute manifestations of the Causticum sort are the product of a rather long period of development. So you will find a patient who has been in a state of grief for some time now—and that grief may have been totally silent—and now is sick. He will seem depressed in his illness. He may not want to live any longer. Like Phosphorus and Pulsatilla, look for the patient to have emotional distress at twilight—at that time, he will become very homesick if he is not at home. The Causticum patient will be very anxious about the future. He will be wistful for what he has lost.

Causticum believes in laughter through tears. Therefore, it is common to the type that they will laugh and cry at the same time. And look for laughter to bring on spasms of pain for the Causticum patient.

The pain in Causticum tends to be accompanied by a feeling of numbness or tingling. The patient may also have a feeling of weakness. While in pain, look for the Causticum type to walk unsteadily, to teeter about as he tries to walk. He falls easily.

The Causticum is prone to back pain, hip pain, rheumatic pains in the limbs, and, especially, neck pain. (I resist the temptation to insist that Causticum has so many pains in the neck because he is constitutionally such a pain in everyone else's neck.) Causticum is perhaps the most common remedy used in cases in which the patient has wrenched his neck, where it is frozen to one side, or where the patient cannot move the neck in either direction.

Causticum is also an amazing remedy for the patient who has lost his voice, whether due to physical or psychological reasons. Physically, the voice is lost to laryngitis. The patient will have a sore throat and will have difficulty swallowing. The throat will feel paralyzed. It will also feel as if it has become internally swollen and that it is now too small. The patient will try empty swallow after empty swallow to alleviate pain and to keep the throat open. The patient will feel scraping pains in the throat. The throat will also burn, and it will feel better from cold drinks.

Causticums may also lose their voices completely, however, for psychological reasons. Rhus Tox and Phosphorus will both commonly lose their voices from overuse. Causticums, however, will lose their voices just when they have something important to say. Unlike Gelsemiums, they are not afraid to speak in public. They climb to the stage without fear, but when they open their mouth to speak, there is no sound at all. In this case, although the patients will feel better by drinking cold water, there is no pain—just no voice.

In home use, think of Causticum, along with Urtica Urens, for the ill effects of burns. It is also an excellent remedy to consider for coughs following colds. The patient will have a cough that is moving deeper and deeper. He will try and try to bring the cough down into his chest to get to the mucus and to get it out. The cough will be made better by cold drinks. It will be much worse when bending forward.

This remedy is also excellent in cases involving bronchitis with the same symptom pattern. It is also valuable for treating patients with asthma brought on by grief.

Finally, although it is not an acute complaint, think of Causticum as the best remedy for arthritis in the hands and fingers. The pains will be worse in cold weather, and also in dry weather. They will be worse from overuse and overwork. This is a leading remedy for carpal tunnel syndrome.

Keynotes: It is an important keynote of the remedy that the patient will be worse in cold, dry weather and better in cloudy, wet, and rainy weather.

It is also keynote that this is a right-sided remedy. Look for right-sided paralysis of the face. Paralysis of a specific part of the face or body is an important keynote. Often the patient will have paralysis of the tongue.

Also keynote are the eruptions on the tip of the patient's nose—not just warts, but any sort of skin eruption.

And Causticum patients will constantly be clearing their throats. They do that more than will any other remedy type.

Aggravations: The Causticum patient is worse in exactly the kind of weather in which the rest of us are best: sunny, dry, and cool. He is also worse in the evening, especially at twilight; worse also in the morning.

The Causticum is worse from the motion of a car, train, boat, or plane.

Ameliorations: The Causticum is better in damp, wet, and rainy weather.

This patient is also better in warm air.

Dosage and Potency: This is another remedy that works very well in 30C. In constitutional cases, higher potencies are used.

While the remedy may be repeated if the symptoms call for it, Causticum works best in a single dose.

Relationships: Causticum is most complementary with Carbo Veg. Rhus Tox, Nux, Antimonium Tartaricum, and Pulsatilla all follow Causticum well and often will complete its action.

Causticum and Phosphorus are totally incompatible. They should never be used in conjunction with each other.

15. CHAMOMILLA

Remedy Source: Vegetable Remedy. Chamomilla is taken from the German chamomile. The plant must be picked when in full flower. The entire plant is used in the creation of the remedy.

Chamomilla was created by Hahnemann.

Situations That Suggest Chamomilla: Pain, especially pain associated with teething and toothache, PMS. Also coughs, colic, and fever; otitis media. The remedy is also useful for the hot flashes that accompany menopause. It is a great remedy for use with those with behavioral problems. Consider it also for neuralgia. It is an excellent remedy for cases involving diarrhea that follow general pain pattern.

Remedy Portrait: The Chamomilla patient is not just an irritable or angry patient; he is a difficult patient, a demanding patient, also a very bratty patient. In fact, the tendency for the Chamomilla patient to be whiny, irritable, and impatient is so strong that the mere fact that a patient is calm or easy to deal with counterindicates this remedy.

The idea here is that the Chamomilla patient is overwhelmed by his pain. And you may stand there and think to yourself that he seems to be reacting far more to this pain than is called for. The Chamomilla will howl or scream and will seem to be so sensitive to pain that he must be faking. No one could be in that much pain from an earache or a toothache.

But Chamomilla patients are. And they become furious when in this pain state. They will want things, demand them, and then refuse them when they are offered. The bottom line is that they don't know what they want. They are frantic and feel that they are no longer in control of themselves, that the pain is in control.

If there is one thing that every Chamomilla wants—especially if the patient is a child—it is to be carried. The Chamomilla child will insist that you carry him and will only be comforted when he is carried. If you put him down even for a moment, the howling and screaming starts again. This is an important keynote of the remedy, especially in children, because the patient may be so young that he can't answer any questions. Just look for those arms to be flailing wildly while the child is demanding to be picked up, only to flail again when the child is put down, and you have a strong indication of the remedy.

Also look at the patient's cheeks. It is keynote of the remedy that the patient will have one red cheek and one pale cheek. If you note this sign, and it is accompanied by the angry nature described above, you have a Chamomilla case.

Another thing to look for in the Chamomilla patient is a spasm of the eyes. The Chamomilla will often spasmodically open and close his eyes. His eyes may also have a yellow tinge to them.

This is the remedy to consider first in cases in which the patient is made worse by drinking coffee. Chamomilla, and not Coffea (taken from coffee), should be considered when ailments come on after drinking coffee, or when the patient is wild, irritable, and sleepless after drinking coffee. The Chamomilla, in fact, will be made worse by drinking any warm liquids. The patient will be worse at night.

This is a remedy to consider in all cases of severe pain that come on at night. It is a remedy for the patient with a toothache, especially if that tooth pain is worse when the patient takes in any warm liquid. And think of this remedy for the period in which a child is teething as well.

Chamomilla is also an excellent remedy to consider in cases of earache that come on at night. The pain will be accompanied by a ringing in the patient's ears. The ears will also feel stopped up. Look for a swelling of the affected part of the ear to accompany the pain. The patient will be frantic with pain.

Chamomilla is a valuable remedy for those with headache. The patient will complain of a one-sided headache. Look for the patient to have sweat on his forehead and scalp during the period of pain. Look for him to bend his head backward in order to alleviate the headache pain.

Chamomilla speaks to an array of digestion troubles as well. The Chamomilla patient will often have a distended abdomen. He will have nausea after drinking warm drinks, especially coffee. Every evening he may have nausea accompanied by sweat. Look for the Chamomilla patient to sweat after he eats or drinks anything.

This is a remedy to consider for acid indigestion and heartburn. The patient will regurgitate his food. He will feel pressure in the stomach, as if there is a stone inside him. Look for all the signs of indigestion to come on after the Chamomilla becomes angry. Such a patient will have many different ailments after anger—headache, colic, and diarrhea chief among them.

Patients who need Chamomilla are given to diarrhea. It is such a strong tendency that the symptom of constipation in a given case will actually counterindicate this remedy. The Chamomilla patient with diarrhea will pass stools that are hot and watery. They will resemble chopped eggs and spinach and will contain undigested foods. And they will leave the Chamomilla feeling a great deal of pain in the anus. Therefore think of Chamomilla as a remedy for those with hemorrhoids, and think of this remedy also for cases of teething children who have diarrhea.

Chamomilla is another rheumatic remedy, but it has the unusual keynote symptom of the patient being better during warm, wet weather. The patient will feel worse, however, from heat in general, and from being in the open air, especially the night air.

The patient will complain of violent pains that force him out of bed at night. The patient will be awakened by pain (this is not limited to rheumatic pains; the Chamomilla is likely to be awakened in the middle of the night by any pain, but especially by pains in the teeth and ears). The patient will have to walk when in pain. This will be true even if the patient feels as if his lower limbs will not support him, as if they are paralyzed. The patient will especially feel that he cannot trust his feet to support him. This is a wonderful remedy for those who suffer lumbago, for those with pain that extends from the lower back into the hips and legs.

Chamomilla patients will have restless sleep at best. They often will sleep with their eyes only partly closed. They will toss and turn in their sleep. They will have vivid dreams. They often are given to terrible nightmares.

Keynotes: This remedy is specifically called for at the stage of teething in early childhood; for children and newborns; for patients who are angry, mean, and cannot give a civil answer to any question.

Chamomilla patients want to be carried. It is the only thing that quiets them. They will pace the floor in anger and pain. They are irritable and fretful. They have a very low tolerance for pain of any sort.

Look to the face for these keynotes: one cheek is hot, the other cold; one is red and the other pale.

Aggravations: From heat. From anger.

The patient will also be aggravated in the evening, especially in the period just before midnight.

The patient will be worse from any draft, worse in open air.

The patient will be worse from drinking coffee. Some will be so sensitive as to be worse from smelling coffee.

Dosage and Potency: Hahnemann himself commented that Chamomilla works best in the 12C potency. It will assist in all general aches and pains that follow the Chamomilla pattern. Higher potencies are useful in more long-term situations and in behavior disorders.

One dose of this remedy will remain effective for up to thirty days. It may, however, be repeated as necessary in the treatment of the patient.

Relationships: Think of Belladonna for use both before and after Chamomilla, especially in childhood diseases that come on quickly, and in cases of teething.

Pulsatilla is also to be considered as a complementary remedy, especially in tearful patients.

Nux Vomica should not be given just before or after Chamomilla because their actions are not compatible.

16. CHINA

Remedy Source: Vegetable Remedy. China is also known as Cinchona. It was the very first remedy in the homeopathic pharmacy. It was created from the bark of the *Cinchona officinalis,* a bark from which the allopathic medicine quinine is also taken. The substance, which was known for centuries for its medicinal qualities, was named *Kina-Kina,* or "bark of barks," by the natives of Peru.

China was created by Samuel Hahnemann.

Situations That Suggest China: Fevers of all sorts, fever with delirium, influenza, and respiratory infections of all sorts, coughs. Also colic: constipation and diarrhea, hemorrhoids. Headache, vertigo, tinnitus and Ménière's disease, deafness. Rheumatism: hip pain, backache. Also food poisoning and indigestion, suffocation, acute asthma, home recovery from strokes, sleep disorders.

Remedy Portrait: In the consideration of this remedy, the first thing you will notice about a China patient is how exhausted he is, how his disease state has depleted his vital force. China is especially indicated in the patient who is depleted due to a loss of what the classic texts call "vital fluids," especially for the patient who has been weakened by a loss of blood.

This is also a remedy specific to the conditions surrounding the patient's recovery from surgery. China is the indicated remedy especially for cases involving much postoperative gas, when the passing of gas does not bring the patient any relief.

The China patient, postoperative or not, will seem apathetic to his condition. He will seem indifferent at best to the suggestions made to him to aid his recovery. In fact, the China patient will often seem to go out of his way to disobey the doctor's orders. He may be passive–aggressive in his approach to all who offer treatment. Look for the patient to seem totally disinterested in his state of health for long periods of time, and then to suddenly burst into tears over his condition. Look for the patient also to toss his head about in a sudden fit of concern.

The China patient will often state that he feels as if his brain is loose in his head, that it will hit the inside of his skull if he moves his head too quickly. The China patient will, therefore, keep his head perfectly still for the most part. He will complain of vertigo, of the sensation that he is falling backward. He will complain of throbbing pains in the head. He will say that he feels as if his skull is about to burst. He will feel better when direct pressure is applied to his head. He will also feel better in a warm room.

Look at the patient's eyes for an indication of the remedy. The patient will have blue rings of color all around the eyes. The white of the patient's eye will often take on a yellow tinge, and it may have black spots on it as well. The patient will complain of black spots in his field of vision as well.

The patient will complain of a ringing in the ears. This ringing may be an acute or a chronic complaint. The patient will have an increase of acuity in hearing accompanying the ringing. Look for the patient to have swelling and redness of the external ear, especially the earlobe. The external ear will also be very sensitive to touch.

Consider this remedy in cases of toothache in which the patient feels better if he clenches his teeth together, applying pressure to the pain. The tongue will be coated with a thick yellow or white film. The patient will complain of a bitter taste in the mouth.

He will also complain of digestive upset. He will report that his stomach feels internally cold, that the region of his stomach is tender. Stomach pains will come on after the patient drinks milk; these will be made worse by eating fruit.

Consider this remedy for the patient with hiccoughs, if the general pattern of symptoms follows the remedy. Also consider it for cases of heartburn and acid indigestion, and also in cases in which the patient vomits, if the vomiting contains undigested food.

In general, the pain and bloating associated with China's indigestion will be improved by movement. The patient, in general, will also have a very slow digestion, which will further weaken him if he eats too much or too often.

China is also for the patient with diarrhea, if, again, the stool contains undigested food. The diarrhea will be painless, and will be made worse by consuming milk or fruit. And it will also become worse if the patient drinks beer. Consider this remedy for cases of diarrhea that are accompanied by flatulence. And consider this remedy for chronic cases of diarrhea that have severely weakened the patient due to dehydration.

Consider China in cases of flu that have weakened the patient, especially for cases in which the patient must raise his head in order to breathe. He will say that he cannot breathe if he holds his head low. The patient's breathing will be slow, just like his digestion. The patient will have a rattling cough. Listen for the sound of rattling mucus in the patient's chest. The patient's heartbeat will be irregular, with strong, solid beats being followed by weak, rapid beats.

China is very sensitive to touch. Both the patient's skin and all the joints in his body will be very sensitive to touch. The patient will complain of terrible pain if he is just lightly touched. And yet firm pressure will alleviate his pain.

The patient will complain of a sensation that a string has been tied around his limbs. He will say that he feels cold. His skin will be covered with sweat. Look for the patient to have one cold hand and one warm hand and for his hands to be sweaty. Look for his joints to be swollen. Look for the patient's limbs to tremble and for the patient to say that his limbs feel numb. The patient will also complain that his joints feel weak, especially in the morning, or when he has been in a sitting postion for too long.

Consider this remedy in cases of fever, especially for long-lasting fevers or fevers of unknown origin. Consider this remedy for fevers that return again and again. The fever will have a set pattern. The patient will be chilly in the morning. This chill will start in the patient's chest. Then the fever will come and go throughout the day. Look for the patient to have night sweats with the fever, and then look for him to awaken very thirsty. The patient's chill will be preceded by thirst. The patient will drink often, but only a little sip at a time, like the Arsenicum patient.

Keynotes: This is a patient who will not want to exercise at all. He will not be willing to even go through the motions of getting well. He will appear to have no interest in getting well. This is an important remedy to consider for those patients who are recovering from surgery, or who are weakened due to the loss of blood or other fluids. Consider this remedy especially in cases of nosebleeds that will not stop, when the patient becomes weakened from the blood loss.

Classic texts state the case as follows: The patient "has no desire to live, but lacks the courage to commit suicide."

The patient will crave sour things. These may be the only things that he craves to eat. He will want liquids, especially in the morning, but will only sip a little at a time.

Consider this remedy in depleted patients who are always catching cold, for patients who become drenched in sweat from the slightest exertion.

Aggravations: The China patient will be worse at night, and worse from the slightest touch, although a firm touch will relieve the patient's pain. He is also worse in wet weather.

The China patient will typically have an aggravation every other day. He will be worse from the loss of fluids from the body and worse from simply bending over.

Ameliorations: The China patient will feel better if he bends over double. He will be better from firm pressure and better from warmth. The patient will be better when not eating.

Dosage and Potency: China works well in standard low-to-middle potencies and should be kept in a 30C potency in the home kit. Higher potencies should be reserved until the lower fail to work. China does not repeat especially well and should only be repeated if absolutely needed.

One dose of China works for seven days.

Relationships: China is often the first remedy needed to begin a patient's complete recovery from debilitating disease. It is followed well by Arsenicum, Phosphoric Acid, and Veraturm, all of which work well for patients with a weakened vital force. Mercurius also follows well after China, as do Arnica, Carbo Veg, Pulsatilla, and Sulphur.

17. CINA

Remedy Source: Vegetable Remedy. The remedy Cina is taken from the *Cina artemisia,* also know as "wormseed." The remedy is taken from the unopened green-yellow flowers of the Artemisia, a plant belonging to the Natural Order Compositae. These unopened flowers are called the plants' "seeds." The mother tincture is prepared from these.

Cina is a remedy created by Hahnemann.

Situations That Suggest Cina: Worms, especially pinworms. Also bronchitis, acute asthma, and fever, coughs and colds, whooping cough. Also strabismus and other vision disorders. Also colic and diarrhea.

Remedy Portrait: We all know that in classical homeopathy we are never treating a disease condition, but always treating a patient with a specific set of symptoms, but the remedy Cina is so specific in its action that it almost defies us not to simply think of it as the worm remedy, rather than the most common remedy for people—especially children—afflicted with worms and dealing with a range of symptoms caused by the presence of worms.

Look for patients needing this remedy to have terrible breath. Look for them to wake up at night feeling hungry and to be unable to return to sleep until they have eaten. (They always tend to be as hungry after they have eaten as they were before.) And look for them to chronically pick their nose. (They also dig their fingers into their ears.) All of these are symptoms of worms and all are symptoms of Cina. As with the yang remedies Apis, Chamomilla, and Belladonna, look for the Cina patient to be nervous and easily startled. Like Chamomilla, they will have a general air of dissatisfaction. They will demand something and then refuse it—or physically throw it—when it is given to them.

Also look for Cina patients to have a specific pain in the region of the navel. The pain will be twisting in nature and will cut in around the navel. They will have abdomens that are distended and hard to the touch. They will complain that they have odd sensations inside their abdomen and that it feels unpleasantly warm and alive in there.

Look for the pains in the abdomen to alternate with a headache. Patients will get into a stooping position to relieve the pain. This position mirrors one that is common in sleeping Cina patients. Look for them to sleep on their hands and knees.

Cina is also an excellent remedy for several eye conditions. The patient will typically have dark circles around his eyes. His eyes will feel tired. He will complain of eyestrain. He will say that it seems as if there is a fog in front of his eyes, or that his eyes are shrouded in gauze. This is an excellent remedy for those who suffer from presbyopia, which usually has its onset in middle age. Look for the patient to need to squint in order to see.

Think of Cina in cases of whooping cough and asthma that come on in especially severe attacks—especially in the autumn and the spring. The patient will swallow after coughing or choking. He will cough when he attempts to breathe. Listen for a gurgling sound that will come from the patient's body after an attack of coughing; it will come from the throat and stomach. Look for the patient's whole body to stiffen from an attack of coughing or gasping.

The Cina patient will not be able to eat enough to feel full. And it is keynote of the remedy that the patient will lose weight while eating more and more. His whole body will have a sour smell, especially his breath, and yet his tongue will be very clean.

This is an angry, ill-tempered patient. And yet, like Pulsatilla, he will want to be rocked. He will want to be held. But other than that motion when they want it, Cina patients do not want to be touched. They will tell you when and how they are to be touched.

As this is a child's remedy for the most part, consider also that the Cina patient will be beset with bedwetting. The condition will be worse during the full moon. Also, the patient will grind his or her teeth while asleep. He will also make chewing motions with his mouth while he is asleep.

Keynotes: The patient will not allow himself to be fussed over. The Cina will not let you brush his hair.

This is an angry patient, one who insists on being in charge, who will constantly tell you what to do and how and when to do it. He will become angry and will feel insulted over the least thing. The Cina is also overly sensitive physically and cannot bear surfaces that are too hard.

That behavior, when coupled with the inexhaustible hunger, is keynote to this remedy.

Aggravations: The patient will be worse during the full moon; also when he is exposed to the sun. The patient also tends to be worse in summer. He will be worse at night, especially in the time just before midnight, when the Cina will become very easily frightened. The Cina is also worse from touch.

Ameliorations: The Cina patient will be better from sleeping on his abdomen; also from motion. He will also feel better if he is allowed to rub his eyes, shake his head, or move in a rocking motion.

Dosage and Potency: Cina is most often used in either the 30C or 200C potencies. The 30C is used in ailments such as whooping cough, the 200C for worms.

One dose holds for two to three weeks. The remedy may be repeated as needed.

Relationships: Cina is considered an excellent remedy to follow Drosera in whooping cough if the first remedy fails to totally cure. It is also used as a follow-up to Phosphorus and Aconite and Spongia in cases of severe cough and loss of voice.

Cina is well followed by Calcarea Carbonica, Silicea, and Ignatia.

18. COCCULUS

Remedy Source: Vegetable Remedy. The remedy is taken from *Cocculus indicus,* or the Indian cockle, a plant from the Natural Order Menispermacae. The plant is a climbing shrub known for its strength and its small round purple berries.

These berries, after having been dried and powdered, are used to create the mother tincture from which the remedy is made.

Cocculus is a remedy of Hahnemann.

Historically, the plant was used as a poison to stun fish in order to make them easier to catch by hand. It was known also for its intoxicating impact upon the human system. *Cocculus indicus* was known to disorient the human sense organs. It was even added to beer to increase its intoxicating properties.

Situations That Suggest Cocculus: Motion sickness, seasickness, nausea, vomiting, fainting. Also lack of sleep, weakness from nursing others, insomnia. Also PMS, menstrual headache, headache, colic. Also rheumatism, numbness, overexertion (mental or physical), paralysis, convulsions. Also illness from anger, anxiety, depression.

Remedy Portrait: The usual portrait of this remedy is the person who is nauseous, vomiting, experiencing vertigo. He will often will have a feeling of paralysis in the tongue and a sensation of hollowness in the head, chest, and abdomen. He will feel that parts of his body have gone to sleep. He will feel weak, often too weak even to speak out loud. He will be aggravated by any form of motion, and will want to lie down. Even the motion of rising up in bed will cause aggravation, and will cause vertigo and nausea. Headache, even migraines, will be brought on by motion. Headaches will be aggravated by the motion of a car or boat.

In other words, the person needing Cocculus may be said to be seasick. Cocculus is of special help for persons who become ill from motion sickness in all its forms. (Nux Vomica is another important remedy for persons in this situation; the two remedies are further related by the anger that is often the basis or concurrent symptom of the nausea.) That is the most common home use for the remedy.

Cocculus, however, is also an excellent remedy for those who have gone without enough sleep for a period of time, especially those who have done so in the service of others, such as nursing a sick relative, and now feel somewhat put upon for having to do so. Again, the Cocculus patient will be somewhat irritable, somewhat angry. The remedy will be of great help in getting this patient back into his natural sleep pattern and in helping him recoup his own energy and let go of his anger.

No matter the quality of the physical symptoms, and no matter their cause—from a boat ride to physical exhaustion—look for the Cocculus patient to be very sensitive emotionally. And his negative emotions will come to the forefront. He will be angry, anxious, or fearful. He may go into deep, quiet depression. But a patient who is upbeat, who seems to be taking the situation in stride, is indicating another remedy.

The physical pains in this remedy are sharp and cramping in quality and may appear in any part of the body. However, abdominal pain is most common. The patient may say that he feels as if his abdomen is filled with sharp stones or broken glass. The abdominal muscles will feel weak. Intestinal gas will abound and there will be a tendency to reflux, which may even make the patient feel as if he cannot breathe. There may be a sensation of cramping in the chest as well. In a case like this, it is common for the patient to have an audible rumbling issuing from the chest. Also very common is a pain in the area of the liver. This pain will be brought on by motion or by anger. The area of the liver will be swollen.

The patient, especially in times of nausea, will be averse to food. He will not be able to bear the sight or smell of food. He will, however, long for cold drinks, often for beer, but the patient will feel worse for eating or drinking anything. If he must drink at all, he should be encouraged to take only the smallest sips.

Again, as with Nux Vomica, look for the patient to feel that his hearing has become very acute. Either that, or he will feel a great reduction in his ability to hear. The ears will feel closed up, especially the right ear.

Women needing this remedy will find that their period has come on too early, and that the flow is very heavy. The flow will be dark. It will be preceded by intense spasmodic cramping. There will be a sensation of clutching in the uterus.

The patient will usually feel too weak to even stand up during the time of her period. As with the general picture, the patient will feel too weak even to talk out loud.

During the period of the PMS, look for the patient to display the anger that is typical of the remedy. It is also common that the patient will be overly concerned about her health. Practitioners report that those needing this remedy will often demand that every conceivable medical test be performed. From their weakened position, they will demand attention.

Keynotes: The general keynote of the remedy is "liver pain and swelling in the region of the liver, worse from anger."

Other keynotes include vertigo, and this is true vertigo, in which the patient experiences the room spinning. There is also a weakness that leaves the patient too weak to talk. The aggravation from motion is keynote. Look for the patient to need to lie down in order to speak, or to in any way deal with his situation.

It is also keynote of the remedy for the patient to feel intoxicated. The Cocculus will often feel as if he has left his body.

Aggravations: The Cocculus patient is made worse by anger, anxiety, or fear. He is worse from any form of excitement; he needs to be calmed. He is worse from any exertion, even from rising up in bed. He is worse from talking.

The patient will be worse from smelling strong odors, which will increase both the vertigo and the nausea. He will especially feel worse from the smell of food cooking, especially fish, eggs, or meat.

He will be worse from eating and drinking, even though he will crave cold drinks. He is worse for motion of any sort—for riding in a boat, car, train, or plane.

The patient is worse when he lies on the back of his head; this tends to increase his vertigo. He is better if his head is turned to the side.

The patient is worse for any loss of sleep.

The general aggravation for the remedy comes on at 11 P.M. Sometimes this will take place at 11 A.M. All those needing this remedy however, will be worse during the hours of darkness, from sunset to sunrise.

Ameliorations: There is very little that one can do to bring about an improvement in this remedy portrait. The patient will be better if he is allowed to lie down. He is also improved by being in a closed room.

Dosage and Potency: The potencies 30C and 200C are most commonly used and are the most effective.

Cocculus works best in a single dose; it does not repeat well. It is best to give a single 30C and follow it, if a second dose is called for, with a single dose of 200C.

One dose of the remedy holds for up to a month.

Relationships: Cocculus is often followed by the remedy Nux Vomica, which will complete the healing process. Other remedies that follow well include: Arsenicum, Ignatia, Lycopodium, Pulsatilla, Rhus Tox, and Sulphur.

19. COFFEA CRUDA

Remedy Source: Vegetable Remedy. The remedy is taken from the unroasted coffee bean. The coffee plant is native to tropical regions, and the remedy is most commonly taken from the plants native to India.

The remedy is taken from a mother tincture created from the seeds of the plant only.

It was created by Hahnemann.

Situations That Suggest Coffea: Nervous excitement, insomnia, anxiety, shock. Also headache, migraine. Also toothache. Also sciatica.

Remedy Portrait: Just think of the effects of a cup of coffee—and not the effects of that nice single cup you had this morning. No, think of the effects of the twentieth cup that the truck driver has had in the middle of the night at some truck stop in the middle of Indiana before he climbs back in the truck to drive on the interstate. Think of the physical and emotional impact of patching yourself together with another and another and another cup of coffee when there is a task that just has to get done. That's the central sensation of the remedy.

The patient will be jittery, anxious. This is the remedy for the situation in which the sensations described above happen naturally, when the patient is overreactive, overly sensitive to everything, to every situation. Think of when you have had a toothache that seemed to have taken over your body. You could not believe that just a little hole in a little tooth in your mouth could so completely overwhelm your entire being. You could not only not stand warm things in your mouth, but it seemed as if your entire body could not stand being warmed. (*Note* that the Coffea toothache is improved by having cold things in the mouth.)

The Coffea patient feels this way, with or without that specific tooth-ache. He cannot bear any sensations, especially not noise. He cannot stand talking or being spoken to. He does not want to answer questions and will become angry when you try to take his case.

The Coffea patient also cannot stand the cold. Now, be aware that he will feel cold, a general, all-encompassing cold. He does not feel chilly, like an Arsenicum does. Instead, his hands and feet will be icy and he will feel cold like he is in a meat locker.

The patient also cannot stand light. He will, during times of great pain, seek places that are both quiet and dark. This will be especially true of those with Coffea headaches. These will often be severe migraines. Look for them to come on very slowly, over time becoming worse and worse until the pain of the headache takes over the patient's entire being.

So this overreaction, this overall sense of excitement, is keynote to the remedy, no matter what other symptoms are present. The Coffea state can come on as easily from overexcitement from joy as from pain. Whatever the cause, the patient is nervous, high-strung, and unable to relax. And yet, the Coffea patient wants, more than anything else, to be able to relax. He is exhausted and totally wired.

Keynotes: This is the patient who is wide awake when he does not wish to be. There is a general exhaustion coupled with a mental restlessness and/or activity that mirrors that of a person who has had too much coffee.

Also look for the patient to quickly alternate extremes of emotion. Therefore, he will laugh one minute and cry the next. Or he will literally weep for joy.

And, as in Chamomilla, it is keynote of this remedy that those needing it cannot stand pain. It seems that their reaction to their pain is out of proportion with the actual pain that they are experiencing.

Aggravations: Almost any sensation, especially noise, light, and touch. Any quick or jarring motion. Any sudden emotion, good or bad.

The Coffea patient is also aggravated especially by having warm liquids in his mouth.

Ameliorations: The Coffea patient will feel better if he just lies down. If he can get some rest.

He is also better if he puts some ice in his mouth and lets it dissolve.

Dosage and Potency: Use Coffea in either the 30C or 200C potencies for best results. And, for best results, use in a single dose. Coffea does not bear repetition well. It may, however, be repeated if absolutely needed, but wait and see.

This is a very quick-acting remedy. Its actions hold for only one or two days, but, as this is a remedy that is usually used to "break a cycle" of pain or exhaustion, this amount of time is often enough.

Relationships: The most complementary remedy for Coffea is Aconite, which makes sense, as both types are hyper and are restless. Either remedy may be used as needed to complete the action of the other.

Coffea is antidoted by Nux and Ignatia. It both antidotes and is antidoted by that other great pain remedy, Chamomilla.

20. COLOCYNTHIS

Remedy Source: Vegetable Remedy. It is taken from the bitter cucumber, or *Colocynth cucumis,* of the Natural Order of Cucurbitacae, which is native to Egypt and Turkey. Also known as the bitter apple. The mother tincture from which the remedy is taken is made from the dried fruit of the plant from which the rind and seeds have been taken.

This is a remedy of Hahnemann.

Situations That Suggest Colcynthis: Colic, diarrhea. Also PMS. Also rheumatic pains, especially sciatica. Also toothache.

Remedy Portrait: Those needing Colocynthis tend to have severe pains in the abdomen. The pain will cause the patient to double over in order to control its severity. The patient may also ball his fist into his abdomen as hard as he can to alleviate the pain. The pains will come in waves, with brief periods of calm in between.

This is the first remedy to think of in cases of colic, and in all cases of abdominal cramp, whether they are caused by the onset of diarrhea or the menstrual cycle (in which women will experience severe pain in the area of the ovaries—pain that is boring in nature). The pain may be brought on by anger or by eating the wrong foods, especially cheese and other dairy products. The patient, whatever the cause, will want his abdomen supported and will feel relieved by the application of pressure.

Abdominal pain may alternate with vertigo, with diarrhea, or with cramps in other areas of the body, most commonly with cramps in the calves. The abdominal cramps will be worse at night and after eating.

All pains in this remedy portrait will be improved by pressure. The sciatic pains of this remedy are shooting in nature. Like lightning, they strike quickly and then there is a period of relief. The pains will travel down the lower left side of the body, from the left hip to the thigh to the knee and below. The patient will say that he feels that his lower body is being tightened in a vise, and yet the patient will find relief when he lies on his painful side—the pressure applied alleviates the pain. The pain is also improved by applications of heat.

Compare this with the portrait of other common remedies for those with sciatica:

Bryonia is commonly used to treat those with sciatica. The pains in these patients will be worse from any sort of motion, but they will find relief by resting and by lying still. They are warm patients in general and want cool air and cool water. They are also very irritable.

Chamomillas will display, like Colocynthis, pain after anger. They will not, however, want to lie on the painful side but will toss about in pain and anger instead.

Rhus Tox patients will not want to lie down at all but will want to keep moving. Their pain increases when they are at rest. Pain will greatly increase during cold and wet weather.

Arsenicum patients will have pain that increases at night, especially at midnight and just after. They are also worse when they are cold, and they are made worse by lying on the painful side. They feel better when they are warm. They feel exhausted from their pain.

Belladonnas will experience pain and inflammations that are worse from any motion and or touch. They are better after rest, better when in a sitting position, and better when warm. Patients will complain of a rush of blood to their head.

Colocynthis patients are, in general, irritable patients. They do not want to be questioned—not even to have their case taken. And they are quite capable of showing you their displeasure. They usually do so by throwing things at your head.

Keynotes: The most important specific keynote of the remedy type is that those needing the remedy will have pain that is severe in nature and comes in waves or spells, during which they must either bend over or apply pressure to the pain in order to survive the spell. The patient may also wish to lie upon the painful side.

While we are dealing with the acute uses of the remedy in this writing, it is important to note that Colocynthis is an important constitutional remedy type as well. The keynote of this constitutional type is that Colocynthis patients have extremely strong opinions and have already made up their minds about nearly every possible topic. They believe in right and wrong and all but refuse to look at any subject from anyone else's point of view. They refuse to allow themselves to be disagreed with publicly. You will often see this behavior pattern even in acute cases.

Dosage and Potency: This remedy is usually considered best in the 200th potency. It is in this potency that it works especially well in cases of pain that also involve insomnia. It may also be given effectively in 30C and in higher potencies.

This remedy holds for a day to a week. It may be repeated as needed and classic texts hold that one dose should be given after all symptoms have cleared in order to finish the case.

Relationship: Mercurius is a complementary remedy in cases involving diarrhea. Also complementary in their actions are Bryonia, Chamomilla, and Staphysagria. Colocynthis and Staphysagria especially are used in association with each other and each follows the other well and completes its action.

Colocynthis is antidoted by Camphora and by Coffea.

21. DROSERA ROTUNDIFOLIA

Remedy Source: Vegetable Remedy. The remedy is taken from the plant known as sundew or moongrass, which belongs to the Natural Order of Droserecae. It is native to Europe and America. The remedy is taken from a mother tincture made from the whole plant that is picked just before flowering.

The remedy was created by Hahnemann, although Tyler gives us the best indication of its uses.

Situations That Suggest Drosera: Coughs: whooping cough and bronchitis, laryngitis, colds and coughs. Also colic, headache, vomiting. Also sciatica. Also anxiety and fear.

Remedy Portrait: This is another excellent remedy to consider in cases of cough, especially when the cough is spasmodic in nature, as with whooping cough. Drosera is a small remedy and truly acute in nature, so it is somewhat lacking in characteristics of persona. But look for the patient to be easily irritated, and look for him to get upset over nothing. Expect to not know just why he is angry with you, but to chalk it up to the acute remedy state. The patient will not want to be alone, but he will tend to be so suspicious of the motives of everyone around him that he is likely to spend a good deal of time alone. Drosera patients are anxious, especially in the evening, and can become fearful, especially of ghosts. They are future-oriented and are one of the remedy types that always seem afraid that something bad is about to happen.

Physically, the remedy tends to dominate with right-sided complaints, although in cases involving vertigo the patient will fall to the left.

Consider Drosera for coughs that are barking in sound. The patient will be hoarse. The cough will be made worse by the patient talking or laughing, especially when he is lying down. The cough will be spasmodic in nature, and gagging and vomiting will likely accompany the cough.

Drosera is the best bet remedy for coughing that comes on after a bout of the measles. It is also an excellent remedy for coughs that come from a tickling sensation, as if there is a feather in the patient's throat.

This is also an excellent little remedy for sore throat and loss of voice in singers and public speakers. A nagging, tickling cough will accompany the voice loss.

The patient may also experience hearing loss during the cough, and may have a sensation of whizzing or blockage in the ears.

Aggravations: The patient will feel worse when talking, singing, or laughing. He will feel worse from warmth and from warm drinks, and worse from eating any sort of acidic food. He will feel worse from cold foods.

The Drosera patient is also worse in the evening and at night, especially after midnight. He will feel worse on lying down and worse from getting up.

Ameliorations: Look for the patient to be better in the open air. Walking will improve the patient's condition.

The patient will also feel better from scratching and from being scratched—he will want his back scratched.

Dosage and Potency: The remedy may be given as needed in low potencies. In the higher potencies of 200C and above, it should be given in a single dose.

One dose of Drosera holds for up to a month.

Relationships: Drosera is complementary to Nux Vomica. Nux often follows and completes the remedy's action. Cina will also often follow Drosera in cases of whooping cough that have severe symptoms. Drosera often follows Sulphur.

22. DULCAMARA

Remedy Source: Vegetable Remedy. Dulcamara is taken from the bittersweet, a climbing shrubby little plant that grows in damp regions. It is native to the United States and to Europe. The plant belongs to the Natural Order of Solanaceae. The remedy is made from the fresh green stems of the plant that are gathered just before flowering.

The remedy was created by Hahnemann.

Situations That Suggest Dulcamara: Colds and flus, tonsillitis, laryngitis, whooping cough, hay fever. Also rheumatic pains, stiff neck, lumbago, sciatica, TMJ, headache. Also herpes. Also stammering. Also mononucleosis. Also warts.

Remedy Portrait: In *The Organon* Samuel Hahnemann wisely advises us all to avoid at all costs having favorite remedies, because we will tend to give that remedy when others are called for. But I just can't help it. Dulcamara is one of my very favorite remedies. No other remedy so well captures the hay fever of those who know that when their neighbor is mowing the grass, that grass will be the last thing they smell for the next few days until the attack of hay fever ends. And no other remedy so well captures the type of allergies that come on in early spring and especially in fall, when the days are hot and sunny and the nights cold and chilly.

And, Hahnemann's advice aside, I don't think that this remedy is given often enough. Dulcamara is a remedy in which the patient is greatly—and I mean greatly—aggravated by damp and especially from cold, damp weather. And no other remedy reacts so strongly to autumn. The Dulcamara responds to the change from summer to autumn not only with physical symptoms but with psychological ones as well. As if Dulcamaras simply cannot bear that winter is coming on, a part of their nature seems to die with the summer.

This can and should be considered a constitutional as well as an acute remedy. Those patients needing this remedy on an ongoing basis seem to be a little high-strung, a little sensitive in nature. They are opinionated and outgoing people. They tend to focus very much on family and the needs of their family, and they tend to talk about their family to others and will offer their views about some rather private family issues.

Physically, only Rhus Tox and Phosphorus can match Dulcamara for sensitivity to weather. Dulcamara can sense any change in weather, especially if the change is from warm to cold, thus the terrible aggravations a Dulcamara endures in the seasons in which the weather changes from hot to cold in the course of a single day. But Dulcamara can also strongly sense when wet weather is coming and will be much worse, not only for the change but during the wet weather as well.

Dulcamara will catch cold easily and will take on other illnesses from catching cold. Look for diarrhea, body aches, and pains (especially low back or neck pain) and conjunctivitis to accompany the cold.

Dulcamara is also an excellent remedy for sinusitis and for conditions that are brought on from the suppressive use of antihistamines. Look for headaches from sinus conditions. Dulcamara is second only to Kali Bi for use with all types of sinus headaches. The Dulcamara headache will tend to follow the same pattern of aggravations as the other aches and pains of the remedy. Therefore, Dulcamara will tend to get a sinus headache when there is a change in weather coming.

And Dulcamara should also always be considered for earaches in the left ear that come on with cold, damp weather; also for all colds and all stoppage of the nostrils in the same pattern.

Think of Dulcamara for cases involving warts on the face and herpes around the mouth if the case follows the general pattern of Dulcamara.

Aggravations: Need I mention again that the patient is worse in cold, damp weather, from changes in the weather, and, especially, at times during the year in which the weather is hot in the day and cold at night?

The patient is also worse from cold air and from becoming chilled. He is worse in the evening, and especially at night. Also worse from rest.

The Dulcamara patient is worse from the suppression of any bodily discharges, especially from suppressed mucus and sweat. This trait is so strong that one could argue that it is the suppression of these discharges that is responsible for the Dulcamara state itself.

Ameliorations: As with Rhus Tox, which Dulcamara can strongly resemble, the patient is better from gentle continuous motion.

Dosage and Potency: Dulcamara may be repeated in the 30C potency or lower. It should be given in a single dose in 200C or higher. One dose holds for a month.

Relationships: Dulcamara is incompatible with Lachesis and Belladonna and should not be given in conjunction with either remedy. However, it works well with five important remedies: Bryonia, Calcarea, Lycopodium, Rhus Tox, and Sepia. Rhus Tox and Sepia, especially, work well either before or after this remedy and each completes the other's action.

Dulcamara is antidoted by Camphora; also by Calcarea and Bryonia.

23. EUPATORIUM PERFOLIATUM

Remedy Source: Vegetable Remedy. Eupatorium Perfoliatum is taken from the plant known as both "boneset" and thoroughwort, a perennial plant with white flowers and leaves that grow at right angles to those that are growing immediately above or below. It belongs to the Natural Order of Coposite and is native to the United States and Canada.

The remedy was proven in 1846 by Williamson and Neidhard.

Situations That Suggest Eupatorium: Influenza, fever, bilious fever, diarrhea, measles. Also ringworm. Also rheumatism. Also hiccup.

Remedy Portrait: This is a small remedy and is very specific in its sphere of action, but it is a very useful remedy when called for.

In general, you are going to see a patient who is in great pain. The pain is aching in nature and the patient will say that he feels as if his bones are broken. (This symptom is so strong that the remedy is sometimes given in actual cases of broken bones.) Most often, these pains will accompany either flu or fever or both. Look for the high fever to be preceded by chills. This will be most common in the early morning hours between 7 and 9 A.M. The patient will be very thirsty during this chilled stage. He may want cold drinks or cold foods such as ice cream.

The patient will be sluggish. He will moan with pain. He will feel that he is being driven out of his mind by the pain. The patient wants to stay very still, but cannot, because he is being driven to restlessness by the pain.

The pain is beating in nature and can affect all the bones in the body. Pain in the back, however, is most common.

This is a great remedy for flus that are accompanied by body aches. You will reach first for Bryonia, since the remedy resembles Eupatorium so much, and since it is a much more common remedy. When Bryonia does not work, think of Eupatorium. This is a deeper pain. And, where the Bryonia patient will want to stay very still, the Eupatorium patient, who knows darned well that motion is only going to increase his pain, cannot manage to stay still, because he is in such pain that he thrashes about. Think of this as Bryonia, squared.

Eupatorium is a remedy that belongs in the home kit during flu season. Often you will have plenty of time to order the remedy at the onset of the season, as soon as you hear that this is a season of a particularly painful flu. Order it in both a high and a low potency and keep it on hand just in case.

Aggravations: Patients will be worse in the morning hours, especially from 7 until 9 A.M. They are also worse from cold air. They are worse from motion, especially the spasmodic motions involved in coughing. They are worse from smelling food and cannot bear the sight or smell of it.

Ameliorations: Patients will feel better if they can manage to vomit. They will also feel better when they sweat.

The patient will also feel better when he has company; conversation will make him feel better.

Dosage and Potency. Have Eupatorium on hand in 30C and 1M. The remedy may be repeated as needed in low potency, but use a single dose in high. One dose will hold for seven days.

Relationship: Eupatorium is complementary to Bryonia. It follows Bryonia well and acts when Bryonia fails.

Eupatorium is followed well by Natrum Mur and Sepia.

24. EUPHRASIA

Remedy Source: Vegetable Remedy. Euphrasia officinalis is taken from an herbal remedy known as eyebright. It is taken from a plant of the Natural Order of Scrophulariacea. The plant is native to Europe.

The remedy Euphrasia is taken from a mother tincture prepared from the whole plants, with the exception of the roots. The plants are gathered during the time of flowering.

The remedy Euphrasia was created by Samuel Hahnemann.

Situations That Suggest Euphrasia: Allergies, hay fever, colds, conjunctivitis, iritis, measles.

Remedy Portrait: This is a small remedy, but one that can be very helpful. Like Allium Cepa, Euphrasia is known primarily as an acute remedy and one that speaks to colds and hay fever. The symptoms are very similar to Allium Cepa's as well, with both the eyes and the nose flowing freely. However, in Euphrasia, the tears coming from the eye irritate the eye, causing redness and itching. The flow from the nose is bland and watery and causes no particular problem other than the flow itself. In this way, the symptoms of Euphrasia are opposite from those of Allium Cepa, and learning which flow irritates what part of the face will guide you quite quickly to the right remedy.

It is the watering of the eyes that is the most important symptom of the remedy. The eyes will water all the time, and will be glued shut in the morning. The margins of the eyes are red and swollen and burning.

Look for the patient to also have fluent flow from the nose, especially in the morning. The patient will sneeze and sneeze upon awakening, and often will also have a violent cough. As the patient coughs, look for a good deal of expectoration. The patient will cough so hard in the morning, trying to bring up mucus, that he may vomit up his breakfast.

In that Euphrasia is known for its impact upon the eye, it is also a very important remedy for iritis and for other inflammatory conditions of the eye. Look for ulceration of the cornea. This is also a leading remedy for acute conjunctivitis.

Eye conditions may be accompanied by headache. The headache will be of a bursting quality, with a sensation of dazzling of the eyes from sunlight.

Think of this remedy also for measles and influenza, in which there is a good deal of watering from the eyes, especially in cold air and windy weather.

Aggravations: The Euphrasia patient is at his worst in the morning. The light of morning increases the symptoms of Euphrasia as the sunlight intensifies. The patient's cough, in particular, will be worse during the day. The cough will be better at night.

The patient is also worse from warmth, especially from being in a warm room. He wants to be outdoors, and, even if his allergy or cold symptoms are made worse outdoors, the patient will feel better when outside.

The Euphrasia patient is also worse from moisture and from damp weather or surroundings. He is particularly aggravated by exposure to warm winds.

The patient is also worse from touch and does not want to be touched.

Ameliorations: The Euphrasia patient is always better at night, or from being in darkness.

He is better from lying down, and better when in bed.

Dosage and Potency: Euphrasia is used in low potencies for colds and allergies. In cases of allergy, potencies of 6C to 12C are most common. The potency 30C is most common for cases of colds.

The remedy Euphrasia is also commonly sold as an eyewash, which is very helpful in cases where the patient's symptoms match the remedy portrait.

While there is not a definitive statement of the remedy's duration, it bears repetition well and may be repeated as needed.

Relationships: Euphrasia is usually the first remedy called upon for a given case. It is followed well and its action completed by Aconite, Calcarea Carbonica, Lycopodium, Mercurius, Nux Vomica, Phosphorus, and Rhus Tox.

25. FERRUM PHOSPHORICUM

Remedy Source: Mineral Remedy. The remedy is taken from the chemical compound of iron and phosphoric acid. The chemical formula is $Fe_3(PO)_2$.

While the remedy was first proved as a homeopathic by J. C. Morgan in 1876, it was one of Schussler's favorite remedies, and much of what we know of the action of the remedy comes from him. In Schussler's cell salts, Ferrum Phos takes the place of some other important remedies that he omitted from his pharmacy: Aconite, Belladonna, and Arnica among them. Schussler notes that Ferrum Phos, like these other remedies, is very helpful in treating problems with the blood, like anemia, and with the circulatory system as a whole.

Situations That Suggest Ferrum Phos: Fevers, colds, coughs, flu, croup, sore throat, also whooping cough, vomiting. Also hemorrhages of all sorts, nosebleeds. Consider also injuries, sprains, rheumatism. And gastritis, dyspepsia, diarrhea, frostbite.

Remedy Portrait: Often we choose to give Ferrum Phos not because of the symptoms that the patient is expressing, but because of a lack of expected symptoms. Take fever for example, as this remedy is a common one for fevers. The fever that Ferrum Phos will help is not the quick and violent fever of Belladonna or Aconite. It is, instead, a fever with no specific symptoms and indicators, perhaps of unknown origin, that has left the patient weakened. It is most common that this fever will be congestive in nature, and may, like Belladonna's, come on from exposure to the sun, or even as an aftereffect of a physical trauma, but most often the fever will just be a simple fever, with no clear symptoms or guides to any given remedy. In this case, give Ferrum Phos.

In fact, this is a major remedy for the first stage of any inflammatory illness; also for hemorrhages, especially nosebleeds, that are also characterless in nature. In general, the patient needing this remedy will display such symptoms as a fever that exhausts the patient and a site-specific inflammation that may impact upon the throat, the stomach, or the lungs most commonly and that further exhausts the patient. But the most important aspect of the remedy is that these symptoms will be vague and general in nature, and will lead you to no specific remedy. In that case, the remedy is Ferrum Phos.

Look for the patient to have a rather high fever, usually at least 102 degrees. And look for him to have a good deal of thirst with the fever. Most often the thirst is for cold things, but a thirst for warm beverages does not counterindicate the remedy selection.

Look also for the patient to report that the majority of his symptoms are on the right side of the body, or begin on the right side and move left. This will be particularly true of the rheumatic symptoms, with the patient reporting right shoulder pain, etc.

The patient's face will be flushed with fever, with red spots on the cheeks being most common. But, again, the opposite may be true, and the patient may present a pallor, which does not counterindicate the remedy.

The illness in Ferrum Phos will most likely begin as a head cold. Look for the fever to develop over time. Look also for a nosebleed to accompany the cold. Look for the patient's mucus to be streaked with blood.

Look for the patient to desire sour things, and to want stimulants of all sorts. He will not want milk or dairy products or meat. Any of these will make the patient nauseous. The patient will be made worse by coffee, although he may specifically crave coffee. The same goes for tea. In fact, although the patient may be hungry, he is made worse in general by eating anything.

The illness is most often accompanied by a headache, which will be made better by cold applications. The pain will be increased by touch, by noise, and by movement. As with Belladonna, the headache can come on from exposure to the sun.

The patient, in general, will be exhausted. He will be drowsy but will have trouble falling asleep. When he does sleep, he will have nightmares. Night sweats are also common.

Ferrum Phos is also a key remedy for those with sore throats. It is of particular importance to singers and public speakers, in that it, like Phosphorus and Rhus Tox, speaks to laryngitis and is accompanied by hoarseness. The throat will feel worse from swallowing, most especially empty swallowing. The sore throat is usually accompanied by thirst. The Eustachian tubes will be blocked and inflamed. The sore throat often will hurt in the ear as well when the patient swallows.

Finally, in that this remedy is similar to Phosphorus, and in that it speaks to blood and circulation, this is a major remedy for use after operations of all sorts. It stops bleeding and promotes healing after an operation.

Keynotes: The keynote for the remedy type is fever in which the patient tosses about. Restlessness is pronounced, although the patient is exhausted.

The patient's pulse will be rapid and shallow. The patient's face will alternate between flushed and pale.

Blood runs through the remedy. Accompanying the fever will be nosebleed or expectoration of pure blood.

Ailments will include rheumatic pains. Shoulder pain is most common, worse on the right side. Look for numbness of the right arm or leg. The patient will feel that the part is numb but has a pulsing sensation running all through it.

The patient is angry, even violent in his fever. He is averse to company and may become hysterical if people enter the room. His emotions change rapidly; his moods shift. The patient may be fearful and forgetful.

The patient is overly sensitive to his own pain.

Look for the patient to feel that he cannot get enough air, that he cannot breathe.

Aggravations: The patient is worse from cold air, and from becoming cold, although his headache will be improved by cold applications.

The patient is worse from eating, worse from standing up, and worse from any strong motion.

The patient will also experience a general aggravation every night, and this aggravation will reach its peak daily from 4 to 6 A.M.

Ameliorations: The patient's pain will be improved by gentle pressure.

The patient will feel better when sitting up and when slowly walking about. He will be in general better when rising.

And the patient will be better if left alone. He will crave solitude.

Dosage and Potency: Schussler recommends that this cell salt be used in the range of 3X to 12X. Classical homeopaths, however, use the remedy in much higher potencies. In inflammatory diseases, the potency 30C is the most usual opening remedy, although all potencies are used, from lowest to highest.

While the length of the action of a single dose is unknown, Ferrum Phos is considered to be a deep and long-acting remedy. While it may be repeated as needed in acute cases, the single dose is considered best for chronic conditions.

Relationships: Ferrum Phos is considered to blend best with the actions specific to the Calcarea and Kali groups of remedies. In colds, flus, and other inflammatory conditions, look for it to work best with Kali Muriaticum.

26. GELSEMIUM

Remedy Source: Vegetable Remedy. The remedy Gelsemium is taken from the plant yellow jessamine (called *chambeli* in Hindi), which is best identified by its beautiful scent. It belongs to the Natural Order Longaniaceae and is native to India, Europe, and North America.

The remedy Gelsemium is made from the roots of the plant, which is picked at the time of flowering.

The remedy was created by Dr. John H. Henry of Philadelphia in 1852.

Situations That Suggest Gelsemium: Influenza, diarrhea, fever, hay fever, laryngitis, upper-respiratory infections. Also stage fright. Also chronic fatigue syndrome, mononucleosis, neuralgia, paralysis. Also headache. Consider also anxiety disorders, vertigo, tremor, insomnia.

Situations That Suggest Gelsemium: When you think of the remedy Gelsemium, you immediately think of weakness, as a general feeling of weakness will be the central issue for the patient or will accompany the more specific symptoms. This weakness will take place on all three planes of existence: mental, emotional, and physical. On the physical level, it will seem as if part of the patient has gone missing, as if he had been secretly drained of his blood or his life force. And, in terms of the emotional weakness of the remedy, it will seem as if the patient has lost his will, as if he has become a coward, too weak and too frightened to fight his way back to health. Mentally, this weakness will be expressed in a dullness, a slowness. Patients will not be able to recall things that they have known well for a long time, or they will not be able to put their information to practical use.

This mental weakness is the basis for the use of the remedy acutely for persons who are experiencing stage fright. When they have to approach the podium, they feel as if their strength is leaving them. Perhaps this happened even sooner, the night before, when they suddenly felt weak, or when—as commonly happens—they suddenly had to run to the bathroom, as their stage fright manifests itself in diarrhea. Look for the patient in need of this remedy to feel paralyzed by his stage fright—paralyzed on all three planes of existence.

Gelsemium is also the remedy to think of when this same paralysis, especially if it is accompanied by diarrhea, manifests itself for the person who has to take a test, or who has some challenge before him that overwhelms him, that paralyzes him. Therefore, any form of test, challenge, or performance, from a job interview to a Broadway opening, can bring on the symptoms of Gelsemium.

The other major use of this remedy acutely has to do with influenza. Where the remedy Bryonia speaks to the general flu with body aches and pains that sends one to bed in a bad mood, and Eupatorium speaks to the deeper, more aching and more exhausting flu, Gelsemium speaks to what we think of as "Southern" flu. Here the patient is not as ill. There are no high fevers or night sweats, but there is general exhaustion. The patient just wants to relax and rest. Such patients are averse to mental activity of any sort, especially work. They do not want to have long conversations or play cards or laugh, like the Sulphur or Phophorus will want to. Nor are they angry and withdrawn, like the Nux Vomica or the Natrum Mur.

Instead, they are happy for a gentle touch and some kind attention, but they will want to lie still in their room (and they will want to be in their own room) and snooze a bit.

It is characteristic of this remedy that the patient will be a bit droopy in general. He is mentally droopy, a little sluggish, a little forgetful. He will also be a bit physically droopy as well. Look for him to slump if he has to either sit or stand up, as if he simply did not have the energy to hold his body up. Look also for his eyelids to droop. His arms and legs will also seems droopy, as if the muscles had been removed.

Gelsemium can be an important constitutional remedy for some very serious illnesses such as multiple sclerosis, and all these illnesses will have at their core this same droopy and weak quality. Gelsemium can also speak to the patient who may have been of another remedy type but who, through chronic conditions or long-lasting illness, has been worn down and exhausted.

But it is important to remember, however, that the Gelsemium will not be beset with terrible aches and pains; indeed, he may seem to be out of touch with just how much pain he may be in. What is terrible about his condition is that he is no longer fully aware or fully able to function on any level.

The headache that is common to Gelsemium comes on from drinking wine. It begins in the back of the head and moves forward. It makes the head feel heavy, as if it cannot be lifted. The headache will be worse at 10 A.M., at which time the patient will describe it as "maddening." The patient may also experience a feeling of vertigo accompanying the headache. He may feel numb. His tongue may feel paralyzed and heavy.

Gelsemium is also an important remedy (along with Arsenicum, Carbo Veg, Lycopodium, Phosphorus, Sulphur, and others) for congestive heart failure. The patient's heart feels as if it will stop beating. The patient will jump up and move about because he will fear that if he stops moving, his heart will stop beating.

This is also a remedy for those with trembling or tremors of all sorts. It is a remedy for those with writer's cramp, for those who experience heaviness and trembling in the legs or arms, for those who experience chills in their bodies that begin in the hands or feet.

Consider the remedy also for those who are sleepless due to anticipation of an upcoming challenge, who are sleepless due to anxiety, and sometimes also sleepless from excitement, such as on Christmas Eve.

Keynotes: Those drooping eyelids are considered keynote. It will be all but impossible for the patient to keep his eyes open.

Another important symptom is that Gelsemium patients tend to lose their voices from fear. Thus the public speaker, if he can get past the bathroom, will walk out on the stage and find that he has lost his voice.

Diarrhea from fright, from anticipation of upcoming events, and from bad news is common. The patient will have no thirst during the diarrhea.

The most important issue in this remedy portrait is the exhaustion itself. Unlike other remedies that speak to exhaustion, Gelsemium is mentally, physically, and emotionally exhausted all at once. You cannot separate one form of exhaustion from the others. Such patients will even have an exhausted expression on their face that will make you hesitate before you disturb them with questions you need answered in order to take their case.

Aggravations: Gelsemiums are aggravated by sun. They are overwhelmed by sunlight. They cannot bear concentrated heat, such as from a fireplace or a gas stove. They are worse in summer heat.

They are also worse for cold, damp weather, especially worse from thunderstorms.

The Gelsemium is worse from any strong emotion—worse from excitement, worse from receiving bad news. The patient is worse from the anticipation of upcoming events; worse for thinking about his condition; worse when faced by public speaking or examinations; worse when confronted by any unusual event in life.

The patient will be at a loss when spoken to and will be worse from being questioned. He will be worse also from tobacco smoke.

Ameliorations: The patient will feel better after urinating; the symptoms of headache will be especially improved by urinating.

The patient will feel better by bending forward and even by wanting to gently rock forward and back, as will Pulsatilla.

The patient will want to close his eyes. The patient is better for closing his eyelids.

The patient is improved by fresh air; also by stimulants.

Dosage and Potency: Gelsemium is given in all potencies, although many practitioners find that it is especially effective in the 1M potency.

It bears repeated doses well and may be given as needed.

One dose of Gelsemium may hold for up to a month.

Relationships: Gelsemium is especially complementary in its effect to the remedy Agentum Nitricum, which is made from silver nitrate. Both are mild remedies, with patients needing them riddled in fear and anticipation of upcoming unpleasant events.

The remedy Ipecac often follows Gelsemium in the treatment of those who have diarrhea.

27. GRAPHITES

Remedy Source: Mineral Remedy. The remedy is taken from "amorphous carbon," or graphite. It is a form of carbon in which there is a quantity of pure lead. Graphite is the material from which the lead in our pencils is taken.

As a carbon-based remedy, it has a good deal in common with the others of its class. This is a psoric remedy related in type and function to Carbo Veg, among many others. Look for the keynote of dysfunction of organs and bodily systems.

This is a remedy created by Hahnemann.

Situations That Suggest Graphites: Digestive dysfunction: diarrhea, constipation, irritable bowel, colic, stomach pain, and cramps. Also skin conditions: psoriasis, eczema, poison ivy, rashes, ulcers, acne. Also worms. Also distortions of the senses: deafness and ear disorders, eye disorders. Also coughs and colds, flu, whooping cough.

Remedy Portrait: Graphites is a constitutional as well as an acute remedy. As a constitutional remedy it speaks especially to what once was called "peasant stock." Those of the type tend to be somewhat heavy, with thick wrists and ankles. Their systems, like those of Sulphur, seem a bit simpler than do those of some other types. As with Sulphur types, it is fairly easy to keep their system in balance. Mentally, they tend to be timid, and can also be very indecisive. They are deeply emotional and can have a strong emotional reaction to music.

In acute treatments, Graphites is most often going to be used in skin conditions of all sorts—for patients with brittle nails; with cracks and fissures in their skin and nails; with rashes and itches of all sorts. Diarrhea commonly will accompany the rash, as will abdominal flatulence and distension. Look also for sweat which stains clothing yellow to accompany skin disorders. Look also for the patient to complain of the sensation—particular to the forehead—of having walked through spiderwebs.

Ailments will come on from simple suppression, as with Sulphur. The patient who has used a cortisone rub for a rash will suddenly develop deep digestive distress. Suppressions of skin conditions and sweat are the most common causes of disease for the type. Something as simple as using an antiperspirant instead of a deodorant can cause terrible distress.

The patient's skin is thick. It tends to be callused and to crack and form fissures, especially on the feet, hands, elbows, and knees. The skin also tends toward all sorts of rashes—toward eczema and psoriasis and herpes. All the rashes itch and the patient will scratch his skin until it bleeds. The itching is always worse when the patient becomes warm, especially from the warmth of the bed.

Ailments also will come on from grief and fear; also from lifting too much weight and stressing out the physical body. This, like Calcarea, is a remedy type that usually moves rather slowly into illness, through emotional or physical stress.

This is also an excellent remedy to consider for the patient who is experiencing diarrhea or, especially, constipation that does not go away and is threatening to become a chronic condition. It is also for irritable bowel syndrome, in which diarrhea and constipation alternate.

Like Calcarea, Graphites tends to be a bit chilly and a bit sluggish. As Calcarea's head will sweat, so will Graphites' feet (as will Sulphur's as well). Graphites' feet tend to be very smelly things.

Food is very important to Graphites, as it is to Calcarea and Sulphur. But where Sulphur uses food as a reward, allowing himself a pizza or a bag of chips at the end of a long day, and Calcarea uses food as an emotional medicine, drowning his fears and sorrows in chocolate cake, Graphites uses food as a physical cure-all. Graphites tends to ailments of the stomach and the digestive tract, after all, and it is his particular blessing and curse that all those ailments are improved by eating. Therefore, the Graphites who awakens in the night with stomach cramps will know to get something to eat so that he can fall back into a peaceful sleep. No wonder the Graphites type tends to be heavy. Patients particularly crave chicken, which they digest very well. While they do like some sweets, sugar does not drive their desires as it does Lycopodium's. Instead, they like heavy and rather bland foods. Potatoes are a particular favorite. They are also thirsty people and like cold drinks of all sorts. They tend to particularly crave beer.

In almost all ailments, look for the Graphites patient to have changes in vision and hearing. The patient will be very sensitive to light. He will suffer a hearing loss or, very commonly, will hear a buzzing or a ringing in the ears. He will actually hear more acutely when surrounded by white noise, such as when he is in an airplane or a car.

Graphites is commonly a remedy for those with conjunctivitis; also with similar discharge from the ears; for cracks in the eyelids and cracks or eruptions behind the ears.

Graphites is also a helpful remedy for those with seasonal allergies or for colds that either will not go away or seem to reoccur over and over again. The sides of the nose tend to crack during these bouts of illness.

Keynotes: The keynote sensation of pain for the remedy type is numbness. This is particularly true in headache. The patient may feel drunk when he has a headache.

The sensation of the spiderweb is unique to Graphites and is a most important guiding symptom.

It is also keynote that the patient will be at his worst first thing in the morning. He may be anxious or sad upon awakening. He will awaken feeling exhausted. He feels that gravity is very heavy indeed when he is in the process of awakening.

Aggravations: The typical Graphites is a chilly person and feels worse when cold. The patient feels especially bad from drafts of cold air.

Graphites patients are also worse upon awakening. They need time to feel up to getting up out of bed and should be allowed these moments of strength gathering.

They are worse from any suppression of the bodily systems, especially from the suppression of rashes and of sweat.

They are worse from light; also worse at night.

They are worse from the heat of the bed, worse from scratching their rashes, and worse from getting their feet wet.

Ameliorations: They are better in dark places, especially if they are allowed to wrap up and feel cozy. They are better after walking in open air, especially if they can come inside and get cozy before they become too cold.

They are also better from warm drinks when they feel exhausted or in pain. They tend to especially like warm milk.

They also feel better after a good cry, especially from music or old movies.

They are better from being touched. They are made better by belching.

Dosage and Potency: This is a remedy that works well in lower potencies. You will get some very good results with 6C. Most often in home use, expect to use these low potencies, 6C to 30C, in skin conditions. The higher potencies should not be used in the skin conditions, as they will greatly aggravate them before improvement sets in. Save the high potencies for chronic digestive conditions. High potencies should be given in a single dose; low potencies may be repeated as needed.

One dose of this very slow-acting remedy holds for up to six weeks.

Relationships: For students of homeopathy, it goes without saying that Graphites would work well with our other great psoric remedies. It will follow well and complete the action of Calcarea, Sulphur, Lycopodium, Sepia, and Pulsatilla.

It is also highly complementary to Hepar Sulph and can follow it well in infections of all sorts.

Graphites is antidoted by Nux and Aconite; also by Arsenicum, which is also a highly complementary remedy in terms of potency and action.

28. HEPAR SULPHURIS

Remedy Source: Animal Remedy. The remedy was created by Hahnemann from sulphuret of lime, also called Hepar Sulphuris Calcareum. It was created by fusing the middle layers of oyster shells (from which Calcarea Carbonica is made) with flower of sulfur (from which Sulphur is made). The two substances are burned together in a crucible in the creation of the remedy.

Alchemists referred to this substance as the "liver of sulfur." Its color was supposed to mimic that of liver. It was used as a folk remedy for itch, rheumatism, gout, and goiter.

Situations That Suggest Hepar Sulph: Abscesses of all sorts, infections, glandular swelling, colds, upper-respiratory infections, pneumonia, sore throats, laryngitis, whooping cough, bronchitis, ear infections, cough, croup, also rheumatism, hip joint disease, joint pain. Also herpes. Also diarrhea and constipation. Also skin disorders, boils, suppuration, eczema, skin ulcers, impetigo, warts.

Remedy Portrait: Here you have a very vulnerable patient. He is in a state of depletion on all three levels: physical, mental, and emotional. The patient will be sensitive to pain on all three levels. The patient needing Hepar

Sulph will feel in pain—physical pain—that seems intense beyond all boundaries of the illness that he is experiencing. It is as if his entire life force is caught up in this pain and is overwhelmed by it. The patient is like a person who has been set adrift in a small boat and who is battling the elements. He feels beset by his environment, by the weather, overwhelmed, and defeated. Look for him to have no strength left to rise up against outside forces.

Historically, this has been the remedy for the condition known as quinsy, which is a sore throat that has become so swollen and painful that it can threaten—or at least seem to threaten—the very life of the patient.

This is almost always a case in which there is a real and active infection present. There will usually be some form of fever, and often the development of pus and a flow of discharge from the body will lead the prescriber to this particular remedy. While in his weakened state, look for the patient to be very sensitive to outside impressions—to any strong weather patterns or changes in weather; to light, to noise, or to chemical odors. Look especially for the patient to be vulnerable to cold. Cold will cut through into the deepest levels of his being.

The patient will often seem agoraphobic. He will not want to leave his home. He will feel safe and protected from outside impressions only when he is in his own home. Often he will not even want to leave his bedroom and will set up his sickbed with almost a bunker mentality. Security will be very important. The patient will need to feel secure in his surroundings and with all the persons, sights, sounds, and smells that come into contact with him.

Look for this patient to be especially sensitive to the pain he is in. Look for the patient to have little or no interest in anything other than this pain. Often the patient will come to believe that the pain will never end. The patient may even contemplate or attempt suicide in order to escape his pain.

The patient will also be filled with fear. He will be especially fearful about physical pain and anything that may increase his pain. Therefore, a visit to the doctor or the dentist will become a terrifying event, even if that visit is necessary in the ultimate removal of the present pain. Often Hepar Sulph patients will not be able to bear any news of pain. They will not be able to watch the news on TV, for instance, because they cannot look at videotape of an auto accident. In the same way, they will often be unable to watch any movie that contains violence.

The quality of pain specific to Hepar Sulph is termed stitching or sticking. Most often, especially in cases of sore throat, the patient will say that he feels as if a splinter is lodged in the painful area.

It is also common to the remedy that the patient will not bear his pain in silence. The Hepar Sulph patient will complain of his pain, will continue to list his woes.

It is also common that, because a real infection is present, the patient will have swollen glands. All the infections will be slow to heal and will drain the patient of his strength. Abscesses, cracked skin, and skin ulcers will be particularly slow to heal. The infection will most commonly take the form of tonsillitis, otitis media, corneal ulcer, whitlow, or abscessed tooth.

Finally, look for this patient to generally be most averse to cold. He will even be unable to bear anything cold that touches only one small part of the body. Look for him to be unwilling to handle a can of cold soda. Look also for the patient to be unable to stick even his hand or foot outside of the warmth of the bed covers. In the same way, the patient will likely want his head covered, and will complain of headache or earache if the head is uncovered. (In all earaches covered by this remedy, expect the child to scream in pain and to grow much worse if he is taken out of doors, especially into windy weather.)

Keynotes: The sensation of a stick being caught in the throat or in any other painful area of the body is keynote of the remedy.

Also keynote of the remedy is the fact that the patient is chilly and is extremely aggravated by cold in any form, especially cold wind. The patient wants no contact with open or moving air.

As with Natrum Mur, it is keynote of this remedy that the middle of the lower lip will be cracked and sore. Look for cracked skin throughout the body.

As with the remedies Mercurius and Silicea, look for every little injury to have the tendency to become infected. The formation of pus is keynote to this remedy as with the other two.

As with Mercurius, sweat is keynote of the remedy. Look for the patient to sweat profusely day and night, without the sweat giving any kind of relief. The perspiration will have a sour smell. The patient will perspire from the slightest exertion.

Although the patient will want to be warm and will want to be covered in order to stay warm and be protected from the air and from cold, he will also have to contend with overly sensitive skin. He will not be able to bear touch, sometimes even the touch of clothing or bed covers. Sometimes the patient will take off his coverings in even the coldest room. The fact that skin sensitivity leads him to this action indicates this remedy.

Aggravations: Cold air; being uncovered; eating or drinking cold things.

Aggravation is brought on by the touch of painful areas of the body by human hands, by clothing, or by bedclothes; also by lying on painful parts of the body and putting the slightest pressure on the painful areas of the body.

Look for the patient to be aggravated by coughing. Coughing forces him to take his hand out from under the covers.

Ameliorations: The patient is improved by warmth; by being wrapped up, covered up warmly, especially around the head.

The patient is improved in damp, cool, overcast weather as long as he himself is indoors and warm.

Dosage and Potency: The potencies 30C and 200C are most common. The potency 200C works best in severe infections. Higher potencies are used in constitutional cases.

Low potencies may be repeated as needed. Higher potencies are used in a single dose.

One dose holds forty to fifty days.

Relationships: Calendula is very complementary to Hepar Sulph and may be used topically while this remedy is taken internally to clear infections of the skin.

Bryonia and Silicea follow well and often complete the action of Hepar Sulph.

29. HYPERICUM

Remedy Source: Vegetable Remedy. The remedy Hypericum Perforatum is taken from the plant Saint-John's-wort. The remedy is made from the whole plant, which must be picked while at full bloom.

The remedy was proven by German homeopath George F. Mueller.

Situations That Suggest Hypericum: Injuries: punctures, lacerations, or contusions involving any part of the body dense with nerves, especially the fingers, tongue, teeth, eyes, and genitalia. Also for injuries to the spine, from sprains to fractures; injuries to the coccyx. For phantom pains of all sorts.

Remedy Portrait: Hypericum is a must-have remedy for the home kit. No other remedy for patients with pain will duplicate the work of Hypericum. This is the first remedy to think of in cases that involve animal bites. It is an important remedy for lacerated wounds. Hypericum will often be used in alternation with Arnica or Calendula in severe physical trauma. This is another remedy that must also be considered strongly in postoperative recovery. It is of special help for those recovering from dental surgery.

Mentally, the Hypericum patient must be described as being "in a fog." This is a drowsy patient, one who will want to fall asleep. This is a patient dealing with shock. He may have the sensation that he is weightless, that he is flying up into the air. He may also, just as he drifts off to sleep, have the frightening sensation of falling to earth from a great height. Look for the Hypericum patient to make mistakes in talking, and especially to make mistakes in writing.

The patient will say that his head feels heavy. Also that it feels cold— but he will say that it feels as if his head is being touched by a cold hand, or as if cold applications were being pressed against it. It will be a phantom external coldness. He may also say that his head feels enlarged or elongated.

Head pain will be located in the top of the head. Hypericum will have a head pain when he is in a warm room. Consider this remedy for the patient with severe head pain, especially pain associated with a mechanical injury to the head. Consider this remedy for patients with toothaches that are accompanied by tearing pains. The pain will usually be worse on the right side of the head. The patient will be sad when he is in pain.

The most important use for Hypericum will be for patients with lacerated wounds, especially when the patient has lost a good deal of blood. It is important also for any injury to a part of the body in which nerves are injured as well as soft tissue, especially for injuries to fingers and toes. This is the first remedy to consider for the patient who has crushed his finger in a car door. But Hypericum has also been used for the treatment of those with gunshot wounds (in which case, it will likely be used in alternation with Calcarea).

It has been stated that Hypericum will not only assist in the treatment of pain, but that it will also greatly heal the treatment of the injury itself. Hypericum (especially when used in alternation with Calendula) has been shown to bring about healing even when tissue has been all but torn off the body. It will help the wound to knit, as Calcarea will help the patient to avoid infection during the healing process.

This is also an excellent remedy for the patient who has pain without physical trauma, for the patient whose pain resides between his shoulders. The pain will be daring in nature. The remedy is also useful for rheumatic pains, especially those in the hands or feet. The patient will complain of a crawling sensation in his hands and feet and a numbness in his limbs. He will say that his limbs feel as if they had been torn away. He will say that all his joints feel bruised. The patient will complain that the pain centers in the coccyx and radiates upward to his spine and down into his legs. Look for the patient to have twitching and jerking of the muscles in affected parts of the body.

Consider this remedy also for cases of acute asthma that occurs during foggy weather. Look for the Hypericum patient to be worse in every way—both in his physical and emotional symptoms—during foggy weather.

The patient will feel nausea but will be thirsty. He may crave alcohol, especially wine. Look at the patient's tongue for an indication of the remedy. The tongue will have a white coating on its base, but will have a clean tip.

Keynotes: This is a remedy for those with physical trauma. It is especially helpful in cases of injury to the nerves and spine; also for injury to the brain. It is for tailbone pain after an injury; for puncture wounds that are very sensitive to the touch; for animal bites and wounds. It is keynote of this remedy that the injuries are much more sensitive and painful than they look. Look for the pains in this remedy to be both sharp and shooting in nature.

Hypericum is also an important remedy in recovery from gunshot wounds, knife wounds, and any form of surgery, particularly dental surgery.

Look for the patient to be confused and somewhat irritable. Look for a loss of memory. Look for fear, particularly fear of falling and fear of heights. The patient will feel as if he is flying, as if he has been taken up high and is going to be dropped. The patient will be anxious.

Aggravations: The patient feels worse from any sort of exertion or from touch, particularly from any touch that jars him.

He is also made worse by any change in weather, especially by the change from dry to damp. He is worse in cold, damp weather, and worse during a fog.

The patient feels worse in a closed, warm room, but also worse when exposed to cold, damp weather. Even the slightest exposure weakens the patient greatly.

Ameliorations: The patient's pains are improved by rubbing the area.

He is better from bending his head back and from lying on his face.

He is also better when lying still, and when lying on the painful side.

Dosage and Potency: Hypericum is often used as an external low-potency rub. This rub is excellent at lessening pain and protecting the wound from infection.

Internally, it may be given in any potency, from lowest to highest, and may be repeated as called for.

This is a quick-acting remedy whose action does not hold for a long period of time. Be prepared to give this remedy frequently until improvement has begun.

Relationships: Hypericum is used most often in conjunction with Arnica or with Calendula, and it combines in action well with either of them. Hypericum will often, taken internally, complete the action begun by Arnica.

30. IGNATIA AMARA

Remedy Source: Vegetable Remedy. Ignatia Amara is taken from the Saint-Ignatius's-bean. The plant is a large shrub or a climbing tree that is native to the islands of the South Pacific. The shrub has fragrant white flowers. The mother tincture is made from the seeds of the shrub.

The remedy was created by Hahnemann.

Situations That Suggest Ignatia: Hysteria, grief, anxiety, compulsive behavior, also acute asthma, chronic fatigue, environmental illness, chronic headaches, and migraine. Also spasms and tics of all sort; depressions, sometimes clinical depression; low back pain.

Remedy Portrait: Let's be very clear about the emotional picture of this remedy. Sometimes it is mistakenly thought of as being the remedy for persons in a deep state of grief. Grief is a natural part of our lives. For the wife who has lost a husband, or the parents who have lost a child, grief is a natural process. And the remedy Ignatia is not indicated for those who are naturally grieving, who are working through the loss of a loved one. No, Ignatia is suggested for those who are trapped in grief, who have already been through the process and who find that they cannot move past their grief. It is for patients for whom grief has become their constant companion and their heavy burden in life. Think of this remedy for those who are not manifesting what the classic texts call "the ill effects of grief and worry," who have undergone a change in behavior and outlook because of their grief, and who are now manifesting physical symptoms as well that match those contained within the remedy picture. To give Ignatia simply because of a loss is like simply giving Arnica because of a bump. While you may sometimes do some good, you will far more often, with your allopathic practice of homeopathy, do nothing at all. (If the picture of Ignatia is not clear, or if you just don't know what to do, consider Rescue Remedy. See that listing at the end of this guide.)

In terms of both the physical and emotional symptoms, look for Ignatia patients to display rapid changes in mood. They will go from laughter to tears in an instant. Ignatia patients will not want to explain the reasons for these changes. They may suddenly leap up and run into the room. You will hear them crying moments later. Ignatia patients anger suddenly and laugh just as suddenly. They sigh a lot.

The key here is that these changes are very quick and the Ignatia keeps everyone else off-balance. You will never know what you said that made the patient angry or made him cry. Therefore, everyone else will be forced to tiptoe around the patient and around the house. This will give the patient, by virtue of his erratic behavior, a kind of control over the actions of those around him.

Erratic is a good word for the physical symptoms as well. This is a remedy picture that is filled with spasms of all sorts. Look for the muscles of the patient's face, particularly, to twitch spasmodically. Look for twitching of the eyelids and of the mouth. Look for the Ignatia to repeatedly bite the inside of his cheeks.

The patient will complain of a sour taste in his mouth. He will also have a good deal of saliva in his mouth. The patient will feel as if he has a lump in his throat. This is a good remedy to remember for the patient with a sore throat. The pain will be characterized by the fact that it will be better when the patient does not swallow. It will also be better when he swallows something solid. The Ignatia's sore throat will be worse from empty swallowing or swallowing liquids.

Ignatias will be made worse by drinking coffee—which upsets their whole system—and worse from tobacco. Just the smell of coffee and/or tobacco may set them off. Consider this remedy for cases of toothache in which the pain is increased when coffee or tobacco is used.

The patient may have a spasmodic cough as well. The cough is dry and comes on in quick fits, quick attacks of coughing, between which the patient sighs. He will say that the fits of coughing only make him feel as if he has to cough more. The cough will be worse in the evening and will irritate the patient's sore throat.

Other aspects of spasm include hiccoughs and colic. The patient will complain of severe pains in the abdomen. He will not want that area of his body to be touched. He will only want to eat acidic things. The colicky pains will be accompanied by a rumbling in the bowels.

Consider this remedy when the patient has a bout of diarrhea that comes on after a fright, when the stool contains a good amount of blood and is very painful to pass. This is also a remedy for the patient with hemorrhoids, especially when he complains of a sensation as if a sharp instrument were moving from within his body in an outward direction.

The spasms will extend into the patient's limbs as well. Look for the patient to have jerking movements in all his limbs as he goes to sleep. And the Ignatia patient will not sleep well. He tends to have insomnia and nightmares often as well.

Keynotes: Hysteria; grief. The patient feels betrayed in love and is trapped in these feelings of betrayal. This is not a remedy for the normal and necessary feelings of grief that we all feel at the loss of love, but it is rather a remedy for those who become trapped in these feelings of grief, loss, and betrayal.

Look for wild changes in mood and behavior. The patient displays spasmodic laughter from grief; also irrational anger.

The symptoms of the remedy contradict themselves and change very quickly. Just as with mental symptoms, in which the patient will go from joy to sorrow to anger in a very short time, the physical symptoms will shift and change as well, seemingly without reason. Symptoms are sudden.

Headaches are pronounced. Patient has headaches that feel as if a nail were being driven out through the side of the head. Headaches are relieved by lying on the painful area.

Look for the patient to bite the inside of his cheek. He will do this either on purpose or by accident. He bites the inside of his cheek each time he eats. He also chews the inside of his cheek nervously.

Aggravations: Consolation. The Ignatia does not want any pity, or any compassion. He wants to be left alone. He will become very angry if consoled, or if told that anyone "understands just what he is going though."

The patient is worse in the presence of strong smells. He cannot bear the odor of perfume, and he may become ill at the smell of coffee or tobacco.

He is worse from alcohol, from tobacco, and from coffee.

He is worse for any strong emotions. The patient feels genuine sorrow after anger. The patient is worse from any touch: mental, emotional, or physical. The Ignatia patient is worse in winter, in cold weather in general.

The patient is overwhelmed by grief and yet is impatient. He will often want to move very quickly but will feel worse from walking too fast.

Ameliorations: The Ignatia patient is better for warmth, and from becoming warm. The patient will relax with warm liquids or in a warm room.

The patient feels better from hard pressure on any area of physical pain. Look for the patient to press his head when he has a headache.

The Ignatia feels better also from walking slowly and if he changes position while either sitting or lying in bed.

Dosage and Potency: While it can be used in all potencies, since the remedy is usually given on the basis of emotional symptoms, it tends to be given in high potency. Potencies of 1M and above are given in cases of prolonged grief.

While the lower potencies can be repeated as needed, high potencies should be given in a single dose.

Ignatia is a fast-working remedy of short duration. One dose is said to hold for up to nine days.

31. IPECACUANHA/IPECAC

Remedy Source: Vegetable Remedy. The remedy Ipecacuanha is taken from Ipecac, a small shrub that grows in moist and shady areas, often deep in the woods. The shrub is native to Brazil. It is of the Natural Order Rabiaceae. The plant is known for its small white flowers.

The remedy is made from the dried roots of the plant, which are made into a mother tincture.

The homeopathic remedy was created by Hahnemann.

Situations That Suggest Ipecac: Nausea and vomiting. Also fevers that reoccur, bronchitis, acute asthma. Also nosebleeds, hemorrhages. Also migraines with nausea and vomiting.

Remedy Portrait: This is a very specific and somewhat small remedy, but it works brilliantly when called upon.

Think of Ipecac basically in three areas of action: (1) for patients with nausea and vomiting; (2) for patients with either asthma or asthmatic bronchitis; and (3) for patients with hemorrhage.

The patient who needs Ipecac will most often have a constant nausea that has completely incapacitated him. The patient will feel as if his stomach is hanging loose within him. Although the patient will likely vomit frequently, he will not feel better after vomiting. It is keynote of this remedy that although the patient will have nausea and vomiting, he will have a totally clean tongue. Look for the tongue to look pink and healthy.

In home use, Ipecac can be particularly helpful for migraines that are accompanied by nausea and vomiting. Look for the patient to have one side of the face both hot and flushed. He will feel the pain of the headache down into his face, his teeth, and even his jaw. And look for the muscles of the patient's neck to be tight during the headache (or during cough).

The nausea and vomiting can come on from causes other than headache: they can be the result of coughing; of hemorrhage, and even childbirth. Look for the nausea to be accompanied by colic and by abdominal cramping. Look for the patient to be unable to bear the smell of cooking food.

In cases involving asthmatic bronchitis, the patient is likely to be a child. Look for the patient to have a rattling cough that comes on during warm, humid weather. Look for the characteristic stiff neck to accompany the cough. Look for the cough to become so severe that it interferes with the patient's ability to breathe. Ipecac is also an excellent remedy for young patients with croup.

In cases involving hemorrhage, uterine hemorrhage is most common. Look for blood to begin to gush suddenly—bright red blood that will not coagulate. Look for the common portrait of nausea, vomiting, and exhaustion to accompany the bleeding, no matter from what part of the body the blood flows.

Keynotes: The combination of nausea and vomiting and the tendency toward hemorrhage is truly keynote of the remedy.

Also keynote is the tendency for the patient to have one side of his face hot, the other cold; also, one hand cold, the other hot.

It is also keynote that the patients who need this remedy will have a very clean, clear, and healthy-looking tongue.

Ipecac patients will also have no thirst.

Aggravations: The patient receives an aggravation from the slightest motion.

The patient is worse in autumn and in winter, and worse in dry weather. He is especially bad during periods of cold nights and hot days.

He feels worse after eating salads, fats, or rich meals; worse after overeating in general.

Ameliorations: The patient feels better when breathing fresh air.

Dosage and Potency: The potency 30C tends to be the best strength to begin with, although higher potencies may be needed in cases of severe nausea and vomiting. In hemorrhages, 30C works best.

It may be repeated as needed. One dose holds for up to a week.

Relationships: Arnica is a complementary remedy and follows Ipecac well. So do Arsenicum, Bryonia, Calcarea Carbonica, Nux Vomica, Phosophorus, and Pulsatilla.

32. KALI BICHROMICUM

Remedy Source: Mineral Remedy. The Kalis are a large group of remedies, all based in part on the substance potassium. Kali Bichromicum is potassium bichromate. Its chemical formula is $K_2Cr_2O_7$. It is a compound of potassium and chromic acid, and is available in salt form at most drugstores.

The remedy was created by Dr. J. Drysdale, a British homeopath. The proving of the remedy was performed and published by the Austrian Society of Homeopaths.

Situations That Suggest Kali Bi: Allergies of all sorts, acute asthma, colds, coughs, sinusitis, postnasal drip, pneumonia, whooping cough. Also sinus headaches, migraines. Also gastritis and diarrhea. Also rheumatic pains, low back pain, neuralgia.

Remedy Portrait: This is a small remedy but one that belongs in every home kit because its use is very specific and commonly needed. Kali Bi is most often called for on an acute basis as the last remedy used in clearing a cold. (Often up to three remedies will be needed to completely clear away cold symptoms: one for the onset of the cold, one for the period of time during which there is a clear discharge from the nose, and one for the final stage of the cold when the discharge becomes colored.) The action of Kali Bi is geared to the cold that will not end, to the time during which the mucus is thick, green, and ropy. It also helps the cough that drags on and on. This cough tends to be somewhat shallow and more annoying than dangerous. The remedy will help the patient to expel the plug of mucus that he has been trying to move, and then be finished with the cough.

The major action of the remedy is on the sinuses. Look for the patient to have a total loss of smell. The patient will also be unable to breathe through his nose. Look for there to be pain and heaviness in the frontal sinuses. Look for the patient to complain of postnasal drip. Often, the patient will feel as if his left nostril is being tickled by a hair or a feather. The patient will snuffle in his attempt to breathe through his nose, but he will usually have to breathe through his mouth.

This is also the major remedy for sinus headaches. It is keynote of the remedy that the pain of the headache will be located in one small area. If asked where it hurts, the patient will point to one specific small spot, usually right above his nose and between his eyes. It is also keynote that the pain of the headache—and, indeed, all physical pains—will move about a good bit. So while they are confined to one spot, that spot will tend to shift about a lot.

This is also a major rheumatic remedy, one that responds to changes in weather. Look for the headaches and sinus conditions, as well as the body aches, to increase during weather changes.

Kali Bi, while acutely a very simple remedy, does have some interesting emotional symptoms as well. In the constitutional state, the Kali type is known for the intensity of his religious feelings. Even in the acute state, the patient may equate his illness with the wrath of God and may ask why he is being punished. Kali Bi patients are intense, and can even be paranoid. They are afraid, and this fear is deepened by their illness. They do not want to be alone and fear what will happen to them if they are left alone. They also fear that they will lose their minds. They worry about being poisoned, and will become quite paranoid about it.

Kali Bi is a major remedy for sleep disorders. Look for the patient to have trouble falling asleep. Look for his fear to grow greater as he approaches sleep, as if the solitary act of sleeping is a fearful thing. Night terrors are common, as is sleepwalking.

This is a right-sided remedy. Look for the patient's symptoms to be worse on the right side of the body. This is particularly true of rheumatic pains, especially sciatica. Look for a general feeling of numbness to run through this remedy.

The Kali Bi's hand will often give him away. Look for the patient to have cold sweat on the hands and feet, although the rest of the body is covered with sticky sweat, which usually precedes a general chilly feeling. The Kali Bi will also wring his hands. Often this will be accompanied by sighing. Like Ignatia, Kali Bi will sigh a good bit.

Often the patient will combine gastric and rheumatic conditions. There can be a good bit of diarrhea with this remedy, and it will be worse in the morning. This diarrhea, or cutting pains in the abdomen, will be improved by eating, but after eating the patient's rheumatic pains will become pronounced. Thus the diarrhea is better after breakfast but the sciatica is worse.

This is an excellent remedy for hay fever and other seasonal allergies. In this remedy's portrait, however, the allergies are more severe, so that they overwhelm the patient's whole being. Look for the characteristic sinus troubles coupled with a sticky, cold sweat that covers the whole body.

Keynotes: The color green is very important to this remedy portrait. Look for all bodily discharges to be green, or greenish-yellow. This is particularly true of any mucus discharge, which is green, thick, and stringy in texture. It can also be true in cases involving diarrhea.

It is also keynote of this remedy that pains occur in small spots. The patient can always tell you exactly where it hurts and, often, the area of the pain will be no larger than his fingertip.

It is also keynote that these pains shift very quickly from one place to another; thus the headache will be over the root of the nose one moment and above the right eye the next. This is true of complex symptoms as well: the patient's gastric symptoms will alternate with headache or allergy or rheumatic symptoms. Look for these changes also to be rapid.

Finally, there is the rather strange minor keynote that the patient will be troubled by the feeling that a part of his body is being tickled by a hair. This is most common either in the nose or on the tongue. He will try and try to remove the hair. This odd sensation, however, can take place anywhere on the body.

Aggravations: The patient, being rheumatic, will be worse in cold, damp air or in cold weather; also during changes from dry to damp weather.

However, the patient is also intolerant of hot weather, especially hot, damp weather, which will make his allergies much worse.

The patient feels worse when drinking alcohol in any form, especially beer. Look for the patient to crave beer, however, which causes diarrhea.

The Kali Bi patient is worse during the morning hours, and may have a crisis in the hour from 2 until 3 A.M. He is worse from sleeping in that his sleep is so disturbed.

And, although some symptoms will be improved by eating, the patient, in general, will be worse for having eaten. Look for the patient's cough to grow much worse after eating.

The patient will also be worse from sitting and, especially, from stooping.

Ameliorations: The Kali Bi patient will be better from heat, and from wrapping up. He will like warm applications on his headache and over the area of the sinuses and will be relieved for these applications.

Kali Bi patients also feel better in the open air in general, although open air may aggravate their gastric complaints.

In that the nights are so difficult for Kali Bi patients, look for them to want to take short naps, and to awaken from these naps feeling much refreshed.

Dosage and Potency: For the most part, the potencies 30C and 200C are the most effective in clearing up the symptoms associated with the remedy. The remedy can be repeated as needed.

Relationships: Kali Bi is a complementary remedy to Arsenicum, and will often be used to complete that remedy's action. Pulsatilla follows the remedy well in allergic conditions and in colds.

33. LACHESIS

Remedy Source: Animal Remedy. The remedy Lachesis is taken from the poison of the surukuku snake, also called *Trigonocephalus lachesis*. The snake is native to South America. It belongs to the Natural Order Ophidia.

The remedy was created by homeopath Constantine Hering.

Situations That Suggest Lachesis: Sore throat, voice loss, swollen throat, swollen glands. Also hay fever, acute asthma. Also varicose veins. Also warts, tumor and ulcers, whitlows. Also menopause. Also Ménière's disease, vertigo. Also bleeding gums. Also amblyopia and vision disorders.

Remedy Portrait: This is an amazing remedy. It is both a very important remedy in the constitutional context and one that has many acute applications. With this remedy, think of the neck and throat region of the body as the snake itself, because almost all illnesses associated with the use of the remedy will either center on symptoms of the neck and/or throat or contain them as an important component of the illness. Most common is the sensation of swelling—of either the internal or external throat. The patient will feel that he cannot swallow liquids, due to either pain or swelling, but he will be able to swallow solids. In some cases, swallowing solid foods will actually improve the pain.

An important keynote of the remedy is that the patient will not be able to tolerate anything around his throat. He will not be able to wear tight collars or turtlenecks. He will not want his throat touched. While this symptom may appear in other parts of the body as well, with a sensation of tightness and a fear of touch, it will nowhere else be as pronounced as in the area of the throat.

Another consideration has to do with the nature of snake poison itself. The impact of the poison is to thin the blood, to remove its coagulation factor. And so the remedy Lachesis, taken from snake poison, will be an important remedy in cases of bleeding, especially when the bleeding will not stop. Therefore, think of Lachesis in nosebleeds that just gush and gush and will not stop. The blood will be thin and dark, with dark particles floating in it. Look for blood in bodily discharges: mucus, stool, and urine. Any small wound will bleed a great deal. This is also true of two other remedies: Phosphorus and Rhus Tox. The Rhus Tox nosebleed can look a good deal like the Lachesis, but the color of the blood in Rhus Tox is much brighter red than in Lachesis. And small wounds in Phosphorus bleed as much as in Lachesis, but the color of the blood again in Phosphorus is bright, bright red and is easy to tell apart from that of Lachesis. It is important to note that Phosphorus and Lachesis are the two remedies most commonly used (along with Staphysagria for pain) in stopping the bleeding from wounds and knife cuts. They are also used in the recovery period after surgery.

It is also an important remedy for toxic states, toxic states of all sorts. The patient has been poisoned environmentally or by his own lifestyle and now his system is broken down. This will happen in the case of an alcoholic. This sort of Lachesis patient will have broken health as well as a multitude of small afflictions, all chronic in nature. You will see diabetes. You will see gangrene, and also blood in the urine. The patient is exhausted.

The pains in this remedy will tend to be dominant on the left side of the body, or will begin on the left side and then move right. As this is a great remedy for females, pain in the left ovary is an important guiding symptom of the type.

The sensations common to the remedy include sudden flashes of heat to any part of the body and sudden rushes of blood to any part of the body. Also, the patient will commonly feel the sensation of a lump in his throat or abdomen. He may also feel this sensation of a lump in the area of the liver, rectum, or bladder.

The color blue is important to Lachesis. Look for the skin of the affected parts of the body to take on a shade of this color. Look for the affected parts to swell also, especially after having been scratched.

There is also a sensation of constriction that is very common to the remedy. This is especially true in the head and the throat. Also look for the patient to tremble—especially the hands will tremble as the whole body is filled with throbbing or hammering pains.

With the sensation of heat and feelings of exhaustion and constriction, and, especially given the fact that this is a common remedy in females, think of Lachesis during the period of menopause, most especially if the physical symptoms are accompanied by wild mood swings.

Think of this remedy first for sore throats that begin on the left side and move right, most especially if the other characteristics of the type are present. This is also an excellent remedy for puncture wounds and bites of all sorts and should be thought of just behind Ledum and Apis as an acute remedy in situations involving any puncture of the skin, most particularly when the skin in the area of the wound turns a shade of blue.

Finally, think of this as a great fever remedy. Look for the patient to be in a stupor. Look for him to mutter and to rave in delirium. Look for the tongue to protrude from the mouth. The patient will crave cold water. Lachesis fevers are most common in the spring and summer months.

Keynotes: Perhaps the most important keynote of the remedy type is that sleep brings the patient aggravation. The Lachesis patient will always feel worse from sleeping at any time of day or night. And so, if you have a patient with a left-sided sore throat, watch to see his disposition upon awakening.

Also keynote is the sense of constriction in the body, especially in the head and throat, and the fact that the Lachesis cannot bear anything to touch his throat. Most patients will not even be able to wear jewelry of any sort around their neck.

Another important keynote of the Lachesis is his method of speech. He will love to talk and talk more than any other remedy type. He not only talks, he orates. Sulphur and Phosphorus also like to talk. And Natrum Mur and Pulsatilla like to gossip, but only Lachesis is Lachesis. He is a fast talker, a wild talker. They are in love with the sound of their own voice. And, as such, this is an important remedy for any condition that has to do with human speech, from stuttering to incoherent muttering. Pay attention to the way in which the patient presents himself verbally and you will spot the Lachesis even before you ask the first question.

Emotionally, jealousy is the keynote. No other remedy, not even Ignatia, can touch Lachesis for feelings of jealousy. Illnesses come on from feelings of jealousy.

Aggravations: Lachesis is a warm-blooded remedy. Lachesis patients are worse in the heat, during the summer, and especially in the summer sun. They are worse when drinking hot beverages. They may feel worse from swallowing liquids of any sort.

Lachesis patients are worse during the spring. The transition from winter to spring is difficult. They are also worse in the high heat of summer, especially on sunny days.

They are worse from any pressure or constriction. They cannot bear tight clothing.

They are worse from sleeping, worse after sleep, and worse from closing their eyes.

Ameliorations: Lachesis feels better after the appearance of any discharge: mucus, urine, or blood.

Dosage and Potency: This remedy is useful in all potencies. For the home kit, keep it in 30C and 1M. It is usually used, in any potency, in a single dose.

One dose of Lachesis holds for thirty days.

Relationships: Lachesis is complementary to Hepar Sulph and Lycopodium. Natrum Mur follows this remedy very well, especially in women's ailments, and often completes the case.

It is antidoted by several remedies, most commonly by Nux and Coffea.

34. LEDUM PALUSTRE

Remedy Source: Vegetable Remedy. The remedy Ledum Palustre is taken from the herb called marsh tea. It is also known as wild rosemary. It is a plant that is quite common in Europe and North America. Note that the plant grows in damp regions. The remedy is made from the whole plant, which is gathered just after flowering has begun.

Ledum is a remedy created by Hahnemann. Dr. Teste later reproved the remedy's actions.

Situations That Suggest Ledum: Puncture wounds from stings and bites. Wounds of all sorts, bruises. Also abscesses of all sorts. Also headaches, sprains, rheumatic pains, nosebleed.

Remedy Portrait: Ledum is a remedy that is very specific in its action and very specific in the picture of its symptoms. Consider this remedy in cases of all wounds, especially puncture wounds (including insect stings and spider bites), in which the affected area of the body has an internal feeling of cold, and yet the affected area will feel better from applications of cold and worse from applications of heat.

As the classic texts say, "There is a general lack of animal heat" that runs throughout the remedy's picture. This sensation of cold may be specific to one part of the body, or it may run through the patient's whole body. Many Ledum patients will have coldness throughout their whole body, but their face will be hot.

Ledum is one of our most important rheumatic remedies as well. Consider this remedy first for cases of rheumatic pains that begin down in the feet and travel upward throughout the body. Consider this remedy when the patient complains about pain and swelling in the ball of the big toe. He will also report that the soles of his feet are so painful that he can put no weight on them.

Ledum is an important remedy for the ankles, for pains that begin in the feet and extend into the ankles. But it is also for the patient with weak ankles who finds that he can very easily sprain his ankles. As is common to the remedy, a sensation of cold will be felt in the patient's ankle, and yet the ankle will be better from cold applications and worse from hot ones. The patient will feel better from putting his feet in cold water.

Another indicator for the remedy is the presence of a red rash, of a rash resembling poison ivy or oak. (Because of this, Ledum is another remedy to be considered as an antidote to Rhus poisoning, to poison ivy rash, if it follows the general remedy picture.) You will especially find this remedy across the patient's forehead and cheeks, and the rash will sting when it is touched. The patient may also have acne of the forehead.

Consider this remedy for the patient who has burning in the nose, who has a spasmodic cough that is accompanied by bloody expectoration. The patient will also complain of a constrictive sensation in the chest. The patient's chest will hurt when it is touched. Consider Ledum in cases of whooping cough that match the remedy's general picture.

The Ledum patient may have vertigo. He will tend to fall to one side or the other when he attempts to walk.

Keynotes: The pains in Ledum are sticking, tearing, throbbing. They are always made worse by motion. They are worse at night, and are worse from the warmth of the bed, just as with the remedy Mercurius. These pains are always improved by the patient putting his feet into ice water.

And yet look for the patient to always complain that he is cold, chilly. There is a lack of animal heat in the patient. Look for the area of the injury to feel cold to the touch. It will also feel cold internally to the patient.

Swelling is also keynote—swelling of the feet up to the knees, and swelling of an ankle, usually the result of a sprain. The patient will be unable to trust his ankles to bear his weight. The ankle and the foot will be easy to sprain, as if the initial injury has permanently weakened the area of the body. Look also for the ball of the big toe to be swollen and painful and for there to be swelling at the point of the injury.

The area of the injury will also be discolored: black and blue. After a time, instead of the color returning to normal, look for the site of the injury to become green.

Aggravations: The patient will be worse from scratching the site of the injury. He will feel worse at night, worse when lying down, and worse from the heat of the bed.

The patient will be worse after eating eggs or drinking wine.

Ameliorations: The patient will be better from cold applications or a cold bath; better from putting his feet into ice water. He will feel better in cool air.

Look for a general improvement in the patient after eating.

Dosage and Potency: All potencies up to 200C are common. The remedy is not usually given in high potencies.

One dose of Ledum is said to last for up to thirty days. It is best given in a single dose.

Relationships: Arnica is usually given first, with Ledum given as the follow-up. The two work very well together.

Aconite may also be given before the remedy in cases of sudden injury and shock. Aconite may also be given after the initial dose of Ledum. Other remedies that follow well include Belladonna, Bryonia, and Rhus Tox.

35. LYCOPODIUM

Remedy Source: Vegetable Remedy. The remedy Lycopodium is taken from the spores of club moss. The spores of the plant are shaped like a wolf's paw, which gives the remedy its name: *lyco* means "wolf" and *podo* means "foot."

Samuel Hahnemann created the remedy.

Situations That Suggest Lycopodium: Male issues: impotence, premature ejaculation; digestive disorders of all sorts: irritable bowel syndrome, colitis, Crohn's disease; eating disorders, especially bulimia. Also diabetes; kidney and urinary disease: kidney stones, urinary tract infection, cystitis; headache and migraine; allergies: rhinitis, acute asthma; infections of all sorts: colds, flu, bronchitis, otitis media, sinusitis; chronic fatigue.

Remedy Portrait: Lycopodium is such an important homeopathic remedy with so many uses that it is almost certain that every patient will, at some time or another, need to make use of this remedy in either the acute or the constitutional context.

Most often when we think of Lycopodium we are dealing with a patient who has some form of digestive upset. Think of this remedy if you have a patient who has indigestion accompanied by flatulence, especially if it comes on after that patient has eaten wheat or fermented foods such as cabbage or beans. The Lycopodium patient will also not be able to tolerate onions, and many will become ill after eating anything with onions, especially raw onions.

The Lycopodium patient is the one who must open the top of his pants after eating. He may go to the table hungry, but after taking only a few mouthfuls of food he feels full. His abdomen will feel swollen and enlarged to the point that it strains against his clothing—this same clothing that was perfectly comfortable only a short while ago. The Lycopodium will not be able to tolerate anything tight against the abdomen, hence the open buttons. The pain in the abdomen will travel from the right to the left. The area of the patient's liver will also be very sensitive and swollen. The patient may also have brown spots on his skin all over his abdomen.

The patient will complain of a sensation of pressure in his stomach that comes on after eating. He will complain of a bitter taste in the mouth. He may also have heartburn and may experience an actual burning sensation in his stomach that lasts for hours. The patient may also have hiccoughs after eating.

And then there is the gas. Perhaps there is no other remedy type that is as gassy as is Lycopodium. It will be as if he is fermenting internally. The patient may become alarmed by the size of the swelling. This swelling may be most pronounced in the area of the upper-left abdomen. And no matter how much gas the patient passes, there is always more, and he still has the sensation of fullness and swelling.

This is an important remedy for cases involving both diarrhea and constipation, and for those with chronic cases of irritable bowel syndrome. The intestines will seem all but inactive at times, and will actively purge at other times. Each bowel movement will seem incomplete, and will leave the patient dissatisfied. Also consider this remedy for those with hemorrhoids, especially chronic ones.

Lycopodium is a right-sided remedy. Most symptoms will be worse on the right side, or will begin on the right side and move to the left. This patient also will traditionally feel worse in the late afternoon, during the period of time between 4 and 8 P.M., although some Lycopodium patients will have aggravations in the morning (again, in the period between 4 and 8 A.M.) as well. These two symptoms are so pronounced that, should they be lacking, they may well counterindicate the remedy selection.

Think of this remedy for colds and flus and sore throats that begin on the right side of the patient's body. The patient will complain of dryness in the throat, but he will not be thirsty. He will feel an inflammation in the throat that is accompanied by stitching pains. These pains will be aggravated each time the patient swallows. The patient will feel better after swallowing warm liquids. Consider this remedy in cases of swollen and inflamed tonsils, when the inflammation begins on the right side.

The patient may have a tickling cough that accompanies or follows the sore throat. The cough will be deep seated, with gray, thick expectoration that may or may not be bloody. The cough will be made worse from any downward movement or motion. The cough will be worse at night.

The patient will feel dryness in the back of his nose as well. His nose will feel stopped up. This is not only an excellent remedy for acute colds, but it is a major remedy—along with Nux—for patients with chronic blockage of the nose, especially when this blockage and snuffling is related to food or environmental allergies. There may be fluent drainage of the nose, or the patient may have crusts of dried mucus forming in his nose. Either way, look for the patient to fan his nostrils in an attempt to breathe.

As part of the cold/flu picture, Lycopodium is an important remedy for ailments of the eyes and ears that accompany respiratory infections. Consider this remedy for the patient with styes in his eyes, and for the patient with conjunctivitis. The patient's eyelids will be red and painful, often with a sensation of dryness running through the eye. The patient will have trouble seeing at night. He will have trouble seeing all of an object and may insist that he can only see half of it. The Lycopodium patient may sleep with his eyes only partly closed.

The patient may have a yellow discharge from his ears after a respiratory infection. He will complain of a sense of fullness and deafness. He will say that every sound echos in his ears. He will say that he hears a humming sound in his ears.

The Lycopodium patient will say that his whole body feels heavy, that his limbs feel numb. He will complain of sweaty feet and also that one foot feels hot and the other cold. (The right foot will usually be the hot one.) He will complain of chills in the limbs, especially in the early evening.

Keynotes: Look for the patient to be intellectually very clear, but to be physically weak. Look for him to think too much about his condition, and to fear the worst from his illness.

While Lycopodium tends toward more chronic conditions than acute illnesses, look for even the acute illnesses to tend to come on rather slowly, to evolve rather than to quickly take hold.

The symptoms of Lycopodium will be strongly right-sided, or the pain will appear on the right and travel to the left. This will be true particularly for symptoms of the throat, chest, abdomen, liver, and ovaries.

Look for the pains to have an aching nature. Look for the patient to equate his pains with pressure.

Look for a strong aggravation to appear like clockwork: the patient will be much worse from 4 until 8 P.M. This symptom is so keynote to the remedy that it has guided many a successful treatment.

The patient will be chilly and irritable. He will not want to be alone but will not want you in the room with him either. The Lycopodium prefers to hear his loved ones in the living room, while he rests alone in the bedroom. The fact that you are in the house and can be summoned if needed is all that Lycopodium needs or wants from you.

Aggravations: Symptoms tend to be worse from 4 until 8 P.M.; in some cases, the aggravation may occur from 4 to 8 A.M., but this is not common.

The patient feels much worse after eating—even the smallest amount of food makes him feel bloated and filled with gas. And yet the patient feels much worse if he skips a meal, and will often get a headache if he does not eat on time. He feels aggravated after eating any food with wheat in it, but his gastric symptoms get worse also after eating onions and, often, dairy. Lycopodium also will be aggravated by cold drinks.

While his headache will be aggravated by warmth, the whole person will be aggravated by cold. The Lycopodium tends to be chilly and tends to get more irritable when cold.

The patient will also be aggravated by sleep and will tend to wake up in a nasty mood. He will also be aggravated by lying or sleeping on his right side.

Amelioration: The Lycopodium patient will feel much better if he loosens his clothing. This is especially true of clothing around the waist. The Lycopodium male will loosen his pants at the end of every meal.

They will be better from warmth in general and specifically from warm drinks.

The Lycopodium also feels better in damp weather.

Dosage and Potency: This remedy is used in all potencies, from lowest to highest. In acute situations, potencies 30C and 200C are most common and may be repeated as needed. High potencies are given in a single dose.

One dose of Lycopodium may last for up to fifty days.

Relationships: Calcarea Carbonica often precedes well and Sulphur follows. Other remedies that follow Lycopodium well include Bryonia, Nux Vomica, Phosphorus, and Pulsatilla.

36. MAGNESIA PHOSPHORICA

Remedy Source: Mineral Remedy. In the creation of this remedy, sulphate of magnesia is dissolved in distilled water. This is then mixed with phosphate of soda that has also been dissolved in distilled water. The mixture is then set aside until crystals are formed. The salt is then triturated into the remedy. The chemical formula of phosphate of magnesia is $Mg\ HPO_4\ 7H_2O$.

The remedy was created by Schussler as part of his biochemical approach to homeopathy.

Situations That Suggest Mag Phos: PMS. Also toothache. Also writer's cramp. Also headache. Also psoriasis. Also anger and paranoia.

Remedy Portrait: In home use, Mag Phos will be used primarily for the cramps that accompany PMS. It can, however, be useful as a general remedy for cramps: for all cramps that are improved by heat, and for all cramps that force the patient to bend forward to alleviate the pain. It is also useful for treating the cramping of muscles with pains that radiate through the whole body. These cramps are made worse by any motion, and by cold air, cold wind, and cold water. They are also made worse if the patient lies down on his back. They are also worse when the patient eats. The cramps will be made better by gentle pressure and general rest. The cramping pains may be so intense that the patient cries out. Look for the patient to be anxious and depressed during the pain.

This is also a great spasm remedy. Hiccups and yawns are important indicators. Think of Mag Phos for writer's cramp and for cramps in the hands that can accompany playing musical instruments and any other precise work. These cramps come in sharp, sudden pains. These patients will say that they feel like lightning has struck their hands. Again, the cramps will be improved by rest and from applications of heat. This is also a remedy filled with tics and twitches. It is an important remedy in Parkinson's disease.

In toothache, Mag Phos speaks to the pains that come on at night. The pains shift rapidly through the teeth. It is very hard for the patient to pinpoint the source of the pain. The pain will be worse after eating and after drinking cold liquids, but better after drinking warm liquids. The pain will also be better when gentle pressure is put on the teeth. This can also be an important remedy in children who are teething, if they follow the general pattern of the remedy.

In headache, Mag Phos again is better for heat and warmth. The headache will typically begin in the back of the head and move forward over the head. The face will be flushed red. Headaches will be worse from 10 until 11 A.M. and again from 4 until 5 P.M. The headaches tend to come on from overwork or emotional exertion.

Mag Phos is also an important remedy for cases of colic. It is a good backup remedy when Colocynthis fails. Here, too, the patient will want to bend forward to stop the pain. Flatulence will accompany the pain. The patient will be better when warm.

In general, the pains common to this remedy will be termed sharp, cutting, stabbing, shooting, and intermittent. During the sudden spell of pain, the patient will be incapacitated. The pains, as they will also in Pulsatilla, will move suddenly and without pattern to other parts of the body. The pains are often accompanied by a feeling of constriction in the painful area.

Mag Phos is a remedy in which the pains dominate on the right side of the body, especially in the head, the ear, and the face; also in the ovaries and the chest. Look for sciatic pains that are improved by this remedy to also dominate on the right side of the body and to be improved by heat.

Keynotes: Simple keynotes here are pains on the right side of the body, pains that are sudden and that suddenly shift, pains that are usually cramping in nature, and pains that are all improved by applications of heat.

Aggravations: The major aggravation is from cold: cold air, especially drafts, and cold water.

The patient will also be aggravated by touch and by any motion.

Ameliorations: The patient will feel better from heat, from bending over double, and from gentle pressure.

Dosage and Potency: As Schussler created the remedy, I feel that I should mention that he used it, along with his other cell salts, in a very low potency, in this case, a 6X. For the home kit, however, it is recommended in 30C potency. It may be repeated as needed. As a matter of fact, in cases of great pain, expect to repeat it a good deal in the first few hours of treatment. Lessen the dosage as improvement begins.

Relationships: Mag Phos works well with the other right-sided remedies, specifically with Bryonia and Lycopodium. But it also works well with Belladonna, which also speaks to the sudden onset of symptoms.

37. MERCURIUS

Remedy Source: Mineral Remedy. There are several remedies based on the metal mercury. For our purposes here, we consider the remedy Mercurius Vivus, which was a remedy devised by Hahnemann himself, although Hering must be given the credit for the actual creation of the remedy.

Situations That Suggest Mercurius: Abscess and infections of all sorts; sinusitis and tonsillitis, colds, ear infections; upper-respiratory infections of all sorts; toothaches. Also acne, eczema. Also colitis and gastroenteritis, ulcerative colitis, sexual disorders, vaginitis. Also phobias, anxiety disorders.

Remedy Portrait: As an acute remedy, Mercurius always suggests that an infection of some sort is present. Look for the patient to have swollen glands under the jawbone. Look for the patient to have a swollen tongue (you will be able to see toothmarks along the sides of the tongue where it has swollen well beyond its normal size). Look for a great increase in saliva, so that the patient's pillow will be soaked every morning. And look for the patient to complain that he has a bad taste in his mouth. He will say that his mouth tastes metallic. The patient's breath will smell terrible.

The pains, in general, will be made worse by the warmth of the bed. The patient will become too hot very easily, but will just as easily become too cold. There will be a very narrow range of temperatures, usually from about 72 to 75 degrees, in which the Mercurius will feel comfortable.

This is also a remedy with discharges. The discharges will come especially from the nose, mouth, and ears and will be yellowish in color. As this is a major remedy for conjunctivitis, look for the yellow discharge from the eyes as well. The patient's face will have a yellow hue as well. The patient will look sick, act sick, and smell sick. The Mercurius patient is smelly. An odor of sickness seems to permeate his entire being.

This is also a remedy for persons with mumps. The patient will have cheeks that are swollen, red, and hot. Look for aching of the facial bones, aching in the jaws. The patient's lips will be dry and cracked.

Mercurius is also a remedy for appendicitis. The patient will want to lie on his back. He will feel very chilly and will complain of stabbing pains. The pains will especially shoot into the right side of the groin.

As this is a remedy that involves infection, look for the patient to be sweaty. Night sweats are especially typical. The perspiration does not in any way relieve the patient of his aches and pains. The sweat will be oily and foul with a strong penetrating odor. Look for the patient to be hot before the sweat, chilly after.

Mercurius is also a major remedy for measles, and for fevers. The skin may be covered with boils and abscesses of all sorts.

This is also a remedy that speaks to the teeth and to toothache. The patient will have gums that are spongy, receded gums, gums that bleed very easily. The mouth will be filled with sores and abscesses. In this case, the tongue will again be swollen, and there will be a good deal of saliva. The patient will also be thirsty, although his mouth is very wet.

Keynotes: The Mercurius patient is strongly aggravated by lying on his right side.

The Mercurius patient is also very sensitive to both cold and heat. The temperature of the room must be within his narrow comfort range.

Look for the Mercurius to be very sensitive to cold, damp weather. He is aggravated by cold, damp weather, especially by cold, damp nights.

Look for the characteristic swelling of the tongue. The patient will say that his mouth tastes metallic. He will have very bad breath.

Notice the smell of the patient. The Mercurius patient smells ill. He has increased perspiration that smells sickly sweet and is oily. Night sweats are very common.

The Mercurius patient is very weak. Look for trembling of the limbs due to general weakness. Look for a trembling of the hands.

Aggravations: The Mercurius patient is worse at night, especially on cold and damp nights that follow warm days; therefore, the Mercurius can have aggravations during the spring and fall.

The Mercurius patient is aggravated by the warmth of the bed and by a warm room, but he also becomes cold very easily.

He is aggravated by his perspiration. It actually will increase the patient's symptoms.

The patient is aggravated by lying on his right side.

Ameliorations: The Mercurius is improved by sleeping, and by long periods of rest.

He is also improved by moderate temperatures and gentle surroundings.

Dosage and Potency: To help clear abscesses, low potencies are suggested. High potencies will bring about the reabsorption of abscesses and are used for severe infections and gastrointestinal ailments.

In severe cases of diarrhea, you may have to give one dose after every stool. In general, the lower potencies may be repeated with some caution. Be careful not to give it too often, but only when truly called for. High potencies are given in a single dose. Chronic conditions are usually treated with one dose as well.

Although this is a powerful remedy, it is brief in its action. One dose holds for one to three days.

Relationships: As Mercurius is a remedy that involves an infection of some sort, it is usually not the first remedy given in a case, but is considered at the end of a case. Mercurius follows Belladonna particularly well. It also often follows Sulphur.

38. NATRUM MURIATICUM

Remedy Source: Mineral Remedy: Natrum Muriaticum is made from sodium chloride, or regular table salt. Because this chemical compound is so common to our environment and is indeed a natural part of our own bodies, the remedy taken from it is one of our most benign and curative. This is one of the most important remedies for both acute and chronic conditions.

Natrum Muriaticum is one of Samuel Hahnemann's first remedies.

Situations That Suggest Natrum Muriaticum: Emotional distress: grief, depression. Also allergies and chemical sensitivities of all sorts: environmental illness, chronic fatigue, hay fever and rhinitis, acute asthma. Also herpes and aphthae; contagious diseases: cold and flus, sore throat, fever and fevers of unknown origins, whooping cough; digestive disorders: dyspepsia, gastritis, constipation, colitis, ulcer; hemorrhoids; edema; joint and muscle pain: low back pain, sciatica; skin conditions: eczema and psoriasis, rash, ringworm and warts; eye troubles: myopia, eyestrain; headaches and migraine.

Remedy Portrait: Among the many uses for Natrum Mur are cases that involve fever, especially intermittent fever; hay fever and colds—Natrum Mur is one of our best remedies for colds that begin with sneezing—headache, especially chronic migraines and headaches that come on from studying and overwork; and digestive ailments that can be traced to an overuse of salt. Among the many chronic conditions for which Natrum Mur is a frequently indicated remedy are thyroid problems, especially hyperthyroidism and diabetes.

Natrum Mur is a grief remedy. It is often considered to be the chronic equivalent of Ignatia. When patients cannot remain at the emotional pitch of Ignatia, they tend to evolve, over time, into the more stoic emotional plateau of Natrum Mur. It is keynote of Natrum Mur that when faced with any pain—emotional or physical—the patient will want to just go and lie down on his bed. He will want to be left alone, and will not want to be consoled by anyone—in fact, this is the single worst thing that anyone can do. Keep this in mind as we take a look at the acute and home uses for Natrum Mur.

This is perhaps the single most useful remedy for colds and for hay fever. Consider this remedy whenever either condition comes on with sneezing as the first symptom. The patient will then experience a flow of mucus from the nose that is like raw egg white in consistency—clear and somewhat thick. In a cold, this flow will last for one to three days; in hay fever, it may last a good bit longer. The patient will have violent attacks of sneezing. He will complain that the inside of his nose hurts, that his nose feels overused and tender. He does not want to touch it or blow it, but the mucus just keeps on flowing. The patient will lose all sense of smell. Listen for the Natrum Mur patient to have the nasal voice of one whose nose is entirely blocked. He will be unable to breathe through his nose at all.

As the cold or allergy continues, the patient will complain of a cough. This cough will seem to come out of the pit of the patient's stomach. The patient will complain of a tickling in the pit of his stomach that makes him feel as if he has to cough. The coughing will bring on an increase of all the patient's aches and pain. The patient will complain that his head aches when he coughs. He will complain of pains in the abdomen when he coughs. This is a remedy that should be considered in all cases of whooping cough in which the patient's eyes stream with tears as the patient coughs.

The eyes give many indications of the remedy. The patient will say that his eyes feel weak and bruised. This is a remedy for those whose eyes feel tired from overwork, for those whose eyes feel weak after they read too much. Look for the patient's eyes to tear and for his eyes to smart from tearing. Look for the patient's eyelids to be swollen. Look for the patient to complain that his sense of vision is diminished. The patient will feel that he cannot bear to look around when he is outdoors in the bright sunshine. He will experience pain in his eyes when he is looking downward. He may say that he sees fiery halos around all objects.

The patient will also complain that he has lost his sense of taste as well. Look to the patient's tongue as an indicator of the remedy. His tongue will have a frothy coating, and will have small bubbles on the sides. The patient will complain that his mouth and throat feel dry. He will say that he has a sensation of numbness in his mouth, particularly in his tongue. This numbness may extend to the patient's lips and even to his nose. Look for the patient's lips to be dry. It is keynote of this remedy that the middle of the patient's lower lip will be cracked.

The Natrum Mur patient will be very thirsty. Natrum Murs are among the thirstiest of patients. They will want cold water. This symptom is so strong that its absence will counterindicate the remedy.

The patient will crave salt. He will not want baked things, especially bread. He will be repulsed by anything that he considers fatty or slimy. This is an excellent remedy to consider in cases of simple indigestion and heartburn. The patient will be hungry and yet will not be sure if he wants to eat. He will still be thirsty. He will complain of a throbbing pain in the pit of his stomach and may experience a cutting pain all across his abdomen.

Consider this remedy for patients who are chronically given to constipation or diarrhea or to both in alternation. Consider this remedy for those who are given to constipation in which the stool is dry and crumbling in nature, but who, from time to time, experience a sudden pinching pain in their abdomen which drives them into the bathroom. This will be followed by a sudden, painless bout of diarrhea. At this time they will have a large evacuation, which will again be followed by a period of constipation.

In the same way, Natrum Mur should be considered for the woman who experiences an irregular period. The patient will experience a bearing-down pain before her period. And that period will mirror the symptoms of elimination: sometimes scanty, with other flows being profuse. The patient will feel hot during the flow of the period.

This is an excellent remedy for the patient with acute or chronic back pain. Think of this remedy for the individual who wants to go and lie down when he has back pain. The patient will want to lie on something very firm, perhaps the floor. He may feel a numbness that extends from his back into his arms or lower extremities.

Also consider Natrum Mur for the patient who experiences cracking in all his joints when he moves, who experiences weakness in his legs, especially in his knees. Consider it also for the patient who has a chronic weakness in the knees or ankles. Consider it for the patient who has injured his ankles or knees in the past and now has a chronic tendency to reinjure the joint. The patient will complain that his legs are cold, but that his head and chest feel congested and hot.

Look at the patient's skin and hair for an indication of the remedy. The patient will have skin that is greasy. His hair will be oily. This is perhaps the most important remedy that we have for those with fever blisters, especially fever blisters that accompany a cold. Think of this remedy for cases of eczema in which the skin is raw, red, and inflamed.

Also look at the patient's hands for an indication of the remedy. Consider Natrum Mur for the patient who has warts on his hands, especially on the palms of the hands. Look for the patient's hands to be hot and sweaty.

Keynotes: Look for the symptoms of Natrum Mur to always follow the sun. As the sun rises over the horizon, the symptoms begin. This is certainly true of the headaches common to the remedy, which will come on while the patient is in bed in the morning. If the Natrum Mur patient is moving into a migraine, he will know it upon awakening.

The symptoms will grow worse as the sun rises in the sky. The patient will begin to feel better as the sun begins to set. By evening, he will be much improved.

In the same way, the Natrum Mur patient is worse for sunshine and better for lying down in a dark and quiet room.

The Natrum Mur patient wants to be alone. He does not wish to be consoled. Often this will be an irritable patient who will fly into tantrums over nothing. The Natrum Mur may also be a weepy patient, one who will cry for no apparent reason.

Look for the patient's face to be shiny and oily; it will look as if it has been greased.

Look for a general loss of taste and smell. Look for a crack in the middle of the lower lip. Also herpes on the lips are very common. This is a major remedy for herpes.

The patient will be very thirsty for cold water. He will also crave salt. The Natrum Mur patient will be averse to bread and to any food that he considers "slimy." Most often this will include oysters. The Natrum Mur patient will sweat while eating.

Aggravations: Look for a general aggravation of all symptoms from 10 until 11 A.M.

The Natrum Mur patient will also be aggravated at the seashore or from sea air. He will also, however, crave the sea and desire to go there.

There is a general aggravation also from the sun and from sitting out in the heat of the sun.

The Natrum Mur will also be aggravated by any mental exertion. And although the patient is weepy, there is an aggravation from crying.

Amelioration: The Natrum Mur will be improved by open air. He is also made better by bathing in cold water. The patient is further improved by skipping regular meals and by lying on his right side.

Dosage and Potency: This is another remedy that was adopted by Schussler in his cell salts. He gave the remedy in 6C potency. But homeopaths make use of Natrum Mur in all potencies, from the very lowest to the highest. Many use this wonderful remedy in 30C and find that potencies lower than this are not as effective.

The low potencies are given as needed. Higher potencies are given in a single dose, and, if they need to be repeated, will work best if another remedy is given before the Natrum Mur is repeated.

One dose of Natrum Mur will hold for up to six weeks.

Relationships: Natrum Mur is complementary in action both to Apis and to Ignatia. In fact, Natrum Mur can often be considered to be the constitutional equivalent of Ignatia. Both Ignatia and Apis should be given before Natrum Mur.

39. NUX VOMICA

Remedy Source: Mineral Remedy. The full name of this remedy is Strychnos Nux Vomica. It is taken from the gray seeds of a tree. These seeds contain strychnine, or rat poison. The seeds are said to be incredibly bitter as well as highly toxic. This tree is related to the Saint-Ignatius's-bean, making Ignatia and Nux Vomica related remedies.

The remedy Nux Vomica was created by Samuel Hahnemann.

Situations That Suggest Nux Vomica: Constipation, most especially chronic constipation; hemorrhoids; influenza. Also diarrhea, colitis, irritable bowel syndrome; high blood pressure; spasms and twitches of all sorts. Sleep disorders: insomnia, nightmares; addictions: coffee, tea, drugs, alcohol, tobacco. Also coughs and colds, acute asthma, chronic fatigue, environmental illness, neuralgic pains.

Remedy Portrait: Nux is a remedy that we are always going to think of first for the patient who is angry, who is irritable; the patient whom we feel that we can never satisfy. Only the Chamomilla patient will be as demandingly difficult and fault-finding as the Nux, but the Chamomilla patient will not be chilly.

The Nux patient will always be chilly. Where the Arsenicum patient—who is another difficult sort, but more fussy than angry—will also be cold, he can get warm if wrapped up enough; the Nux patient never can get warm. The Lycopodium patient will be chilly and will be demanding, but he, too, can finally get warm. Not Nux. The Nux patient will not become warm even if he is covered up from head to toe, not even if there is a fire roaring in the fireplace. Our classic texts tell us of homeopaths who, when they are taken into a patient's room and find that patient in bed with the covers pulled up to his nose, know what remedy to give without asking a question. Nux will not be able to bear even the slightest movement of air, as this will aggravate his sensation of cold.

These two symptoms are so classic to the type that the lack of either or both almost completely counterindicates the remedy.

Picture the sensations of a hangover and you pretty much have the picture of Nux. It is, in fact, perhaps our first choice of a remedy for those with a hangover. The Nux patient feels toxic. As one text puts it, "Nux alway seems to be out of tune; inharmonious spasmodic action." Indeed, the Nux never seems in tune with his environment or with anyone or anything in it. This is among our most sensitive remedies. The patient will be both physically and emotionally sensitive.

The Nux patient will be, as stated above, very sensitive to temperature. He cannot bear cold. He will also be oversensitive to noise. The patient will have a very keen sense of hearing and loud noises will likely cause the patient physical pain. They will also make the patient very angry. Look for the patient to be very sensitive to smells as well. Even if his nose feels constantly blocked and snuffly, the Nux will be very sensitive to the smells of perfumes and flowers. He may become angry at these smells, or may feel as if he will faint after smelling them. The smell of perfume may stay lodged in the patient's nose for several days. The patient will also be very sensitive to light. He will not be able to bear bright lights, especially in the morning. He will not be able to stand the morning sun. This condition will be worse if the patient drinks alcohol or smokes tobacco—which will also make all the patient's other senses more sensitive as well.

The Nux will also be emotionally sensitive. He will be suspicious of anything that someone says about him. He will ask, "What did you mean by that?" He will find fault with everything that everyone does. Look for the patient to be very impatient as well. Look for him to complain that time is passing too slowly. This is not a patient who wants to take to his bed and rest and get well.

Consider this remedy for cases of headache in which the patient complains of a pain either in the back of his head or over his eyes. The patient will say that it feels as if there is a nail being pounded into his head. He will complain of vertigo accompanying his headache. He may want to press his head against a wall or anything else hard in order to get relief. Of course, we should consider this remedy first for headaches that come on after drinking alcohol. The patient's headache will be made much worse by light, especially sunlight.

Consider Nux for colds that come on slowly, that start with a sensation of blockage and stuffiness in the patient's nose. The patient will then begin to feel chilly and to display the emotional portrait of the remedy. Consider Nux for colds that come on after the patient has been exposed to cold weather; when the patient, although chilly, experiences an increase of cold symptoms when he is in a warm place. Look for the flow of mucus to alternate sides of the nose. Or look for the patient to have a copious flow during the day, but a dry, stopped-up nose at night.

The patient will say that his ears itch, and that the itching extends into his Eustachian tubes. He will be driven crazy by the itching in his ears, and by the accompanying stopped-up sensation.

The patient will also report that his throat feels raw. He will say that the soreness is worse in the morning, that he feels his throat is tight. He will complain that when he swallows the pain extends into his ears.

Consider Nux as well for cases of cough, especially if the patient reports that his cough feels as if it is tearing something loose inside his chest. He may complain that his cough brings on a headache. The cough will be dry but hacking. The patient may have trouble breathing. Look for his breathing to be very shallow, and for a deep breath to bring on a cough and headache. This is an excellent remedy for cases of asthma, especially those in which the asthma is worse in the morning or after the patient eats.

The Nux patient will almost always feel discomfort after eating. The Nux will be nauseous every morning, will awaken with a sour taste in his mouth and a sensation of a weight in his stomach. Consider this remedy for cases of dyspepsia and heartburn, especially when the region of the patient's stomach is very sensitive to touch; when the patient becomes very tense and angry if he thinks you are going to touch his stomach.

Nux may be a very belchy patient. He may also be very flatulent. Nux patients crave fats, and they love to eat meat. He also craves coffee, which he cannot deal with at all well. And, of course, he craves tobacco and alcohol, both of which are hightly toxic to his system.

Among the most important uses for the remedy Nux are cases of constipation, especially chronic constipation. Expect constipation to accompany every other symptom in the Nux case. Again, the patient who is not constipated is likely not in need of Nux. The patient will have the urge to move his bowels. He will try again and again, and may strain a good bit, but he will not produce a stool. The patient will complain that his rectum feels tight, that it feels constricted.

Consider this remedy particularly in cases of stubborn constipation for which the patient has already taken a good deal of allopathic medicines. (In fact, Nux is considered our "universal antidote." It is often the best choice for a remedy for a case in which a patient has been taking a good deal of allopathic medicine in the treatment of any condition. It is also used to antidote the actions of poorly selected or used homeopathic remedies as well.) Consider this remedy also for conditions that alternate between diarrhea and constipation when the patient has used allopathic drugs to purge his system. Finally, consider this remedy for cases of irritable bowel syndrome that fit the physical and emotion portrait of the remedy.

Finally, consider Nux for cases of lumbago in which the patient complains of a burning sensation in the lower part of his spine. This pain will come on at or around 3 A.M., while the patient is asleep. (The Nux has many difficulties with the issue of sleep. He may have insomnia and only be able to sleep as the sun begins to rise. Or he may have a fretful sleep, with dreams of exertion and business. Often the Nux will awaken as this critical time of 3 A.M. for no apparent reason and will not be able to sleep again until sunrise.) He will complain of numbness accompanying the pain. The patient will be worse if he is in a sitting position.

This numbness and sensation of paralysis may spread to the patient's legs. The remedy type is particularly given to cramps in the calves. Look for the patient to feel weak in the morning, to feel that both his arms and legs are very weak at that time. Look for him to drag his feet when he walks.

Keynotes: All Nux patients are filled with twitches, spasms, and tics. Look especially for them to have a facial tic, usually with an eye that twitches. Most of their pains will have to do with spasms. These are most common in the intestines, which will go into painful states of colic.

Nux Vomica is perhaps our coldest remedy. While other remedies are chilly, most, like Arsenicum, will become warm by an open fire or under a down comforter. Nux patients, however, will remain cold from September until June. Look for them to wear hats to keep their heads covered and their body heat in. They may even want to wear these hats indoors.

Because they are so cold, Nux patients cannot bear any moving air. Look for the Nux driver to want to keep the heater on in the car and to refuse to let anyone open a window even the slightest crack.

This feeling of coldness is just one of the many ways in which Nux Vomica patients show their sensitivity. They are emotionally sensitive and show it by looking for an argument. They are also physically sensitive— mostly to cold, but also to noise and to light. Nux patients cannot bear being bothered by noise; it gives them a headache.

Nux is angry. Even in simple illnesses, even with the slightest cold, the patient is impatient and angry.

Finally, it is keynote of the remedy that illnesses, even colds, come on slowly, and sometimes seem as if they will never fully form. Thus, you have the patient who has had a cold coming on for more than a week, and who finally impatiently waits for the illness to come on so that it can be gone. In this way, you will find an odd combination in Nux Vomica: he is impatient and sluggish at the same time. It is a major remedy for chronic fatigue, but the way in which Nux handles chronic fatigue is to rage against his weakness. Often his method of becoming sick will show the slow breakdown of his system, as his diet, his lifestyle, and his core anger finally add up to a toxic system that simply can no longer function.

Aggravations: From any mental exertion. The Nux type, once he yields to illness, will not want to think, will not want to work.

There is a general aggravation in the morning. The patient may awaken at 3 or 4 A.M. and be unable to sleep again until sunrise, when he falls into a deep sleep.

Also there is an aggravation of all symptoms in dry weather. Nux is happier in damp weather.

There are aggravations from noise, from light, and from strong odors, which will make him feel as if he is about to faint; also aggravations from spicy foods, alcohol, and drugs, all of which he craves.

Finally, Nux is aggravated by touch, especially by touch that jars him.

Ameliorations: The patient will be made better by lying down and by being allowed to rest for a long period of time. He is also improved in the evening, and feels better in damp or wet weather.

Dosage and Potency: Nux is most commonly given in the potency 30C, but it may be used in all potencies from lowest to highest. It is usually not given in mother tincture, due to the poisonous nature of the substance. Lower potencies are suggested in drug or alcohol abuse, in headaches, in digestive disturbances, and in headaches. Low potencies are also useful for nausea in pregnancy. Higher potencies are better for chronic conditions, especially in chronic constipation.

In all potencies, Nux Vomica works best in a single dose and should only be repeated if necessary. The dose should be given at bedtime.

Relationships: Nux Vomica is considered to be complementary to Sulphur and is often given as a follow-up remedy to Sulphur. The remedies Bryonia, Calcarea Carbonica, Carbo Veg, and Rhus Tox all follow Nux well. Sulphur may also be used as a follow-up to Nux.

In that the two remedies are so similar, Ignatia is incompatible with Nux and the two remedies should never be used back to back.

40. PETROLEUM

Remedy Source: Mineral Remedy. This remedy is the homeopathic petroleum byproduct. It is taken from coal oil or rock oil, from the underground rock in which oil is found. It is to be found across the globe, especially in the Middle East.

The remedy was created by Hahnemann.

Situations That Suggest Petroleum: motion sickness, vertigo. Also allergies. Also skin disorders: psoriasis, eczema. Also toothache, headache. Also digestive disorders: constipation, diarrhea, ulcer. Also rheumatism, strains and sprains, TMJ. Also frostbite, chapped skin.

Remedy Portrait: There is really only one use that this remedy is put to from the home kit: motion sickness. Perhaps more than any other remedy, Petroleum is useful for ailments that come on from riding on ships, in cars, or in planes.

This motion sickness will largely consist of vertigo and nausea. Vomiting is likely to occur.

But Petroleum has other uses from the home kit as well. Consider it also for the following symptoms:

It is a valuable remedy for those with headache. The headache will typically begin at the back of the head and extend forward to the forehead. The headache will affect the vision, which is commonly blurred with this specific headache. Vertigo will accompany the headache.

Think of this remedy also for diarrhea that comes on in the daytime. It will also come on in stormy weather. The diarrhea will be accompanied by that same sense of vertigo and by a gnawing pain in the stomach. This pain is relieved only by eating. The Petroleum patient will want to eat constantly, even if other ailments are increased by eating, because it settles this gnawing pain.

Think of this remedy also for chapped skin in the winter, especially for chapped hands. Look for cracks on the ends of the fingers and on the backs of hands. It is a great remedy for people who get chapped skin every winter, for those who get frostbite easily.

Keynotes: The gnawing pain that is relieved by eating is keynote. Even the patient who is suffering from motion sickness may want to eat in order to settle this pain. He may feel that he needs to eat, even if the idea of the food itself repulses him.

The sensation of vertigo accompanying the other symptoms is also keynote, especially headache and motion sickness with vertigo.

The Petroleum patient also will tend toward skin conditions only in the winter. These conditions will clear themselves in warm weather. The Petroleum patient is worse, in general, in winter.

The Petroleum patient will also be worse both before and during a thunderstorm.

Aggravations: Motion, of car, plane, or, especially, boat. The Petroleum is also worse in winter and before and during thunderstorms. They are irritable patients who are worse from any aggravation. They are also worse from any mental labor.

Now, it is important to note that, ultimately, Petroleum patients are worse from eating. They often will feel that they have to eat, but the small improvement that they receive is soon offset by a general aggravation of symptoms. They feel particularly bad after eating cabbage.

They are worse in the damp, especially when cold and damp are combined.

Ameliorations: Petroleum patients feel better in warm, dry weather. They are improved by lying down, but only if the head is elevated high.

Dosage and Potency: The most common dosage is 30C, which usually does the trick just fine. It may be repeated as needed.

This is a long-acting remedy. One dose holds for up to six weeks.

Relationships: Petroleum is complementary in action to Sepia. It is also used successfully both before and after Pulsatilla, Bryonia, Lycopodium, and Calcarea. It is antidoted by Nux and Phosphorus.

41. PHOSPHORUS

Remedy Source: Mineral Remedy. Phosphorus is created from the element phosphorus. The element is known for its pale yellow color and its distinctive odor. Like sulfur, phosphorus is found in regions surrounding volcanoes.

Samuel Hahnemann created the homeopathic remedy Phosphorus.

Situations That Suggest Phosphorus: Upper-respiratory illnesses: acute asthma, colds and flus, sore throats, influenza, bronchitis, respiratory infections of all sorts; chronic otitis, tinnitis. Also chronic laryngitis; preacher's throat; skin disorders: ichthyosis, skin ulcers, eczema, psoriasis; Also headache; vertigo; Ménière's disease; arthritis; rheumatism; neuralgia. Also: phobias; eye and vision troubles: epistaxis; pyorrhea, with easily bleeding gums; excessive bleeding from dental procedures; excessive bleeding after any operation.

Remedy Portrait: Consider this remedy for the patient—particularly for the patient who is a child—who is given to frequent upper-respiratory infections, especially when those ailments start in the throat and move swiftly to the ear or the chest. The Phosphorus patient is known for a weakness in the respiratory system. The young patient who is constitutionally Phosphorus will have an underdeveloped chest, a very narrow rib cage. This patient will also be given to frequent, even chronic ear infections as well.

The patient who is in an acute Phosphorus state will be given to symptoms in the ear. It is as if the ear is the steam valve to the patient's body, and infections that would otherwise go more deeply into the system, into the patient's chest and lungs, will instead play out in the ears. The patient will complain that he has diminished hearing during a cold or flu; he will complain especially of being deaf to the sound of the human voice.

The patient's own voice will likely also be affected. Consider Phosphorus in cases of hoarseness that are worse at night. This is the leading remedy (along with Rhus Tox) for loss of voice due to overuse. The classic texts call it "Preacher's Throat." The patient will lose his voice in the evening. He will complain that his throat feels raw. The patient will say that his voice box is very painful.

A cough may accompany the loss of voice. This is a major remedy for patients with cough. The patient may say that he has a sweetish taste in his mouth that comes on when he coughs. The cough will be hard and dry. The cough will cause the patient's throat to hurt. The patient will complain of a tightness or a congestion in his chest and lungs. His lungs will burn. (Phosphorus, along with Arsenicum and Sulphur, form the "burn trio" of remedies. Look for all the aches and pains in the remedy picture to be accompanied by a burning sensation.) The cough and associated pain will be made worse when the patient is in a cold room, especially when he goes from a warm room into a cold place. It will also be aggravated by the patient talking or, especially, laughing. The cough may also be brought on by the presence of a stranger in the patient's sick room. And the Phosphorus patient will be very sensitive to smell during his illness. His cough may be brought on by various odors, especially by the smell of flowers and perfume.

The Phosphorus cough can go deeper than this. The patient will complain that he has stitches in his chest, and a sensation of weight upon his chest every time he tries to breathe. The patient will have great difficulty in breathing. He will feel a sensation of heat and burning all through his lungs. The patient will be unable to breathe if he lies on his left side. (It is keynote of this remedy that all symptoms will be made worse from the patient lying on his left side. The Phosphorus patient sleeps on his right side.) The patient's whole body will tremble when he coughs.

The Phosphorus patient's cough may be accompanied by expectoration. This expectoration will be bloody, or blood-streaked. (Even the nasal discharge associated with a simple cold will be bloody or blood-streaked.

The classic texts say that the Phosphorus' handkerchief will always be bloody.)

Blood is an important aspect of this remedy picture. It is keynote of this remedy that every little wound will bleed profusely. The blood will be bright red. This is one of the remedies to consider, along with China and Rhus Tox, for the patient with a nosebleed that will not stop. Phosphorus was also a remedy given in homeopathic hospitals in order to stop the bleeding after surgery. It should be considered a remedy for the patient in postoperative recovery.

The patient's emotions will give a clue to the need for the remedy. The Phosphorus patient is among our most sensitive. He will be sensitive to all aspects of his environment—to light, touch, taste, and smell—but also to the aesthetic nature of his environment, to color and to sound. He will also be very sensitive to the emotions of those around him and will have a strong response to the emotions of others. Fearful parents will make their Phosphorus child all the sicker from their fear. The Phosphorus patient may become psychic in his sensitivity. Yet even with this state of emotional sensitivity, the Phosphorus patient will not want to be alone. He will literally become sicker if he is left alone. He will recover faster if he is surrounded by those he loves and who love him. He wants to be cared for. He wants to be made to laugh.

The Phosphorus patient—unless very sick—will be a somewhat restless patient. He will want magazines and books and movies on TV. He will want to be waited on. He will want gifts. Look for him to become excited, even overly excited, very easily; and look for that state of excitement to be accompanied by a sensation of heat in the body.

If Phosphorus patients are very ill, they will show the opposite. They become apathetic patients. They become very depressed and are easily angered. They will become frightened and startled very easily, especially by noises or light. They will become convinced that they will die if they are left alone.

This Phosphorus state of oversensitivity will be displayed in the physical body as well. No other remedy, with the possible exception of Rhus Tox, is so sensitive to changes of weather or environment as is Phosphorus. This will be true in either the acute or the constitutional state. Patients will be worse from any change in the weather, but especially when the weather is changing to cold and wet. They will be worse from an oncoming thunderstorm and they will also be worse during that storm. Many Phosphorus patients will experience fear during a thunderstorm; others will just experience an increase of their physical symptoms. Look for aches and pains, colds and flus, and, especially, headaches all associated with changes in the weather.

The Phosphorus headache will be accompanied by vertigo. Patients will complain of a sensation that the skin on their forehead is stretched too tight. They will complain of an itching and burning in their head. The back of their head will feel cold and their spine will feel hot. This heat up the spine is another keynote of the remedy and will occur in association with many other symptoms.

Phosphorus should also be considered in cases of rheumatic pains in the body, aches and pains that come on with every change in the weather. Patients will complain of a sensation of numbness and paralysis that spreads from their fingertips outward. They will say that their hands and arms feel numb. This same numbness may spread from the toes as well.

Patients will complain of a general weakness. They will tend to drop things. All the joints in their body may suddenly give way. Patients may feel a special weakness in their elbows and shoulders.

They will also complain of a pain in their back. The pain may center in between the patients' shoulder blades. They will feel heat and burning in this area. They will say that their back hurts so much that it feels as if it is broken. Look for patients to have a good bit of sweat running up and down their spine, which accompanies both this pain and the sensation of heat in the spine. Phosphorus patients are, generally speaking, rather sweaty and will sweat very easily as well, but the back will be the sweatiest part of their body. (This will also be true of the night sweats that accompany Phosphorus patients, especially when they are in a state of fever. This will be accompanied by a weak but rapid pulse.)

In digestive disorders, look for Phosphorus patients to complain of the characteristic burning sensation running all throughout their organs of digestion and elimination.

Phosphorus patients will have pain in their stomach that is burning in nature and improved by eating or drinking cold things. They will be especially thirsty for cold water, but the improvement that the cold food or liquid brings on may be very short-lasting, as Phosphorus patients may vomit up the food or drink as soon as it is warmed in their stomach. They may throw up undigested food. They will belch up much gas after every meal. Phosphorus patients will want cold things, especially ice cream, and will be nauseated by warm foods and drinks. (This remedy should, along with Natrum Mur, be considered for patients who have become chronically ill from eating too much salt.)

The Phosphorus patient will complain of pains in the stomach. The stomach will be painful when he walks, or when it is touched. He will also feel pain in his abdomen—sharp, cutting pain. The patient will also say that his abdomen feels cold inside.

The Phosphorus patient will pass a stool that is long and narrow and hard, like the stool a dog passes. The stools will be very foul-smelling and accompanied by a great deal of foul-smelling gas. The patient will feel the urge to pass a stool every time he lies on his left side.

This is also a remedy to consider for cases of diarrhea, especially when the diarrhea is painless and copious. Look for the diarrhea to be green and to contain a good amount of mucus. Look for the mucus to be bloody as well. The patient will be left exhausted by the diarrhea.

Keynotes: The Phosphorus patient is a very sensitive patient. All his senses will be heightened. He will be sensitive to all external sensations—to light, to color, to smell, and to sound.

Look for the Phosphorus to be fidgety, to want to move continually, to want to touch things, and to look at things. Look for him to use up whatever energy he has very quickly, and then to be totally exhausted.

Sleep is the great refuge for Phosphorus and the Phosphorus patient will be greatly improved by sleeping. He will tend to have vivid dreams, and whether he remembers the specific dream or not, look for him to remember the impression of the dream. The Phosphorus patient may dream of fire.

It is keynote of the remedy that Phosphorus patients bleed a great deal from every little cut. And there may be a problem in stopping the bleeding. The blood will be bright red. The patients tend toward nosebleeds.

It is also keynote that Phosphorus can be hard of hearing when it comes to the human voice. He may hear everything else just fine, but not be able to hear a human speaking directly to him.

It is also keynote that the Phosphorus patient will have a hard time at sunset. Even if his physical symptoms are not aggravated at this time, the Phosphorus patient will become depressed.

And the Phosphorus patient cannot sleep on his left side. He usually will choose to sleep on his right side only and will not be able to sleep in any other position.

Aggravations: The Phosphorous patient will suffer aggravation from lying on the left or on the painful side.

The Phosphorus patient is also aggravated by thunderstorm. He may become very excited or fearful during the storm. He may suffer an aggravation during the approach of the storm. The Phosphorus patient is often referred to as being a "human barometer," and will experience aggravations at changes in the barometric pressure.

The patient is also aggravated from weather changes that go from hot to cold or from cold to hot.

The Phosphorus patient is also aggravated in the evening, especially at sunset, but at any time up until midnight.

Ameliorations: Although some Phosphorus patients will be afraid of the dark, they are better at night, and better in darkness.

The Phosphorus patient will also be improved by lying on his left side.

The Phosphorus patient wants to be touched and will be improved in every way by touching or rubbing.

And the Phosphorus patient will be improved by ingesting cold drinks and cold food, which he craves, especially ice cream.

Dosage and Potency: Phosphorus works best in potencies of 30C and above. It should not be given in too low a potency or in too many doses.

As with any other remedy, Phosphorus should only be given in a single dose. It may be repeated as needed.

One dose of Phosphorus is said to hold for up to forty days.

Relationships: Phosphorus is complementary to Arsenicum. Either may be used in chronic cases to complete the action of the other.

Sulphur is also a similar remedy to Phosphorus and is often used either before or after the remedy.

Other remedies that follow Phosphorus well include Carbo Veg and Rhus Tox.

42. PHYTOLACCA

Remedy Source: Vegetable Remedy. Phytolacca, the remedy, is taken from *Phytolacca decandra,* a plant known for its greenish white flowers and for its fruit, which are small, dark purple berries that grow in clusters. The plant belongs to the Natural Order of Phytolaccacae. It is commonly called poke root.

The remedy may be made either by working with the roots that are dug up during the winter, or by working with the fresh summer fruit.

The remedy was created by Hale.

Situations That Suggest Phytolacca: diseases and disorders of the breast: pains associated with breastfeeding, pain in the nipples. Also mumps, general infections with enlarged glands, tonsillitis, sore throat, acute asthma. Also vision disorders, diplopia. Also diarrhea. Also rheumatism, sciatica. Also ringworm, warts, boils. Also toothache, mercury poisoning.

Remedy Portrait: Phytolacca is often called "vegetable mercury," because it so strongly mimics the action of the remedy Mercurius and its symptoms. Also consider Phytolacca the most important remedy in the treatment of mercury poisoning in all of its various forms, including dental fillings. Phytolacca is also a remedy for those who have inhaled various forms of poison gas.

In the home, you are most often going to use Phytolacca in cases that are similar to the infections present in Mercurius. Look for swelling of the glands throughout the body, especially the glands in the breasts. Phytolacca is an excellent condition for many different ailments of the breast, especially mastitis. The patient will have a pain that radiates from her nipple. She will have increased tenderness in the breasts, which may be swollen, or feel heavy and/or hard. This is an excellent remedy for the pains that may be associated with nursing. The woman will feel pain as the child nurses and the pain will travel throughout her body.

Think of this remedy for rheumatic pains that travel throughout the body like electrical currents. The pains will be worse in the morning. The inflamed joints, particularly the finger joints, will look shiny and swollen. It is also very common for the Phytolacca patient to have pain in the right shoulder. He will feel stiff in the shoulder. He will be unable to lift his right arm.

In general, look for the Phytolacca patient to complain of pains throughout the entire body. He feels sore. Pain appears suddenly, especially in the eyes, neck, and shoulders. The area of the kidney may also be very painful; again, the pain will be electric and aching in character and will appear suddenly.

The color associated with the remedy is bluish-red. Areas of pain and infection will show this color, and they will be shiny.

This is an excellent remedy for sore throats; they will be right-sided. The patient will want liquids—warm liquids will make the pain worse, cold liquids will ameliorate the pain. The sore throat may be so painful that it will drain the patient of his vital force. This is the remedy for quinsy, for tonsillitis. The patient will lose weight from the impact of the sore throat. Most often, the patient will lose all appetite, although it is possible that his appetite may increase so much that he cannot be satisfied.

You will commonly find that the Phytolacca patient will appear strangely indifferent in his illness. He will often seem not to care whether he gets well or not. Also, he will not care about the things that used to matter to him. You will see a fastidious housekeeper suddenly not care whether the house is neat or not. You will see an excellent businessperson suddenly not care a bit about his business. Also you will see a patient who no longer cares about his personal habits, or about personal hygiene. In some cases, he may not even care if his pajamas are open and his body is exposed.

Look into the patient's throat. It will give you all the needed information. The Phytolacca throat is dark red or blue/red. The patient will complain of shooting pains that extend into the ears. He will say that he cannot swallow anything that is hot. His tonsils will be swollen. He will have pain at the root of the tongue and he will tell you of a sensation of a lump in the throat. He will tell you that this lump feels like a burning ball of pain. These are the most common indicators that will lead you to this remedy.

Keynotes: While Phytolacca's pains are increased when the weather is cold, the patient himself is worse from heat. He will want cold drinks.

It is keynote of the type that they will have mucus flow from one nostril. They will say that their sinuses feel heavy.

The intense pain at the root of the tongue is keynote, as is the general quality of pain as electrical and aching. The sensation of a burning ball or lump in the throat is also keynote of the type.

Aggravations: The patient will be worse from sunset to sunrise. (True of Mercurius as well.)

Worse when it rains and worse from cold, damp weather.

Worse from hot drinks.

Worse from motion.

Worse from swallowing.

Ameliorations: The patient will be better when lying down. He will feel better after bathing.

Dosage and Potency: Phytolacca works best in the 200C potency. You may need a higher potency in cases involving infections.

The tincture is used externally on tender or painful breasts.

The remedy may be repeated as needed.

Relationships: Most complementary in action is Silicea. Silicea is an excellent follow-up to speed recovery after severe illness.

This remedy is antidoted by coffee; also by Belladonna and Sulphur.

43. PODOPHYLLUM

Remedy Source: Vegetable Remedy. The remedy is taken from the may-apple or "duck's foot," a plant that bears a single flower, followed by a large yellow fruit. The plant is from the Natural Order Barberidaceae. The plant is native to the United States, where it is known to grow in damp and shady places. The remedy is made from the root of the plant, which is gathered just prior to the ripening of the fruit.

The plant was known to have medicinal properties in that it was used by Native Americans for centuries to cause diarrhea to expel worms from the body. As a remedy it was first proven in 1846 by Dr. Williamson, a Philadelphia homeopath.

Situations That Suggest Podophyllum: Diarrhea. Also digestive disorders: acid stomach, gagging. Also headache, whooping cough.

Remedy Portrait: This is a small remedy, but a good one for the home kit. As Ferrum Phos is the best general remedy for those with fever but who lack specific symptoms, so, too, is Podophyllum the best remedy to think of in cases that involve diarrhea that is persistent and lacking in specific or striking symptoms.

These patients will have rumbling in the abdomen. They will feel weak and sick, especially after an attack of diarrhea. They will rub their abdomen in hopes that it will relieve their discomfort. Look for the diarrhea to come on in the early morning. The patient will have a red face during and just before the bout of diarrhea. His cheeks will be red and shiny. (*Note:* Podophyllum is an excellent remedy for those children who have diarrhea at the time of teething. The red, shiny face is a keynote symptom in the selection of the remedy.) The first symptom will usually be a gurgling in the abdomen. The patient will have to run to the bathroom. The stool will gush out. The diarrhea is painless, but leaves the patients exhausted.

Podophyllum should also be thought of in cases in which diarrhea alternates with constipation. It is also an important remedy for cases of diarrhea that come on in summer (along with Bryonia).

Keynotes: The patient will want to drink large quantities of water. The patient will continually rub the region of the liver and abdomen. The patient will alternate periods in which he feels very hot and very cold.

This is a right-sided remedy, especially affecting the right ovary and the right side of the throat.

Aggravations: The patient is worse from 2 until 4 A.M. and throughout the early morning in general. Fevers are worse at 7 A.M., which is a common time for the onset of diarrhea as well.

The patient is also worse in warm weather, and, in general, during the summer months.

Ameliorations: The patient will be better in the evening.

Dosage and Potency: Keep it in the home kit in 30C dosage. It repeats well, so don't hesitate to use it as needed.

One dose can hold for up to a month.

Relationships: Podophyllum is complementary to Sulphur, another good general remedy for those with diarrhea. Each follows the other well. Podophyllum is antidoted by Nux.

44. PULSATILLA

Remedy Source: Vegetable Remedy. Pulsatilla is created from the anemone, or windflower. This flowering plant is also called the pasqueflower because it blooms during the Easter season each year. The violet-purple flowers have been traditionally used in the creation of dye used to color Easter eggs.

Pulsatilla is a remedy created by Hahnemann.

Situations That Suggest Pulsatilla: Women's health issues: PMS, pregnancy, menopause, puberty, uterine prolapse, labor pains; allergies and respiratory complaints: hay fever, acute asthma, bronchitis, sinusitis, colds and flus in their later stage. Also mumps, measles, conjunctivitis, chicken pox; eye troubles: obstructed tear duct, cataract, styes. Also heart palpitations and vertigo; digestive troubles: heartburn, diarrhea; mental anguish: fear, depression, hysteria. Also pain.

Remedy Portrait: You can pretty much expect the Pulsatilla patient to be weepy and somewhat clingy and needy, and you can expect the Pulsatilla to lack thirst, even during fever, and you can expect the Pulsatilla to be chilly but worse in a warm room and better in the open air. Changeability is what you can expect most about the Pulsatilla patient. Everything in Pulsatilla's physical condition changes as much as his moods. In fact, no other patient, not even Ignatia, changes moods as quickly, and no other patient will have symptoms that shift so suddenly and without apparent reason. Pulsatilla is known as the best remedy for pains of unknown cause and for traveling pain that courses throughout the body without rhyme or reason.

These then are the core symptoms of the Pulsatilla: the patient is chilly, has no thirst, is moody, and has a symptom picture that is erratic and ever-changing. Add to this the frequent presence of a yellow discharge of almost any sort and a craving for open air, and you pretty much have the whole picture.

Pulsatilla is one of our most frequently used remedies, both in acute and in constitutional cases. In the acute case, it is often used as a remedy for those who are in the final stage of a cold. The mucus has changed from being clear to being yellow or yellow-green. The mucus is not ropy, as it will be in a Kali Bi case, but will instead be like a cloud, without form. The mucus will be especially abundant in the morning, and it will likely flow more from the patient's right nostril than from the left. The patient will totally lose the sense of smell and the ability to breathe through the nose. He will complain that the bones of the nose are sore or that he has a pressing pain at the root of the nose.

This same yellow-colored discharge will likely come from the patient's eyes as well. This remedy is one of the best for cases of conjunctivitis that accompany a cold. The patient will experience itching and burning in the eyes, which will tear; the tears will contain the yellow mucus. The patient's eyes will be glued shut by the discharge each night during sleep.

The patient may also cough up this same mucus, although it will tend to be more greenish than yellowish in this case. The patient will complain of a bitter taste in his mouth that accompanies the expectoration.

If a fever accompanies the illness, look for the patient to have no thirst at all during that fever. And look for the patient to be chilly, even when in a warm place, although warm applications will make the patient feel much worse. The patient will tend to be hot with fever during the night, and chilly during the daytime, especially in the late afternoon. Or he may have heat in specific parts of the body and coldness in other parts. Look for the patient to have sweat only on one side of his body. Headache, nausea, or diarrhea may accompany the fever.

The patient may also suffer from a cough. This dry cough will be worse during the evening and especially during the night when the patient is asleep. The patient will be awakened by the cough and will have to sit up in bed in order to breathe. Look for the cough to be loose in the daytime, especially in the morning, but dry at night.

The Pulsatilla sleep state will often reveal the remedy. Many of Pulsatilla's troubles will come on when the patient lies down to go to sleep. These patients will be especially restless during the first part of the night, in the first stages of sleep, even if they have been drowsy all evening long. Look for Pulsatilla to want to sleep with many pillows, to want his head raised when he sleeps. And look for him to sleep with his hands up over his head. The Pulsatilla who tries to sleep with his head low, lying down perfectly flat, is likely to induce a fit of suffocation.

The Pulsatilla patient will likely experience this feeling of suffocation, of difficulty in breathing, in association with any sort of other symptom. Look for a shortness of breath to accompany any sort of anxiety or fear, and look for palpitations to accompany the shortness of breath. Look for this feeling of suffocation to be especially pronounced when the patient is in a warm, closed room. The Pulsatilla patient will crave the cool air, and will need the door or window open in order to breathe.

This is an important remedy for cases of indigestion of all sorts. And here the patient's tongue will be an excellent source of information. Look for the Pulsatilla's tongue to be covered with a thick mucus. And look for it to be colored either yellow or white. Look for the Pulsatilla to also have a crack in the lower lip, and for the lips in general to be very dry. (The Natrum Mur will have this same characteristic dryness of the lips and the crack in the middle of the lower lip, but the Natrum will be a very thirsty patient, while the Pulsatilla will have no thirst, even though his mouth will be very dry.)

The Pulsatilla will complain of a greasy taste in his mouth, and will have a deep aversion to any food that is greasy or fatty, especially butter. These foods will make the patient nauseous. The Pulsatilla will also be averse to warm foods and drinks. Look for him to crave cold things, especially sorbets and fruits of all sorts. The Pulsatilla may complain that his sense of taste is diminished.

This is a fine remedy in cases of heartburn, especially cases in which the patient feels that he must loosen his clothing after every meal. (In this way, the Pulsatilla may resemble the Lycopodium, who also feels this discomfort after eating. Note that the Lycopodium feels this immediately after eating, while the Pulsatilla does not feel discomfort for an hour or two after eating. In this way, the Pulsatilla resembles the Nux more than he does the Lycopodium, although the emotional symptoms of the remedies make it very easy to tell the Pulsatilla and the Nux apart.)

This is an excellent remedy to consider in cases of water brash—cases in which the flavor of the food eaten pushes back up into the patient's mouth; also when the a bitter taste pushes into the back of the patient's mouth. Look for the Pulsatilla to have bad breathe from his indigestion, especially in the morning.

Pulsatilla should be considered in cases of diarrhea, especially when it is worse at night, or comes on after eating fruit. No two stools will be alike. There may be blood or mucus in the stool. The patient may even pass two or three normal stools in a day, or some that are normal and some that are very loose.

The Pulsatilla patient will have an increased desire for urination as well, especially when the patient is lying down. The patient may also leak urine when he coughs, also when he passes gas. Look for the patient to complain of a pain in his bladder after he urinates.

Pulsatilla is also among our rheumatic remedies. This is the first remedy to consider in cases of pains in the patient's limbs that move or change suddenly for no reason. The patient feels pain in the knees or hips especially and he may feel numbness in the limbs. This numbness will be accompanied by restlessness and sleeplessness. Look for the patient to be chilly when in pain. Look for the pains to be worse in the night.

Keynotes: It is keynote of Pulsatilla that the case itself may make no sense. The patient is not usually helpful in relating his symptoms, and may be too emotional to give you any information. The pains and symptoms will twist and turn, and shift as quickly as the patient's moods. This, rather than being a confusion of the case, is actually a solid indicator of the remedy.

It is also keynote that the patient will experience an aggravation—emotional, physical, or both—at sunset. The light of twilight brings out all that is melancholic in his nature.

Further, it is keynote that the patient will lack thirst. Especially in patients with fever this can be a solid guiding symptom.

Look for patients to want to be outdoors in the open air. They will want to go for a walk in the fresh air. Look for them to feel faint if they must stay in a closed, stuffy room.

The Pulsatilla patient may be a sweaty patient, but the sweat will be only on one side of the body. One side of the body will tend to be hot, while the other will be cold. This one-sidedness is common to the remedy. You may find one-sided headaches as well as other aches and pains.

Emotionally, look for the patient to be very needy. He will also tend to be timid, to be somewhat whiny, and to not want to be alone. He wants to be taken care of. Little children will want to be rocked in a rocking chair. Adults will rock themselves back and forth as they sit on the edge of the bed.

Aggravations: The patient will be much worse in a warm, closed room. He will also feel worse in the sun. He will feel better with the window open, or if he can sit outside in the shade.

The patient is worse, in general, after eating, especially from eating or drinking warm things. He becomes worse if he eats too much. Pulsatilla patients should be encouraged to eat very light meals composed of foods that are cool and crisp.

Aggravation time for the Pulsatilla is at twilight, and then again just before midnight. Look for all the symptoms to be worse at these times.

Pulsatilla patients will need to keep their heads high. Even when they are in bed, they will need several pillows to support their head. They are aggravated if they are forced to have their head low. They are aggravated if they lie on their left side or on the painless side. They may also be aggravated from having their feet hang down.

Pulsatilla patients are worse from getting wet and from wet weather. Look for them also to be aggravated on first motion, such as when they first get up out of bed. As they slowly move, this aggravation will cease.

Amelioration: Pulsatilla patients are better in cool, open air; better in the shade. They are also better for cold applications to the painful area.

The Pulsatilla is better from slow, gentle motions; better for walking slowly; better for a change of positions.

The patient is also better if allowed to lie with head up and feet raised.

Finally, the Pulsatilla is better from being rubbed, from pressure on the painful area.

Dosage and Potency: Pulsatilla is used in all potencies from lowest to highest.

In acute conditions, be prepared to repeat the remedy as needed. In chronic cases, the remedy works best in a single dose.

Clarke tells us that one dose of Pulsatilla will act for up to forty days.

Relationships: Pulsatilla is most complementary in action with the Kali remedies, and with the basic remedy Silicea.

It is very often called for in cases that also involve Arsenicum, in that both speak to allergic conditions that also involve gastric complaints.

Graphites is a remedy that particularly follows Pulsatilla well in cases of chronic digestive disorders.

45. RHUS TOXICODENDRON

Remedy Source: Vegetable Remedy. Rhus Toxicodendron is taken from poison ivy, and is also known as snow rose. The leaves of the plant are used in the creation of the remedy. They must be gathered at sunset just before the flowering stage.

This remedy was created by Hahnemann.

Situations That Suggest Rhus Tox: Joint and muscle pain: low back pain, connective tissue disease, torticolis, tendonitis, sciatica, housemaid's knee, lumbago, sprains and strains of all sorts; physical trauma; rheumatism and rheumatoid arthritis. Also herpes and shingles; poison ivy and poison oak; smallpox and chicken pox; measles; laryngitis and preacher's throat; skin conditions: rash, warts, wen, scarlatina, abscesses, acne rosacea; fevers of unknown origin; hemorrhages of all sorts.

Remedy Portrait: There is perhaps no better remedy for those with pain than Rhus Tox. Certainly it is a valuable member of the homeopathic pharmacy. Often Rhus is used in combination with Arnica, completing Arnica's action in healing patients with strains and sprains of all sort. But, as with any other homeopathic remedy, we must match the patient to the Rhus Tox and the Rhus Tox to the patient.

The most important aspect of the remedy is the feature that has caused Rhus Tox to be referred to as being the "rusty hinge remedy." After a period of quiet or rest, the Rhus Tox patient feels as if the joints have stiffened and have become painful. The first motion that the patient takes after rest will be the most difficult and painful. He will have to move around a bit before he can say he is warmed up and the pain begins to subside. After he warms up, he will want to move more. And the Rhus Tox will have the tendency to overdo the movement and thereby cause the pain to begin again.

Rhus Tox belongs to Nash's "restless trio," along with Aconite and Arsenicum. This is because many Rhus patients will feel that they have to keep moving in order to stop the pain from coming back, as well as the stiffness in their joints that is almost as painful. The Rhus Tox patients will also feel as if their skin has shrunk, that it has grown too tight for their body. This sensation can also only be held in check if the patient continues slow, steady movement as a method of avoiding pain. Therefore, Rhus patients always say that they want to be up out of bed, that they want to be moving.

There is also no more rheumatic remedy than Rhus Tox. Only Phosphorus comes close to being as reactive to the weather environment as Rhus is. The Rhus patient is worse from any change in the weather from dry to wet. The patient will feel worse from becoming wet, especially from becoming cold and wet. This is a patient who cannot bear cold, wet weather.

Consider this remedy for any sort of injury that results in the "rusty hinge" syndrome, especially for injuries in which the patient has strained his muscles by lifting too much weight or by lifting an object incorrectly. Consider this remedy first for the patient whose back is in spasm after too much lifting that stresses the muscles. The patient will feel stiffness and pain in the back. The pain will be made better by motion, or from lying on something hard. It will be worse if the patient stays in a sitting position. The patient will be worse in the cold.

Consider this remedy for any form of pain that involves a swelling of joints accompanied by a sensation of heat. The joints will also be red. This is our major remedy for cases of arthritis pain, particularly rheumatoid arthritis.

The patient may complain of pain in many parts of the body, and all will respond to Rhus as long as they follow the picture of the remedy. The patient will say that he is worse at night, and especially worse in cold, damp weather. He will complain of a sensation of numbness and a loss of muscular power. Look especially for the patient to have pain in the back, in the nape of the neck, and in the knee joint. The patient may also experience pain in the hands and wrists—consider this remedy for cases of carpal tunnel syndrome—as well as in the feet. The patient will say that his feet tingle and feel numb. Rhus is also perhaps the first remedy to think of in cases of sciatica, in which the patient's limbs feel stiff, even paralyzed.

Think of the poison ivy rash to get an indication of the remedy. In fact, Rhus Tox will of course be a leading remedy for those with the poison ivy rash, for those whose skin has broken out in a red and intensely itching rash. Again, the patient will say that he feels as if his skin has shrunk, that it is too tight. And, again, the patient will be made better by warm applications, from the heat of a shower, and he will be worse from the cold. He will be made especially worse by the combination of cold and wet.

The redness of the rash will carry through to other parts of the symptom picture as well. Look for the affected part of the Rhus patient's body to have a red coloring. Any rash will be bright red, as will any affected joint. And it is keynote of the remedy that the patient's tongue will have a bright red triangular tip. Even the tip of the patient's nose may be swollen and red. This will be particularly true in patients with nosebleed. Consider Rhus Tox especially for the patient who suffers nosebleeds often, or whose nosebleeds are long-lasting. The patient will get a nosebleed when stooping.

Rhus Tox is an important remedy for those with flu, for those with ailments involving body aches. The patient will have fever, a fever in which the patient alternates between chills and heat. During the chill stage, the patient will say that he feels as if cold water has been poured all over his body. During the heat stage, the patient will stretch his muscles, stretch all his limbs. Through all stages of fever, the patient will be restless, will have to keep changing positions in order to be comfortable. If the patient lies still too long, he will feel the characteristic stiffness returning and will therefore keep tossing and turning in bed. Look for the patient with fever to have a tongue that is dry and brown-colored. The fever may be accompanied by diarrhea.

The Rhus patient may feel terrible pains in his abdomen. These pains are only relieved when the patient lies down and presses on the abdomen. The pain will be so great that the Rhus will have to walk bent over. He will be unable to straighten up. The colic will be accompanied by flatulence. The patient will have rumbling from the gas that will worsen when he first moves, but will disappear as he keeps walking. The pain and gas will be worse if the patient eats.

The patient will likely lose his appetite altogether. He will complain of a bitter taste in his mouth and of nausea and vertigo. All symptoms will worsen if the patient eats anything, yet the patient is very thirsty. He will say that his mouth feels very dry and that he must have liquids. The Rhus patient may crave either cold or warm beverages. He may crave warm liquids if a sore throat accompanies the other symptoms. He may crave milk as well.

Rhus Tox should be strongly considered for the patient who has diarrhea, especially if the stool contains blood and mucus—especially red mucus. The diarrhea will be sudden and painless, but will have a terrible odor. The stool will be frothy.

Look at the patient's face and head for indications of the remedy. The patient will say that his head feels too heavy. He will complain of headache pain that centers in the back of the head. He may have to lean his head backward to obtain relief. The patient's head will be very sensitive. He will want nothing to touch his head. Head sensitivity and pain will be worse when the patient awakens from a rest.

The patient's face will look red. His eyes will be red and swollen. Consider this remedy for all inflammations of the eye, especially those that involve a discharge of yellow pus. Consider it also for those cases in which the patient's eyes gush hot tears when he first opens them after resting.

This is also an important remedy for inflammations of the ear. The patient will complain that it seems as if there is some object lodged in his ear. The ear will also discharge yellow pus. The external ear will be swollen and red, especially the lobe.

The patient will complain of pain in the jaw. The jaw will crack every time the patient chews. This is an excellent remedy to keep in mind for cases of TMJ. The patient will also feel that his cheekbones are overly sensitive. He will feel that his teeth are sensitive and that they are loose. He will also say that his teeth feel as if they have grown to be too long. Again, look at the patient's tongue. In general, it will be red and cracked in the center. Or you may find it coated yellow, but the tip of the tongue will be red.

Consider this remedy for cases of sore throat, especially if, like the patient's back, his throat is sore from overuse of his voice. This is an excellent remedy for sore throats in actors, teachers, and singers. The pain will be worse at night and better from warm liquids. Look for the throat to be very red.

Also consider this remedy for those who suffer from palpitations. The patient will complain of palpitation accompanied by a sensation of numbness in the left arm. Consider this remedy especially for palpitations that come on from overwork and from strain. The patient will feel the palpitations and a general sense of weakness even when he is sitting still. The patient's pulse will be quick but very weak.

Exertion is the key to so much of this remedy. This is for the patient who feels that he cannot stop, that he must keep moving, even if this continued stress moves him into even deeper pain. Even in his sleep, the Rhus Tox patient will dream of exertion. He will fall into a deep, heavy sleep, and then will dream of rowing a boat all night long.

Keynotes: I think that I can safely say that, more than any other remedy, Rhus Tox is affected by the weather and by changes in the weather. The patient will be deeply aggravated by wet weather, whether the physical condition at hand is a sore throat or chronic arthritis. He will likely also be able to predict a change in the weather that is yet to come.

It is also keynote that the pains in Rhus Tox are worse on first motion. This is the "rusty hinge" remedy that squeaks loudest when it is first moved. Thus the Rhus gets out of bed in the morning in agony, but as he moves about slowly and warms up, he begins to feel much better. It is also keynote that this improvement will have limits—that, after the Rhus has moved about too much, the pain will return and will be even worse.

It is also keynote that the Rhus patient is a restless patient. He will always want to keep moving and never be willing to just sit or lie still. This can be an important guiding symptom.

The Rhus patient, who is very aggravated by cold, wet weather, will be dramatically improved by taking a hot shower. He will say that he feels as if his skin is tightening around him, especially if he suffers from poison ivy itself, and that only a hot shower makes his skin feel better. The hot water will improve him in every way. Only Phosphorus wants to take a hot shower as badly as does a Rhus Tox patient.

A typical symptom as well is the Rhus Tox tongue. Look for the patient to have a tongue that is dry, sore, and cracked. Look for it to have a triangular red tip.

Aggravations: The Rhus Tox is worse for rest, better for gentle motion.

Rhus Tox patients are worse at night, especially after midnight. They are also worse before storms, which will aggravate their entire system. They are worse in cold, wet, rainy weather.

The Rhus Tox patient is worse on first motion, worse on beginning to move after resting. It is as if during rest his entire body tightens itself up.

The Rhus Tox patient also feels worse when drinking cold water. He will be improved by imbibing warm liquids. In this way, you can tell him apart from the Phosphorus patient, who will need cold water.

Ameliorations: Rhus Tox patients are better from continuous gentle motion, and from moving their painful parts. Stretching improves their conditions. They are better when changing positions, and may seek to change them constantly.

They are better in warm, dry weather and are better from warm applications to the body.

Dosage and Potency: Rhus Tox can be given in any potency, although the 30C and 200C potencies are most common. And it may be repeated as called for. In acute cases of pain, strain, or sprain, high potencies may be required and in multiple doses.

In general, though, as usual, the remedy is repeated in lower doses in acute situations, but acts best in single doses for chronic conditions.

Those who are highly susceptible to poison ivy may want to use Rhus Tox preventatively. If the remedy is taken at least a month before the poison ivy season, a single dose of 200C will usually be effective, but if the patient already has the rash, do not give it in a high potency, as it will cause the rash to express itself and cover the whole body. The remedy must be given in a very low potency, like a 6X.

Rhus Tox is a quick-acting remedy. One dose acts for one to seven days.

Relationships: Rhus Tox is complementary to both Bryonia and Calcarea Carbonica, both of which share the rheumatic disposition and the sensitivity to weather changes.

Rhus may, at times, be similar to Phosphorus as well, but the two remedies are not complementary in their actions and do not work particularly well together, although the patients needing these two remedies may seem similar.

The remedies that do work well before or after Rhus Tox include Bryonia, Calcarea, Nux, and Sulphur.

46. RUMEX CRISPUS

Remedy Source: Vegetable Remedy. The remedy is taken from the plant called both yellowdock and curled dock. The plant is considered a weed. It is native to Britain and belongs to the Natural Order of Polygonacae. The plant was brought to the New World from England. It now grows wild in North America, where it is also considered to be a weed.

Rumex was created by Dr. H. A. Houghton, who was a student of the

Hahnemann Medical College in Philadelphia. He created the remedy in 1852. The remedy was prepared from the roots of the plant and made into a mother tincture.

Situations That Suggest Rumex: Cough, bronchitis, acute asthma, colds, sore throat. Also indigestion, diarrhea. Also tender feet.

Remedy Portrait: This is a very minor but very handy remedy. This is the homeopathic remedy that will be of the most help for the patient who has a nagging, tickling little cough that seems as if it will never go away.

Therefore, Rumex is often the last remedy given in a cold. The rest of the illness has gone, but the slight cough goes on and on. There will be a rawness in the throat that is worse in the open air. And there will tend to be still a good deal of mucus, especially in the upper airways. The cough is the body's method of removing this mucus from the body. The mucus in the larynx will tend to be thick and hard to move.

The cough will be so troubling that patients will want to cover their mouths to keep from coughing. They will not want to laugh or to speak because they know it will lead to coughing. They will often pull their bedclothes up over their mouths to keep from coughing. It is as if all their strength and will is wrapped up in keeping them from coughing.

The cough will be shallow and will issue from the pit of the throat. There will likely be a sensation of tickling that is constant. A cough can be triggered by touching the pit of the patient's throat. The cough will occur in spasms and will make the patient feel as if he cannot breathe. It will keep him from breathing. It will be made worse by the application of pressure, by talking, and, especially, by breathing deeply or breathing in cool air. The cough will grow worse if the patient moves from a warm room to a cold room, or a cold room to a warm room.

The cough may have a barking sound to it. It will be worse at 11 P.M., 2 A.M., and 5 A.M.

In general, look for the pain of Rumex to be constantly shifting and changing. There will be sharp pains; neuralgias. The mucous membranes will be especially affected: the larynx, the trachea, the bowels, and the pit of the throat. These areas can feel dry, and very sensitive. Headaches are also common. Look for a darting pain to shoot through the left side of the head. The headache will be worse from coughing, and upon waking in the morning. There will also likely be pain in the right jaw upon waking.

Look for the patient to feel that his nose is too dry. Although there may be a good deal of mucus from the nose, the patient will feel that it is dry and irritated. The inside of the nose will itch. The patient will want to pick his nose.

Look for enlarged lymph glands. Look for glands to be very sensitive.

Look for the patient's tongue to have a burning sensation. Look for the patient to complain of tooth pain upon awakening in the morning.

Look for the patient to be very hungry and to want to eat, but to feel worse from eating anything. Eating meat causes an aggravation. This remedy is given for chronic gastritis. Look for the patient to complain of aching pains in the pit of the stomach. There will be a good deal of belching. The patient will feel better from this belching.

Patients will have to settle for short naps, as they will be awakened frequently by their cough. They become suddenly sleepy, and fall asleep very quickly. They will dream of danger and trouble.

Keynotes: The nagging, shallow cough is keynote, as is the tendency of the patient to be aggravated by inhaling cool air. The cough being aggravated by moving from room to room is also keynote.

Intense itching, especially in mucous membranes, is keynote to the remedy portrait.

Aggravations: The patient will be worse from any contact with cool air, especially from inhaling cool air. He feels worse when there is a change in temperature from cool to hot, or from hot to cool.

The patient is made worse from deep breathing, or from any irregularity in breathing, such as laughing or talking loudly. He feels worse when lying on his left side.

The patient is worse in the evening and at night. Times of aggravation are 3:30 and 11 P.M. and 2 and 5 P.M. The patient will also be worse in the morning upon awakening.

The patient will also be made worse by any motion, and by riding in a car or train, or anything that jostles him.

The patient feels worse after eating.

Ameliorations: The patient is better from being covered, especially from covering his mouth; also his head.

The patient feels better when lying on his right side.

The patient feels better after a discharge of mucus.

Dosage and Potency: Rumex works best in lower potencies. Potency 30C is most common and most effective.

It is a short-acting remedy, with one dose lasting as little as a day or as much as a week. It may be repeated in acute situations as needed.

Relationships: Calcarea Carbonica often follows Rumex in helping the patient to regain his strength.

Phosophorus also may follow Rumex in clearing the chronic cough.

47. RUTA GRAVEOLENS

Remedy Source: Vegetable Remedy. Ruta is created from the common garden plant rue, also called bitterwort. The remedy is created from the whole plant. The remedy Ruta was proven by Hahnemann.

Situations That Suggest Ruta: Injuries, specifically injuries to the muscles and connective tissue. Also colds and coughs, allergies, asthma. Also eye pain and strain. Consider for constipation and worms.

Remedy Portrait: Two apparently unconnected conditions combine in the picture of the remedy Ruta: eyestrain and hip pain. No other remedy speaks so well to either, or especially to both.

Consider this remedy for the patient who gets a headache from eyestrain, who gets a headache after straining to read or after doing close work like sewing. (Natrum Mur would be the other remedy to consider in this situation, if the patient's eyes water from the strain.) The patient will say that his eyes feel weary, that they feel hot and heavy in his head. The patient may experience a sensation of pressure over the eyebrows. He may also complain of a headache that feels as if it is caused by a nail being driven into the head. (Because of the nature of this headache, so similar to that of Nux, Ruta is another remedy to consider in cases of headaches that are brought on by the consumption of alcohol.)

Ruta has two odd symptoms that have to do with the face. Look for the patient to have sweat on his nose, especially on the root of his nose, and it will usually be accompanied by nosebleed.

And the Ruta patient will experience a cramp in the tongue. This will make it difficult for him to speak and will cause him embarrassment. The patient will have a woody taste in his mouth. He will likely also have a swollen tongue.

The other major use of this remedy is for cases of lumbago in which the patient's backache is better from pressure. The patient will feel better if he lies down on his back. The pain will be worse in the morning and in cold, wet weather.

Think of Ruta first in cases of hip and limb pain in which the patient has difficulty getting up out of a chair. He may have trouble getting in and, especially, out of a car as well. This motion of rising up from a sitting position is the worst for the Ruta patient. He will say that his spine and lower limbs feel bruised. (In fact, this sensation of bruising pain will accompany nearly every symptom in Ruta.) The sensation of pain will center in the small of the back and through the loins. The patient feels as if his legs will give out under him if he tries to put his weight on them.

The patient's tendons may also be sore. The patient will say that he feels as if his muscles and tendons have been shortened. The patient will complain that his hamstrings feel shortened. He feels the need to stretch, but stretching brings on pain.

Think of Ruta for patients who experience pain and weakness in their wrists and hands. The patient will complain of a shrinking sensation in the fingers, that his fingers feel shortened. In the same way, the patient may feel the same sensation of pain and of shrinking in his feet and ankles.

The Ruta patient may also suffer from the aches and pains associated with bursitis. The patient will be worse when he is out in the open air, especially when he is walking. The patient will complain that all his joints crack and feel both stiff and numb.

The Ruta patient may feel symptoms in the chest as well. He may complain of a sensation of weakness in the chest. Consider this remedy strongly for cases of mechanical injury to the patient's chest. He may suffer shortness of breath. Look for the patient to have a cough, and to cough up a thick, yellow expectoration.

The patient may also experience constipation that will likely alternate with diarrhea. Look for stools that contain mucus and perhaps a little blood. During the constipation stage, the patient will have to strain to pass a stool. The patient will feel the urge to pass a stool but will be unable to do so. In general, the patient will have constipation and then will experience a sharp pain in the abdomen. This pain will be the sign that he is in for a bout of diarrhea.

Finally, consider the symptoms that will characterize the skin of the Ruta patient. The patient will complain that his skin is sensitive and is easily chafed. This chafing will be brought on by walking or riding. The patient's skin will also be very itchy. The itch may drive the patient to distraction. And look for the Ruta to have warts. Ruta is a leading remedy for those who have flat and painful warts on the palms of their hands.

Keynotes: Ruta is a helpful remedy for situations in which the patient is experiencing lameness after sprains or strains of the wrists or ankles. It is characteristic of this remedy that the pains experienced in these parts of the body blend a bruised sensation with numbness and tingling.

The situation that will usually indicate Ruta is when the patient feels that his legs will give out under him when he tries to rise up out of a chair or especially out of a car. It will take the patient several attempts before he can get up.

Look for a general weakness in the hips and thighs. Look for the patient to say that his hamstrings feel shortened or weak.

It is also a peculiar symptom of this remedy that the sensation of itching will change location after it has been scratched.

The patient will be restless, as with Rhus Tox. Look for him to change positions often.

This is a major remedy for the eyes and for eyestrain. The eyes will feel like balls of fire. This can be brought on by overworking the eyes reading in too little light or from close work like sewing.

Aggravations: The patient will be worse in cold, damp weather. He will feel worse when he becomes cold.

Look for physical pains to increase when the patient lies down at night. He will have an aggravation from rest.

The patient feels worse from any form of overexertion. He is worse when stooping or sitting up.

Ameliorations: Ruta patients feel better during the daytime, especially in the morning.

They are better when slowly moving about, when in a warm room, and when applying warm things to the pain.

In cases involving backache, the patient feels better lying down on something hard and applying pressure to the pain.

Dosage and Potency: Ruta is most often used in the 30C and 200C potencies and may be repeated as needed.

One dose of the remedy acts for up to a month.

Relationships: Ruta is most complementary in its actions with the Calcarea remedies, especially with Calcarea Phosphoricum.

It is often used to complete cases that have been started with Arnica. The two remedies work well with each other, especially if the case has been opened by Arnica. It is also used to follow Symphytum in cases that involve injury to bones.

Ruta may be followed most commonly by Calcarea Carbonica, Lycopodium, or Pulsatilla.

48. SABADILLA

Remedy Source: Vegetable Remedy: Taken from *Sabadilla officinarum,* also known as the cevadilla and the asagracea. The plant is native to Mexico. It is part of the Colchicum family of plants, the Natural Order of Melanthaceae. The remedy is taken from the seeds of the plant.

Sabadilla is a remedy created by Hahnemann.

Situations That Suggest Sabadilla: seasonal allergy, hay fever. Also colds and coughs, sore throat. Also toothache. Also earache. Also lice, worms, tapeworm.

Remedy Portrait: Sabadilla is perhaps the first remedy to be thought of for cases that involve general and typical seasonal allergies. The most important symptom will be the sneeze. The patient will produce sneezes that are like explosions. Everyone in the room will jump when the Sabadilla sneezes.

And once he starts sneezing, look for the patient to keep on sneezing. If Allium Cepa and Euphrasia—other leading remedies for seasonal allergies—are like snipers with rifles, Sabadilla is like a sniper with an Uzi. The Sabadilla patient will sneeze ten, twelve times in a row. The patient's throat will be raw from the sneezing. His eyes will be red and burning. Look for his eyelids to be rimmed red as well. There will be a great deal of tearing as well. The patient will cry from sneezing, but the tears will not be in steady flow, as with Allium Cepa and Euphrasia.

The nose will have copious flow. As the sneezes come spasmodically, look for the nose to run like a bursting dam. The patient will complain of a tickling sensation in the nose. The nose will itch internally. And when the patient is not sneezing, his nose will feel uncomfortably dry. The patient will also be oversensitive to smells. Smells—most especially the smell of flowers—will trigger the spasms of sneezing. Another common trigger is the smell of garlic. The odor of cooking in general may trigger some Sabadilla patients. Some patients will be so sensitive that even thinking about the trigger smell will bring on an attack.

The Sabadilla patient will wheeze when he breathes, like an asthma patient. He will have attacks of coughing that are as overwhelming as the sneezing. He will not be able to breathe in deeply. Look for the patient to have rapid and shallow breathing.

After an attack of sneezing or coughing, it is quite common for the Sabadilla to pass blood from his mouth or nose or both. This again will be a spasmodic response. A large amount of bright red blood will flow out very quickly and then stop.

The patient will complain of a sweet taste in his mouth, sometimes sweetish-metallic. The mouth itself will feel burnt. The tip of the tongue will be painful, again as if burnt. The patient will not want to drink—the idea of liquids, hot or cold, in his mouth is painful to him. Look for the patient not to be able to stick out his tongue if his symptoms are accompanied by a sore throat. Worst of all, the patient will complain of soft palate itch. Only one other remedy (a remedy specific to fall allergies and hay fever) has as much itching of the soft palate: Wyethia.

The patient will be hungry, or, often, he will not feel hungry until he takes the first bite of food and then he will eat and eat and eat. He will want things that are both hot and spicy. It will make his throat less sore and will help to open his sinuses and ears. He also craves sweets, and he also is likely to want milk. The patient will be averse to coffee and other stimulants.

The patient will complain of a sensation of deafness. His ears will feel pressurized and full. He may hear noises in his head, particularly buzzing and humming noises. His ears may itch as well. A burning sensation may accompany the itching. This burning and itching may alternate between the anus and the ears.

For years the cevadilla seed was used to kill lice and worms. The remedy Sabadilla serves the same function. Look for the patient with worms to be constipated. He will complain of itching, burning, and a crawling sensation in the anus. This will alternate with itching in the ears and/or the nose. Like most worm-infested patients, the Sabadilla patient will likely be a nose picker. He will also dig his fingers into his ears.

Look for the worm-infested Sabadilla to also experience a burning sensation when passing stools. The stools will be small, broken, and hard. Look for headaches in the patient with worms to be very common.

Finally, think of Sabadilla in cases that involve tonsillitis. Look for the pain to be left-sided, or to move from the left side to the right. Look for the patient to refuse cold things, but to feel better when drinking hot beverages. And look for the sensation of the pain and the patient's generalities to follow the pattern of the type.

Emotionally, Sabadillas are caught up in fear. They have a jumpy sort of anxiety and fear about themselves. They will commonly have fears about their health. They will get strange ideas, such as that one side of their body is larger or longer than the other. They will feel that one area of their body, the right leg perhaps, or the head, has been stretched out of shape.

But the most important mental characteristic of the type is that this remedy, in general, will follow the following pattern: if the patient thinks about a pain or a symptom, he will instantly physically manifest that symptom. Therefore, if he worries about sneezing, he will sneeze, but if you can keep his mind off his own health, he will do much better all the way around.

Keynotes: Alternation is keynote. Physical symptoms alternate between complete dryness and total flow. Also itching and burning alternates between the anus and the nose or ears.

The peculiar mental symptom is also keynote that the patient need only think about his symptoms and the catalyst to his symptoms to bring the physical symptoms on.

Aggravations: The attacks of symptoms tend to come on in Sabadilla at the same time every day. The specific time of day will vary from patient to patient. But the general aggravation period for the type is from 4 until 8 P.M.

They are worse during the period of the new and the full moon.

They are made worse by certain smells, usually flowers. Sabadilla is one of the remedies that is most reactive to specific smells. In this way, the remedy resembles Nux.

Ameliorations: Sabadillas are better in the open air. Even if the allergy symptoms increase, patients will in general be better when they are in the open air.

They are better when ingesting warm foods and/or drinks, also better when they are wrapped up and kept warm.

Dosage and Potency: Sabadilla works best in 30C generally, but 200C is excellent for ending an allergy attack. It is a remedy of short duration and will have to be repeated as needed.

Relationships: Sabadilla is complementary to Sepia. It is well followed in cases of seasonal allergy by Arsenicum and by Nux.

49. SEPIA

Remedy Source: Animal Remedy. Sepia is taken from cuttlefish ink. As a substance, it is used in the tinting of photographs and as a coloring agent.

This remedy was created by Hahnemann for the treatment of a patient who used the cuttlefish ink in his work as an artist. Hahnmenn originally thought of the remedy as specific to this case. It has, however, become one of our most important and most widely used remedies.

Situations That Suggest Sepia: Pregnancy, puberty in women, menopause, ailments associated with menstruation. Also schizophrenia, rage, ailments from betrayal. Also baldness. Also skin conditions: seborrhea, liver spots, eczema, ringworm, psoriasis, varicose veins. Also liver disease: jaundice. Also herpes. Also sciatica. Also incontinence, ailments of the bladder.

Remedy Portrait: Sepia is often thought of as being primarily a women's remedy, and a remedy for women in menopause. While it is true that as a constitutional remedy Sepia is more often indicated for women than it is for men, as an acute remedy it should not be thought of as being gender-specific.

If there are two symptoms that are most characteristic of the remedy, they have to do with the sensations of pain associated with the remedy and with the color of the patient's skin.

The patient will likely have skin that has a yellow tinge to it—it will be sepia-toned. The skin will itch, and this itching will not be relieved by scratching. The itch will be particular to the bends of the patient's elbows and knees. The patient's feet will also give a clue to the remedy. Look for the patient's feet to be sweaty. The toes will be especially sweaty, and the sweat will be very smelly. (The patient will feel better in every way when his feet are sweating. He will, in fact, be better for sweating in general.) Sepia is a remedy to keep in mind for eruptions of the skin as well. Consider it for cases of ringworm; also for herpes, especially for herpes eruptions on the patient's mouth, lips, and nose.

The pains experienced by the Sepia patient will have a downward motion and a downward pressure. There will be a general sensation of increased gravity to the patient.

This is a patient who may be given to vertigo. These patients will complain of a sensation of heaviness to their head. They will also complain that they feel as if something were lodged inside their head and rolling about in there. (This sensation of a weight somewhere within the body, blocking things and moving about, is also common to Sepia.) The headache will be centered either within the head or in the forehead. The patient will complain of a stinging pain. Nausea and even vomiting may accompany the headache pain, as well as flatulence. This is a remedy to keep in mind for the woman patient who is having headaches with hot flashes during menopause.

Sepia is a major remedy, in both the acute and the chronic context, to consider for many female health issues. Here, too, the patient will complain of a pushing down or bearing-down sensation within the area of the pelvis. The area of the pelvis will feel very heavy. The patient will cross her legs to alleviate the pain.

Consider Sepia for the female patient whose monthly period comes late or comes irregularly, for the period that is too scanty or is accompanied by sharp clutching pains in addition to the bearing-down sensation. This is an excellent remedy to consider during the time of menopause. The patient will experience sudden flashes of heat that are accompanied by sweat. The patient will sweat from the least motion. And yet, other than during the flashes of sudden heat, this is a chilly patient. There will be a general lack of vital heat. The patient will become thirsty when chilled, especially toward nighttime.

Consider this remedy also for the woman who experiences vaginal pain from sex. And think of this remedy first for the patient who once was interested in sex and now wants nothing to do with it, for the patient who suddenly is suspicious of men and who suddenly dislikes men, especially her husband. (Natrum Mur will share this symptom.)

Also think of Sepia for the pregnant woman who is experiencing morning sickness. (Sepia is most commonly called for in female patients at times of great hormone shift.)

Like the woman with morning sickness, the Sepia will feel nausea. This nausea will be most pronounced in the morning before the patient has eaten anything. The sight or smell of food nauseates the patient. If these patients eat, they may vomit up everything that they have eaten. All foods will taste too salty. These patients will feel worse from consuming milk or any dairy product. They will become nauseous particularly from fatty or greasy foods. They may crave sour things, especially vinegar and pickles. Consider this remedy in all cases of indigestion in which patients have burning pain in the pit of their stomach that is accompanied by sour belching and a bloated abdomen. The indigestion will be worse if the patient lies down. (It is true in general for Sepia patients that everything will be worse if they lie down.)

This sensation of nausea will extend into the patient's abdomen. This is a flatulent patient who will experience discomfort and sensitivity in the liver region. The pain will be improved if the patient lies on his right side. Look for the patient to complain of a bearing-down sensation in his abdomen as well. Look for the Sepia to complain of headache accompanied by flatulence.

The Sepia may feel the sensation of a stone or a ball in the abdomen, but this will more commonly be felt in the rectum. The Sepia is usually a constipated patient. He will have hard, large stools that are often bloody. If the patient strains at his stool, he will feel a terrible pain that will extend upward.

Look at the patient's tongue. The Sepia patient will have a tongue that is coated white—although the female Sepia will have a clean tongue during her period. Look for a swollen and cracked lower lip. (Natrum Mur shares this symptom.)

Consider this remedy for the patient who has a thick greenish discharge from the nose, making this another remedy to consider, along with Pulsatilla and Kali Bi, for the final stages of a cold. The patient's nose will also be filled with plugs and crusts of dried yellow-green mucus. Consider this remedy, along with Thuja, for the patient who has chronic sinusitis, and who especially suffers from postnasal drip.

Look for the patient to have a yellow tinge to his face. In chronic cases, the patient's face may have a brown caste to the cheeks and nose. The area around the patient's mouth especially will be yellowed.

Sepia is another remedy in which the patient experiences a pain in the back. The patient will complain of a sensation of weakness in the small of the back and also a chill, especially between the shoulder blades.

Sepia patients will complain that their limbs, especially their lower limbs, feel lame and stiff. Their limbs feel too short. They will also say that their legs feel too heavy, and that their legs feel chilly. Like Rhus Tox, Sepias will like to exercise in order to keep their limbs moving. They also like exercise, especially dancing, in that it allows them to sweat and they feel better when sweating. Finally, exercise helps the Sepia to build a sensation of vital heat.

Although I mention the emotional symptoms last, it does not mean that they are not important. I do this because the emotional ones will be less apparent in the acute case. But look for the Sepia to be an indifferent remedy. Patients will not much care about what is going on around them. They will be particularly indifferent to their family, their loved ones. Those that they have, until now, loved suddenly seem to be unimportant. Sepia will be an irritable and fault-finding remedy, and yet these patients will not want to be alone—they dread it. Sepia patients are sad; they feel disappointed; they feel that things are not fair, and that life has been unfair particularly to them. This is keynote: Look for patients to cry when they talk about their own symptoms. Their own suffering is a cause for great sorrow. But note that their sorrow will be displayed on an angry face, one that does not want to be comforted. Sepia patients do not want your consolation.

Keynotes: Look for the characteristic yellowing of the skin, and for the brown tinge across the cheeks and nose. The Sepia is sepia toned.

Also look for Sepias to experience the pressing-down and bearing-down pains common to the type. And look for them to complain of an increased sensation of gravity, that they and everything in their environment has become too heavy. Sepias will also likely have the sensation of a stone or ball lodged somewhere in their body.

This is a sweaty patient, one who sweats very easily, especially on the feet and legs. And yet this is a chilly patient. Like Pulsatilla, the Sepia is chilly even in a warm room.

Finally, these patients will cry when they tell you their symptoms, again like the Pulsatilla. But the Pulsatilla patients will want to be rocked and comforted. The Sepias may cry, but they do not want to be touched or comforted. The Natrum Murs, who also do not want to be comforted, will never cry when they tell you their symptoms. They cry when they are alone in their room.

Aggravations: Patients are worse from cold, especially from cold, wet air and weather.

They feel worse while driving.

They feel worse if awakened for any reason during the early part of their night's sleep.

Female Sepias are worse at any time of life when there is a hormonal shift, especially just before their period (PMS), during and just after pregnancy, and during menopause.

Ameliorations: Sepias feel better when they are active and moving about, especially when these motions exhaust them. They feel better when swimming, dancing, or exercising.

In general, they are better when they are busy, when their bodies and minds are occupied. They are happiest when they have a successful career.

They also feel better when they drink cold things.

Dosage and Potency: Sepia is most often used in the 30C potency. It does not repeat well, and, if repetition is needed, it should be given in the next higher potency.

One dose holds for up to two months.

Relationships: Sepia is most complementary to Ignatia and Natrum Mur. All together, they form a triad of remedies—first Ignatia, then Natrum Mur, and finally Sepia. Sepia is also complementary to Nux and to Sulphur; also Sabadilla.

Sepia is incompatible with Lachesis and Pulsatilla.

It is antidoted by Rhus Tox and Aconite.

50. SILICEA

Remedy Source: Mineral Remedy. This remedy is made from quartz or flint (silica). The chemical formula for the silicic oxide is SiO_2. The substance is ground into a fine powder that is mixed with mild sugar and dissolved in alcohol.

This is a remedy created by Hahnemann.

Situations That Suggest Silicea: Bone disease: hip-joint disease, weak ankles, TMJ and jawbone disease; rickets; housemaid's knee. Also malabsorption and other digestive disorders: food allergies. Also splinters and other foreign objects in the skin. Also swollen glands, general infections, abscesses, boils, keloids. Also toothache and tooth decay. Also rheumatism and neuralgia. Also sinusitis and allergies.

Remedy Portrait: This remedy, especially in patients who are children—for whom the remedy works well—can be thought of as almost a skinny version of Calcarea Carbonica. Just as the Calcarea is depleted and slow to heal, the Silicea is exhausted, all but beaten by his disease, and very, very slow to recover. (This symptom is so pronounced that Silicea should be considered in all cases in which the patient seems unable to recover from an ailment that others would push aside quickly and easily. It is also to be considered in cases in which acute illness reccurs.) Both will be sweaty. Both will have digestive upsets and allergies to foods. Both will often go from one acute illness to another, seemingly without end. But the Calcarea is a heavyset patient and is flabby and exhausted. The Silicea most often is a skinny patient. Often, the Silicea is a child who suffers from failure to thrive.

The classic texts begin their study of Silicea with the statement, "Imperfect assimilation and consequent defective nutrition." This is our leading remedy, along with Calcarea, Sulphur, Lycopodium, and Arsenicum, for the patient who is not able to make the proper use of the food he eats, or digest common and simple foods. In the case of Silicea, however, this defective nutrition is coupled with what the texts call "exaggerated reflexes"—that is, this is an overly sensitive patient. Like Phosphorus, Siliceas will have a deep sensitivity to their surroundings, including the weather. And they will also somewhat share their sensitivity with the aesthetics of the environment as well. Like Mercurius, Siliceas will be very susceptible to changes in weather.

This is, even as an acute remedy, a remedy for patients with ailments that come on slowly, that develop over time. The remedy will be counterindicated by a situation that comes on quickly. Think of Silcea, however, for many acute situations: for sore throats, especially for cases of what the old texts call "quinsy," a sore throat that is so painful that it drains the patient of his vital force. Think of Silicea for abscesses of all sores, spasm, headaches; for digestive disorders of all types. All of these, and many more acute ailments, will have one thing in common: the patient will have a sensation of chilliness—deep coldness, really, in most cases—just before the onset of symptoms. The Silicea is one of our chilliest patients. Like Arsenicum, such patients are cold because they are depleted of vital force. They will want to be wrapped up, and they will want to wear warm clothing. Siliceas will want to sit right by the fire. They will feel worse from any contact with cold. They will avoid drafts. They will even be afraid of the cold. These are patients who dread the winter and are likely to be sick throughout the winter. They are patients who will especially feel the cold in their hands and feet. They will feel that their feet are especially vulnerable and they will do whatever they must to keep their feet warm and dry. Silicea patients whose feet get cold and wet will likely panic. It is likely that their condition will become a great deal worse.

Finally, consider this remedy in any case in which pus is present. The Silicea patients, like Mercurius patients, will produce pus easily. It may ooze from their eyes, their ears, or any infected point on their body. Abscesses will form virtually anywhere on their body, as will boils. This is the remedy to consider in cases in which the skin has not healed correctly, in which infections become reinfected and scars suddenly become painful. Consider this remedy for patients who have keloids; also for the patient for whom every injury will become a pus-producing infection.

Consider this remedy for the patient with a long-lasting cold, or for the patient with simple allergies. The patient will have a fetid discharge from his ears as well as his nose. The patient will complain that his nose itches. Look for the patient's nose to have crusts and blocks in it of dried mucus and blood. Look for the nose to bleed when these crusts are removed. The patient will say that his nose is sensitive. It may also be somewhat swollen.

The patient will also complain of itch and stuffiness in the ears. He will say that he hears a roaring sound in his ears. The patient will be very sensitive to noise and will startle very easily from noise.

The patient will also be very sensitive to light, especially to daylight. The patient will complain of a sharp pain in the eyes if he suddenly has to look at light. He may actually be dazzled by light. Consider Silicea for the patient with conjunctivitis that accompanies a cold; also for patients who suffer from styes; also for patients who suffer infections in the eyes as a result of mechanical injury.

Expect the Silicea, like the Calcarea, to have head sweats. The Silicea patient will have sweat that begins on the back of the head and extends down the neck. The Calcarea will sweat all over his head. The Silicea will, unlike the Arsenicum, want his head covered. He will want it wrapped up tight. The Silicea often suffers from vertigo, which is either brought on or made worse by the patient looking upward. He will get both vertigo and headache if he does not eat on time, like Lycopodium.

It is keynote to this remedy type that the patient will feel as if he has a hair on his tongue. This is a remedy for those with toothache, especially if the tooth is abscessed. The pain will be worse from cold water and from contact with anything cold.

Consider this remedy for cases of sore throat, especially when it is accompanied by a swelling of the glands under the chin. The throat pain will be worse when the patient swallows. Like Phosphorus, this is a remedy for the patient whose cold either begins in the throat or very quickly moves to the throat, chest, or ears. This is also, like Phosphorus, a remedy to keep in mind for the child who is given to frequent ear infections, who seems to have one infection after another.

Because this is a remedy of defective nutrition, we can expect many symptoms having to do with digestion and elimination, and Silicea does not disappoint. Look for these patients to have little appetite. They will be disgusted by food, especially by meat. He will be nauseous, and the nausea will increase if he tries to eat any warm food. The Silicea patient will crave liquids however, but, like the Phosphorus, he may vomit soon after he drinks.

The patients will complain of a feeling of pressure in the pit of their stomach. They may have vomiting and/or belching after eating anything. The pain will extend into the patient's abdomen. The patient will also feel a chill in the abdomen. This is a remedy for those with colic, especially if the pains of colic are accompanied by a sensation of chill and are improved by the external application of heat.

The patient will say that he feels as if his intestines are frozen, or that they are paralyzed. And yet, you will hear a good deal of rumbling and gurgling in the bowels, as with Thuja. This is a good remedy to consider in cases of constipation. The patient will have to strain to pass a stool. He will say that he feels as if the stool will only partially move from his body, only to draw it back in. Consider this remedy also for women patients who have constipation each month with their period.

This is a remedy to consider for sciatica—for the patient with pains in his hips, legs, and, especially, feet. The patient will complain of leg cramps, especially in his calves. He will feel as if he has lost muscle power in his legs. He will have icy cold and sweaty feet. He will also have cold, sweaty hands. The patient's hands will also tremble, especially if he tries to lift something.

The patient's back gives us an indication for the emotional makeup of the patient. It is said to be for the patient who has had an injury to the spine, who must keep his spine warm. As this is a remedy for those with bone pain and bone disease of all sorts, it is also the remedy for those with a weak spine.

Emotionally, the Silicea is rather spineless. These patients, whose remedy is taken from pure flint, are said to lack grit. They will not have much fight in them; they are yielding to others and will go out of their way to avoid conflict. They are, however, quietly willful. These are the passive-aggressive patients who will never argue with their physician, but once the physician has gone will do whatever they wanted to do in the first place.

Keynotes: Silicea types are usually easy to spot. They are shy, even timid. In the acute context, they will have been drained of sufficient life force that they will have lost their ability to fight as well as their ability to heal. They resist making decisions and refuse to be drawn into confrontations. They feel chilly. They feel weak. They always seem to be sick. This sickness is most apparent in their skin, which is sickly looking.

Aggravations: Patients are worse in cold and damp. They are even worse from bathing, and from becoming cold after a hot bath.

They feel worse when drinking milk and are allergic to dairy products.

They are worse when offered emotional support and consolation, as they do not know how to absorb it.

They are worse from putting their body weight on the painful side or parts.

They are worse during the period of the new moon.

They are exhausted from the sex act, and are worse after sex itself.

Ameliorations: Silicea patients are improved by becoming warm. They are better sitting under a warm cover and better in a warm room. They are improved by covering their head.

They also feel better when they urinate.

Dosage and Potency: Silicea works well in the 30C potency; also very good in 12C. It is a slow-acting and long-acting remedy. One dose holds for six weeks to two months.

This remedy works well for skin conditions. Create the remedy Aqua Silicea by dissolving the pellets in pure water. Then apply it to the skin, the infected area, the scar tissue, or the splinter (homeopathic literature is filled with stories of World War II shrapnel coming out of bodies when the patients are given Silicea) directly. The same remedy may be taken internally and externally at the same time if in the same potency.

In acute uses, Silicea is repeated as needed in low potencies. In constitutional care, a single high-potency dose is used.

Relationships: As you would expect, Silicea is complementary to Thuja; also Sulphur and Calcarea. It is considered a deeper level of Pulsatilla, which is the equivalent remedy from the vegetable sphere.

Silicea is antidoted by Hepar Sulph and by Camphora.

51. SPIGELIA

Remedy Source: Vegetable Remedy. Spigelia is created from *Spigelia anthelmia,* the pinkroot or Indian pink. This plant is native to North and South America. The remedy is taken from the dried whole plant.

The remedy was created by Hahnemann.

Situations That Suggest Spigelia: Anxiety attacks, depression, eating disorders. Also stammering. Also worms. Also eye pains and vision disorders, iritis. Also tinnitus. Also toothache and headache. Also rheumatism and TMJ.

Remedy Overview: This is another small remedy that is very appropriate to the home kit. Most often, cases needing this remedy will involve the presence of worms in the patient's body.

The remedy also speaks very often to patients who have chronic nasal discharge. Postnasal drip is also common. The mucus will be thick and bland. It will trickle out or down the nose. It will be accompanied by itching.

This remedy speaks to a good deal of itching in the body. As with other remedies of the sort, look for anal and rectal itching.

This is also a major remedy to consider in patients who are anemic. They will be totally exhausted. They will also tend toward rheumatic aches and pains in addition to their anemia.

This is another remedy in which, no matter how great the patient's appetite, no matter how much he eats, he does not seem to be able to maintain his weight. Although he is hungry, expect the patient to say that all food tastes bad, that nothing seems to smell or taste right.

The patient will be greatly aggravated by the smell of tobacco in any form. He also cannot tolerate the smell or taste of coffee. He will have a great thirst.

Spigelia is, by the way, a major remedy for eating disorders. As Arsenicum is a common remedy for those with anorexia, Spigelia is common for those with bulimia, which is accompanied by great thirst.

The eyes of the Spigelia patient will give you many indications of the type. The patient will have severe pain all around and in his eyes. He will complain of great pressure in and around his eyes. He will say that his eyes feel too large for his skull. He will get rheumatic pains in his skull and in and around his eyes.

As with the pain in the area of the eyes, the Spigelia will have a tendency toward pains that are stabbing in nature. He will say that it feels as if he has needles sticking in various areas of the body. In addition to the eyes, he will have these pains most commonly in the head (with headaches beginning at sunrise, growing worse until noon, and then lessening until they finally end at sunset), the heart, the teeth, and the navel. For many patients of this type, the region of the navel is the most painful one.

In addition to the needlelike pain, Spigelias will say that they are very chilly. And, unlike most chilly patients, Spigelias will literally shudder from the chill. The chill may be in specific parts of the body or throughout. The chill may or may not accompany pain.

As with the headache, all the aches and pains of the type will increase with sunshine and decrease and end with sunset. The patients will all also have a tendency toward feelings of anxiety. They are restless and are greatly concerned with their personal future. This is a remedy filled with gloom and doom. Look for Spigelia patients to stare fixedly at a specific object as they brood over their dark future.

In that the pains of the type are needlelike in nature, no other remedy type is as afraid of needles as is Spigelia. He will be terrified of needles and pins, of any sharp and pointed object. Because of this, when he is in a suicidal mood, he will often brood over knives and ice picks and other sharp things.

The Spigelia will usually have overly sensitive skin. He will not want to be touched. This is another remedy that has swollen glands, and these glands will also be very sensitive to touch, and very painful when touched. The Spigelia type will often have bad skin. His face and back will typically have red eruptions. These, too, are very painful when touched.

This is an important remedy for ailments of the heart and the region of the heart. Palpitations are common. The palpitations will be so violent that they will be audible. The patient will experience pressing pains that will radiate into the throat and arms. Commonly, the pressure will be accompanied by needlelike pains and numbness. The left arm is especially given to numbness.

Aggravations: The Spigelia patient will be made worse by any motion or noise. He also feels worse when touched. He is especially aggravated by any shaking or jostling motion.

Ameliorations: The patient will feel better when lying on his right side; also when lying down with his head high.

The Spigelia headache will be improved by cold applications or a cold shower.

Dosage and Potency: This is a remedy that is almost always given in the 30C potency. It does not work well in 200C and above.

While it can be repeated, it works best in a single dose.

Relationships: Spigelia is complementary with Aconite. In conditions following the pattern of the remedy, it follows Aconite well and completes its action.

Calcarea follows Spigelia well, as do Arsenicum, Rhus Tox, and Sepia.

Spigelia is antidoted by Camphora.

52. SPONGIA TOSTA

Remedy Source: Animal Remedy. If I asked you where you thought this remedy was taken from, and you decided to make a joke of it, you would likely say from toasted sponge. And you would be right.

Spongia Tosta is taken from roasted sponge. It must be a natural sponge, from the Natural Order of Coelenterata. This is the sort of natural sponge that is sold in stores for use in the shower.

Hahnemann got the idea for the remedy, he said, from an alchemist, Arnold Von Villanova, who used the sponge itself, toasted, ground, and mixed with other substances, for the treatment of goiter. This was in the thirteenth century. The use of sponge as a folk remedy had fallen into disuse until revived by Hahnemann.

Situations That Suggest Spongia: Cough, colds, croup, acute asthma, bronchitis, laryngitis. Also rheumatism, rheumatic fever, whooping cough. Also worms.

Remedy Portrait: In home use, this is a very specific remedy. It is the greatest blessing for parents of children who are suffering from croup.

This is the remedy for the patient, usually a child, who is coughing and coughing and coughing. It is a very dry cough, often termed "as dry as a bone." The cough sounds like someone is sawing wood.

This is the remedy for dry asthma, for coughing that is accompanied by anxiety and difficult breathing. The patient will have a fear of suffocation. He will fear that he will die from his cough.

The patient will experience a good deal of flow from the nose. Or the mucus flow will alternate with stoppage. The patient will hold his nostrils wide open in an attempt to breathe. He will move his nostrils in a fanlike motion as he attempts to breathe.

Wheezing may accompany coughing. The cough will be dry, barking, and croupy. The patient's larynx will be very sensitive to touch. The patient will have trouble breathing, may pant in his attempt to breathe. The patient may throw his head back in his attempt to breathe. Breathing is particularly difficult during the times of the full moon.

The cough will be made worse by dry, cold winds and also by fresh air. It will be improved by eating and drinking. Swallowing, in general, will make the cough better and make the patient feel better. He will be unable to cough up his mucus, and will instead swallow it and will feel better. He will be better after swallowing warm food and drink.

The patient will feel heavy. He will feel exhausted. For the parent who has to lift the child, the child will seem like dead weight. The patient will become exhausted by doing the simplest things. He will have to lie down and rest to recover from the exhaustion. The patient will also feel a bit stiff, especially in the lower part of the body, which may also feel numb.

Many of the patient's symptoms will center upon the area of the chest. He will feel weak in his chest. He will feel so weak that he is unable to talk. There will also often be a feeling of pressure on the chest that is worse when the patient lies down. He will feel as if there is a weight on his chest. There may be shooting pains in the chest as well, a sensation of rawness or burning.

The patient, especially if an adult, may be anxious about his heart and may have many symptoms centering in the heart area. He may feel pain in the heart that accompanies the coughing. The patient may experience rapid heart palpitations and may feel that he cannot lie down because of these palpitations, which will actually be improved if the patient does lie down. The patient may get a feeling of faintness as well as anxious sweat. The heart will surge and will feel as if it is about to pound its way out of the chest. The patient's pulse will be hard and full, or else very feeble.

The patient may also feel a rush of blood to the head accompanied by a congestive headache that will be worse in the forehead and worse when coughing. The headache may be accompanied by a severe itching of the scalp.

Look for the patient's limbs to be numb. The numbness will run throughout the lower part of the body. The thighs will be numb and cold. The patient will have pain in the knees, especially when rising.

Keynotes: The cough itself is keynote of the remedy. It is dry, sibilant, and sounds like barking or like sawing wood. The cough makes the patient restless and fearful.

Look for great dryness of the mucous membranes and all air passages: the throat, the trachea, the larynx, and the bronchi are all dry. In an attempt to breathe, the patient will wheeze, pant, make whistling sounds, and make ringing coughs. All symptoms are made worse by cold, especially cold water.

The patient will be anxious, restless, and fearful. He is afraid of suffocating. Any sort of mental or emotional excitement aggravates his cough.

Palpitations are common to the remedy portrait. The palpitations are characterized by violent pain and difficult respiration; the patient gasps in an attempt to breathe. The palpitations come on suddenly after midnight and awaken the patient, causing panic and fear of death from suffocation.

Aggravations: The patient will be aggravated at midnight; also after midnight until 3 A.M.

The patient is aggravated by lying down with his head low. He also feels worse when lying on his right side or when stooping.

The patient will sleep into aggravation and is worse for sleeping, as is the remedy Lachesis.

The patient is worse from cold, dry wind and from fresh air. Also from a too-warm room and from any sudden change in atmosphere or weather.

The patient feels worse when touched or when any pressure is applied to a painful area. He is worse during the period of the full moon.

Ameliorations: The patient's condition is improved by the motion of lying down. He feels better from any descending motion or from bending forward.

The patient's cough will be improved by eating or drinking warm things.

Dosage and Potency: Low potencies are most common, beginning with the 6C potency. Spongia is given in all potencies, but the 30C is most common and quite helpful in cases of croup. In home use, it is seldom called for in potencies above 200C.

Spongia bears repetition well and may be given as needed.

This is a fairly deep-acting acute remedy. It is seldom to be considered a constitutional, even in cases in which the patient has repeated acute episodes.

One dose of the remedy holds for twenty to thirty days.

Relationships: Spongia often follows Aconite in situations like croup that come on very suddenly, and in which the patient is very anxious, restless, and fearful. Spongia may also follow Hepar Sulph in cases of croup.

Carbo Veg is a great follow-up remedy for Spongia. In both cases, the patient will feel as if he cannot get enough air, that he cannot breathe. Both cases have the characteristic fanlike motions of the nostrils as the patient attempts to breathe.

Other remedies that may follow Spongia include Bryonia, Hepar Sulph, Nux Vomica, Rhus Tox, and Pulsatilla.

53. STAPHYSAGRIA

Remedy Source: Vegetable Remedy. The remedy is taken from the plant known as stavesacre. It grows to be about a foot high, and its flowers are spur-shaped, which gives the plant its name. The seeds have a bitter and burning taste. It is from the ripe seeds of the plant that the remedy is made.

The remedy was created by Samuel Hahnemann.

Situations That Suggest Staphysagria: Backaches, connective tissue disease, teething pains, toothache, cut wounds. Also hip-joint disease, neuralgia, neck pain and stiffness, leg pain. Also headache, tics. Eye problems: styes. Also a treatment for sexual abuse, rape. Also warts and eczema.

Remedy Portrait: It was either Louella Parsons or Hedda Hopper who asked actor Montgomery Clift to answer the question, "What is life?" He answered, "I've been knifed," giving perhaps the best single Staphysagria answer of all time. It gives us the two central issues of the remedy picture: the sense of having been wronged, and the pain and suffering associated with a clean cut.

Like Ignatia, Staphysagria is an acute remedy for people who have been harmed, who have, through no fault of their own, been mistreated. They have undergone some form of betrayal. They know that they have been wronged and they feel angry about it—righteously indignant, in fact—but they do not know what to do about their anger. Some will be very angry. Others will deny their anger and hold it deep within, seeming to be nice, calm people. Either way, righteous indignation is the key. Staphysagria is a useful remedy for victims of child abuse and rape. Like Ignatia, Staphysagria can be considered an acute remedy, even if the event that caused the anger happened some time ago. The patient has been frozen in his emotional trauma. Just as Arnica can clear a case involving the chronic effects of an acute mechanical injury, so, too, can Staphysagria clear the effects of a long-term emotional injury, even if that injury happened long ago.

The Staphysagria patient will be given to quick and violent outbursts of passion and/or anger. He will care very deeply about what other people think. He can be humiliated very easily, if he believes that others think ill of him. Until he has sorted through his trauma, he will find it difficult to know what he wants. Like Chamomilla, this is a remedy for those who demand things only to discard them just as soon as they get them. The wanting is all, the having is unimportant.

The Staphysagria patient tends to have very low self-esteem. He may even experience some memory loss about what has happened to him.

The physical ailments in Staphysagria may come on from suppressed anger and from the combination of anger and humiliation. The patient have been made to feel both worthless and powerless. Think of Staphysagria as a remedy for the patient who has experienced sexual or emotional abuse. Think of this remedy for the patient who has been raped. This is also commonly a remedy for children of alcoholics.

In the realm of acute treatment of physical complaints, Staphysagria also has important uses. This is perhaps our most important remedy for the recovery period after an operation. Hypericum is used in the treatment of nerve pain associated with a puncture and Phosphorus is helpful in stopping bleeding, but Staphysagria is used in treating the shock and pain that can be associated with any sort of cut wound, as well as for the loss of blood.

This concept of cutting pain and Staphysagria is so pronounced that it is to be considered a remedy for any pain that is cutting in nature. Indeed, all the ailments that are treated by the remedy can be associated with cutting pains: toothache and colic among them.

The patient with toothache who needs Staphysagria will have spongy gums that bleed easily. He will feel as if his teeth are crumbling in his mouth. This patient will be overwhelmed by the pain of the toothache. Consider this remedy for toothache associated with tooth decay. Also consider this remedy for women patients who suffer toothache with their monthly period.

The toothache may be accompanied by a sore throat that hurts into the patient's ear when he swallows. The toothache itself may extend into the patient's ears.

This is an excellent remedy to consider for patients with colic, especially for colic pains that are brought on by anger. The patient will be flatulent, and the gas passed will be hot. The patient will have a swollen abdomen and will complain of a rolling pain throughout the abdomen. Consider this remedy in cases of irritable bowel syndrome and colitis that is brought on by anger.

Staphysagria should also be considered in all cases of irritable bladder, especially in young married women. This is also an excellent remedy for the male patient who feels a burning sensation that accompanies his inability to urinate. He will complain of pressure in the bladder, of the sensation that he cannot empty his bladder. The remedy is also useful for cases of cystitis.

Think of Staphysagria for cases of eczema that are also triggered by anger. The patient will be much better when the cause of his anger is removed. Think of Staphysagria also for eczema on the patient's head, face—especially the ears—and all over his body. The skin will have thick scabs that itch violently.

Keynotes: It is common to Staphysagria people that they are sleepy. They will appear to never quite be fully awake and alert during the day, and yet they are sleepless at night. Look for this insomnia to be accompanied by a higher-than-usual sex drive and many sexual thoughts and fantasies.

Staphysagria patients are unrefreshed by sleep. They will take a nap in the daytime, particularly in the afternoon, and will awaken feeling worse than before they went to sleep.

Look for Staphysagria patients to be somewhat haughty, even prideful. Look for them to take offense easily and to wonder about the hidden meanings of all statements made to them.

Aggravations: Anger causes aggravation. It doesn't matter whether the patient himself is angry or whether anger is directed toward him. Staphysagria patients cannot deal with any sort of anger or outburst. They also cannot bear to be made to feel stupid. They are easily vexed. They are worse if they feel humiliated.

The patient will be worse from sex, and especially from sexual excess. Male patients especially will be given to masturbation and will be made worse by it. Staphysagria patients will often have dyspepsia after sex.

They feel worse when they come into contact with tobacco in any form.

Their symptoms tend to be worse at night. They feel worse after sleeping.

Ameliorations: Staphysagria patients improved by warmth and rest. They are better after they have eaten breakfast.

Dosage and Potency: The remedy is used in its tincture form for the external treatment of lice.

For physical pains, it is most commonly used in the 30C and 200C potencies, although all potencies may be used. For emotional situations, it is best used in the 200C or 1M potencies and above.

The remedy bears repetition well.

One dose of Staphysagria holds for up to one month.

Relationships: The remedy Causticum, with its need for all things to be fair to all people, is most similar to Staphysagria. And Causticum may at times be considered the constitutional for Staphysagria, as Natrum Mur is the constitutional for Ignatia.

Staphysagria often is used to clear away suppressed anger and to clear the way for other remedies to complete the case. Remedies that follow well include Calcarea Carbonica, Ignatia, Lycopodium, Nux Vomica, Pulsatilla, and Rhus Tox.

54. SULPHUR

Remedy Source: Mineral Remedy. The remedy Sulphur is created from the element of the same name. It is also called brimstone. The substance occurs naturally as a brittle crystalline mineral that is found near volcanos.

Hahnemann, who first proved the drug as a homeopathic remedy, notes that the substance was used curatively for at least two thousand years.

Situations That Suggest Sulphur: Skin conditions of all sorts: acne, eczema, rash, herpes, measles, chicken pox, psoriasis, ringworm, worms; allergies:

particularly food allergies; colds, flu, sore throat, acute asthma; digestive disorders: irritable bowel syndrome, constipation, diarrhea, ulcer, rectal fissure. Also mental disorders: depression, mania, dementia, anxiety; functional disorders of all sorts: chronic fatigue syndrome, arthritis. Also pregnancy and menopause, menstrual troubles. Also headaches, migraines, and inflammatory conditions; alcohol abuse; sleep disorders, especially sleeplessness; vertigo.

Remedy Portrait: Like the biblical fire and brimstone, those needing the remedy Sulphur will be beset with symptoms that burn, as if they had been cast into the Lake of Fire. And along with that burning sensation, the patient will be beset by itch. The patient who experiences a combination of itching and burning almost anywhere on the body may well be in need of the remedy Sulphur. In the home, Sulphur will be called upon for cases of cold, flus, sore throats, allergies, skin conditions, indigestion, and smelly armpits—for everything from chronic fatigue to hangnails. It is one of the most used remedies in the home kit. It is an essential tool of all three levels of homeopathic care: acute, constitutional, and transformational.

No matter the circumstances that call for treatment, there are certain symptoms that will nearly always be present in the Sulphur case. Look for the patient to have an aggravation in the later morning, usually at or around 11 A.M. The patient with low blood sugar will suddenly need to eat at this time, and will usually want to eat a candy bar or a doughnut. This patient and others may feel faint at this time, may have a spell of low energy. Patients with fever will experience chills as well as exhaustion at this time. But every Sulphur patient will have some aggravation of symptoms at this time. (Sometimes the Sulphur patient will have his aggravation at 11 P.M. and may have to eat something before he goes to sleep. Keep an eye out for this as well.)

In general, the Sulphur patient is aggravated by heat. Sulphurs will complain that this sensation of heat runs through their whole body, but it is centered in their head. Sweat and heat are combined symptoms for Sulphurs. Their whole body may be covered with sweat, but it is more common for Sulphurs to sweat on only one side; or it is possible for patients to have sweat and heat in specific areas of the body: they may have a hot, sweaty head. Or it is possible for the sweat to be located only on the patient's neck. This patient will have hot, sweaty hands and/or feet. The sensation of heat will be accompanied by a throbbing sensation in specific areas of the body. Look for Sulphurs to want to remove or loosen clothing because of a general sensation of heat. Sulphurs cannot bear to get too hot in bed. Look for them to stick their feet out from under the covers in order to get cool so as to be able to sleep comfortably. Sulphur patients are also given to night sweats, but their sweat will not bring them relief. Their sweat may have a strong, sulfurish smell, like that of rotten eggs.

Along with the heat and sweat, look for the Sulphur patient to experience burning pains. It completes the "burn trio" with Arsenicum and Phosphorus pains. In each of these remedies, all symptoms will have burning sensation. In the case of Sulphur, the burning pains will be accompanied by the sensations of heat and sweat.

This will especially be true of the Sulphur's head. The patient will complain of a constant sensation of heat in his head, especially on the top of his head. Sulphur's headaches will usually be centered in the forehead. The patient will complain of heat and pressure and a burning sensation in the forehead. He will experience vertigo with the headache. The headache may extend to the vertex, the top of the head, or into the temples. The vertex will be the center of the sensation of heat for the patient's whole body. Consider this remedy for the patient who has a hot head and cold feet. Also consider this remedy for the patient who has a headache— particularly a sick or migraine headache—on a regular cycle. The classic texts refer to patients with headaches every Sunday (this is actually quite common, as the Sulphur type will become sick when he stops working or when his regular schedule is changed—he will become sick on Sunday because it is the day that he lets his guard down, in the same way he typically will become sick when he goes on vacation), but consider this remedy for the patient who has a headache every other day, or every fourth day, or on any other regular cycle. Look for this cycle in other ailments as well, especially for Sulphur cases of digestive disorder.

The Sulphur patient's skin will be a strong indicator of the remedy. Look for him to have skin that is not only hot and sweaty but also red. It is most common for the Sulphur to have red skin across the cheeks and nose, or to have a red face (especially during headache), but the Sulphur may have redness of the skin in any affected area of the body. Consider Sulphur for virtually any rash, especially when the patient's general condition matches the remedy picture. The rash will be red, it will be hot, and it will be itchy. Any itch that a Sulphur patient experiences will be made worse by heat of any kind, but especially by the heat of the bed. Sulphur patients will be driven all but crazy by the itch and heat that they feel when in bed. They will kick off their covers in order to sleep.

The rash will be itchy and will be burning in character if the patient scratches it. The rash will also be sensitive to air, wind, and washing. The rash will be much worse if the patient washes it. The Sulphur patient will always feel worse from bathing as well. In acute ailments, even colds and flus, you may find that the patient does not want to bathe. Sheer laziness is not the cause; the patient will actually experience aggravation from bathing.

Consider Sulphur for such diverse conditions of the skin as eczema, boils, acne and pimples, even abscesses and ulcers of all sorts. Look for the skin conditions—especially in chronic cases—to alternate with other conditions, especially with digestive disorders and with respiratory troubles, especially asthma. Especially in chronic cases, expect the Sulphur's skin to look unhealthy. And consider this remedy, along with Silicea, for skin conditions that do not readily heal.

In respiratory infections, the Sulphur will continue with the same combination of symptoms: burning, sweating, and heat. The patient's eyes will be red and hot. The patient will complain of burning in the eyes and a sensation that there is sand or glass in the eye. This is a remedy to consider in cases of ulceration of the margins of the eyelids. It is also a remedy to consider in any case in which the patient complains of a bursting sensation in the eyeball, especially if it is associated with burning and heat. Look for the eyes to water and tear, and for the tears to seem somewhat oily or thick.

The patient will also complain of a sensation of heat in the ears. He will complain of throbbing and congestion. The patient's external ear will be very red and hot to the touch. The patient will insist that when he moves his head he can feel water sloshing around inside his ear. He will alternate between deafness and very acute hearing. He will complain of a whizzing or hissing sound in his ears. Look for the patient's ears to discharge on a regular cycle, usually once a week or on every eighth day.

Look at the patient's face for indications of the remedy. The patient will have red cheeks, and a red band across the nose. He may also have the large red, swollen nose that we associate with W. C. Fields. (Sulphur is a major remedy for alcoholism and the Sulphur who drinks will almost always exhibit this symptom of the swollen nose, often a red nose with very purple veins in it.) The patient's lips will be bright red. The upper lip may be swollen. They lips may appear rough, dry, and cracked. The patient will complain of a sensation of dryness and burning in the lips and mouth.

The Sulphur patient will have gums that bleed easily, as will Rhus Tox and Phosphorus. The Sulphur's gums will also be red and swollen. The patient may complain of a throbbing sensation in the gums and of extreme sensitivity in the teeth. Look for shooting and throbbing pains in the patient's teeth. The patient may also grind his teeth, especially when he is asleep. The patient's tongue will be coated white, with a red tip and red borders. This is an important remedy to consider for cases of thrush, for any case involving aphthae.

The patient's nose will have a constant flow of mucus and it will be watery in nature. The patient's nose may also be filled with crusts of dried mucus that will bleed when removed. The patient will sneeze constantly. He will sneeze more and will have more nasal discharge when he is outdoors (the Sulphur's nose will become blocked when he goes indoors), yet the patient will as a whole feel better while the sun is out and may stay outside in spite of his worsened nasal symptoms.

It is an important symptom of Sulphur that the patient may have a blocked nose, but his sense of smell remains acute, especially for specific smells. Sulphurs will be sensitive to particular smells. Some will be sensitive to perfumes, others to chemical smells, especially gasoline and other petroleum products. These smells will stay in the patient's nose long after he has actually smelled them. Perhaps for days and weeks afterward, the patient will insist that all he can smell is that perfume or chemical. Sulphurs will also tend to smell imaginary odors. They will insist that they can smell something that no one else can smell. They will also be unaware of their own unpleasant body odor, or they will be hyperaware of their own scent and in despair as to what to do about it. Often, Sulphur patients will smell like the brimstone that is associated with the remedy. It will often be part of the remedy's picture or a necessary part of the healing process as they sweat out their toxins. Either way, there will be little or nothing that patients can do about it, as it is a smell that cannot be washed away. And Sulphur patients who cannot tolerate the smell of perfume will be unable to cover it over with artificial scents.

Consider Sulphur for any cold or flu that has the picture of the remedy present, but especially consider Sulphur for cases of seasonal allergy that are attended by the overall sensation of heat or burning or sweat and of nasal symptoms as listed above. There is perhaps, with the exception of Natrum Mur and Sabadilla, no remedy that is as valuable for those who suffer from seasonal allergies as Sulphur.

Sulphur is also considered, like Calcarea, to be a general tonic remedy. It is the first remedy considered in cases in which the indicated remedy does not work, or works only for a short time. The classic texts suggest that a dose or two of Sulphur will help any other remedy work more effectively.

Sulphur is a major remedy for all sorts of digestive disorders as well, especially when the disorders are associated with a poor diet or with food allergies. Sulphurs will tend, either in the acute or chronic case, to be drawn to salty, sweet, and greasy foods. They love fast foods. They tend either to think that everything is too salty, like a Natrum Mur, or to feel that there is never enough salt on anything. They tend either to crave meat or to be totally averse to it. They will become ill from milk and usually will not like it at all. They tend to crave sweet things of all sorts, and to become ill from eating them. (Sulphur is perhaps the most important remedy to consider for patients with low blood sugar.) And they crave cold drinks, especially sweet and bubbly drinks, like sodas of all sorts, and cold alcoholic beverages, especially beer. They tend to like any drink that causes them to belch. Sulphur patients are belchy patients who feel better from their belching. They may belch just for the pure joy of it.

The Sulphur's belch may taste like rotten eggs; it may be smelly as well. Sulphur patients will especially be belchy if they have drunk milk or eaten any dairy product.

The Sulphur patient has great thirst. He will complain of burning and heat in the throat that will be made better by drinking liquids, especially cold liquids. His sore throat will also feel better from eating salty things, especially potato chips. The patient will have a voice that is deepened by the sore throat. He will have redness of the external as well as the internal throat. He will have a cough that tends to be dry, except in the morning when it is loose and the chest rattles with mucus.

This is a remedy that should be strongly considered for the patient with acid indigestion. The Sulphur patient will have a great deal of stomach acid. He will feel a burning sensation in the stomach if he eats anything he shouldn't, and, as Sulphur patients tend to pretty much always eat things they shouldn't, this burning sensation is pretty much ongoing. The Sulphur patient will feel an improvement in the burning pressure in his stomach if he eats something—this will be especially true at 11 A.M. or P.M., at which time the Sulphur's digestive complaints will be accompanied by a fainting sensation. The Sulphur patient may vomit and may feel very nauseous. Consider Sulphur an important remedy for pregnant women who have morning sickness.

The Sulphur's abdomen will be very sensitive to pressure; it will also feel heavy. There may also be the sensation of a ball or lump in the patient's abdomen, as with Sepia. The patient may also complain of the sensation of something alive and moving in the abdomen, as will the Thuja patient. Consider this remedy for the patient who is colicky, especially for the colicky baby. Consider this remedy if the patient has cramping pain in the abdomen that comes on after eating, and that forces the patient to bend double to get relief. The pain will center in the area of the patient's navel. Consider this remedy for the patient who has a large, swollen abdomen, especially if it is accompanied by thin or emaciated limbs, especially arms. Sulphur is the remedy of choice for children and teens who grow quickly and run to a hot body temperature and have large abdomens and thin arms.

The Sulphur patient will complain of burning and itching in the anus. It is an important symptom of this remedy that the patient will be driven out of bed in the morning by diarrhea. He will be awakened by the urging. The diarrhea will be painless and quickly expelled. The patient's anus will be red. The Sulphur will have diarrhea from drinking milk or eating any dairy product. Look for the diarrhea to be accompanied by a good deal of sweating.

This is an important remedy for patients with hemorrhoids that are associated with burning, itching, and redness of the anus; for external hemorrhoids that are red, swollen, and sore.

Sulphur is also an important remedy to consider in cases of chronic digestive disorder—for the patient who alternates between constipation and diarrhea, for those with irritable bowel syndrome, for those whose poor diet has stressed their organs of digestion and elimination. Consider it also for gassy patients, when the gas is hot and smelly—it smells like rotten eggs.

Consider this remedy for the patient with kidney pain as well, especially the patient who experiences itching and burning pain in the left kidney. (Sulphur is primarily considered to be a left-sided remedy, although its symptoms may appear anywhere and everywhere in the body.) The patient may have pus in his urine. And the urine itself may cause the parts of the body through which it passes to burn and ache. Look for the patient to pass a good deal of clear, watery urine, and look for him to urinate involuntarily when he passes gas. (The patient will also urinate when he coughs or laughs.)

Sulphur is an important pain remedy as well. It is a rheumatic remedy and may be considered for any rheumatic pain, even arthritic pain, that is accompanied by a sensation of heat and burning. The affected joints will be swollen and red. They will also feel stiff. Especially the patient's knees and ankles will feel stiff. Patients will complain of numbness of the arms, especially of the left arm. They may also complain of numbness in their hands, especially in their fingers. This is an important remedy for patients with whitlows, ulcers around the fingernails, that are hot and burning and stinging and throbbing. The patient's hands will alternate between being hot and dry and hot and sweaty. The skin on the palms of their hands may be rough and cracked. The patient may complain that his hands tighten up painfully, that the muscles of his hands contract painfully when he tries to lift anything.

The patient will feel a sensation of heat in the feet, especially in the soles. The patient will have feet that are hot and sweaty and smelly.

The Sulphur patient will have trouble straightening up. He is aggravated by standing and will not want to stand or walk upright. He will slump, lean, rock—anything other than stand up straight. He will also walk in a slump. He will feel that his body is too heavy to hold upright.

This sensation of heaviness will be felt all through the body, but especially in the patient's shoulders. He will thrust his shoulders forward. It is all but impossible for the Sulphur to push his shoulders back into an upright position.

In terms of respiration, the Sulphur will need open or cool air in order to feel that he can breathe. He often feel as if he is suffocating, especially at night. He will have to sleep with a fan on or with the windows open.

Consider Sulphur for the patient who has a loose cough in association with a cold. The mucus that is coughed up will be greenish. He will expel mucus most copiously in the late morning.

Consider Sulphur also for cases of asthma that come on after a cold; also for cases of chronic asthma that follow the Sulphur picture. Consider Sulphur for the patient who has a violent cough accompanied by a headache, for the cough that grows worse when the patient lies on his back. This is also a remedy for those with pneumonia, especially when it centers in the left lung.

Mentally and emotionally, Sulphur patients will be crabby but will want company, especially company that will get their mind off their troubles. They will want to watch TV, play cards, read magazines, or gossip. They will also want to talk about conspiracy theories and cosmic philosophies. Only the Lachesis patient will be more talkative.

Sulphur patients are selfish patients. They will run their caretakers ragged if given the chance. They will love to be waited on, and will want to be given gifts when they feel ill. They will not, however, want flowers. They want books, movies on tape, or candy—especially candy.

Keynotes: The fact that the Sulphur will have an aggravation at 11 A.M. (and sometimes at 11 P.M.) is a common keynote. This will be a period of low blood sugar, during which the Sulphur will demand something to eat. He will usually want a doughnut or a candy bar at this time of day.

It is keynote that the Sulphur patient will be sloppy, will look and smell unwashed even if he has just bathed. This can be true even in simple colds, but it is more often the case that the Sulphur patient, who will feel averse to water, simply will not take a shower and will choose instead to walk around in his pajamas until late afternoon, with his hair standing on end from having slept on it last night, and with three days' growth of beard.

Sulphur patients are hot, sweaty, and sloppy. They do not want to be bothered with any details, or with any form of work. Often they are not very sick but choose to use an illness as a reason to throw themselves down in front of the television set with a bag of potato chips by their side.

Look for Sulphur patients to crave junk food. They want salt, fat, and sugar. They want French fries and hamburgers and pizza. They want cold soda or cold beer to drink.

Sulphur patients are thirsty. They will want cold liquids of all sorts, especially ones that sparkling, sweet, or alcoholic. If there are no cold liquids, they will drink anyway, drink whatever you have. They will drink straight from the kitchen faucet if they have to.

It is also important to note that Sulphur is considered a general tonic remedy and is often given in a single dose when the remedy that seems to be called for has failed to work. Often, with that single dose, the suggested remedy will then begin its action.

Aggravations: Sulphur patients are aggravated by standing up straight. Look for Sulphur patients to want to sit, lie down, or slump. They do not want to stand up straight or stand still.

They are worse for the warmth of the bed. Look for patients to stick their feet out from under the bed covers because they cannot stand the amount of heat that has been built up under the covers.

They feel worse for bathing and will not want to get up and take a shower.

They feel worse when they are in a warm room. They will want a cool room, and will even more want to be outside.

They will feel worse when riding in a car but better when walking.

They are made worse by unpleasant odors. Often Sulphur patients will complain of a bad smell that is "stuck in their nose." They may even be offended by the smell of their own body, but they still will not want to bathe.

Ameliorations: Sulphur patients will be better in dry, warm weather. They love sunshine and love the summer.

They are better when lying on their right side.

They are better when in the open air, and better when in motion, as opposed to being at rest.

Dosage and Potency: The 12C potency is usually considered to be the best place to start for this remedy. The potency can be raised as needed. This potency is a good one to begin with in acute situations, and is raised, most commonly, to 30C and 200C. Higher potencies are most often used in chronic conditions.

The high potency will set off a chain reaction that will express from the body whatever has been suppressed. For this reason, the 1M potency and above should be used with caution, as it may set off a powerful aggravation.

The lower potencies may be repeated as needed in acute situations; the high potencies work best in a single dose.

One dose acts for up to two months.

Relationships: Sulphur is considered to be the constitutional for Aconite. It follows Aconite well in emergency situations, and often completes the action that Aconite has begun. Nux Vomica is another complementary remedy for Sulphur and it is used to complete cases—especially those involving chronic digestive symptoms—that Sulphur has begun.

Other remedies that follow Sulphur well include Calcarea Carbonica and Psorinum. Lycopodium precedes Sulphur well, but should never directly follow it.

55. SYMPHYTUM

Remedy Source: Vegetable Remedy. Symphytum is taken from the herbal remedy comfrey, also known as knit-bone and boneset. It is from the Natural Order Boraginaceae. The roots of the plant have been used for centuries as both an external plaster and an internal remedy for physical trauma to the bones.

The remedy is taken from a tincture created from the whole plant, which is picked in autumn just before the flowering stage.

Situations That Suggest Symphytum: Sprains, wounds, broken bones, backache. Also swollen glands, painful breasts. Also hernia, abscesses of all kinds.

Remedy Portrait: Symphytum is a small remedy, but one that is very important in its sphere of action. There is no better remedy to use in cases of fractures of any sort. In fact, Symphytum is so quick in its action and so effective in its cure that it is important that the remedy not be given until the bone is set, because it may actually cause an unset bone to heal incorrectly.

Symphytum is most often given after Arnica in cases of injuries to bone. The Arnica will begin the healing process, while Symphytum will speed the knitting of the bones.

This is also an excellent remedy for the eye, and specifically for injuries to the eye from blunt instruments. Where Belladonna will usually be the remedy of choice for a blow from a sharp instrument, or for a scratch to the cornea, Symphytum is the remedy to think of for a black eye (along with Ledum, if the eye is cold and squishy to the touch). After the blow, the eyelid will twitch, or there may be an involuntary closing of the eyelid.

This is the remedy also for blows to the face—injuries to the face from punches or from blunt instruments. The wound will be swollen, and the swelling will be hard and red.

Consider Symphytum also for backaches that come on from sexual excess or from violent motion of any sort.

Symphytum is an excellent remedy for headaches. The headache will move from the occiput to the top of the head to the forehead. It will extend down the bone of the nose. It will usually be associated with the trauma to the head or face.

Keynotes: The Symphytum patient will feel that when he closes his eye he must close it over a raised patch or elevation. The eye itself will feel enlarged and it will seem to swell out as the eyelid is closed.

The Symphytum patient will complain that his ears are closed up.

Look for the patient's skin to feel cold to the touch.

Aggravations: The patient will be made worse by any motion, especially any strong motion. He will feel worse when touched.

Ameliorations: The patient will be better for rest and for cool applications on injured parts.

Dosage and Potency: Symphytum traditionally is given in low potencies, with 30C and 200C most common.

It bears repetition well and may be repeated as needed until the trauma is fully healed.

One dose of the remedy may hold for up to one month.

Relationships: Most often, Symphytum will be given as a follow-up remedy to Arnica. In cases of sprain, it may be used either before, or most usually after, Rhus Tox or Ruta.

56. THUJA OCCIDENTALIS

Remedy Source: Vegetable Remedy: Thuja is taken from the arbor vitae, which is also called the white cedar. It was known in ancient days as the Tree of Life. It was considered a sacred plant, and its branches were dried and burned as incense in holy places.

The remedy was created by Hahnemann.

Situations That Suggest Thuja: Digestive disorders: diarrhea and constipation, irritable bowel syndrome. Also herpes zoster, warts, polyps. Also allergy, acute asthma, sinusitis, colds, postnasal drip. Also bone disease and rickets. Also rheumatism and sciatica. Also toothache and tooth decay.

Remedy Portrait: In the acute setting, it is most commonly used, as are Pulsatilla and Kali Bi, as a remedy for the patient who is in the last stages of a cold, when the mucus associated with a cold has turned thick and green. Consider this remedy when the mucus is mixed with blood and/or pus, when the patient complains of a sensation of pressure in the root of the nose. Consider it also—and this is important—when the patient says that his teeth hurt every time he blows his nose.

Thuja is a major remedy for sinusitis, especially for chronic sinusitis. A feature of this ailment will be that the patient will have tooth pain from sinus pressure. He will feel the pain most often in more than one tooth, perhaps even in all the teeth on one side of his head. (Toothache may, of course, actually be due to decay as well. The patient will have tooth decay low on the tooth, next to the gums. He will complain of sensitivity in all his teeth during toothache.)

Thuja should be considered in all cases of chronic sinus disorder, especially when it is associated with postnasal drip, as well as a sensation of pressure and pain in the front sinuses.

Thuja should be considered, along with Kali Bi, a major remedy for those with sinus headache. The patient will say that he feels as if a nail is being driven into his head. And the headache will begin or be worse on the left side of the head.

Consider Thuja as well for conjunctivitis that occurs with a cold. The patient's eyes will be be glued together each night by a green pus, and yet the eyes will be dry. Look for dry scales on the patient's eyelids. The eye itself will look inflamed. The white of the eye will take on a red or reddish blue color. Also consider Thuja for cases of styes.

And Thuja may also be considered for ear pain, and especially for cases of middle ear infection, especially for those given to chronic middle ear infection. The patient will complain of a sensation of congestion and throbbing in the ear. There will be a lot of green pus discharged. The patient will hear creaking and crackling sounds in his ears. Thuja is especially indicated for infections of the left ear.

In digestive disorders, Thuja offers some unique symptoms. Although patients usually will lose their appetite altogether, they will still be thirsty. They will crave cold water and tea—hot or iced. Thuja patients are great tea drinkers, and, the classic texts note, some of their chronic symptoms come on from drinking too much tea. It is an important symptom of the type that the Thuja will drink and drink and you will audibly know that the liquid is falling into his stomach. It will make a great sound as it goes down into the stomach.

This is a remedy filled with rumbling. The patient's bowels will rumble loudly. The rumbling may precede or accompany colic. The patient will have terrible cramps in the abdomen, and flatulence, which will also rumble through his intestines. The patient's abdomen will be distended—and it is keynote of the remedy that the distension will occur in specific spots, that the abdomen will be distended here and there. The patient may insist that it feels as if there were something alive and moving in his abdomen. (This is a remedy for false pregnancy.) Sulphur shares this symptom with Thuja.

Consider Thuja in cases of diarrhea, especially for chronic diarrhea, diarrhea that is worse after breakfast. The stool will be forcibly expelled from the body. The movement of the stool will be accompanied by a loud gurgling sound.

Thuja should also be considered for those with constipation, for stubborn, chronic constipation that is accompanied by severe rectal pain. (The other remedy to consider for this is Silicea.) This is also an excellent remedy for those with hemorrhoids. The hemorrhoids will be accompanied by stitching, burning pains in the patient's anus. The pains will be worse when the patient is in a sitting position. They may be so severe that the patient cannot sit at all. Again, the patient may have a sensation of something living and moving about in his anus and rectum.

In that this is a major, if not the major, remedy for those with gonorrhea, there are some important urinary symptoms associated with this remedy. It is keynote of the remedy that the patient's stream of urine will be split in two. The patient may experience great pain after urinating. He may suddenly have the urge to urinate, and may not be able to control the flow of urine. This is also a major remedy for genital warts.

It is in fact a remedy to consider for warts of all kinds; for many different skin growths, including skin tags and fibroid tumors of all sorts. The Thuja patient will chronically be given to freckles and all kinds of blotches. Look for him to have skin that is dry and covered in brown spots. Thuja, along with Natrum Mur and Rhus Tox, is a major remedy for herpes, especially for genital herpes.

Thuja patients will have fingernails and toenails that are soft and brittle; they may be peeled away. Thuja patients are given to swollen glands throughout the body. Their glands may be chronically swollen and sensitive. They are given to rashes of all sorts. The areas of skin that are covered with clothing are especially vulnerable to eruptions of all sorts. The rashes will be made worse by scratching.

This is a left-sided remedy. The Thuja patient's skin is very sensitive to touch. He tends to be a sweaty patient as well. The Thuja's head especially will tend to be both sweaty and greasy. The patient will tend to have a greasy face as well. His sweat has a distinctive garlic-honey smell, sort of sweet and rancid at the same time.

Thuja is also an important remedy for those with fever, especially for chronic fevers or fevers that reoccur. The patient will have a chill that begins in the area of the thighs or in the genital region. He will sweat only on the uncovered parts of the body, especially on the head. Night sweats are common in cases involving fever. The patient will also feel a sudden flow of blood into their head, a congestion of blood, such as in Belladonna. The patient will say that his head throbs. The patient will have restless sleep or insomnia accompanying the fever.

This is also an important pain remedy; it is another rheumatic remedy. The Thuja patient is vulnerable to cold, damp air, especially to night air. He will say that he feels as if his body is made of glass or wood, that he feels as if his body, especially his limbs, is fragile and will break into a thousand pieces if he is not careful. He will feel especially fragile when walking.

Look for the Thuja patient to have muscular trembling and twitching. Look for the joints to crack. Look especially for the fingers to be swollen and red and painful. The patient will say that he feels as if his hands are dead.

Thuja patients startle easily. They may suddenly feel as if they are being watched, as if there is a stranger at their side. They are also very sensitive. They will be especially sensitive to music, which may actually make them weep.

Keynotes: Keynote of this remedy is the sensation that something is alive in the patient's abdomen; the sensation that the patient is made of glass or a very fragile material; the sensation, especially upon falling asleep, that the patient will fly out of his body and not be able to get back in.

Also it is keynote that the patient will have very fixed ideas—the feeling that something is alive inside is one of these ideas; another is that someone is following him, that there is someone at his side. The patient turns but finds no one there, and yet he does not give up this idea. He will walk around and around in a circle in his room. He will also feel that his body or his blood is toxic, that it has been poisoned and there is nothing he can do about it.

The Thuja patient is very depressed. He may even be suicidal. He will cry easily, especially from hearing music.

Aggravations: There will be aggravation at night and in the afternoon— at 3 A.M. and 3 P.M. There will be aggravation also from damp, especially from cold, damp air.

Thuja patients are also aggravated if they breathe in too deeply. They also feel worse from talking.

They do not handle drugs well and their entire system will be aggravated from drugs of any sort as well as from alcohol. Thuja tends to crave both, but both are highly toxic to the system and will especially aggravate the Thuja's emotional symptoms.

Ameliorations: Thuja patients will feel better if they can lie down on their back, or on the painful side of the body.

They want to be covered or dressed warmly. They are better when they are warm.

Dosage and Potency: Thuja is known for its rather wild aggravations, which can be very long-lasting. Therefore, it is always wise to start with a low potency whenever there is any doubt. It is commonly begun in a 12C potency, which is a good potency for the home kit. While it may be repeated in lower potencies, it is given in a single dose in potencies over 30C.

Relationships: Thuja is an excellent follow-up remedy for cases that have been opened by Sulphur. It completes Sulphur's healing action.

It is also complementary to the remedies Arsenicum and Silicea.

Thuja is antidoted by Camphora.

57. URTICA URENS

Remedy Source: Vegetable Remedy. Urtica Urens is created from the stinging nettle, a plant native to northern Europe. The stinging nettle and the related common nettle have both been considered medicinal herbs and are both ingested and brewed into teas. They are used as herbal treatments for inflammatory diseases of all sorts, particularly whooping cough.

Urtica Urens was popularized as a homeopathic remedy through the work of Burnett.

Situations That Suggest Urtica: Burns, scalds, and fevers; sore throat; whooping cough; rheumatism; kidney stones; puncture wounds: insect bites and stings; chicken pox; worms.

Remedy Portrait: Urtica Urens is a small remedy but an important one for patients with burns, scalds, or fevers; also for patients with sunburns. Also consider this remedy for cases of frostbite that follow the general picture of the remedy, for cases in which the patient's skin takes on a purple/red color from exposure to cold, damp air, especially when the patient's hands or feet become purple, swollen, and take on stinging pains from the exposure to cold and especially when that exposure is to snow. There will be both burning and stinging pains in the exposed area.

In cases of burns and scalds, the patient will complain of an intense burning of the skin that is accompanied by itching. Think of this remedy in cases of first-degree burns. In that the remedy is taken from the "stinging nettle," look for the patient to complain of a stinging sensation in the skin. The affected area of the skin will be made worse by bathing, and especially worse by applications of cold water. Look for the skin to have raised red patches that are very painful. The burning sensation, however, will be only felt in the patient's skin—it will not be felt internally, as it will with Sulphur. Consider this remedy also for hives and for chicken pox, in which the skin both burns and itches. Also think of Uritca for conditions such as prickly heat, especially for rashes that return at the same time every year. (The treatment of the rash associated with Urica Urens is very important. If the rash is suppressed—treated by allopathic means—the patient may take on chronic digestive disorders, especially chronic diarrhea. The patient may also vomit from the suppression of skin conditions of any sort.) Urica is a rheumatic remedy. It should be considered for states that alternate rheumatic pain with burning and itching of the skin.

The rheumatic pains common to the type will center in the patient's arms, especially in the right arm. The patient will complain of constant pain in the area of the deltoid muscle. He will not be able to rotate his arm inward. He will not be able to put on a coat. He will report that his whole right arm feels bruised.

The patient will also have ankle pain—pain in both ankles that is accompanied by swelling and redness. The patient will also suffer from pains in the hands. The patient's fingers will be red, sore, and swollen. Both the ankles and the hands may be covered by raised red patches that itch and burn.

In cases of fever, look for the Urtica Urens patient to experience heat in the body that is accompanied by soreness in the abdomen. The patient may have swelling in the region of the abdomen as well. Night sweats will accompany fever, as will vertigo. There will be a fever with a general sensation of heat and soreness—a bruised feeling—all over the patient's body.

The patient may have diarrhea, especially chronic diarrhea that contains a great deal of mucus. The mucus will resemble bits of boiled egg white. The stool itself will be green-colored. The patient will experience a great deal of itching and burning in the anus. He will usually feel dissatisfied by his stool, as if there is still more matter to be removed from the system. Along with Cina, Urtica Urens should be considered a remedy for those with worms. It is specific to infestations of pinworms.

This is also a remedy for the patient with hemorrhoids. The patient will complain of burning and itching in the anus. The anus will also feel raw after the patient passes a stool.

The Urtica Urens patient may also have vertigo, especially vertigo that is associated with headache and a general tenderness and swelling in the area of the liver and the spleen.

Urtica Urens is also considered a solid remedy for those with whooping cough. The patient will pass a frothy expectoration. It is for cases of whooping cough in which there is only a small amount of expectoration. Look for the patient to say that the left side of his chest is very sore, constantly sore and tender, that it feels bruised, as if he had been struck on the left side of the chest. The right side of the chest will hurt only from time to time, usually after the patient has been coughing. (Women needing this remedy will often complain of pain in the breast. The pain will be ongoing in the left breast, sporadic in the right breast.) The patient may cough up blood.

This bruised feeling is common to the remedy. The patient may also complain that his eyeballs feel bruised, that he feels as if someone had hit him in the eye. The patient may also experience the sensation of sand in his eyes. He will feel that his eyes are sore and weak. He may have trouble reading, or will feel that reading makes his eye pain worse. The patient will get drowsy when he reads.

This eye pain may extend into headache. Urtica Urens patients will feel headaches that begin in their eyes and extend upward, or they will feel headache pains over their eyes. The pain will be dull and aching. Look for the headache pain to be accompanied by swelling and pain in the region of the liver and the spleen.

Like Calendula and Hypericum, Urtica is used both internally and externally. In external uses—for burns, scalds, sunburns, and the like—Urtica Urens works best if used as Aqua Urtica Urens, created by dissolving the pellets of appropriate potency in pure water and then applying this water to the affected parts of the body. The remedy may be taken orally and used topically at the same time.

For the patient with a burn, look for him to be worse after sleep, and, again, much worse from the application of water to the area of the burn.

Keynotes: Look for the patient to feel as if there is sand in his eyes, as if he had received a blow to the eye.

Look for the muscles of the right arm specifically to feel bruised. The feeling in this arm will be burning in nature. This burning sensation is most common to all the pains in this remedy. Pains will also be characterized as stinging, itching, and sore.

Aggravations: The patient will feel worse from cold air, especially from cold, moist air. He will feel worse from bathing in cool water and worse from cold applications.

The patient feels worse when he is touched, and worse when lying on his arm.

The patient will be made worse by any exertion, by any strong motion.

The sensations of burning will be aggravated by sleep.

Ameliorations: The patient's condition is improved by rest, improved by lying down.

Dosage and Potency: The potency 30C is the most often used. The remedy bears repetition well and may be repeated as needed.

Relationships: Like most remedies that involve physical trauma, Urtica is commonly used either before or after Arnica.

58. VALERIANA

Remedy Source: Vegetable Remedy. The remedy is taken from *Valeriana officinalis,* which is a small bush that grows two to four feet high. It belongs to the Natural Order of Valerianaceae. The plant is native to Europe, where it grows by the banks of streams and rivers.

The plant is known for its slender roots, which look like fingers. The remedy is taken from the roots of the valeriana.

This is a remedy created by Hahnemann.

Situations That Suggest Valeriana: Hysteria, nervous collapse. Also insomnia, toothache, headache. Also sciatica. Also menopause.

Remedy Portrait: This is an excellent little remedy to have on hand in the home kit for moments of nervous excitement or an anxiety attack. It will calm the most intense patient. The remedy Valeriana is taken from the same source as the allopathic drug Valium and has much the same action in the human system, without the suppression and the emotional addiction of the allopathic drug.

Valeriana is similar to Ignatia in much of its emotional character. Look for the patient to be very changeable in mood. He will plunge from the highest peaks of joy to the darkest depths of sorrow or anger in seconds and you will not know why or what you did to cause such a change.

Often a feeling of lightness, of floating, will accompany the patient's change of moods. Often a physical pain—commonly, earache—will also accompany mood swings. The patient will be made very nervous by noises. He wants quiet. And he may actually even have auditory illusions. He will insist that he has heard the phone ring, or the doorbell, or some other kind of ringing sound.

In the same way, Valeriana commonly will see things that are not there. He will see animals or people in his room at night. (Illusions will usually happen only at night.) Or he will see sparks of light in front of his eyes.

Along with the mood swings, with the wild emotions, expect the patient to exhibit emotional flatulence. Valeriana types become very gassy when anxious or angry. They will also likely experience nerve pain. Pains will travel very quickly throughout their body. They will move and change as swiftly as the emotions.

An important keynote of the type is that the Valeriana type will have a pain in the heel. This pain will tend to occur when the patient is sitting. It, like all the type's sciatic pains, will be made worse by rest and made better by walking. Valeriana types want to keep walking—this not only helps their physical pains, but it drains them of their emotional energy and helps them to calm down. Thus, they will pace; they will walk the floor long into the night.

For the patient who is in hysterics, and who seems incapable of giving you any solid answers to help you with a drug diagnosis, Valeriana and Rescue Remedy will usually be your best bets for acute treatment.

Keynotes: The pain in the heel is keynote to the type. No other remedy of this hysterical sort has such a pain, or has a pain that is improved by walking. The pain is usually in the right heel, but it may also appear in the left.

The other important keynote is a sensation. The patient will have a sensation of a string hanging down the throat. This can cause choking, especially when the patient is falling asleep. The patient will report severe nausea in association with this keynote symptom.

Aggravations: The patient will be made worse, by sitting or resting in general.

Expect the patient to be worse, especially emotionally, at night.

The patient will be made worse by any excitement, or by any sudden sight or sound. Things need to be very quiet and calm around him.

Ameliorations: The patient is better when walking, when moving freely.

The patient is better when painful parts are rubbed.

Dosage and Potency: Keep it on hand in the 200C potency. It is a very short-acting remedy. It may be repeated as needed.

Relationships: Valeriana will be a good stopgap remedy, but it will usually not be curative in and of itself. Both Pulsatilla and Phosphorus follow the remedy very well and complete its action.

Valeriana is antidoted by Camphora.

59. VERATRUM ALBUM

Remedy Source: Vegetable Remedy. The remedy was created from the white hellebore, of the Natural Order of Melanthacae. It is native to Europe, and is especially found in the Alps. It is a small plant with white flowers. The plant is picked just before flowering.

The remedy was created by Hahnemann.

Situations That Suggest Veratrum: Coughs, colds, bronchitis, fevers, whooping cough. Also digestive troubles: constipation and diarrhea, colic. Also acute asthma. Also sunstroke. Also recovery from childbirth.

Remedy Portrait: This remedy will mirror Arsenicum Album in nearly every use; in fact, it is the vegetable-based remedy that is the equal of Arsenicum's mineral base.

Therefore, we are going to think of Veratrum in cases in which the patient's condition includes exhaustion, chill, and fever; also severe flus and food poisonings; also cases of unchecked diarrhea.

The Veratrum patient is manic. He looks to the future, as do Arsenicums, and is looking ahead to a bleak future. In cases of Veratrum mental disorders, these are the patients who take to the streets with a milk crate to stand on and a sign that says that the end is near. In their manic state, they are quite certain that something terrible is just about to happen.

Veratrum patients will talk a lot. They will talk loudly. Consider this remedy for patients who rave and have fever, and who are generally quite melancholy in their behavior. They are depressed, and they show it. They want to tear things, destroy things. They will pray out loud. And they will curse you as their caregiver. They may also sing to themselves or whistle or laugh for no reason.

Like Arsenicum, these patients will likely be in a state of collapse. They are very cold. Even their breath will feel cold. The tip of the nose will also be very cold. Their skin will take on a blue tinge, especially about the lips. Look for a cold sweat on the forehead. And look for vomiting.

This is a major remedy for vomiting. The vomit will be profuse. There will be violent retching accompanying the vomiting. Even when there is nothing left to vomit, the patient will continue to retch.

The patient will faint. This is one of our best remedies for those who faint. Look again for that cold sweat on the forehead. Look for the patient to faint from the slightest exertion, or from the terrible ordeal of vomiting or diarrhea. They will also faint at the sight of their own blood.

Given all this, it may seem odd that Veratrum patients should be very hungry, and yet they usually are. They will crave ice water (which, as with Phosphorus, they will tend to throw up as soon as it becomes warmed in their stomach). They will want cold drinks and sour drinks. They want juice. They will especially seem to want lemonade. This is one way to tell them apart quickly from Arsenicum. Although both remedies love lemons, Arsenicum will want hot drinks, especially hot tea with lemon, while Veratrum wants cold drinks, especially ice cold lemonade, even though it disagrees with their system. Also, Veratrum will drink a great deal of the lemonade very quickly, while Arsenicum will slowly sip their tea.

Veratrum patients will also tend to want milk and milk products, which do better in their system than does lemonade and fruit juice. They will also want meat, which they digest well. Veratrum patients may also want potatoes, but these disagree with their systems.

Veratrum patients will also experience a good many aches and pains. Often they will suffer rheumatic and sciatic pains. The pains will strike quickly and will have a lightning–like quality. Veratrum patients will often have sudden cramps in their calves that accompany diarrhea. Look for Veratrum patients to have trouble walking. They tend to feel as if heavy weights are attached to their legs and feet. Look for them to have feet that are icy cold.

Keynotes: The total picture of coldness is keynote: cold feet, nose, and hands; even the patient's breath is cold. The Veratrum patient yearns for warmth.

Also keynote is the patient's manic behavior, his high verbal skills, and his abusive language. Top it off with the notion that the end of the world (if only his own specific world) is near.

Aggravations: Veratrum patients will be worse from any contact with cold, damp air. They are worse during foggy weather, during cloudy weather, and during any change in the weather.

They are worse from even the slightest motion.

They are worse while passing a stool, and while sweating.

The Veratrum patient is worse from eating, especially from eating fruits, fatty foods, cabbage, peas, and potatoes; also from drinking beer and tea.

Ameliorations: Veratrum patients are better when lying down, when walking about slowly, and when they are covered up and warm.

They are better from eating warm foods.

Dosage and Potency: This remedy is most commonly used in 30C potency. For cases involving emotional distress, use 200C. It may be repeated as needed.

One dose will hold for three weeks.

Relationships: Arnica is the most complementary remedy. Veratrum follows Arnica well in clearing up the ill effects of physical trauma.

It also follows Arsenicum well and completes its action.

Other complementary remedies include Carbo Veg and Ipecac.

Veratrum is antidoted by Arsenicum and by Camphora.

60. RESCUE REMEDY

Remedy Source: Vegetable Remedy. Rescue Remedy is not a classical homeopathic remedy, or one that follows Hahnemann's methods of creation or use. Rescue Remedy is the creation of Edward Bach, who, after a lifetime as first an allopathic and then a homeopathic physician, established his own method of treatment with the Bach flower remedies.

Rescue Remedy is a combination of five of Bach's floral essences. It is made up of: star of Bethlehem, which is included to work with shock, either physical or emotional, and to keep that shock from moving deeper into the patient's system; rock rose, for panic and trauma; impatiens, for intense emotions and inner tension; cherry plum, for fear, most especially for fear of losing one's self and losing control; and clematis, again for shock, which creates in the patient a dream state in which he is not totally awake and aware of what is happening to him. Clematis is particularly good if the patient has the tendency to lose consciousness.

Remedy Portrait: The patient who needs Rescue Remedy is one who has received a trauma of either a physical or emotional nature. Thus the person who has been mugged, the person who has been in an accident or a near miss, and the person who has just lost his job all need Rescue.

The remedy is created in combination, which by all standards would make it other than a classical homeopathic remedy. But Bach's floral essences, while created from mother tinctures just like Hahnemann's remedies, are used by a philosophy that is very different from Hahnemann's. Bach's remedies are given on the basis of mood, on the emotional state of the patient, with little or no interest taken in the physical condition. So we will look at our patient and decide whether or not he seems to be in shock, whether or not in our estimation he is in need of rescue. If he is, give him Rescue Remedy.

Rescue Remedy is also wonderful to use to prevent illness if we know that we are going into a stressful situation. Therefore, if we know that we are going to have to give a speech in front of a large audience, or if we are going to have to take an important test, or if we are going to have to take a stressful subway ride we may want to take Rescue Remedy in advance to help us face the situation. It is also excellent when give before, during, and after visits to the doctor or dentist. It is excellent for people who suffer panic attacks or any sort of emotional trauma. It is wonderful for patients who become speechless from panic or who tremble from it.

Also, in that the remedy is given based only on emotional need, it is an excellent remedy for our pets—for the dog who is afraid of thunderstorms, or the cat with separation anxiety. A little Rescue Remedy in the animal's drinking water can have wonderful results.

Keynotes: Look for the patient to be a bit glassy-eyed, or to have a frantic look on his face. Look for trembling; look for the patient to be speechless, have dry mouth, or speak without making sense.

Aggravations and Ameliorations: In that Bach's remedies are used in a method different from Hahnemann's, there are no set aggravations or ameliorations, although, typically, the patient will be better for getting rest, having quiet, and being touched gently.

Dosage and Potency: The potency of Rescue Remedy is set by the mixture itself in the concentrate's bottle. It is created in liquid form, in an alcohol base.

To use the remedy, you may simply put a couple drops of the concentrate under the patient's tongue, or, more effectively, you may take four or five drops of the concentrate and put it in some water. The patient should sit quietly and sip the water.

If the patient is unconscious, the Rescue Remedy may be placed on his lips, or may be placed on the pressure points on the wrists and the wrists rubbed together. Persons who do not wish to use an alcohol-based remedy may use the remedy topically in the same manner.

Rescue Remedy is also available in a salve. The topical preparation is wonderful for any physical injury, from cuts and scrapes to puncture wounds and other forms of torn tissue. The salve is very soothing and may be used on broken or unbroken skin. It can also be used to speed the healing of rashes, acne, and other skin conditions.

Rescue Remedy, like all other Bach remedies, may be used as needed. You cannot use the remedy too often. It may also be placed in food or drink of any sort in order to provide help.

The patient who takes Rescue Remedy will not feel drugged. He will not feel separated from himself, and he will not be put to sleep. Quite the opposite, actually. The patient who takes Rescue Remedy will be brought totally back into his body and will become more alert and more able to handle the situation at hand. No harm can ever be created by taking Rescue Remedy.

Relationship: Rescue Remedy is made up of very low-potency floral essences, most of which are little more than mother tinctures. And yet, they must in their preparation be considered to be homeopathic remedies. Therefore they must be used carefully in combination with other remedies.

Bach remedies in general do not blend well with Hahnemann's. This is because they are too similar in their actions and will therefore interfere with each other. Therefore, in acute situations especially, one must decide early on which sort of remedy one thinks will be of the most help, Hahnemann's or Bach's. In other words, Rescue Remedy will not combine well with Arnica or any other acute homeopathic remedy. In fact, you may do more harm than good by combining these therapies.

Beginning students of homeopathy especially would do very well to make use of Rescue Remedy, both internally and externally. Not only is it easier to select when one is just learning the homeopathic pharmacy, but it is a surprisingly effective remedy. Many cases have been brought to a very successful conclusion just by the use of Rescue Remedy. And many people who will not take Hahnemann's more dynamic remedies will happily take Bach's gentle and loving preparations.

Section III

Appendices

On Taking the Acute Case

On Potency and Doses

On Diet During Treatment

On Caring for the Remedies

On Antidoting Specific
Remedies

Suggested Repertories and
Materia Medicas

A Brief Glossary of
Homeopathic Terms

On Taking the Acute Case

Case Taking: A Structure

The problem that many of us have in selecting the appropriate remedy in an acute situation is that we fail to behave in a homeopathic manner. Whether the case is acute or chronic, it is taken in basically the same manner.

We need to find out how the patient has shifted in his move from health to illness. We need not only an understanding of the physical symptoms of that illness but also a feel for how the person shifted emotionally. Remember, homeopathy involves wholeness, and the remedy that speaks to the whole person—in an acute or a chronic situation—is the remedy that will have the most impact upon that person's health.

So the first thing we need do is to list the symptoms as the person is experiencing them. And we need then to find out the same information about each of the symptoms. Say the person has a sore throat, a headache, and a runny nose. We are going to go after the same information about each.

Sensation. How does it hurt? Is the pain burning in character, or throbbing? What is the specific nature of the discomfort? Try not to put words in the patient's mouth. Just ask the patient the question and record the answer.

Location. Where does it hurt? And please be specific. A headache is almost bound to involve the head. But where in the head? In what specific spot did the pain begin? Has the pain traveled? If so, where did it move and when did it move there? As you likely know by now, some remedies are specific to parts or sides of the body. If we know the specific location of the symptom, it will rule out some remedies and suggest others.

Duration. When did the pain begin? How long has this been going on? I also like at this point to try to find out if the patient has had anything like this before. Is there a pattern to this symptom? Does the patient get it every week, every month, every spring? When the pain comes on, how long does it last?

Modalities. What makes the pain feel better? What makes it feel worse? And what makes the person as a whole feel better or worse? Is there a position in which the patient's body is most comfortable? Is there a best and/or worst time of day for the symptoms and for the person as a whole? Is the patient thirsty? For what? Is he hungry? For what? Does he want to be alone, or does he want to be with people? These are all the modalities of the case and they will often be most useful in helping you locate the correct remedy.

Also, it is important to find out what else the patient already has done for his illness, what other homeopathic, herbal, or allopathic remedies that he already might have tried. And find out if he is under constitutional treatment, because unless the acute condition is particularly difficult, or even threatening, it is best to just stay with the constitutional treatment rather than to go on to an acute remedy. (*Note*: Sometimes an acute illness, particularly a cold, can be the action of a constitutional remedy as it begins to open up a case. In a situation such as this, it is important not to treat the cold, but to let it carry on through its natural healing process.)

In a chronic/constitutional situation, a case taking can take over an hour and the research that follows can take a full day. In an acute situation, however, it is generally not necessary to go as deeply into either the medical history or the homeopathic repertorization of the case. So, while the case is still being correctly taken, a remedy can be selected with some assurance in just minutes. The more time that you spend in learning the remedies themselves—materia medica study—and in learning how to repertorize a case, the more effective you will become in selecting remedies.

Some situations are, of course, easier than others. A skinned knee is easier to treat than is a cold. And a cold is easier than a headache. But remember to try to resist the temptation to treat the illness. Many of us start out our lives in homeopathy thinking that if a bruise occurs, then the remedy is Arnica. Arnica is the remedy for bruises. Hopefully, after reading this guide, you are now aware that there are several remedies for bruises, not just Arnica. And yet, truthfully, there are only several remedies for bruises. And the fact of the bruise allows you to rule out many dozens of remedies. So while we are treating the person with the bruise and not the bruise itself, in an acute situation the actual illness does play a far more important role than it does in a constitutional situation. We are more concerned with the physical in acute situations, and while this is not homeopathy at its best and finest, it is a true and competent practice of homeopathy.

So, to sum up, learn the remedies. There is no getting around this and that is why I keep repeating the sentence. Remember that until Kent came up with the concept of a repertory, practitioners had to learn their materia medica. They had to recognize the needed remedy because there was nowhere to go to get help.

Today, we have numerous guides like this one. We even have computer software. But these tools can do nothing but give you a few suggestions for a given situation. In reality, if you cannot recognize Belladonna and tell the difference between it and Ferrum Phos, then no matter how many books you have, you will be stuck when you face the choice between the two. So learn the remedies.

Case Taking: A Format

Many practitioners of homeopathy begin case taking with a form to be filled out as the patient is speaking. This form, when well completed, will aid in your ability to organize the patient's words for your own repertorization process. Whether the case involves acute or chronic illness, the form printed on the pages following will allow you to place the information received in a manner by which it can most easily be repertorized.

Included here are two different forms of my own creation that I have found to be helpful in acute situations.

First, there is the Patient Form, which speaks to the general symptoms of the patient when looked on as a whole, what makes the patient feel better, what makes him feel worse, his cravings and aversions, etc.

Second is the Symptom Form, which takes a detailed look at one specific symptom and its connection to any other symptoms that the patient might also be experiencing.

Together, these forms give a complete look at a case. While only one Patient Form would be needed, expect to use three, four, or more Symptom Forms for the sake of complete information.

Patient Form

Name:

Age: *Date:*

OBJECTIVE INFORMATION:
Initial Observations:

Diagnostics:

    Tongue:

    Pulse:

    Countenance:

    Body:

SUBJECTIVE INFORMATION:
Generalities:

1. What symptom(s) of illness are you presently experiencing?

2. Is there one symptom that troubles you more than the others?

3. Other than specific aches and pains, what else has changed since the onset of the illness?

General Modalities:

4. Is there a time of day when you feel best or have the most energy? Is there a worst time of day?

5. As a whole being, is there anything that makes you feel better? That makes you feel worse?

6. How is your appetite? Is there anything you crave? Anything that you can't stand right now?

7. How thirsty are you? For what are you thirsty?

8. How has your sleep changed during this illness?

9. How do you feel about company? Do you want to be alone or be taken care of?

10. What has your mood been like during this illness?

PHYSICIAN RESPONSE:

Drug Diagnosis:

Differential Diagnosis:

Disease Diagnosis (if any):

Potency of Remedy Used:

Dosage of Remedy Used:

Patient's Response to Remedy:

Case Closure:

Notes:

Symptom Form

Name: Date:

Symptom discussed on this form:

Duration:

1. When did the symptom first appear?

2. What were the circumstances that surrounded the onset of this symptom?

Location:

3. What is the location of the symptom (where does it hurt)?

4. How has the location changed or shifted since the onset of the symptom?

Sensation:

5. How does the symptom feel to you?

6. What is the quality of the pain associated with the symptom?

7. How has the sensation of pain changed or shifted since onset?

Modalities:

8. What makes the symptom feel better? Feel worse?

9. At what time of day is the symptom at its worst? At its best?

Concomitants:

10. Are there any other symptoms that link to this one? Other aches and pains that alternate with this one?

Treatments:

11. What other forms of treatment or medicine have you already used in treating this symptom?

12. Are you presently taking any form of medicine on a regular basis for any other illness? Are you under any type of treatment for any other illness?

Notes and Observations:

On Potency and Doses

B Y NOW, I HOPE you have noticed one thing—that the same few remedies are used over and over again homeopathically for a great number of ailments. That and the fact that whatever illness a remedy is being used for, the keynote attributes of that remedy will carry over. Bryonia will never want to move. And Nux Vomica will always be irritable.

So, to know how to treat acutely, you must first know how to treat constitutionally—that is, you must know the remedies not as a collection of symptoms but rather as persons, some angry and some sad, some restless and some exhausted. If you can spend the time with the materia medica to learn the sixty remedies listed early on in this text, you will have the ability to help out many persons who are acting out the symptoms of the remedies in their own lives.

Potency

Now, just a word about potency. I have largely ignored the whole thing up to now because there are so many who swear by low potencies and so many who will only use high ones and therefore someone will get angry no matter what I write. So I can only say that both work—low potencies, high potencies. Like anything else, they must match the illness. If the person is very ill but the vital force is still strong, use a high potency. It will work better and faster. But if the illness is slight, or if the person is very weak, you should go low. All in all, it's always safer to start low and move up. This adheres to Kent's methods of working, in which he started with the lowest potencies and moved upward. In this way, he was able to stoke the vital force of the patient gradually, without upsetting that vital force and causing severe aggravations. Some people work by aggravations; me, I avoid them.

Often, however, you are forced to use whatever is on hand. Therefore, I always suggest that you have both a high and a low potency of important remedies on hand at all times—say a 30C and a 1M. Then you are covered. Most kits that you can buy today are available in 30C, and this is a good basic potency. In fact, for acute care, you can pretty much say that when in doubt, give 30C—with the exception of the elderly (always start lower here, especially for those who do not regularly take any form of medicine) and those who are especially weak.

In constitutional care, the potency of the remedy is much more important. In acute situations, think low or high. If 6C is your only low potency, then use it. If you only have 200C, then it will have to do. Remember, when in doubt call your practitioner.

It is a good idea to invest in an acute kit for home. They are available from all homeopathic pharmacies and most good health food stores carry them as well. In buying a kit you will save about half the cost of buying remedies separately. Then all you need do is supplement your kit with higher potencies specific to your needs. If you have a baby who has not yet teethed, then getting some high-potency teething remedies is a good idea. Arnica in high potency is always a good idea in any home, as usually are Rhus Tox, Sulphur, Phosphorus, and Arsenicum. All you need to do is a bit of work in individualizing your home kit.

Doses

I often tell students that more cases are ruined by not knowing when to stop giving the remedy than by all other causes put together.

We have to judge when to give the second dose of any acutely selected remedy by two criteria: the urgency of the case and the impact of the first dose.

Homeopathic remedies are always given as needed. If one dose clears the case—if the patient's overall energy improves and the symptoms of illness fall away—then by all means do not give a second dose. If the first dose seems to help some, then watch for a return of symptoms and a falling off of the overall energy, and then give a second dose.

In some emergencies, you may have to give more than one remedy or give the remedy more often than you usually would. In a situation, for instance, that combines physical trauma with shock. In this sort of case, you might give these remedies as often as every few minutes until you see a clear indication of improvement (often the patient will fall into a gentle sleep). Remember, though, in emergencies, saving the life and getting to the emergency room is of paramount importance. Hahnemann will forgive you for breaking the laws of cure.

The same holds for acute illnesses to an extent. Here, it is best to give just one remedy, but you may give a 30C every fifteen minutes for the first hour (or until you see improvement, whichever comes first) and then repeat the remedy in one or two hours. Once the remedy is "set in" and begins to work, however, please go back to the notion of "as needed."

If a remedy must be repeated often (and by this I mean more than three or four times a day), it is a clear sign that the potency needs to be higher for a cure to take place. But, if all you have is 30C and 1M, it is best to continue on that 30C for a while and not go jumping right up to 1M. Think of potency like *The Price Is Right*: you want to be the closest without going over.

But back to doses for one last moment. To conclude, homeopathic remedies are truly to be given as needed. When there is improvement in the overall condition of the patient, stop giving the remedy, whatever the remedy is, whatever the potency that was used. Do not give it again until you need to give it again. As long as the patient continues to improve, you do not need to give it. As with the microdoses of homeopathics, so, too, with the number of doses of a remedy given: in homeopathy, less indeed is more.

Finally, it is important that you know your limits. Unless you are in a situation in which money or geography keeps you from a professional's office, start small. Learn to remove the pebbles in people's shoes before you attempt to get the boulders off their backs.

And study your materia medica and your repertory. The more you learn about the remedies themselves, the less often you will have to open any guide. The more you learn about yourself and the people you love, the less you will have to seek outside guidance. Learn to think and live with the philosophy of healing and the philosophy of homeopathy. And also learn the practical basics of the appropriate uses of the homeopathic remedies in acute situations.

On Diet During Treatment

MOST OF US WISH that there were just one diet, one range of foods that are nourishing to us all. But while there are some things that we can be sure should not be included in any diet—cigarettes, for example—most substances can differ greatly in their impact upon the individual system.

Take alcohol, for instance. Some of us feel much better if we have a glass of wine with dinner; others just get a headache. And much has been made of coffee, especially when it comes to homeopathic treatment. The truth is that some of us can tolerate coffee much better than others. And while it is true that some of us can antidote our homeopathic treatment by drinking a cup of coffee, it is also true that others can drink cup after cup without any mishap. In fact, many millions could take their remedy dissolved in a cup of coffee and still get its full impact.

A good rule of thumb is this: the foods, chemicals, and what-have-you to which you are very sensitive or to which you know you are allergic should be avoided during treatment. Therefore, the person who will be strung out and awake for two days if he has a single cup of coffee should certainly avoid coffee during treatment. But the person who is already drinking coffee every morning has a system that is already infused with caffeine and will have no interference with his remedy.

So the more you can eat and drink what you like without becoming ill, the more you will be able to eat and drink during treatment. The more careful you be about what you eat, the more careful you should be during treatment.

Hahnemann and Diet

In aphorism #263 of *The Organon,* Hahnemann writes that "the cravings of the acutely ill patient with regard to edible delectables and drinks is, for the most part, for things that give palliative relief." In other words, the patient who is acutely ill should usually be trusted to desire the things that will help his condition. The patient who wants cold water for a sore throat should be given the cold water.

Hahnemann continues, "These are not, however, actually of a medicinal nature and they are only appropriate for the current need. The slight obstacles which this gratification, held within moderate bounds, could perhaps put in the way of the thorough removal of the disease are amply made up for—indeed outweighed—by the power of the homeopathically fitting medicine and the life principle unleashed by it, and by the refreshment afforded the patient through the gratification of his cravings."

This is an important statement for our consideration if we are to enact the role of the physician. The patient may want ice cream, something that he usually does not eat. He may, for instance, never have dairy, or never have sugar, but here he wants ice cream and he wants it badly. Hahnemann tells us two things. First, he says that the cravings will be palliative. They will help the patient with the pain of his condition, but they are not truly medicinal. While the cravings will be a catalyst to a short-term relief, they will not be a strong enough catalyst to be considered medicines. Therefore, they will not represent an obstacle to the patient's natural ability to heal.

Second, these weak catalysts will not in any way interfere with the power of the remedies. You can give them along with the remedies without fear of obstacle to the homeopathic cure.

Therefore, Hahnemann is telling us that the acute patient needs to be trusted and needs to be coddled a bit. Give him the treat that will lighten his heart and lessen his pain.

Now, when it comes to the patient who is chronically ill, the opposite applies. This is the patient who will usually crave exactly the wrong thing, who will want foods and drinks that will work against his progress.

About the diet of the chronically ill Hahnemann writes in the lengthy footnote to aphorism #260:

Patients with chronic diseases should avoid the following: Coffee; fine Chinese tea and other herb teas; beers adulterated with medicinal vegetable substances not suitable for the state of the patient; so-called fine liqueurs prepared with medicinal spices; all kinds of punch; spiced chocolate; many kinds of colognes and perfumes; strongly scented flowers in the room; medicinally compounded tooth powders and tooth spirits (mouthwashes); perfumed sachets; highly seasoned foods and sauces; spiced cakes and frozen goods (ices and ice creams) prepared with medicinal matters (e.g. coffee, vanilla, etc.); raw medicinal herbs on soups; vegetable dishes with herbs, roots or sprouting stalks (such as asparagus with long green tips); hop sprouts and all vegetables possessing powers (celery, parsley, sorrel, tarragon, all kinds of onions, etc.); old cheeses and meats which are putrid; foods which have medicinal side effects (e.g. the meat and fat of pigs, ducks and geese; all-too-young veal; sour foods; all kinds of salads).

Hahnemann also warns here of the overuse of salt and sugar, and of living in rooms that are overheated. He also warns that the chronically ill patient who makes only "passive movement (through riding, driving, swinging)" only encourages his ailment. Hahnemann encourages exercise and fresh air whenever possible.

As can be seen, the environment was as important to Hahnemann as was the diet. The chronically ill patient must especially avoid overwhelming smells, but he must avoid as well any other aspects or his diet or lifestyle that undermine his vital force.

Even in the case of the patient who is acutely ill, Hahnemann considers the patient's environment. In aphorism #263, he writes: "In acute disease, the temperature of the room and the warmth or coolness of the bed coverings must be arranged entirely according to the wishes of the patient." As with the environment, therefore, we are, as with diet, to trust the patient who is acutely ill. He will be drawn to physical sensations that will assist in his cure. Therefore, the patient who wants to lie still should lie still. And the patient who want to be moving should be allowed to move. In a like manner, the patient who wants the window open must have the window open. And the patient who wants the flowers removed from the room should have them removed.

Homeopaths and Diet

Below, I have put together a diet based on the work of Johnson in his classic home guide. It is included here for those who want a specific and rather complete outline of foods allowable for those under homeopathic treatment. Given all that is included above, this is obviously a diet set up more for the patient who is chronically ill than for the one with acute illness. It is strict, but it does give a good outline to follow.

So don't panic when you read the lists below. Just try to keep in mind that Hahnemann, when he treated people, tried to get them to live as healthfully as possible during treatment. He wanted them to eat very simply, with as few spices and medicine substances in their diet as possible. And, further, he wanted them, even if they were quite ill, to get as much exercise and fresh air as possible. He did not believe that people should take to their beds for very long, but felt that you had to do what you could to recover from your illness. Therefore, if the only motion you could make toward exercise was to wiggle your toe, he fully expected to see that toe wiggling.

So give consideration to the diet as outlined below. It comes from several of our homeopathic giants: Pulte, Boericke, and Johnson among them. They have good advice to give. But my advice is simpler: keep the foods simple and easily digested. Avoid complex foods while under homeopathic treatment. That will make the recovery simpler and faster and you can get back to your rich French sauces before you know it.

Articles of Diet Allowed During Homeopathic Treatment

In his 1882 *Homeopathic Family Guide,* I. D. Johnson gives the following structure for a diet while under homeopathic treatment. While I am not nearly as strict as he is on the subject, I still find it a helpful format to follow.

DRINK—Pure fresh water is preferable to all other drinks. Weak black tea is fine in most cases. Avoid milk and all other dairy. Avoid coffee. Avoid herbal teas unless you are sure that the herbs included in the mix are not medicinal and will not interfere with treatment.

FRUIT—All kinds of ripe fruits not of an acid quality, such as apples, pears, peaches, plums, grapes, raspberries, strawberries, blackberries, sweet cherries, sweet oranges, melons, and cantaloupes are fine as long as you are sure that they will not disagree with the patient's digestion.

VEGETABLES—Peas, beans, lima beans, asparagus, squashes, carrots, and broccoli are fine for most patients. Other vegetables, like the night-shades—tomatoes, bell peppers, and eggplant—often will disagree, as will cabbage and Brussels sprouts.

BREAD—Bread made of rye flour is preferable. Wheat can often cause problems, as can other grains. Breads made from rice flour are usually well digested. In fact, rice is the grain that will cause the least digestive upset in most patients.

MEATS—Tender lean beef, chicken, and turkey are usually fine for patients who eat meat, although in acute or inflammatory diseases, animal proteins are seldom a good idea.

FISH—Fresh fish, such as perch, rock, sea bass, mackerel, shad, and small creek fish, are fine, as are tuna steak and salmon. Avoid shellfish of any sort.

The meals should be taken at regular intervals, the food well masticated, and not eaten hurriedly. Long fasting or eating between meals should be scrupulously avoided. Do not take food very hot or cold, not when greatly exhausted.

Articles of Diet Forbidden During Homeopathic Treatment

The following articles of diet should be avoided while under homeopathic treatment, not only on account of the injurious effect which they have upon the system, but because they antidote the effects of the medicine.

DRINKS—All alcoholic and fermented beverages, coffee, green tea, herb teas, and all natural and artificial mineral waters should be avoided.

FRUITS—Pineapples, cranberries, and all kinds of nuts and fruits not mentioned on the allowed list.

VEGETABLES—Salads, pickles, spices, parsley, celery, radishes, horse-radish, onions, all kinds of peppers, catsup, mustard, nutmeg, and ginger should all be avoided.

BREAD—You should avoid cakes prepared with much fat or with aromatics, pastry, pies, honey, and all kinds of confectionery; also baked goods that have icing or contain a good deal of sugar.

MEATS—Liver should be avoided. Completely avoid pork and all pork products; also dairy products, especially cheese and butter. Ice cream should be avoided, and fruit ices substituted.

FISH—All shellfish should be avoided.

All perfumes, minted toothpaste, and other cosmetics should be dispensed with during treatment. As it is important to keep your diet as simple as possible, it is also important to keep your environment as simple as possible. Therefore, avoid all chemical cleaners and all room sprays and other aromatics. Keep the sick room as well ventilated as the patient's condition will allow and keep the patient warm and comfortable.

On Caring for
the Remedies

GAIN, PEOPLE WHO ARE COMING into homeopathy today are always upset to read that, for generations, practitioners insisted that homeopathic remedies should be stored only in amber glass tubes with cork tops and that those tubes should themselves be stored in wooden boxes constructed especially for that purpose. And, while it is true that remedies stored in plastic tubes will not retain their potency as well as those stored in glass, the plastic-stored remedies will still stay potent for years longer than their supposed expiration date (as listed by law on the bottle).

But we still have to store the remedies well if we are to be able to count on them in times of need. They should be well out of bright sun, and away from extremes of temperature. Therefore, they should never be left in the glove compartment of the car for very long.

They do best if stored in a box of some sort, either on the shelf in the closet or under the bed, unless you have mothballs in that closet or under the bed, as strong scents, like that of mothballs (highly toxic to you as well as to the remedies), will totally destroy the potency of your remedies. Again, the following was adapted from the work of the master homeopaths of the last century, especially I. D. Johnson in his *Homeopathic Family Guide*. But their advice is as good today as when they gave it.

Directions for Preserving the Purity of Homeopathic Medicines

1. The medicines should be kept in tightly sealed vials, especially in glass vials with cork tops that will best preserve the remedies in potency. It is also a good idea that if you are going to store a large number of remedies, and especially if you have children in the home, you keep them in a wooden chest constructed for the purpose, with a lock and key to keep it safe from tiny hands. The remedies are best preserved if kept away from the sun or from any strong light.

2. Keep the chest in a dry place, not too warm, away from strong light and all strong-smelling substances, such as camphor, coffee, tobacco, etc. This is very important. It is also important that the remedies be kept away from places that are too cold as well.

3. Use one vial for one medicine. Never empty the contents of one vial into another which has had different medicines in it; do not change the corks from one bottle to another. The effect may be to change or destroy the medicine's potency.

4. Every medicine should be carefully labeled. Should you no longer be able to read the remedy name or potency, throw the vial away.

5. If you are going to dissolve the remedy in water, never prepare the solution without first being assured that the glass and spoon are perfectly clean, and, if it be necessary to prepare two at a time, have a separate spoon for each glass, and be careful to keep them apart.

6. Take the medicine from the vial by dropping the pellet into the vial's cap, onto a small piece of paper, or onto a clean silver spoon. If the dose is for you, and if your hands are totally clean, then you may drop it into your palm, but it is not the best way to take the medicine.

7. Be sure to reseal the vial just as soon as the remedy has been taken from it. Keep the vial tightly sealed.

8. If you are carrying your remedy around with you in a purse or a pocket and the lid accidentally comes off and the remedy spills, throw the pellets out. Try not to touch the pellets as you throw them away.

9. Remedies that have been dissolved in pure water should be used topically or taken internally in that form. It is never a good idea to add the liquid to other liquids or foods, as they may interfere with the remedy's actions.

10. Never give a homeopathic remedy of any sort without the patient's understanding and consent. Sometimes it is very tempting to give a remedy "for his own good," but, truly, no good can ever come from such a treatment.

On Antidoting
Specific Remedies

I N LISTING THOSE REMEDIES and substances which will likely antidote the actions of specific homeopathic remedies, I have capitalized the names of the remedies, while leaving the names of substances in lower case. But it is important to remember that the substances from which remedies are taken are likely to antidote if the remedy is listed as an antidote. Therefore, if I have listed Chamomilla as an antidote to a remedy's action, then it is very likely that chamomile is also an antidote and that the cup of chamomile tea you are taking in the evening to help you sleep is interfering with the potency of your remedy. Keep this in mind as you look over this list.

For more specific information concerning the antidoting of individual remedies, see the materia medica section of this guide. And, for those remedies listed for which no specific antidotes have been found, consider using the "general" homeopathic antidotes of either coffee or camphor. Hahnemann himself used camphor, and would rub it into the pulse points of the patient's wrists and then would have the patient breathe in the fumes in order to blunt the action of the remedy. Rescue Remedy is listed as having no remedy known; this is because Bach, the inventor of this remedy, felt that his floral essences neither had nor needed antidoting.

Remedies and Antidotes

1. Aconitum Napellus: camphor, coffee, wine, Camphora, Nux
2. Allium Cepa: Arnica, Chamomilla, Veratrum
3. Antimonium Tartaricum: Hepar Sulph, Mercurius, Pulsatilla
4. Apis Mellifica: Ipecac, Urtica Urens, Lachesis, Ledum
5. Arnica Montana: camphor, Camphora, Ignatia, Ipecac
6. Arsenicum Album: China, Hepar Sulph, Nux, Ipecac, Veratrum
7. Belladonna: coffee, Coffea, Hepar Sulph, Pulsatilla
8. Bellis Perennis: none found
9. Bryonia Alba: Aconite, Chamomilla, Ignatia, Nux, Aconite
10. Calcarea Carbonica: Camphora, Sulphur
11. Calendula Officinalis: Rheum (rhubarb)
12. Camphora: Opium
13. Carbo Vegetabilis: camphor, Arsenicum, Camphora, Lachesis
14. Causticum: coffee, Coffea, Nux
15. Chamomilla: Aconite, Coffea, Ignatia, Nux, Pulsatilla
16. China: Arnica, Arsenicum, Belladonna, Bryonia, Calcarea, Ipecac, Lachesis, Lycopodium, Nux, Pulsatilla, Sulphur
17. Cina/Cinchona: Ipecac, Veratrum
18. Cocculus: camphor, Camphora, Chamomilla, Coffea, Nux
19. Coffea Cruda: Aconite, Chamomilla, Nux
20. Colocynthis: camphor, Camphora, Coffea, Chamomilla
21. Drosera Rotundifolia: camphor, Camphora
22. Dulcamara: camphor, Camphora, Ipecac, Mercurius
23. Eupatorium Perfoliatum: none found
24. Euphrasia: camphor, Camphora, Causticum, Pulsatilla
25. Ferrum Phosphoricum: none known
26. Gelsemium: coffee, Natrum Mur, Coffea, Nux
27. Graphites: wine, Arsenicum, Nux
28. Hepar Sulphuris: camphor, vinegar, Belladonna, Camphora
29. Hypericum: Arsenicum, Chamomilla
30. Ignatia Amara: Pulsatilla, Chamomilla, Arnica, vinegar
31. Ipecacuanha/Ipecac: Arnica, Arsenicum
32. Kali Bichromicum: Arsenicum, Lachesis, Pulsatilla
33. Lachesis: Arsenicum, Belladonna, Nux, Rhus Tox
34. Ledum Palustre: camphor, Camphora, Rhus Tox
35. Lycopodium: camphor, Camphora, Pulsatilla
36. Magnesia Phosphorica: Belladonna, Gelsemium, Lachesis

37. Mercurius: camphor, iodine, Arnica, Belladonna, Camphora, Hepar Sulph
38. Natrum Muriaticum: Arsenicum, Camphora
39. Nux Vomica: Aconite, Camphora, Coffea, Pulsatilla
40. Petroleum: Aconite, Nux
41. Phosphorus: camphor, coffee, Camphora, Coffea, Nux
42. Phytolacca: coffee, Belladonna, Coffea, Ignatia
43. Podophyllum: Nux
44. Pulsatilla: coffee, Chamomilla, Coffea, Ignatia, Nux
45. Rhus Toxicodendron: camphor, coffee, Belladonna, Bryonia, Camphor, Coffea
46. Rumex Crispus: camphor, Belladonna, Camphora, Lachesis, Phosphorus
47. Ruta Graveolens: camphor, Camphora
48. Sabadilla: camphor, Camphora, Pulsatilla
49. Sepia: vinegar, Aconite
50. Silicea: camphor, Camphora, Hepar Sulph
51. Spigelia: camphor, gold, Camphor
52. Spongia Tosta: camphor, Camphora
53. Staphysagria: camphor, Camphora
54. Sulphur: camphor, Aconite, Camphora, Mercurius, Nux, Pulsatilla
55. Symphytum: none listed
56. Thuja Occidentalis: camphor, Camphora, Pulsatilla
57. Urtica Urens: Rumex
58. Valeriana: camphor, coffee, Belladonna, Camphora, Coffea, Pulsatilla, Mercurius
59. Veratrum Album: camphor, coffee, Aconite, Arsenicum, Camphora, Coffea
60. Rescue Remedy: none known

Suggested Repertories and Materia Medicas

ALTHOUGH I HOPE that this guide will be of great help to you and your family for years to come, I do not say that it is the only work you will ever need in dealing with acute situations homeopathically. It cannot and will not take the place of a good repertory or materia medica. It is now and always has been my particular fear that people who pick up guides like this stay frozen at this level and do not tend to move on to the "real" books on homeopathy. Don't let that be the case. The repertory and the materia medica are the first second-level works on understanding and using homeopathy. A guide like this one, or any of the many paperbacks available on the subject, is below that. It is third level. The first level? Hahnemann's own work, *The Organon of Medicine*. Anyone who seriously wants to understand what homeopathy is all about has to read and study this book. Everything else is just writing about what Hahnemann had already written. This is *the* book on homeopathy.

To help you in finding all these books for your own use, I list below the information on two repertories and two materia medicas that is necessary for you to order them. Now, please note that there are many different repertories and materia medicas on the market, especially now that homeopathy is becoming more popular. So you may want to look at and consider a few others. Those listed here are basic works that are generally available at a fairly low cost. You can easily spend hundreds of dollars on books on homeopathy. In addition, I list the best of the versions of *The*

Organon available with the hope that you will make an extra investment in this important work.

(And, while you are looking for books to get you started, don't forget my own first book on the subject, *Homeopathy, Healing, and You,* published by St. Martin's Press, 175 Fifth Avenue, New York, NY 10010-7848. Buy the book; I could use the money.)

Repertories

Repertory of the Homeopathic Materia Medica with Word Index, by J. T. Kent. Published by B. Jain Publishers, Ltd, 1921 Chuna Mandi, Street 10th, New Delhi-110055 India. It can be ordered through many American companies and is available at many health food stores. The Indian edition is suggested over the British because the Indian runs around $20 and the British is $65 for the same book. This is the basic homeopathic repertory and is a must for all students of homeopathy.

Homeopathic Medical Repertory, A Modern Alphabatical Repertory, by Robin Murphy, N.D. Published by the Hahnemann Academy of North America, 60 Talisman Drive, Suite 4028, Pagosa Springs, CO 81157. This repertory is more expensive—about $85—but many people prefer it because of its alphabetical structure.

Materia Medicas

Pocket Manual of Homeopathic Materia Medica, by William Boericke, M.D. Published by B. Jain Publishers, Ltd, New Delhi, India. Again, this is the cheapest and easiest to get of all the materia medicas. It will run you about $20.

Desktop Guide to Keynotes and Confirmatory Symptoms, by Roger Morrison, M.D. Published by Hahnemann Clinic Publishing, 828 San Pablo Avenue, Albany, CA 94706. This book, like Murphy's, is more expensive (I think that I paid about $65 for it), but it will be very helpful to you if you really want to work with homeopathic remedies.

The Organon

The Organon of the Medical Art, by Samuel Hahnemann, edited and annotated by Wenda Brewster O'Reilly, Ph.D. Published by Birdcage Books, PO Box 2289, Redmond, WA 98073-2289. Because this is a very small company, let me also give you the phone number: 206/285-4737. This edition is rather expensive, about $55, but it is easily the best translation available. And if there is one book on homeopathy that is worth whatever it costs, this is it. No homeopathic library is complete without it.

A Brief Glossary of Homeopathic Terms

WHILE CERTAINLY FAR from complete, the following are some of the common terms that you will find once you break down and try to learn to use a materia medica and repertory. You will quickly see that the medical language contained in these is largely archaic. It will be very helpful to you if you can lay your hands on an old, out-of-print medical dictionary at a book sale. Failing this, I have put together a brief glossary to be of some help.

I have included general terms that you are most likely to see as well as those medical terms that have now passed from the common use. Finally, I include terms that for the homeopath have a meaning different from the usual and cultural.

ABASIA—Lack of ability to walk. Condition is in place, although the patient's coordination and muscle power are not lacking.

ABIOSIS—Death.

ABLEPSIA—Lack of ability to see. Blindness.

ABSCESS—A collection of pus in a specific part of the body, caused by disintegration of tissue.

ABULIA—Loss of will. The patient will feel an inability to make decisions or direct his own life. Also spelled "Aboulia."

ACAMPSIA—Stiffness or inflexibility in any of the limbs

ACANTHA—The spine, considered in whole or part.

ACOMIA—Baldness; also used as a term for alopecia.

ACOUSIA—Any condition related to the sense of hearing.

ACUTE—As applied to disease, one that is manifest by violent symptoms, terminating in a few days, overwhelming the body's usual balance of health.

ADDUCT—Movement of sensation or symptoms to the midpoint or midline of the body, or any part of the body.

ADIPOSA—Body fat.

ADIPSIA—A lack of thirst.

ADYNAMIA—Weakness, related to a loss of vital force, also called "asthenia."

ADYNAMIC—A lack of vital force.

AFEBRILE—A lack of fever.

AGGLUTINATION—The adhesive union of substances; tissue stuck together by secretions.

AGGRAVATION—An increase in or worsening of symptoms or a response to a homeopathic remedy that temporarily causes an increase of symptoms; referred to by the symbol <.

AGNOSIA—Lack of ability to recognize familiar persons, places, or things.

AGUE—Most often will refer to a fever, especially one that is accompanied by spells of chill and/or heat. May refer to the chill itself, especially if the patient shivers in chill.

ALEXIA—The lack of ability to read in cases in which the patient is literate. May be referred to as "word-blindness."

ALIMENT—Every substance or fluid which is capable of affording nourishment.

ALVINE—Relating to the area of the abdomen and the intestines.

ALVINE FLUX—Diarrhea.

AMASESIS—Lack of ability to chew.

AMATIVE—Sexually passionate.

AMBUSTION—Either a scald or a burn.

AMELIORATION—A decrease of symptoms or general improvement in the patient's condition due to any outside catalyst or homeopathic remedy; referred to by the symbol >.

AMENORRHEA—Absence of or abnormal lack of menses.

AMORPHOUS—Having no set shape, no specific form.

ANAKUSIS—The total lack of ability to hear; deafness.

ANALEPSIS—The restoration of the patient to a condition of health.

ANALEPTIC—A catalyst that moves the patient to a state of health.

ANALGESIA—Absence of pain.

ANAMNESIS—Term referring to memory and the act of remembering. It is used to refer to the case taking, to the remembering of a life history on the part of the patient.

ANAPEIRATIC—Onset of symptoms from the overuse of parts of the body. State of pain from overusing limbs.

ANAPHIA—A change in or loss of the sense of touch.

ANCHYLOSIS—Unusual immobility of a joint.

ANEMIA—A deficiency in red blood cells or hemoglobin that results in a condition of general weakness.

ANERGIC—Lacking in energy; weak.

ANESIS—A disease in a state of remission.

ANESTHESIA—A loss of sensation; also a general state of confusion, weakness, and insensibility. Also refers to the induced state in which a patient has a general loss of ability to feel or perceive pain.

ANEURYSM—A pulsating tumor formed by the stretching of the walls of a vein or artery.

ANGINA—A sore throat, with difficulty swallowing; also refers to the more common meaning of a severe pain in the region of the heart.

ANGINA PECTORIS—Spasmodic pain in the chest due to heart disease.

ANGOR—Restlessness.

ANOSMIA—Loss of sense of smell.

ANTALGIC—Any catalyst that results in a lessening or of loss of pain.

ANTERIOR—The front part of the body; also the forward or front part of any organ of the body.

ANTIDOTE—Term used to denote a medicinal agent that has the power of modifying or neutralizing the effects of another medicine previously administered, or counteracting a poison.

APERIENT—Any catalyst that brings about a gentle laxative result.

APHASIA—Loss of the ability to speak.

APHONIA—Loss of voice.

APHTHAE—Small white sores on the skin or mucous membranes; canker sores.

APHTHOUS—A superficial ulcer.

APOSIA—Loss of or lack of a feeling of thirst.

APOSTEMS—Abcesses of any sort or in any location.

APRAXIA—Lack of ability to perform specific movements; lack of fine coordination.

APROSEXIA—Lack of ability to concentrate or to give full attention.

APYREXIA—An end to fever; absence of fever.

ASEPSIS—Lack of or absence of harmful bacteria in the system.

ASPHYXIA—State in which, although patient is alive, the pulsation of the heart cannot be perceived.

ASPHYXIATION—Suffocation.

ASSIMILATION—The conversion of food into nourishment.

ASTHENIA—A state of extreme debility; any state of general weakness.

ATAXIA—Loss of muscular coordination.

ATELECTASIS—A collapsed or partially collapsed lung.

ATELIA—The incomplete development of any part of the mind or the body.

ATHELIA—Lack of or absence of nipples.

ATONY—A weakness or deficiency of muscle power.

ATTRITION—The wearing away on anything from the process of friction.

AUTOINTOXICATION—A toxic state of the body created by the accumulation of waste products in the system.

AXILLA—Armpit.

BALBUTIES—Stammering or stuttering language.

BEAL—Any boil or pustule, especially those that have become infected or pus-filled.

BIBULOUS—Anything with the ability to absorb water or other liquids.

BILIOUS—Refers to any disease which comes about from the presence of too much bile in the system.

BLEB—A large soft blister.

BLENNORRHEA—Any free discharge of mucus from the vagina or urethra.

BLEPHAROPHTHALMIA—Any inflamation of the eyeballs or the eyelids.

BLEPHAROPTOSIS—A drooping of the upper eyelid.

BLEPHAROSPASM—Involuntary winking, usually spasmodic in nature.

BRACHIAL—Anything that is of or belonging to the arm.

BUBO—Enlarged lymphatic gland in the groin or armpit as part of a disease state; any abscess.

BUCCAL—Anything pertaining to the cheek, or the area of the cheek.

BUCCULA—A double chin.

BUGANTIA—Chilblains.

BULIMIA—An appetite that cannot be satisfied; animal hunger.

BYSIS—Cotton; also called "lint."

CALLOSITES—Calluses.

CALMANT—Any catalyst that calms the patient; a sedative.

CALOR—Heat in any part of the body that suggests inflammatory disease.

CANCRUM—Canker sores.

CANITIES—The process of hair turning gray.

CANTHUS—Either corner or side of the eye; the meeting of the upper and lower eyelids.

CARBUNCLE—Deep, pus-filled infection in the skin; more serious than an abscess.

CARDIOGMUS—Diseases of the heart.

CARIES—Decay (usually used in reference to bone or teeth).

CAROTID—General term for anything to do with the heart.

CATAMENIA—Menstruation.

CATARRH—General term for any increase in production of and flow of mucus; an inflammation of the mucous membranes with ongoing nasal flow, sinus infection.

CECITIS—Appendicitis.

CEPHALEA—Any head pain.

CERVIX—The term in general means "necklike" and will be used to refer to the neck in general and to the back of the neck; also the lower portion of the uterus.

CHILBLAINS—Pain, swelling, and itching of parts of the body over-exposed to cold.

CHOANAE—Rear openings of the nose; also called the "posterior nares."

CHOREA—Neurological condition resulting in irregular involuntary movements and motions, especially of the face and/or the limbs; "Saint Vitus' dance."

CHRONIC—The term applied to diseases which are of long-standing, and usually do not involve the occurence of fever.

CICATRICES—Scars of all sorts.

CINESIA—Symptoms brought on by movement; motion sickness.

CLAVICLE—The collarbone.

CLAVUS—A corn on the toe.

COCTION—Digestion.

COLIC—Any spasm or cramping pain; especially in the region of the abdomen; also called "gripe."

COMA—An inclination to sleep, lethargic drowsiness; a pronounced state of sleep.

COMA VIGIL—An inclination but inability to sleep.

COMMISSURE—The point of joining in the lips, eyelids, or labia.

COMPLEMENTARY REMEDY——A remedy whose actions are in harmony with those of another; a remedy that completes the actions of another.

CONDYLOMATA—Warts (as part of the Sycotic miasm); any wart or wart-like growth.

CONFLUENT—Running together, or joining together, usually associated with eruptions of the skin.

CONSTRINGING—Shrinking.

COPHOSIS—Deafness.

COPIOPIA—Exhaustion of the eyes; weakness of vision from overwork.

COPIOUS—A great deal or amount of something, such as mucus.

CORYZA—A head cold, acute condition only.

COSTAL—The ribs or the area of the ribs.

COSTIVE—Constipated; in a state of general congestion or constipation.

COXAGRIA—Pain in the hip joint or the area of the hip joint.

CRUELS—Herpes zoster.

CUBITAL—Pertaining to the forearm.

CUTANEOUS—Pertaining to the skin.

CUTICLE—The thin, insensitive membrane that covers the skin.

CUTIS—The skin itself; the true skin, under the cuticle.

DECUBITIS—A bedsore.

DENTAGRA—Toothache.

DENTITION—Teething, the period of time in childhood when the teeth begin to grow.

DERMOID—Having the appearance of or similar to skin; skinlike.

DESQUAMATION—Shedding or peeling of skin, usually involving scales.

DIAPHORESIS—Perspiration.

DICHROTISM—Any condition that presents two qualities at the same time.

DICROTIC—The condition of having two heartbeats.

DIPLEGIA—Stiffness or paralysis of two contrasting body parts on two sides of the body.

DIPLOPIA—Double vision.

DIURESIS—Literally, a "double" amount of urine; to urinate a great amount at a given time.

DOSSIL—A wad; therefore, a "dossil of lint" is a cotton ball.

DROPSY—A swelling of an area of the body that involves an accumulation of fluid, usually clear or yellow; skin most often will become hardened in the surrounding area.

DYSECOIA—Difficulty in hearing.

DYSMENORRHOEA—Difficulty with menstruation.

DYSNOEA—Difficulty with breathing.

DYSPHAGIA—Difficulty with swallowing.

DYSURIA—Difficulty with urination.

ECCHYMOSIS—A bruise, especially a large bruise that is black and blue in appearance.

ECCOPROTIC—Any laxative.

ECCRITIC—Anything that promotes the flow of waste matter from the body.

ECMNESIA—Loss of short-term memory.

ECTAL—The outer or external part of the body.

EFFUVIA—The giving off of noxious or toxic fumes.

EGESTA—Solid body waste; feces.

EMESIS—Vomiting.

EMETIC—Any catalyst that causes vomiting.

EMPYEMA—Usually, the presence of pus in the area around the lungs; may also be pus in any cavity of the body.

ENCOPRESIS—The involuntary passing of stool.

ENERVATE—To exhaust or weaken.

ENTERORRHEA—Diarrhea.

ENURESIS—The inability to control the flow of urine; incontinence.

EPHIALTES—Nightmare.

EPISTAXIS—Nosebleed.

ERRHINE—Any catalyst that brings about a mucus discharge from the nose.

ERUCTATIONS—Belches.

ESTAVATE—To lie dormant.

EUCRASIA—A state of total health and well-being.

EVETICS—The process of creating health in the human system.

EXTIRPATION—The utter and complete removal of a part or organ of the body.

FAG—Fatigue.

FARINACEOUS FOOD—Food taken from starchy things, from flour or grain (farina).

FAUCES—The cavity behind the tongue at the entrance to the throat.

FEBRILE—Feverish; in a state of fever.

FELON—Abscess of the fingertip, near the nail (also "whitlow").

FIBROID—A tumor made up of muscular fibers.

FISTULA—An ulcer of sorts; a strange or abnormal connection from one body cavity to another, or to the surface of the body.

FLATUS—Intestinal gas.

FLEXION—The bending of a part of the body.

FLUX—Menstrual flow; any flow that cleanses a part of the body.

FOETIDA—Foul-smelling.

FOMENTATION—Partial bathing, to promote sweating.

FORAMEN—An opening in a body part, especially a bone.

FOSSA—A cavity growing or occurring in any part of the body.

GAIT—The manner in which a patient walks.

GALD—Any painful swelling in any part of the body; a blister.

GASTRALGIA—Stomachache; any discomfort in the region of the stomach.

GENU—The knee.

GIDDINESS—Vertigo.

GINGIVAL—Pertaining to the gums.

GLABELLA—The space of the forehead between the eyebrows and above the root of the nose.

GLAIRY—Like the white of an egg.

GLEETY—The chronic gonorrheal discharge.

GLOTTIS—Inflammation of the tongue.

GONITIS—Any inflammation of the knee.

GRACILE—Slim; anything that may be considered slender and graceful.

GRAVEDO—The front sinuses.

GRIPPE—Abdominal colic; stomachache.

GULLET—The throat.

GUTTUR—The throat.

HAWKING—Harsh sound in the throat, clearing the throat.

HECTIC—Illnesses with the symptom of reoccurring fever twice a day, at noon and night; anything that is habitual.

HEMATEMESIS—Vomiting blood.

HEMAXIS—Bloodletting.

HEPATIC—Referring to the liver or the area of the liver.

HIDROSE—Excessive perspiration.

HYDROGOGUE—Any catalyst that causes a loss of fluids from the human system.

HYDROPHOBIA—"Fear of water"; rabies.

HYPOCHONDRIA—Section of the abdomen below the ribs.

HYPOGASTRIUM—Lower middle section of the abdomen, below the navel.

IATROGENIC—A disease state created by medical treatments or drugs; an artificial disease state.

ICHOR—Fluid discharge from a wound or an ulcer.

ICHTHYOSIS—Scaling of the skin of the body.

ICTERUS—Yellowing of the skin; usually associated with jaundice.

IDIOPATHIC—Any disease which is in no way related to any other complaint present in the human system; any disease of unknown origin.

INCUBUS—Nightmare.

INDOLENT—Sluggish and inactive; also, a condition without pain.

INDOLENTHIDROSIS PEDUM—Excessive foot perspiration.

INDURATION—A hard spot on the body, associated with the hardening of a tissue or specific part of the body.

INGUINAL—Referring to the groin or the area of the groin.

INSENSIBILITY—Unconsciousness.

KELOID—Fibrous tissue that forms at the site of a scar.

LACHRYMAL—Belonging to tears; crying.

LANCINATING PAIN—Pain that is sharp in nature, sharp and cutting.

LAVE—To bathe.

LENTICULAR—Skin marking like a freckle.

LEUCORRHOEA—Discharge from vagina that is white or yellow.

LIENTERIC—Diarrhea with undigested food in it.

LIVOR—Any black-and-blue area of the skin; any ashen area of the skin.

LUPUS—Tuberculosis of the skin.

MALUM—Any disease.

MARASMUS—A wasting away, especially from malnutrition; any sudden weight loss, especially in children.

MEATUS—The opening or canal to any part of the body, such as the "meatus of the ear"; that which separates the internal from the external.

MEGRIM—A migraine headache, especially one that is one-sided and over the temple area.

METASTASIS—Translation of a disease from one area of the body to another.

MICTURITION—Urination.

MORTIFICATION—Loss of vital force in any part of the body.

NARES—The nostrils

NASUS—The nose.

NATES—The buttocks.

NEURALGIA—Any nerve pain; pain of throbbing or stabbing nature.

NEURASTHENIC—Exhaustion in "high-strung" patients; nervous breakdown.

NEURITIS—Degeneration of a nerve, associated with the lack of symptoms or sensations.

NISIS—Contraction of the abdominal muscles in passing stool or urine; also, any struggle or special effort.

NODE—Any swollen gland, a bump on the body, usually delicate to the touch.

NOSOLOGY—The classification of diseases.

NOSTRUMS—Applied to all "quack" medicines, which are known only to their inventor and whose ingredients are held a deep secret.

NYCTALGIA—Night pain, especially the pain in the bones at night.

OCCIPITAL—Of the occiput, the back of the head.

ONANISM—Masturbation; also, incomplete coition, withdrawal of the penis during intercourse.

ORCHITIS—Inflammation of the testis.

OS—A specific bone; sometimes used to refer to a body cavity.

OSTEALGIA—Pain in a bone.

OTALGIA—Earache.

PALLIATIVES—Medicines that only relieve pain without curing disease.

PAROXYSM—Sudden intensification of symptoms.

PATHOGENETIC—The term applied to the impact of medicine upon any healthy person.

PATULOUS—Any condition that is spreading.

PAVOR—Fear or terror; "*pavor nocturnus*" is a term for nightmares.

PERNIO—Chilblains.

PHTHISIS—Any wasting away of the body, specifically belonging to tuberculosis.

PICA—A craving or desire to eat substances (dirt, chalk, plaster . . .) not normally eaten.

POLLEX—The thumb or first finger.

POLYSARCA—Overweight; obesity.

POLYURIA—The passing of a large amount of urine.

PORTAL—Referring to the liver.

POSOLOGY—The method or science of determining the dosages of medicine.

PRESENESCENCE—The process of growing old.

PROLAPSUS—Downward displacement of any hollow organ, usually the uterus or rectum.

PRONE—The body lying face-down.

PROSTRATION—Extreme exhaustion.

PROUD FLESH—Any wart or fig wart.

PRURIENT—Lustful; having sexual thoughts and fantasies.

PTOSIS—The prolapse or falling down of organs of the body; especially, drooping upper eyelids.

PTYALISM—Salivation.

PURULENT—Having the appearance of pus.

PUSTULES—Raised, pus-filled lesions on the skin.

PYEMESIS—Vomiting pus.

PYREXIA—Fever.

QUARTAN—Any condition that occurs every fourth day.

QUIESCENT—Anything that is dormant or still.

QUINSY—Tonsillitis; any inflammatory sore throat.

QUINTAN—Any condition that occurs every fifth day.

QUOTIDIAN—Any condition that occurs daily.

RACHIALGIA—Pain in the spine or region of the spine.

RAPTUS—A sudden attack or seizure.

RAUCEDO—Hoarseness.

RAUCITAS—Hoarseness.

REDOLENT—Exuding a specific and pervading odor.

REMITTENT—A form of fever in which the symptoms subside somewhat for a time and then reoccur.

REPURCUSSED—Driven in.

RHACOMA—Chafing.

RIGORS—Chill accompanied by shivers.

RISUS—Laughter.

ROSACEA—A rose-colored rash, to be considered in cases of rubeola.

RUBEOLA—Measles.

RUBOR—Redness.

RUCTUS—A belch.

SALIVANT—Any catalyst that increases the flow of saliva.

SAPORIFIC—Any catalyst that produces a taste or flavor.

SCROFULOUS—Pus-filled abscesses of tubercular origin.

SCURF—Dandruff, or any other exfoliations of cuticle.

SEPTIC—The presence of any toxins or infections in the human system.

SINGULTUS—Hiccup.

SNUFFLES—Obstruction of the nose, especially in young children.

SPECIFIC—A remedy that may always be considered appropriate and curative to a specific condition.

STASIS—Stagnation of the blood or of any other bodily fluid.

STHENIC—Strong and active; sometimes used to refer to excessive force.

SUDORIFIC—That which causes sweating.

SUGGILATION—A bruise.

SUPPURATING—Producing pus; that which causes pus to be deposited in tumors.

SURDITY—Deafness.

SWASHING—A noisy, watery, slushing sound when you touch a part of the body.

SYCOMA—A fig wart; any soft tumor on the body.

SYNCOPE—Fainting or swooning.

SYNDESMOS—A ligament.

SYNOCHA—A long continued fever state.

SYNTAXIS—A joint.

SYNTEXIS—A wasting away of the body; sudden weight loss.

SYRYGMUS—Any ringing in the ears.

TABES—The gradual wasting away of the body; gradual but steady weight loss.

TALALGIA—A pain in the heel.

TENESMUS—Ineffectual straining at stool or urination.

TERTIAN—Conditions that occur every third day; also used for conditions that occur every forty-eight hours.

TETTERS—Rash, usually moist or oozing rashes; especially, herpes, eczema, and psoriasis.

THYMION—Any wart.

TINEA—Any fungal skin condition; especially ringworm.

TINNITUS—Ringing in the ears.

TORMINA—Pain in the abdomen; "the gripe."

TORPENT—Any catalyst that causes a senstion of numbness.

TORPER—The state of being drunk; a drunkard.

TORPID—Anything that is sluggish or inactive.

TORPOR—State of numbness; deficient sensation, sluggishness.

TOXEMIA—Poisoning of the blood.

TREMULOUS—Shaky.

TUBERCLES—The small, round nodules produced in tuberculosis.

TURBID—Having a cloudy or muddy appearance.

TYMPANIC—Anything that can be said to be drumlike in appearance and character.

TYMPANITIC—The distended state of the abdomen, with a drumlike quality.

TYMPANITIS—Middle ear infection.

TYMPANUM—Eardrum.

ULCUS—Any ulcer.

UMBILICUS—The navel.

UNGUENTA—Any ointment.

URANIST—A pervert; a person of perverted sexual habits.

URETIC—Anything relating to urine and to the excretion of urine from the human body.

URTICARA—Hives, nettle rash.

VACCINOSIS—Any disease state brought on from being vaccinated.

VAGITUS—The crying out of an infant; the fussing sounds from an infant.

VARICELLA—Chicken pox.

VARIOLA—Smallpox.

VARIOLOID—Any node resembling smallpox.

VARIX—An enlarged artery or vein.

VAS—A vessel.

VAULT—The rear of the throat.

VELUM PALATI—The soft palate.

VENERY—Sexual intercourse.

VERIFORM—Anything with a wormlike shape or character.

VERMIFUGE—Any catalyst that removes worms or other parasites from the human system.

VERRUCA—A wart.

VERTEX—The top of the head.

VESICAL—Pertaining to the bladder or the area of the bladder.

VESICLES—Small blisters.

VETA—Mountain sickness; sickness from heights in general.

VIRUS—Any contagion or poison, any environmental toxin.

VIVES—Enlargement of the glands behind the ears.

VOLA—The palms of the hand or the soles of the feet.

VOX—The human voice.

VULNUS—Any wound.

WATER BRASH—Heartburn with the regurgitation of sour fluids into the mouth.

WEAL—Hives.

WEN—Sebaceous cyst; any cyst containing oily or fatty matter.

WHITLOW—Abscess of the fingertip near the nail (also "felon").

WRY NECK—A stiff neck; torticollis.

XEROSIS—A dryness of the skin that occurs gradually as a human grows older.

XEROSTOMIA—A dry mouth.

ZONA—Herpes Zoster.

ZOSTER—Herpes zoster, shingles, skin blisters that form along the course of nerves.

ZYMOTIC—Infectious disease; also refers to the disease process itself in which disease was seen to "ferment" in the system.

ZYOMIS—Any infectious disease that is due to fungus.

Acknowledgments

As already mentioned within the text, the works of two homeopaths of the last century, I. D. Johnson and John A. Tarbell, were of great help. And I want to acknowledge also the writings of Richard Hughes, of all people, in his *Manuel of Therapeutics,* as well as the works of Pulte, Hempel, Ruddock, Burt, and Verdi, and that oddity, *Malan's Family Guide.* I also want to acknowledge Humphrey for his patent-medicine approach to family homeopathy; also Ribot & Shedd and Talcott, for their early works on the uses of homeopathics for mental and emotional states; and Curtis & Lillie, for their tiny little book on the home use of remedies. Other sources of information include H. C. Allen for his Key Notes; T. S. Iyer for his home guide to the use of homeopathics; Constantine Hering for his *Homeopathic Domestic Physician*; and Clarke for his own writings on the practice of homeopathy. I must also acknowledge K. N. Mathur for the wonderful *Systematic Materia Medica,* a volume filled with excellent guidance. Francisco Eizayaga must also be acknowledged, as well as Jay Yasgur and his dictionary of homeopathic medical terminology—and M. L. Tyler for her *Homeopathic Drug Pictures.*

Also, as always, Boericke's Materia Medica proved an invaluable resource, as did our modern Materia Medicas created by Roger Morrison, whose *Desktop Guide* is of daily use in my household, and Robin Murphy, whose Materia Medica and Repertory are both excellent tools to the practice of homeopathy. Certainly Kent must also be acknowledged, both for his groundbreaking Repertory and for his lectures and collected writings.

Since I am something of a junkie where homeopathic books are concerned, I am sure that I left someone very important out. If so, I am sorry. But let me also acknowledge my own teachers in this field: S. K. Bannerjea, whose Memorizer is wonderful and wacky; Pearlyn Goodman-Herrick, my first teacher; and Pramilla Vishvanath. And I want to especially acknowledge Edward Whitmont for his contributions to homeopathy, especially for *The Alchemy of Healing*. Finally, I want to acknowledge the contribution of Harry Coulter, a one-of-a-kind teacher and writer, whose life has enriched us all. This book is dedicated to him.

More than any other source, the twenty years I have spent studying the materia medica and using the remedies themselves have served as the basis of the information enclosed here. This book began as a series of class notes that I put together to better help my students understand the philosophy and practice of homeopathy. Over time, they grew to be study guides, and now these notes are collected into this volume. I do this because it is important that we have access to information on homeopathy. It is especially important, in my opinion, that we have information from the homeopathic masters of the last two centuries. I hope that I have given them voice here, and that my voice sings in harmony with theirs.

Acknowledgment must also be paid to my agent, Bob Silverstein, who manages to calm me in even the greatest moments of stress, and to my editor, Jennifer Weis, whose voice on the telephone was always the voice of reason.